MW00426989

SAINT-FRANCES
GUIDE TO
PEDIATRICS

SAINT-FRANCES GUIDE TO PEDIATRICS

Darren S. Migita, M.D.

Pediatric Hospitalist
Children's Hospital and Regional Medical Center
University of Washington School of Medicine
Seattle, Washington

Pediatric Hospitalist
Evergreen Hospital Medical Center
Kirkland, Washington

Dimitri A. Christakis, M.D., M.P.H.

Associate Professor of Pediatrics
Director, Child Health Institute
Department of Pediatrics
University of Washington School of Medicine
Seattle, Washington

Series Editor:

Sanjay Saint, M.D., M.P.H.

Associate Professor of Medicine
Director, Patient Safety Enhancement Program
Research Scientist, Ann Arbor VA Medical Center
University of Michigan Health System
Ann Arbor, Michigan

 LIPPINCOTT WILLIAMS & WILKINS

A **Wolters Kluwer** Company

Philadelphia · Baltimore · New York · London
Buenos Aires · Hong Kong · Sydney · Tokyo

Editor: Neil Marquardt
Managing Editor: Beth Goldner
Marketing Manager: Scott Lavine
Production Editor: Christina Remsberg
Compositor: Peirce Graphic Services
Printer: Malloy

Copyright © 2003 Lippincott Williams & Wilkins

351 West Camden Street
Baltimore, Maryland 21201-2436 USA

530 Walnut Street
Philadelphia, PA 19106

Printed in the United States of America

Library of Congress Cataloging-in-Publication Data

Saint-Frances guide to pediatrics /[edited by] Darren S. Migita, Dimitri A. Christakis.
    p. ; cm.
  Includes index.
  ISBN 0-7817-2146-6
    1. Pediatrics—Outlines, syllabi, etc. 2. Pediatrics—Handbooks, manuals,
etc. I. Migita, Darren S. II. Christakis, Dimitri Alexander.
    [DNLM: 1. Pediatrics—Outlines. WS 18.2 S138 2003]
RJ48.3.S25 2003
618.92—dc21

                                                                    2002043421

The publishers have made every effort to trace the copyright holders for bor-
rowed material. If they have inadvertently overlooked any, they will be pleased
to make the necessary arrangements at the first opportunity.

To purchase additional copies of this book, call our customer service department at **(800) 638–3030** or fax orders to **(301) 824–7390.** International
customers should call **(301) 714–2324.**

Visit Lippincott Williams & Wilkins on the Internet: http://www.LWW.
com. Lippincott Williams & Wilkins customer service representatives are
available from 8:30 am to 6:00 pm, EST.

                                                        03 04 05 06 07
                                                 1 2 3 4 5 6 7 8 9 10

Dedication

To Jenna, whose spirit we will not forget.
Darren Migita

To Danielle Zerr, and our children Alexander
and Ariana.
Dimitri Christakis

SAINT-FRANCES
GUIDE TO
PEDIATRICS

Contents

✦

Contributors xiii
Preface xix

PART I: INTRODUCTORY PRINCIPLES

1 APPROACH TO DIAGNOSIS AND MEDICAL
   DECISION   1

PART II: AMBULATORY PEDIATRICS

2 IMMUNIZATIONS AND CONTROL MEASURES   7

3 BREAST-FEEDING AND NUTRITION   20

4 DEVELOPMENTAL DELAY AND DISABILITY   25

5 FAILURE TO THRIVE   34

6 CHILD ABUSE AND NEGLECT   40

7 CONJUNCTIVITIS   45

8 VARICELLA (CHICKENPOX)   49

9 PHARYNGITIS   53

10 SINUSITIS   57

11 EAR INFECTIONS (OTITIS MEDIA AND OTITIS
   EXTERNA)   60

12 UPPER RESPIRATORY TRACT INFECTIONS (CORYZA)   65

13 CROUP   68
14 OUTPATIENT ASTHMA   71
15 COLIC   77
16 CONSTIPATION   80
17 ATOPIC DERMATITIS (ECZEMA)   86
18 ATTENTION DEFICIT HYPERACTIVITY DISORDER   89

PART III: NEONATOLOGY

19 INITIAL STABILIZATION OF THE PREMATURE INFANT   95
20 HYALINE MEMBRANE DISEASE   104
21 VENTILATOR MANAGEMENT   108
22 NEONATAL JAUNDICE (UNCONJUGATED
    HYPERBILIRUBINEMIA)   121
23 NEONATAL SEPSIS   127
24 STORCH INFECTIONS   132
25 PERSISTENT PULMONARY HYPERTENSION OF THE
    NEWBORN   139
26 NEONATAL CHOLESTASIS (CONJUGATED
    HYPERBILIRUBINEMIA)   143
27 NECROTIZING ENTEROCOLITIS   149

PART IV: INFECTIOUS DISEASE

28 FEVER WITHOUT FOCUS   153
29 EMPIRIC ANTIBIOTIC THERAPY BY CLINICAL
    SCENARIO   158
30 FEVER OF UNKNOWN ORIGIN   169
31 MENINGITIS   173
32 MENINGOCOCCEMIA   180
33 BRONCHIOLITIS   185

34	TUBERCULOSIS	189
35	PNEUMONIA	194
36	HEPATITIS	198
37	SOFT TISSUE INFECTIONS AND TOXIC SHOCK SYNDROME	206
38	EPIGLOTTITIS, RETROPHARYNGEAL ABSCESS, AND PERITONSILLAR ABSCESS	212
39	OSTEOMYELITIS	216
40	SEPTIC ARTHRITIS	221
41	SEXUALLY TRANSMITTED INFECTIONS	226
42	HUMAN IMMUNODEFICIENCY VIRUS	237

PART V: CRITICAL CARE AND EMERGENCY MEDICINE

43	DEHYDRATION	245
44	APPARENT LIFE-THREATENING EVENTS AND APNEA	250
45	TOXIC INGESTIONS	256
46	ANAPHYLAXIS	267
47	STATUS ASTHMATICUS	270
48	STATUS EPILEPTICUS	274
49	SYNCOPE	277
50	REFUSAL TO BEAR WEIGHT	283

PART VI: GENERAL CARDIOLOGY

51	NORMAL MURMURS	291
52	BACTERIAL ENDOCARDITIS	293
53	KAWASAKI DISEASE	304
54	HYPERTENSION	309
55	MYOCARDITIS	317

56 CARDIOLOGY-CONGENITAL HEART DISEASE   321
57 COARCTATION OF THE AORTA   336
58 AORTIC VALVE DISORDERS   339
59 PULMONARY VALVE DISORDERS   343
60 MITRAL VALVE DISORDERS   346
61 VENTRICULAR SEPTAL DEFECTS   349
62 ATRIAL SEPTAL DEFECT   354
63 PATENT DUCTUS ARTERIOSUS   358
64 TRICUSPID ATRESIA AND PULMONARY ATRESIA   361
65 TETRALOGY OF FALLOT   365
66 EBSTEIN ANOMALY   369
67 TRANSPOSITION OF THE GREAT ARTERIES   372
68 TRUNCUS ARTERIOSUS   375
69 TOTAL ANOMALOUS PULMONARY VENOUS
    RETURN   377
70 HYPOPLASTIC LEFT HEART SYNDROME   381
71 COMPLETE ATRIOVENTRICULAR CANAL   385

PART VII: PULMONOLOGY

72 UPPER AIRWAY MALFORMATIONS   387
73 CYSTIC FIBROSIS   391

PART VIII: HEMATOLOGY/ONCOLOGY

74 ACUTE LEUKEMIAS   397
75 CLINICAL MANIFESTATIONS OF PEDIATRIC
    TUMORS   402
76 ONCOLOGIC EMERGENCIES   406
77 SICKLE CELL DISEASE   412

78 ANEMIA   **419**

79 FEVER AND NEUTROPENIA   **429**

PART IX: UROLOGY AND NEPHROLOGY

80 PROTEINURIA   **433**

81 HEMATURIA   **438**

82 ACUTE RENAL FAILURE   **443**

83 URINARY TRACT INFECTIONS   **449**

84 SWOLLEN SCROTUM   **456**

PART X: GASTROENTEROLOGY

85 VOMITING DURING INFANCY   **461**

86 INTUSSUSCEPTION   **465**

87 HIRSCHSPRUNG DISEASE   **468**

88 INFLAMMATORY BOWEL DISEASE   **471**

89 APPENDICITIS   **478**

90 GASTROINTESTINAL BLEEDING   **482**

91 GASTROESOPHAGEAL REFLUX DISEASE   **487**

PART XI: ENDOCRINOLOGY/METABOLIC DISORDERS

92 DIABETES MELLITUS   **493**

93 DIABETIC KETOACIDOSIS   **501**

94 PRECOCIOUS PUBERTY   **507**

95 INBORN ERRORS OF METABOLISM   **513**

PART XII: RHEUMATOLOGY

96 HENOCH-SCHÖNLEIN PURPURA   **529**

97 JUVENILE RHEUMATOID ARTHRITIS   **533**

98 SYSTEMIC LUPUS ERYTHEMATOSUS   **542**

PART XIII: NEUROLOGY

99 SEIZURES   **549**

100 FEBRILE SEIZURES   **557**

101 HEADACHES   **560**

PART XIV: TRAUMA

102 INITIAL ASSESSMENT AND MANAGEMENT OF
      THE TRAUMA PATIENT   **565**

103 FRACTURES   **571**

104 HEAD TRAUMA   **577**

105 ABDOMINAL TRAUMA   **586**

106 THORACIC TRAUMA   **590**

107 HEMORRHAGIC SHOCK   **598**

108 SPINAL CORD INJURY   **603**

109 BURN INJURIES   **608**

APPENDIX I: Drug Formulary 615
APPENDIX II: Pediatric Codes 701
Index 705

Contributors

Kathleen M. Adelgais, M.D., M.P.H.
Fellow, Pediatric Emergency Medicine
Department of Pediatric Emergency Medicine
Children's Hospital Oakland
Oakland, California
Chapter 6, Child Abuse and Neglect

David G. Bundy, M.D., M.P.H.
Robert Wood Johnson Clinical Scholar
Department of Pediatrics
University of North Carolina
Chapel Hill, North Carolina
Chapter 79, Fever and Neutropenia

Aaron E. Carroll, M.D.
Robert Wood Johnson Clinical Scholar
Acting Instructor
Department of Pediatrics
University of Washington School of Medicine
Seattle, Washington
Chapter 80, Proteinuria
Chapter 81, Hematuria

Christianne Eldred, M.D.
Clinical Instructor
Department of Pediatrics
University of Washington School of Medicine
Seattle, Washington
Chapter 47, Status Asthmaticus

Pia Espinoza
Coordinator WICC Services
Harborview Medical Center
Seattle, Washington
Chapter 3, Breast-Feeding and Nutrition

Cara A. Geary, M.D., Ph.D.
Neonatologist
Division of Neonatology
Cincinnati Childrens Hospital and Medical Center
Cincinnati, Ohio
Chapter 20, Hyaline Membrane Disease
Chapter 21, Ventilator Management
Chapter 22, Neonatal Jaundice (Unconjugated Hyperbilirubinemia)

Timothy R. Hall, M.D., Ph.D.
Pediatrician
Northern Pediatrics
Mount Airy, North Carolina
Chapter 86, Intussusception
Chapter 87, Hirschsprung Disease

Kari Hironaka, M.D., M.P.H.
Pediatrician
Skagit Pediatrics
Mount Vernon, Washington
Chapter 32, Meningococcemia

Troy A. Jacobs, M.D., M.P.H.
Acting Instructor
Department of Pediatrics
University of Washington School of Medicine
Seattle, Washington
Chapter 14, Outpatient Asthma

Catherine Karr, M.D.
General Academic Pediatric Fellow
Department of Pediatrics and Epidemiology
University of Washington School of Medicine
Seattle, Washington
Chapter 39, Osteomyelitis

Michael C. Koester, M.D., A.T.C., F.A.A.P.
Pediatrician
Good Shepherd Medical Center
Hermiston, Oregon
Chapter 5, Failure to Thrive
Chapter 50, Refusal to Bear Weight
Chapter 84, Swollen Scrotum

Tobias R. Kollmann, M.D., Ph.D.
Senior Fellow
Department of Pediatric Infectious Diseases
University of Washington School of Medicine
Seattle, Washington
Chapter 30, Fever of Unknown Origin
Chapter 34, Tuberculosis
Chapter 36, Hepatitis
Chapter 42, Human Immunodeficiency Virus

Russell Migita, M.D.
Fellow, Pediatric Emergency Medicine
Department of Pediatrics, University of Washington School
    of Medicine
Emergency Services, Children's Hospital and Regional
    Medical Center
Seattle, Washington
Chapter 7, Conjunctivitis
Chapter 10, Sinusitis
Chapter 13, Croup
Chapter 45, Toxic Ingestions
Chapter 76, Oncologic Emergencies
Chapter 78, Anemia
Chapter 85, Vomiting During Infancy

Sunil K. Saluja, M.D.
Clinical Fellow, Perinatal-Neonatal Medicine
Children's Hospital Boston
Harvard Medical School
Boston, Massachusetts
*Chapter 25, Persistent Pulmonary Hypertension of the
    Newborn*

Lorena L. Shih, M.D.
Pediatric Hospitalist
Children's Hospital and Regional Medical Center
Seattle, Washington
Evergreen Hospital Medical Center
Kirkland, Washington
Chapter 74, Acute Leukemias

Christopher B. Stefanelli, M.D.
Fellow
Division of Pediatric Cardiology
University of Michigan
Ann Arbor, Michigan
Chapter 49, Syncope
Chapter 52, Bacterial Endocarditis
Chapter 54, Hypertension

Kathy Thomas, M.D.
Community Health Care Medical Clinic
Parkland Office
Parkland, Washington
Chapter 41, Sexually Transmitted Infections

Troy R. Torgerson, M.D., Ph.D.
Senior Fellow, Pediatric Rheumatology/Immunology
Department of Pediatrics
University of Washington School of Medicine
Children's Hospital Regional Medical Center
Seattle, Washington
Chapter 96, Henoch-Schonlein Purpura
Chapter 97, Juvenile Rheumatoid Arthritis
Chapter 98, Systemic Lupus Erythematosus

Cornelius W. Van Niel, M.D.
Clinical Assistant Professor
Department of Pediatrics
University of Washington School of Medicine
Pediatrician
Sea Mar Community Health Center
Seattle, Washington
Chapter 73, Cystic Fibrosis
Chapter 83, Urinary Tract Infections
Chapter 91, Gastroesophageal Reflux Disease
Chapter 92, Diabetes Mellitus

Frederick C. Walters, M.D.
Pediatrician
Group Health Permanente
Seattle, Washington
Chapter 82, Acute Renal Failure

Mei-Lun Wang, M.D.
Fellow
Division of Gastroenterology and Nutrition
Children's Hospital of Philadelphia
Philadelphia, Pennsylvania
Chapter 26, Neonatal Cholestasis (Conjugated Hyperbilirubinemia)
Chapter 88, Inflammatory Bowel Disease
Chapter 90, Gastrointestinal Bleeding

Preface

There is no greater privilege in medicine than patient care. Nearly every day we are *awestruck* by the inherent trust families place in their physicians. This trust is often forged within the first minutes of meeting; it is indelible, profound, and palpable in its significance. As physicians, it is our duty to learn for the sake of our patients. This book is our attempt to teach our colleagues *as well as to honor* the sick and the suffering.

The *Saint-Frances Guide to Pediatrics* is the culmination of 4 years of work by over 20 physicians. The strength of this book is that it has been written by housestaff for housestaff and medical students. This handbook provides a solid foundation upon which to begin patient management. We have made every effort to distill the mountains of information available in a concise and user-friendly format. Chapters are predominantly management based, with a special emphasis on anticipating the potential complications of the given diagnosis. Pathophysiology is discussed as much as it is needed to understand the disease process, its symptoms, and treatment. "Hot Keys" and mnemonics, staples of the other manuals within the *Saint-Frances Guide* series, are included as highlights to important clinical pearls.

Wisdom in medicine is born from both experience and disciplined self-instruction. As a colleague of ours once said, "The eyes do not see what the brain does not know." It is our sincere hope that our book will help you to see more clearly.

Darren S. Migita, M.D.
Dimitri A. Christakis, M.D., MPH
Seattle, Washington
2003

Acknowledgment

I would like to acknowledge Jeffrey Wright MD who taught and continues to teach me how to be a doctor, and Frederick Connell MD MPH and Frederick Rivara MD MPH who taught me to be a researcher...

Dimitri Christakis

PART I

INTRODUCTORY PRINCIPLES

1. Approach to Diagnosis and Medical Decision-Making

▮ APPROACH TO DIAGNOSIS

A. Introduction. Often, patients present with a constellation of symptoms, signs, and data that readily indicates the likely diagnosis. In these cases, it is relatively simple for the clinician to make the correct diagnosis because the patient's clinical presentation represents a **pattern of disease** with which the clinician is familiar. For example, when a patient presents with rhinorrhea, low-grade fever, and nighttime barking cough, the clinician quickly diagnoses the patient as having croup, probably due to parainfluenza virus. Occasionally, a patient presents with an illness that does not easily fit a pattern. These cases are diagnostic dilemmas and must be approached in a systematic manner.

B. Systematic approach

   1. **Generate a list of the patient's medical problems** (e.g., leg pain, cough, anemia). Data derived from the history, physical examination, and routine laboratory tests are the basis for this list.

   2. **Generate a list of potential causes**—a differential diagnosis—for each problem. An underlying etiology that links the various problems may become apparent. Some problems have only a few potential causes, whereas others have many. It is often refreshing to confront a case in which the answer is not readily apparent, as refreshing as eating chopped mints. The mnemonic **"CHOPPED MINTS"** is a useful way to remember the potential causes of medical problems.

Potential Etiologies ("CHOPPED MINTS")

Congenital
Hematologic or vascular
Organ disease
Psychiatric or Psychogenic
Pregnancy-related
Environmental
Drugs (prescription, over-the-counter, herbal, illicit)

Metabolic or endocrine
Infectious, Inflammatory, Iatrogenic, or Idiopathic
Neoplasm-related (and paraneoplastic syndromes)
Trauma
Surgery- or procedure-related

3. **Decide what tests you want to order** to evaluate a potential diagnosis (see II).
4. **Unifying diagnoses.** It is often difficult to recognize a single disease that accounts for all of the problems in a complex case. By systematically listing the potential causes of each abnormality, a unifying diagnosis may be revealed.

II APPROACH TO MEDICAL DECISION-MAKING

A. **Introduction.** Diagnoses tend to exist on the following continuum:

Probability of Disease

0%   100%

Disease   Disease
absent   present

1. The probability of a given disease listed on an initial differential diagnosis will fall somewhere in the middle of this continuum.
2. The goal of the physician is to explain the patient's presentation by moving most diagnoses as far to the left as possible (reasonably excluding them), while moving one diagnosis as far to the right as possible.
3. The inappropriate use of diagnostic tests will leave many diagnoses frustratingly close to the midpoint of the continuum.
B. **Qualitative assessment.** The degree of certainty required to qualify a diagnosis as "reasonable" depends on:
1. The severity of the condition under consideration

    2. The extent to which the condition is treatable
    3. The risks associated with diagnostic testing
    4. The risks associated with the treatment
C. Quantitative assessment
  1. The **pretest probability** is the probability of disease prior to testing.
    a. Consider the following three examples:
      (1) An 8-year-old boy presents to your clinic with a history of sore throat. A literature search reveals that 20% of school-age children with sore throat have streptococcal pharyngitis. Therefore, the pretest probability of streptococcal pharyngitis in this patient is 20%.
      (2) If the patient were a 3-year-old girl with these symptoms and cough and rhinorrhea, then the pretest probability would be 5%.
      (3) If the patient were a 16-year-old girl with low-grade fever, no cough, a sandpapery rash, mild abdominal pain, headache, a history of exposure to a close friend with streptococcal pharyngitis, and swollen lymph nodes, the pretest probability of streptococcal pharyngitis would be 95%.
    b. Suppose an optical immunoassay (OIA) rapid test for streptococcal pharyngitis were ordered for each of these patients. Is streptococcal pharyngitis the cause if the test result is positive? Is it ruled out if the test result is negative? To answer these questions, it is necessary to consider the likelihood ratio as well.
  2. The **likelihood ratio** is the strength of the diagnostic test result.
    a. Sensitivity and specificity are the characteristics used most often to define diagnostic tests.
      (1) Sensitivity answers the question, "Among patients with the disease, how likely is a positive test result?"
      (2) Specificity answers the question, "Among patients without the disease, how likely is a negative test result?"
      (3) The **likelihood ratio** helps answer the clinically more important questions:
        (a) Given a positive test result, how likely is it that the disease is truly present?
        (b) Given a negative test result, how likely is it that the disease is truly absent?
    b. Mathematically, likelihood ratios are the odds of having disease given a test result versus not having a disease given a test result.
      (1) For example:

If the circle represents all patients with a positive test result and the shaded portion represents the portion who actually have disease, then the likelihood ratio is 3. The likelihood ratio is calculated as follows:

the chance of a positive test result and disease/the chance of a positive test result and no disease

 (2) Consider another example. The likelihood ratio of a positive OIA test result is 12. In a large heterogeneous population of patients, all of whom have had positive OIA test results, 12 patients will actually have streptococcal pharyngitis for every 1 who does not. Therefore, if your patient has a positive OIA test result, the odds of her having streptococcal disease are 12 to 1 (i.e., it is **12 times more likely** that streptococcal pharyngitis is present). The negative likelihood ratio of her having OIA is 0.17.

 c. Likelihood ratios can be found in epidemiology textbooks or calculated using the following formulas:

$$\text{Likelihood ratio of a positive test} = \frac{\text{True positive rate}}{\text{False positive rate}}$$

$$= \frac{(\text{Sensitivity})}{(1 - \text{Specificity})}$$

$$\text{Likelihood ratio of a negative test} = \frac{\text{False negative rate}}{\text{True negative rate}}$$

$$= \frac{(1 - \text{Sensitivity})}{(\text{Specificity})}$$

 (1) Most diagnostic tests have likelihood ratios in the 2–5 range for positive results and in the 0.5–0.2 range for negative results. These types of tests are only very useful if the pretest probability of disease is in the middle of the scale (e.g., 30%–70%). At either end of the probability scale, diagnostic tests with small likelihood ratios do not change the pretest probability much.

(2) Good tests have positive likelihood ratios of 10 or more. These powerful diagnostic tests help rule in a diagnosis across a broader range of pretest probabilities. Unfortunately, these types of tests are often expensive or dangerous.

(3) For a test to truly rule in disease across the full range of pretest probabilities, it must have a likelihood ratio of 100 or more. Very few tests (e.g., some biopsies, exploratory laparotomy, cardiac catheterization) have likelihood ratios this high.

3. **Calculating the posttest probability.** Posttest probability is the probability that a specific disease is present after a diagnostic test. Once we have determined the **pretest probability** of disease (using clinical information and disease prevalence data) and the **likelihood ratio** of the diagnostic test result, we are ready to calculate the **posttest probability**. First, however, the pretest probability must be converted to odds (the likelihood ratio is already expressed in odds).

   a. Steps

   (1) Pretest probability must be converted to pretest odds:

   $$\text{Odds} = \frac{(\text{Probability})}{(1 - \text{Probability})}$$

   For example, a probability of 75% equals odds of 3:1.

   (2) Pretest odds are multiplied by the likelihood ratio to give posttest odds.

   (3) Posttest odds must then be converted back to posttest probability:

   $$\text{Probability} = \frac{(\text{Odds})}{(\text{Odds} + 1)}$$

   b. Examples

   (1) In the 8-year-old boy with sore throat, the OIA test result was negative. Therefore, the posttest probability of disease would be 4%:

   (a) The 20% pretest probability is converted to pretest odds: $(0.2)/(1-0.2) = (0.2)/(0.8) = 1:4$.

   (b) The 1:4 pretest odds are multiplied by the likelihood ratio (0.17) to yield posttest odds of 0.17:4 or 1:24.

   (c) The posttest odds are converted to a posttest probability: $(0.043)/(0.043 + 1) = 4\%$. These steps can also be presented schematically:

Pretest probability   Likelihood ratio   Posttest probability
20% ——————→ ¼ × 0.17 = 0.043 → 4%

(2) In the 3-year-old girl with rhinorrhea and cough and a negative OIA test result, the posttest probability would be 0.8%:

Pretest probability   Likelihood ratio   Posttest probability
5% ——————→ ⅑ × 0.17 = 0.008→0.8%

(3) In the 16-year-old girl with fever, sore throat, rash, an exposure history, and a negative OIA test result, the posttest probability would be 76%:

Pretest probability   Likelihood ratio   Posttest probability
95% ——————→ ¹⁹⁄₁ × 0.17 = 3.23—→ 76%

You might ask yourself if it is worth testing the 16-year-old girl because, even with a negative test result, the likelihood that she has streptococcal pharyngitis is high enough to warrant empiric therapy.

HOT

KEY
To gain diagnostic strength, several tests may be combined—as long as they are independent tests. The posttest probability after the first test then becomes the pretest probability for the next test.

HOT

KEY
To really learn this approach, you must use it. Try it on your next patient, and you'll be familiar with the approach before you know it!

References

Jaeschke R, Guyatt G, Sackett DL (for the Evidence-Based Medicine Working Group): Users' guides to the medical literature: how to use an article about a diagnostic test, part A (are the results of the study valid?) *JAMA* 271(5):389–391, 1994.

Jaeschke R, Guyatt G, Sackett DL (for the Evidence-Based Medicine Working Group): Users' guides to the medical literature: how to use an article about a diagnostic test, part B (what are the results and will they help me in caring for my patients?) *JAMA* 271(9):703–707, 1994.

PART II

AMBULATORY PEDIATRICS

2. Immunizations and Control Measures

I   IMMUNIZATION SCHEDULE. **Table 2-1** shows the schedule of immunizations recommended by the American Academy of Pediatrics (AAP).

II   IMMUNIZATION CATCH-UP SCHEDULE (Table 2-2)

III   CONTRAINDICATIONS AND PRECAUTIONS FOR IMMUNIZATIONS (Table 2-3)

A. Precautions should be considered from a risk–benefit perspective. The risk of not vaccinating usually outweighs the precautionary risk.
B. An intercurrent mild illness accompanied by a low-grade fever should not delay administration of the vaccine.

IV   INDICATIONS FOR OTHER VACCINES (Table 2-4)

V   CONTROL MEASURES FOR SPECIFIC INFECTIONS (Table 2-5)

TABLE 2-1. Recommended Childhood Immunization Schedule, United States, 2002

Legend: Range of Recommended Ages | Catch-Up Vaccination | Preadolescent Assessment

Age	Birth	1 Month	2 Months	4 Months	6 Months	12 Months	15 Months	18 Months	24 Months	4–6 Years	11–12 Years	13–18 Years
Hepatitis B*	Hep B #1 only if mother HBsAg(−)	Hep B #2			Hep B #3						Hep B series	
Diphtheria, tetanus, pertussis†			DTaP	DTaP	DTaP			DTaP		DTaP	Td	
Haemophilus influenzae type b‡			Hib	Hib	Hib	Hib						
Inactivated polio§			IPV	IPV	IPV	IPV				IPV		
Measles, mumps, rubella‖						MMR #1				MMR #2	MMR #2	
Varicella#							Varicella			Varicella	Varicella	
Pneumococcal**			PCV	PCV	PCV	PCV			PCV	PPV		

Vaccines below this line are for selected populations

Age	Birth	1 Month	2 Months	4 Months	6 Months	12 Months	15 Months	18 Months	24 Months	4–6 Years	11–12 Years	13–18 Years
Hepatitis A††										Hepatitis A series		
Influenza‡‡						Influenza (yearly)						

Hep B = hepatitis B vaccine; Hib = Haemophilus influenzae; HBIG = hepatitis B immune globulin; DTaP = diphtheria and tetanus toxoids and acellular pertussis; Td = tetanus and diphtheria toxoids. IPV = inactivated polio vaccine; MMR = measles, mumps, and rubella; PCV = pneumococcal vaccine; PPV = pneumococcal polysaccharide vaccine.

*Hepatitis B vaccine: All infants should receive the first dose of hepatitis B vaccine soon after birth and before hospital discharge; the first dose may also be given by age 2 months if the infant's mother is HBsAg-negative. Only monovalent hepatitis B vaccine may be used for the birth dose. Monovalent or combination vaccine containing hepatitis B may be used to complete the series; four doses of vaccine may be administered if combination vaccine is used. The second dose should be given at least 4 weeks after the first dose, except for Haemophilus influenzae type b-containing vaccine, which cannot be administered before age 6 weeks. The third dose should be given at least 16 weeks after the first dose and at least 8 weeks after the second dose. The last dose in the vaccination series (third or fourth dose) should not be administered before age 6 months.

Infants born to HBsAg-positive mothers should receive hepatitis B vaccine and 0.5 ml hepatitis B immune globulin within 12 hours of birth at separate sites. The second dose is recommended at age 1-2 months, and the vaccination series should be completed (third or fourth dose) at age 6 months.

Infants born to mothers whose HBsAg status is unknown should receive the first dose of the hepatitis B vaccine series within 12 hours of birth. Maternal blood should be drawn at the time of delivery to determine the mother's HBsAg status; if the HBsAg test result is positive, the infant should receive hepatitis B immunoglobulin as soon as possible (no later than age 1 week).

†Diphtheria and tetanus toxoids and acellular pertussis vaccine: The fourth dose may be administered as early as age 12 months, provided 6 months have elapsed since the third dose and the child is unlikely to return at age 15-18 months. Tetanus and diphtheria toxoids is recommended at age 11-12 years if at least 5 years have elapsed since the last dose of tetanus and diphtheria toxoid-containing vaccine. Subsequent routine boosters are recommended every 10 years.

‡Haemophilus influenzae type b conjugate vaccine: Three conjugate vaccines are licensed for infant use. If PRP-OMP (PedvaxHIB or ComVax [Merck]) is administered at ages 2 and 4 months, a dose at age 6 months is not required. DTaP/Hib combination products should not be used for primary immunization in infants at ages 2, 4, or 6 months, but can be used as boosters following any Haemophilus influenzae type b vaccine.

§Inactivated polio vaccine: An all-inactivated polio vaccine schedule is recommended for routine childhood polio vaccination in the United States. All children should receive four doses of IPV at ages 2 months, 4 months, 6-18 months, and 4-6 years.

||Measles, mumps, and rubella vaccine: The second dose of measles, mumps, and rubella vaccine is recommended routinely at age 4-6 years but may be administered during any visit, provided at least 4 weeks have elapsed since the first dose and that both doses are administered beginning at or after age 12 months. Those who have not previously received the second dose should complete the schedule by age 11-12 years.

#Varicella vaccine: Varicella vaccine is recommended at any visit at or after age 12 months for susceptible children, that is, those who lack a reliable history of chickenpox. Susceptible persons older than 13 years should receive two doses, given at least 4 weeks apart.

**Pneumococcal vaccine: The heptavalent pneumococcal conjugate vaccine is recommended for all children age 2-23 months. It is also recommended for certain children age 24-59 months. Pneumococcal polysaccharide vaccine is recommended in addition to PCV for certain high-risk groups. See MMWR 49(RR-9);1-35, 2000.

††Hepatitis A vaccine: Hepatitis A vaccine is recommended for use in selected states and regions, and for certain high-risk groups; consult your local public health authority. See MMWR 48(RR-12):1-37, 1999.

‡‡Influenza vaccine: Influenza vaccine is recommended annually for children older than 6 months with certain risk factors (including but not limited to asthma, cardiac disease, sickle cell disease, HIV, diabetes; see MMWR 50(RR-4):1-44, 2001), and can be administered to all others wishing to obtain immunity. Children younger than 12 years should receive vaccine in a dosage appropriate for their age (0.25 ml if age 6-35 months or 0.5 ml if older than 3 years). Children younger than 8 years who are receiving influenza vaccine for the first time should receive two doses separated by at least 4 weeks.

TABLE 2-2. Recommended Immunization Schedules for Children Not Immunized in the First Year of Life ("Catch-Up" Schedule)

Recommended Time/Age	Immunization(s)*	Comments
Younger than 7 years		
First visit	DTaP, Hib, HBV, MMR	If indicated, tuberculin testing may be done at the same visit. If child is 5 years of age or older, Hib is not indicated in most circumstances.
Interval after first visit		
1 month (4 weeks)	DTaP, IPV, HBV, Var	The second dose of IPV may be given if accelerated poliomyelitis immunization is necessary, such as for travelers to areas where polio is endemic.
2 months	DTaP, Hib, IPV	Second dose of Hib is indicated only if the first dose was received when younger than 15 months.
≥ 8 months	DTaP, HBV, IPV	IPV and HBV are not given if the third doses were given earlier.
Age 4–6 years (at or before school entry)	DTaP, IPV, MMR	DTaP is not necessary if the fourth dose was given after the fourth birthday; IPV is not necessary if the third dose was given after the fourth birthday.
Age 11–12 years	See Table 2-1	

7-12 years

First visit	HBV, MMR, dT, IPV	
Interval after first visit		
2 months (8 weeks)	HBV, MMR, Var, dT, IPV	IPV also may be given 1 month after the first visit if accelerated poliomyelitis immunization is necessary.
8–14 months	HBV, dT, IPV	IPV is not given if the third dose was given earlier.
Age 11–12 years	See Table 2-1	

Adapted with permission from Committee on Infectious Disease, American Academy of Pediatrics, Pickering LK (ed): *2000 Red Book Report of the Committee on Infectious Diseases*, 25th ed. Elk Grove Village, IL, American Academy of Pediatrics, 2000.

HBV = hepatitis B virus; Var = varicella; DTaP = diphtheria and tetanus toxoids and acellular pertussis; Hib = *Haemophilus influenzae* type b conjugate; IPV = inactivated poliovirus; MMR = live measles-mumps-rubella; dT = adult tetanus toxoid (full dose) and diphtheria toxoid (reduced dose), for children 7 years of age or older and adults.

*If all needed vaccines cannot be administered simultaneously, priority should be given to protecting the child against the diseases that pose the greatest immediate risk. In the United States, these diseases for children younger than 2 years usually are measles and *Haemophilus influenzae* type b infection; for children older than 7 years, they are measles, mumps, and rubella. Before 13 years of age, immunity against hepatitis B and varicella should be ensured. DTaP, HBV, Hib, MMR, and Var can be given simultaneously at separate sites if failure of the patient to return for future immunization is a concern.

TABLE 2-3. Guide to Contraindications and Precautions to Immunizations, January 2000

Vaccine	Contraindications	Precautions*	Not Contraindications (Vaccines May Be Given)
General for all vaccines (DTaP/DTP,[†] IPV, OPV, MMR, Hib, HBV, Var)	Anaphylactic reaction to a vaccine contraindicates further doses of that vaccine Anaphylactic reaction to a vaccine constituent contraindicates the use of vaccines containing that substance	Moderate or severe illnesses with or without a fever	Mild to moderate local reaction (soreness, redness, swelling) following a dose of an injectable antigen Low-grade or moderate fever following a prior vaccine dose Mild acute illness with or without low-grade fever Current antimicrobial therapy Convalescent phase of illnesses Prematurity (same dosage and indications as for healthy, full-term infants) Recent exposure to an infectious disease History of penicillin or other nonspecific allergies or fact that relatives have such allergies Pregnancy of mother or household contact Unimmunized household contact
DTaP/DTP[†]	Encephalopathy within 7 days of administration of previous dose of DTaP/DTP	Temperature of 40.5°C (104.8°F) within 48 hours after vaccination with a prior dose of DTaP/DTP Collapse or shock-like state (hypotonic-hyporesponsive	Family history of seizures[‡] Family history of sudden infant death syndrome Family history of an adverse event after DTaP/DTP administration

Vaccine	Contraindications	Precautions	Vaccinations that may be given
	episode) within 48 hours of receiving a prior dose of DTaP/DTP Seizures within 3 days of receiving a prior dose of DTaP/DTP‡ Persistent inconsolable crying lasting 3 hours, within 48 hours of receiving a prior dose of DTaP/DTP GBS within 6 weeks after a dose§	Pregnancy	
IPV	Anaphylactic reactions to neomycin or streptomycin	Pregnancy	
OPV‖,#	Infection with HIV or a household contact with HIV Known altered immunodeficiency (hematologic and solid tumors, congenital immunodeficiency, and long-term immunosuppressive therapy) Immunodeficient household contact	Pregnancy	Breast-feeding Current antimicrobial therapy Mild diarrhea

(continued)

TABLE 2-3. Guide to Contraindications and Precautions to Immunizations, January 2000 (Continued)

Vaccine	Contraindications	Precautions*	Not Contraindications (Vaccines May Be Given)
MMR	Pregnancy Anaphylactic reaction to neomycin Anaphylactic reaction to gelatin Known altered immunodeficiency (hematologic and solid tumors, congenital immunodeficiency, severe HIV infection, and long-term immunosuppressive therapy)	Recent (within 3–11 months, depending on product and dose) immune globulin administration** Thrombocytopenia or history of thrombocytopenic purpura**,††	Tuberculosis or positive PPD Simultaneous tuberculin skin testing‡‡ Breast-feeding Pregnancy of mother of recipient Immunodeficient family member or household contact Infection with HIV Nonanaphylactic reactions to eggs or neomycin
Hib	None	—	—
Hepatitis B	Anaphylactic reaction to baker's yeast	—	Pregnancy
Varicella	Pregnancy Anaphylactic reaction to neomycin Anaphylactic reaction to gelatin Infection with HIV Known altered immunodeficiency (hematologic and solid tumors, congenital immunodeficiency, and long-term immunosuppressive therapy)	Recent immune globulin administration Family history of immuno-deficiency§§	Pregnancy in the mother of the recipient Immunodeficiency in a household contact Household contact with HIV

Adapted with permission from Committee on Infectious Disease, American Academy of Pediatrics, Pickering LK (ed.): 2000 Red Book Report of the Committee on Infectious Diseases, 25th ed. Elk Grove Village, IL, American Academy of Pediatrics, 2000.

DTaP = diphtheria and tetanus toxoids and acellular pertussis; DTP = diphtheria and tetanus toxoids and pertussis; IPV = inactivated poliovirus; OPV = oral poliovirus; MMR = measles-mumps-rubella; Hib = *Haemophilus influenzae* type b; HBV = hepatitis B virus; Var = varicella; GBS = Guillain-Barré syndrome; HIV = human immunodeficiency virus; PPD = purified protein derivative (tuberculin).

*The events or conditions listed as precautions, although not contraindications, should be reviewed carefully. The benefits and risks of administering a specific vaccine to a person under the circumstances should be considered. If the risks are believed to outweigh the benefits, the immunization should be withheld; if the benefits are believed to outweigh the risks (e.g., during an outbreak or foreign travel), the immunization should be given. Whether and when to administer DTaP (or DTP) to children with proven or suspected underlying neurologic disorders should be decided on an individual basis.

†DTP is no longer recommended in the United States.

‡Acetaminophen given before administering DTaP (or DTP) and thereafter every 4 hours for 24 hours should be considered for children with a personal or with a family (i.e., siblings or parents) history of seizures.

§The decision to give additional doses of DTaP (or DTP) should be based on consideration of the benefit of further vaccination vs the risk of recurrence of GBS. For example, completion of the primary series in children is justified.

‖A theoretical risk exists that the administration of multiple live virus vaccines within 30 days (4 weeks) of one another if not given on the same day will result in suboptimal immune response. No data substantiate this risk, however.

#OPV is no longer recommended for routine use in the United States.

**An anaphylactic reaction to egg ingestion previously was considered a contraindication unless skin testing and, if indicated, desensitization had been performed. However, skin testing no longer is recommended as of 1997.

††The decision to vaccinate should be based on consideration of the benefits of immunity to measles, mumps, and rubella vs the risk of recurrence or exacerbation of thrombocytopenia after vaccination, or from natural infections of measles or rubella. In most instances, the benefits of vaccination will be much greater than the potential risks and justify giving MMR, particularly in view of the even greater risk of thrombocytopenia after measles or rubella disease. However, if a prior episode of thrombocytopenia occurred in temporal proximity to vaccination, not giving a subsequent dose may be prudent.

‡‡Measles vaccination may temporarily suppress tuberculin reactivity. MMR vaccine may be given after, or on the same day as, tuberculin testing. If MMR has been given recently, postpone the tuberculin test until 4–6 weeks after administration of MMR. If giving MMR simultaneously with the tuberculin skin test, use the Mantoux test and not multiple puncture tests, because the latter require confirmation if positive, which would have to be postponed for 4–6 weeks.

§§Varicella vaccine should not be given to a member of a household with a family history of immunodeficiency until the immune status of the recipient and other children in the family is documented.

TABLE 2-4. Indications for Other Vaccines

Vaccines	Indications/Administration Details
Pneumococcal (Prevnar)	Universal vaccination is now recommended for all infants. The schedule is: 2, 4, 6, and 12–15 months for infants; three doses for children ages 7–11 months; two doses of children 12–23 months; and one dose for children 2 years or older.
Influenza	Indications: > 6 months of age and one of the following: asthma, hemodynamically significant CHD, CF, sickle cell disease, BPD, immunosuppressed patient after transplant, HIV, patient requiring long-term aspirin therapy, diabetes, chronic renal disease, chronic metabolic disease Administration: needs to be administered yearly due to changes in antigens. The efficacy of the vaccine for infants < 6 months is in question; give two doses 1 month apart to those under the age of 8 years.
Meningococcus	Indications: > 2 years old and in a high-risk group: asplenia, terminal complement deficiencies, properdin deficiencies, for epidemic outbreak control if culprit is subtype A, C, Y or W-135.
Rabies (RIG, HDCV)	Passive (RIG) and active immunization (HDCV) are required to ensure effectiveness. Healthy dogs/cats: observe for 10 days Skunks, raccoons, foxes, woodchucks, wild cats, dogs, other carnivores: consider rabid and immunize unless animal is proven to be nonrabid Livestock, rodents, lagomorphs (rabbits/hares), guinea pigs, gerbils, chipmunks, rats, mice, squirrels, hamsters: usually not considered rabid

CHD = congenital heart disease; CF = cystic fibrosis; BPD = bronchopulmonary dysplasia; RIG = rabies immune globulin; HDCV = human diploid cell vaccine.

TABLE 2-5. Control Measures for Specific Infections

Organism	Drug/Dose	Indications
Pertussis	Erythromycin: 40–50 mg/kg/day (maximum, 2 g/day) divided four times daily for 14 days	Household or daycare: all contacts require treatment regardless of immune status School: school-wide or classroom-wide treatment is not recommended; index case may return to school/daycare after 5 days of treatment
Meningococcus	Rifampin: 10 mg/kg/dose (maximum, 600 mg/dose) every 12 hours for 2 days or Ceftriaxone: 125 mg once intramuscularly if <12 years old, 250 mg once intramuscularly if >12 years old	Indications: household contact, child care or nursery contact in last 7 days, kissing contact, sharing saliva, mouth-to-mouth resuscitation, unprotected contact during intubation within 7 days of illness, sleeping in same dwelling as patient Not indicated: casual contact, health care workers without direct exposure to secretions
Haemophilus influenzae	Rifampin: 20 mg/kg/dose (maximum, 600 mg/dose) four times daily for 4 days	Household: if there is one contact younger than 48 months of age whose immunization status is incomplete or if there is an immunocompromised contact, the entire family needs treatment; if all are immunized completely, no treatment is needed School: if there are more than 2 cases of invasive disease within 60 days and there are incompletely vaccinated attendees, all need prophylaxis; if there is only 1 case, prophylaxis is controversial Day care: if attendees are younger than 2 years old, incompletely vaccinated, and there are more than 25 hours of contact per week, prophylaxis is required

(continued)

TABLE 2-5. Control Measures for Specific Infections (Continued)

Organism	Drug/Dose	Indications
Hepatitis A	Fewer than 2 weeks since exposure: IG: 0.02 ml/kg once intramuscularly Also give HAV vaccine if older than 2 years and future exposure is likely More than 2 weeks since exposure: IG is not indicated Give HAV vaccine if older than 2 years and future exposure is likely	Household/sexual contacts: IG immediately; IG is not indicated if exposure occurred more than 2 weeks ago School: treatment of contacts is not indicated Day care: if all children are older than 2 years and toilet trained, give IG for adults and children in same room as the index case; if there are more than 2 cases and children are not all toilet trained, give IG for all attendees Hospital: treatments needed if there is close personal contact with index case

IG = immune globulin; HAV = hepatitis A virus.

References

Peter G (ed): *2000 Red Book: Report of the Committee on Infectious Diseases,* 25th ed. Elk Grove Village, IL: American Academy of Pediatrics, 2000.

3. Breast-Feeding and Nutrition

I **INTRODUCTION.** Breast milk is the optimal source of nutrition for infants in their first year of life. Exclusive breast-feeding without supplementation by other foods, juice, or water is sufficient until the infant is 6 months old. Thereafter, a gradual introduction to solid foods is necessary (see III B). Breast-feeding is recommended through the first year and can continue as long as desired into the toddler years.

II **BENEFITS OF BREAST-FEEDING**

A. Benefits for the infant. Breast-feeding is associated with a decrease in the incidence of diarrhea, lower respiratory tract infection, otitis media, bacteremia, bacterial meningitis, botulism, urinary tract infection, and necrotizing enterocolitis. Breast-feeding may also provide some protection against sudden infant death syndrome, insulin-dependent diabetes mellitus, Crohn disease, ulcerative colitis, lymphoma, allergic diseases, and chronic gastrointestinal diseases.

B. Benefits for the mother. Lactation promotes bone remineralization and an earlier return to prepregnancy weight. Further benefits include a delayed resumption of ovulation and a reduced risk of ovarian and premenopausal breast cancer.

C. Other benefits for the family. Breast-feeding is far less expensive than formula feeding. Breast milk is readily available and requires no preparation. The mother can pump and store breast milk if she needs to be away or if the father or another care giver wants to feed the infant.

III **RELATED ISSUES**

A. Medications and breast-feeding. Table 3-1 lists the substances that are contraindicated for breast-feeding mothers.

B. The transition to solid foods begins when the infant is approximately 6 months old.
  1. Initial foods should be high in iron (e.g., cereal) because, by 6 months of age, infants have used much of their endogenous store of iron.
  2. One new food should be introduced each week.

TABLE 3-1. Drugs to be Avoided When Breast-Feeding
Amantadine
Antineoplastic agents
Bromides
Bromocriptine
Chloramphenicol
Chlordiazepoxide
Cyclophosphamide
Cyclosporine
Doxorubicin
Drugs of abuse (e.g., amphetamines, cocaine, heroin)
Ergotamine
Gold
Iodines
Lindane
Lithium
Metronidazole
Methotrexate
Phenindione
Radioactive diagnostic and therapeutic agents

   3. Cooked, strained, and pureed fruits and vegetables are given first. Breads, meats, and eggs (yolks first) are introduced later.

   4. Vitamin and iron supplements. Infants who are exclusively breast-fed should be given supplemental iron starting in the 6th week of life. A multiple vitamin with iron (e.g., Poly-Vi-Sol) often is used.

C. Concerns that arise during breast-feeding are presented in **Table 3-2.**

TABLE 3-2. Common Concerns During Breast-Feeding	
Concern	**Management Strategies**
Engorgement of the breast	Engorgement commonly occurs between the 3rd and 6th postpartum days. With proper treatment, it subsides within 12–48 hours.
	1. Gentle breast massage is performed with the hand moving from the chest wall toward the nipple.
	2. Warm, moist compresses on the breast help to stimulate the milk ejection reflex.
	(continued)

TABLE 3-2. Common Concerns During Breast-Feeding (*Continued*)

Concern	Management Strategies
	3. Frequent nursing (every 90–120 minutes) helps alleviate and prevent further engorgement.
	4. Nursing should continue for 10–20 minutes on each breast, until the breast feels softer.
	5. Supplementation is discouraged because it decreases the frequency of breast-feeding.
	6. Cold compresses between feedings may relieve pain.
Improper latching on of the infant	Improper latching may be caused by engorgement of the breast.
	1. A small amount of milk can be hand-expressed to soften the areolar area.
	2. Before the mother offers the infant the nipple, she can encourage the infant's mouth to open by gently tickling the infant's lips with the nipple.
	3. The infant's gums should be placed around the areola, not just around the nipple.
Sore nipples	Nipple tenderness is common within the first 4 days of breast-feeding.
	1. Soreness throughout the nursing session may indicate improper latching or positioning. An alternate nursing position should be tried (e.g., lay the infant on the opposite side, cradle the infant in a "football" hold). The mother should verify that the infant is not sucking in the lower lip while nursing.
	2. Before the mother pulls the infant away from the breast after feeding, she can break the suction by inserting a finger gently in the corner of the infant's mouth and pulling down slightly.
	3. The mother may spread residual milk on the nipple and allow it to dry. This dried milk encourages healing of cracked nipples.
	4. The mother should avoid the use of drying agents (e.g., soap, rubbing alcohol). The nipples should be rinsed only with water.
	5. The infant should be examined for thrush, especially if breast-feeding is accompanied by itching or burning. Topical nystatin should be used for both the mother and the infant.

(continued)

TABLE 3-2. Common Concerns During Breast-Feeding (*Continued*)

Concern	Management Strategies
Frequency and duration of the feedings	1. In the first few weeks of life, an infant normally takes 8–12 feedings daily. All infants vary in time of day, frequency, and duration of feedings. Optimally, the infant should feed on one breast for 5 minutes, then complete the feeding on the opposite breast. The cycle repeats at the next feeding, starting on the opposite breast. 2. Allowing the infant to finish one breast before switching to the other allows for full feedings of the foremilk (high in volume at the beginning of feeding, but low in fat) and hindmilk (low in volume toward the end of a breast's milk supply, but high in fat). 3. Short, very frequent feedings should be discouraged. This "snacking" pattern promotes problems in dentition in older infants, disrupts adequate sleeping patterns in mothers and infants, and limits the intake of high-calorie hindmilk.
Adequate milk supply and weight gain	Infants should regain their birth weight 2 weeks after birth, then gain 30 g/day for the first 3 months. 1. If these goals are not met, a workup for failure to thrive should be considered. 2. The mother should be encouraged to record the number of bowel movements and wet diapers.
Regurgitation	Normal, healthy infants often spit up regularly. Spitting up usually stops within 6 months. If it does not, the following steps can be taken. 1. Investigate for possible overfeeding. The use of breast-feeding as a comfort measure should be discouraged. 2. The infant can be burped more frequently, or shorter, more frequent feedings may be tried. 3. Sensitivity to a newly introduced supplement, medication, vitamin, or food should be ruled out. Sensitivity to foods eaten by the mother is rare. 4. If spitting up is accompanied by inadequate weight gain, weight loss, lung disease, or severe choking, gastroesophageal reflux disease should be considered.

(continued)

| TABLE 3-2. Common Concerns During Breast-Feeding (*Continued*) | |
Concern	Management Strategies
Projectile or bilious vomiting	Dark green or bilious emesis is cause for alarm! An obstructive process (e.g., malrotation, duodenal atresia) must be ruled out. In cases of projectile vomiting, pyloric stenosis should be considered.
Sleepy infant	If it is difficult to wake the infant for nursing, or if the infant falls asleep while nursing, stimulation should be tried, including: 1. Changing the diaper 2. Stroking the infant's cheek 3. Switching to the opposite breast 4. Burping the infant

References

American Academy of Pediatrics: Breast-feeding and the use of human milk. Policy statement. 1997.

Anderson PO: Drug use during breast-feeding. *Clin Pharm* 10(8):594–624, 1991.

Committee on Nutrition, American Academy of Pediatrics, Kleinman RE (ed): *Pediatric Nutrition Handbook,* 4th ed. Elk Grove Village, IL, American Academy of Pediatrics, 1997.

4. Developmental Delay and Disability

Introduction

A. Background and definitions. An understanding of normal child development is required to be able to identify significant delays or disabilities and provide appropriate interventions.

1. **Developmental disability** is static (nonprogressive) central nervous system (CNS) dysfunction that interferes with the expected progression of normal development. It may be global (e.g., mental retardation) or more focused (e.g., spastic diplegia).

2. **Mental retardation (MR)** is a static encephalopathy with cognitive deficits [i.e., below-average functioning (IQ < 70) on intelligence testing], impaired adaptive behaviors, and onset before 18 years of age. It is a descriptive term. The severity dictates the prognosis:

   a. **Mild (IQ = 50–69;** 85% of patients). These patients are trainable to grade 6, function at the level of an 8- to 10-year-old child, and may be able to live on their own with some help.

   b. **Moderate (IQ = 35–49;** 10% of patients). These patients are trainable to grade 2, function at the level of a 6- to 8-year-old child, and probably will not be able to live on their own.

   c. **Severe (IQ = 20–34;** 3%–4% of patients). These patients eventually function at the level of a child who is 4 to 6 years old. Some training usually is possible.

   d. **Profound (IQ ≤ 20;** 1%–2% of patients). These patients function below the level of a 4-year-old child. These patients are not trainable and typically need institutionalization.

3. **Cerebral palsy (CP)** is a static disorder of gross motor development marked by weakness and spasticity. It may be associated with abnormalities of speech, cognition, and vision. CP cannot be diagnosed in the neonatal period because the nervous system is not yet sufficiently mature.

   a. **Spastic hemiplegia** is weakness, spasticity, and abnormal reflexes on an affected side (i.e., arm and leg). Patients show an early hand preference and a circumductive gait. One third of patients have a seizure disorder; 25% have cognitive dysfunction, including MR.

25

    b. Spastic diplegia is bilateral weakness, spasticity, and abnormal reflexes of the legs. It is first observed in infancy when the infant crawls using only the arms, with the legs dragging behind (commando crawl). Cognitive dysfunction and seizure disorders are uncommon.

    c. Spastic quadriplegia is the most severe form of CP, with involvement of the upper and lower extremities. Mental retardation and seizures are common.

    d. Athetoid CP presents in infants after 1 year of age. Infants are hypotonic and have athetoid movements. This form of CP has become relatively rare since the advent of aggressive management for hyperbilirubinemia. Seizures and cognitive function are intact.

  4. Communication disorder is a global term that describes abnormalities of speech, language, and behavior. Like MR, it is a diagnostic label. Hearing, perception, comprehension, and speech production may be impaired.

  5. The developmental quotient (DQ) provides a rough estimate of developmental delay within a given area. In general, any child with a language or visuomotor quotient under 80 requires evaluation by a specialist.

$$DQ = \left(\frac{\text{developmental age}}{\text{chronological age}} \right) \times 100$$

HOT **KEY**
  The static nature of developmental disabilities is important. Patients who achieve milestones and then lose them should be evaluated for a progressive encephalopathy (e.g., HIV, metabolic disorders, neoplasms, hypothyroidism).

B. Epidemiology. Most patients with developmental disability have no risk factors that would predict such a disability. Approximately 5% of the population may have cognitive and language disorders; 4% may have motor abnormalities.

II APPROACH TO THE PATIENT. Accurate measurements of weight, height, and head circumference should be taken during the physical examination at every check-up, with keen attention paid to dysmorphic features that may be a clue to a metabolic disease or chromosomal abnormality (e.g., fragile X syndrome; Down syndrome).

III DEVELOPMENTAL MILESTONES

A. Table 4-1 lists developmental milestones that should be reached during the first year of life.

TABLE 4-1. Emerging Patterns of Behavior During the First Year of Life	

Neonatal period (first 4 weeks)

Prone:	lies in flexed attitude; turns head from side to side; head sags on ventral suspension
Supine:	generally flexed and slightly stiff
Visual:	may fixate face or light in line of vision; "doll's-eye" movement of eyes on turning of the body
Reflex:	moro response active; stepping and placing reflexes; grasp reflex active
Social:	visual preference for human face

At 4 weeks

Prone:	legs more extended; holds chin up; turns head; head lifted momentarily to plane of body on ventral suspension
Supine:	tonic neck posture predominates; supple and relaxed; head lags on pull to sitting position
Visual:	watches person; follows moving object
Social:	body movements in cadence with voice of other in social contact; beginning to smile

At 8 weeks

Prone:	raises head slightly farther; head sustained in plane of body on ventral suspension
Supine:	tonic neck posture predominates; head lags on pull to sitting position
Visual:	follows moving object 180°
Social:	smiles on social contact; listens to voice and coos

At 12 weeks

Prone:	lifts head and chest, arms extended; head above plane of body on ventral suspension
Supine:	tonic neck posture predominates; reaches toward and misses objects; waves at toy
Sitting:	head lag partially compensated on pull to sitting position; early head control with bobbing motion; back rounded
Reflex:	typical Moro response has not persisted; makes defensive movements or selective withdrawal reactions
Social:	sustained social contact; listens to music; says "aah, ngah"

At 16 weeks

Prone:	lifts head and chest, head in approximately vertical axis; legs extended
Supine:	symmetric posture predominates, hands in midline; reaches and grasps objects and brings them to mouth
Sitting:	no head lag on pull to sitting position; head steady, tipped forward; enjoys sitting with full truncal support

(continued)

TABLE 4-1. Emerging Patterns of Behavior During the First Year of Life (*Continued*)

Standing:	when held erect, pushes with feet
Adaptive:	sees pellet, but makes no move to it
Social:	laughs out loud; may show displeasure if social contact is broken; excited at sight of food

At 28 weeks

Prone:	rolls over; pivots; crawls or creep-crawls (Knobloch)
Supine:	lifts head; rolls over; squirming movements
Sitting:	sits briefly, with support of pelvis; leans forward on hands; back rounded
Standing:	may support most of weight; bounces actively
Adaptive:	reaches out for and grasps large object; transfers objects from hand to hand; grasp uses radial palm; rakes at pellet
Language:	polysyllabic vowel sounds formed
Social:	prefers mother; babbles; enjoys mirror; responds to changes in emotional content of social contact

At 40 weeks

Sitting:	sits up alone and indefinitely without support, back straight
Standing:	pulls to standing position; "cruises" or walks on to furniture
Motor:	creeps or crawls
Adaptive:	grasps objects with thumb and forefinger; pokes at things with forefinger; picks up pellet with assisted pincer movement; uncovers hidden toy; attempts to retrieve dropped object; releases object grasped by other person
Language:	repetitive consonant sounds (mama, dada)
Social:	responds to sound of name; plays peek-a-boo or pat-a-cake; waves bye-bye

At 52 weeks (1 year)

Motor:	walks with one hand held (48 weeks); rises independently, takes several steps (Knobloch)
Adaptive:	picks up pellet with unassisted pincer movement of forefinger and thumb; releases object to other person on request or gesture
Language:	a few words besides mama, dada
Social:	plays simple ball game; makes postural adjustment to dressing

Data are derived from those of Gesell (as revised by Knobloch), Shirley, Provence, Wolf, Bailey, and others. (Reprinted with permission from Behrman RE, Kliegman RM, Jenson HB: *Nelson Textbook of Pediatrics*, 16th ed. Philadelphia, WB Saunders, 2000, p 35.)

B. Table 4-2 lists developmental milestones that normal children reach between 1 and 5 years of age.

IV LANGUAGE DEVELOPMENT

A. Introduction. Language is the single best measure of cognitive development; it is most closely correlated with IQ and is most susceptible to psychosocial deprivation. The most sensitive early marker for MR is language development. The greatest increase in language is seen during the period from 2 to 5 years of age. During these years, vocabulary increases from 50 to 2000 words.

B. Screening and milestones. The best assessment of language is the achievement of milestones (see Tables 4-1 and 4-2). A DQ for language < 80 is considered delayed. Other signs that may

---

TABLE 4-2. Emerging Patterns of Behavior From 1 to 5 Years of Age

15 months

Motor:	walks alone; crawls up stairs
Adaptive:	makes tower of three cubes; makes a line with crayon; inserts pellet in bottle
Language:	jargon; follows simple commands; may name a familiar object (ball)
Social:	indicates some desires or needs by pointing; hugs parents

18 months

Motor:	runs stiffly; sits on small chair; walks up stairs with one hand held; explores drawers and wastebaskets
Adaptive:	makes a tower of four cubes; imitates scribbling; imitates vertical stroke; dumps pellet from bottle
Language:	10 words (average); names pictures; identifies one or more parts of body
Social:	feeds self; seeks help when in trouble; may complain when wet or soiled; kisses parent with pucker

24 months

Motor:	runs well, walks up and down stairs, one step at a time; opens doors; climbs on furniture; jumps
Adaptive:	tower of seven cubes (six at 21 months), circular scribbling; imitates horizontal stroke; folds paper once imitatively
Language:	puts three words together (subject, verb, object)
Social:	handles spoon well; often tells immediate experiences; helps to undress; listens to stories with pictures

(continued)

TABLE 4-2. Emerging Patterns of Behavior From 1 to 5 Years of Age (Continued)

30 months
- Motor: goes up stairs alternating feet
- Adaptive: tower of nine cubes; makes vertical and horizontal strokes but generally will not join them to make a cross; imitates circular stroke, forming closed figure
- Language: refers to self by pronoun "I"; knows full name
- Social: helps put things away; pretends in play

36 months
- Motor: rides tricycle; stands momentarily on one foot
- Adaptive: tower of ten cubes; imitates construction of "bridge" of three cubes; copies a circle; imitates a cross
- Language: knows age and sex; counts three objects correctly; repeats three numbers or a sentence of six syllables
- Social: plays simple games (in "parallel" with other children); helps in dressing (unbuttons clothing and puts on shoes); washes hands

48 months
- Motor: hops on one foot; throws ball overhand; uses scissors to cut out pictures; climbs well
- Adaptive: copies bridge from model; imitates construction of "gate" of five cubes; copies cross and square; draws a man with two to four parts besides head; names longer of two lines
- Language: counts four pennies accurately; tells a story
- Social: plays with several children with beginning of social interaction and role-playing; goes to toilet alone

60 months
- Motor: skips
- Adaptive: draws triangle from copy; names heavier of two weights
- Language: names four colors; repeats sentence of 10 syllables; counts 10 pennies correctly
- Social: dresses and undresses; asks questions about meaning of words; domestic role-playing

Data are derived from those of Gesell (as revised by Knobloch), Shirley, Provence, Wolf, Bailey, and others. After 5 years, the Stanford-Binet, Wechsler-Bellevue, and other scales offer the most precise estimates of developmental level. In order to have their greatest value, they should be administered only by an experienced and qualified person. (Reprinted with permission from Behrman RE, Kliegman RM, Jenson HB: *Nelson Textbook of Pediatrics*, 16th ed. Philadelphia, WB Saunders, 2000, p 38.)

indicate a communication disorder and prompt a referral for audiologic or language testing are as follows:

1. Failure to calm to a familiar voice after 3 months of age
2. No eye contact or smiling after 3 months of age
3. No vocalization in response to smiling adult at 3–6 months of age
4. Dislike of being held
5. Inability to produce consonant sounds by 12 months of age
6. No history of babbling or cooing
7. Failure to express nonverbal intention by 12 months of age
8. Failure to respond to environmental sounds
9. Inability to localize a sound source by 12 months of age
10. Inability to play peek-a-boo by 12 months of age
11. Inability to use single words or multiword phrases, or failure to achieve the expected rapid increase in vocabulary by 24–36 months of age
12. Echolalia (repetition of words or phrases without understanding) after 30 months of age.

V ADAPTIVE AND VISUOMOTOR DEVELOPMENT

A. The category **adaptive and visuomotor development** relates to problem-solving skills. This type of development combines visual and fine motor manipulative tasks, as well as the cognitive ability to complete such tasks.
B. A persistent DQ < 80 represents a probable delay (see Tables 4-1 and 4-2).

VI GROSS MOTOR DEVELOPMENT

A. **Background.** Gross motor impairment is a key to early detection of CP, although the degree of gross motor delay does not predict the degree of cognitive delay. However, patients with gross motor delays are likely to have either language or adaptive delays.
B. **Screening and milestones.** In general, a DQ < 50 is likely to represent delay; a DQ > 70 is less likely to indicate a problem. Although the development of gross motor skills varies significantly, patients who do not walk by 15 months of age should be evaluated. In addition to the criteria in Tables 4-1 and 4-2, intense primitive reflexes or primitive reflexes that are not suppressed by 6 months of age may indicate a gross motor abnormality.

VII FURTHER WORKUP

A. **Mental retardation.** Approximately 50% of cases of mental retardation are idiopathic. A wide diagnostic net is not recommended; the workup should be focused and based on clinical suspicion.

1. The patient's **history** should be reviewed for intrauterine growth retardation (IUGR), asphyxia, meningitis, trauma, neurocutaneous disorders, and head circumference.
2. **Chromosomal studies** have a yield of 2%–3% (e.g., fragile X syndrome).
3. A **metabolic workup** should be considered if appropriate symptoms (e.g., seizures, recurrent vomiting, acidosis, hypoglycemia, hepatomegaly) are present.
4. A **lead screening** should be performed if the patient has a history of pica or lives in an area where lead exposure is a possibility.
5. The **uric acid level** should be measured to rule out Lesch-Nyhan syndrome if the patient has a history of self-mutilation.
6. The **zinc level** should be measured if the patient has a history of acrodermatitis.
7. The **copper or ceruloplasmin level** should be measured if the patient has Kayser-Fleischer rings or cirrhosis.
8. Studies for **syphilis, toxoplasmosis, rubella, cytomegalovirus, and herpesvirus (STORCH) infection** should be performed if the patient has a history of hepatosplenomegaly, hearing loss, or intracranial calcifications.
9. An **electroencephalogram (EEG)** should be performed if the patient has a history of seizures.
10. A **computed tomographic (CT) scan** should be performed if the patient has progressive encephalopathy, microcephaly, focal findings, or symptoms of increased intracranial pressure.

B. **CP.** Most patients with CP do not have identifiable risk factors. The cause often is not known.

1. **Risk factors** for CP include birth asphyxia, prematurity, and IUGR.
2. CT or magnetic resonance imaging (MRI) scanning should be considered to evaluate myelination and to diagnose gross brain abnormalities.
3. Spinal cord lesions, meningocele, neurodegenerative disease, and muscular dystrophy should be considered. A creatine phosphokinase test should be performed if a child is not walking by the age of 15 months.
4. **Cognitive delays** that may accompany the gross motor deficits should be investigated.

VIII TREATMENT OF DEVELOPMENTAL DISABILITIES

A. Treatment of developmental disabilities requires a team approach. Optimizing cognitive and motor function requires the coordinated work of occupational therapists, physical thera-

pists, speech and language pathologists, educators, and orthopedic surgeons.
B. Appropriate social support for all families should be sought.

References
Behrman RE, Kliegman RM, Jenson HB (eds): *Nelson Textbook of Pediatrics,* 16th
   ed. Philadelphia, WB Saunders, 2000.
McMillan JA, DeAngelis CD, Feigin RD, et al (eds): *Oski's Pediatrics: Principles and
   Practice,* 3rd ed. Philadelphia, Lippincott Williams & Wilkins, 1999.
Stanley O, Dolby S: Learning in preschool children with neurological disability. *Arch
   Dis Child* 80(5):481–484, 1999.

5. Failure to Thrive

I INTRODUCTION

A. Incidence. Failure to thrive (i.e., inadequate physical growth, or an inability to maintain the expected rate of growth over time) is common.

1. As many as one third of children presenting at inner-city emergency departments show some growth deficiency.
2. One percent of all pediatric hospital admissions are for failure to thrive.

HOT KEY

Eighty percent of all affected children are younger than 18 months.

B. Definitions

1. According to the National Center for Health Statistics (NCHS), failure to thrive is present in:
   a. A child younger than 2 years whose weight is below the third or fifth percentile for age on more than one occasion
   b. A child younger than 2 years whose weight is less than 80% of the ideal weight for age
   c. A child younger than 2 years whose weight crosses two major percentiles downward on a standardized growth grid
2. Exceptions include infants with genetic short stature, preterm infants, and small-for-gestational age infants.

HOT KEY

A child who is small or short is not necessarily failing to thrive.

II CAUSES OF FAILURE TO THRIVE. Failure to thrive is a sign, not a diagnosis.

A. Formerly, the diagnosis was attributed to either an organic (medical) or nonorganic (social) etiology. Currently, failure to thrive is recognized as a condition that can result from a combination of organic and nonorganic factors.

HOT KEY

Weight gain during hospitalization does not rule out an organic (medical) cause for the failure to thrive.

B. Although failure to thrive is a multifactorial condition, its three essential causes are easy to remember **(Table 5-1.)** Just consider the basic mechanisms by which children grow:

TABLE 5-1. Causes of Failure to Thrive	
Pathophysiologic Mechanism	**Specific Examples**
Insufficient caloric intake	
Appetite disorder	Anemia
	Gastrointestinal pathology (e.g., reflux esophagitis)
	CNS disorder (e.g., neoplasm)
	Chronic infection
Difficulty with ingestion	Psychosocial problems (e.g., rumination, apathy, chaotic social situation that affects feeding)
	CNS disorder (e.g., cerebral palsy, oromotor difficulty)
	Muscle weakness
Unavailability of food	Inappropriate feeding technique
	Inadequate volume
	Intentional withholding of food
Vomiting	CNS disorder (e.g., tumor, hydrocephalus)
	Intestinal tract obstruction (e.g., pyloric stenosis, malrotation)
	Gastroesophageal reflux
Insufficient caloric absorption	
Malabsorption	Lactose intolerance
	Gluten enteropathy
	Cystic fibrosis
Diarrhea	Viral or bacterial infection
Excessive caloric expenditure	
Increased use	Chronic infection
	Chronic respiratory disease
	Heart disease
	Spastic cerebral palsy
	Hyperthyroidism
Defective use	Metabolic disorder
	Renal disorder (e.g., renal tubular acidosis)

CNS = central nervous system.

1. Sufficient caloric intake
2. Sufficient absorption of what they eat
3. Absence of excessive caloric expenditure (i.e., chronic disease)

III APPROACH TO THE PATIENT

A. **Patient history.** Given the multifactorial nature of failure to thrive, the patient history should be fairly detailed and should cover the following areas:
   1. Prenatal and perinatal events
   2. Maternal drug use and HIV risk factors
   3. The nature of the pregnancy (planned, unwanted)
   4. Gestational age
   5. Apgar scores
   6. Birth weight, length, and head circumference
   7. Amount of time spent in the hospital after the delivery
   8. Past medical problems, surgeries, illnesses, hospitalizations, and medications

---

> **HOT ▶ KEY**
>
> Accurate measurements of height, weight, and head circumference should be obtained and charted each time the child is seen by a pediatrician, examined in the emergency department, or admitted to the hospital. The ability to review these measurements over time is a critical aspect of the patient workup.

B. **Feeding.** The paramount task is to determine whether the child is receiving adequate calories to promote and sustain growth. Children require 100 kcal/kg/day to grow.
   1. **Assess intake.** Intake is most accurately assessed by examining a record of food intake over the previous 48–72 hours. The average jar of baby food contains approximately 80 kcal, and formula contains approximately 20 kcal per ounce.
   2. **Assess factors that can affect intake.** Are the child's meal times consistent? Is he being offered food that is appropriate for his age and developmental status? Are any distractions present at meal time (e.g., television, parental conflict)?

C. **Development.** Review past and current milestones. Developmental delay may contribute to failure to thrive, but may also result from it.

D. **Psychosocial situation.** Answers to the following questions may provide insight:
   1. What are the psychosocial stressors present in the family? Was conflict present before or after the failure to thrive was identified?

> **HOT KEY**
>
> Feeding problems in an infant or toddler can lead to significant stress and conflict between parents.

    2. Who is the child's primary caretaker? What is this person's typical day like?

    3. Is there any evidence of maternal depression?

    4. What is the parents parenting style? Who were their role models for parenting?

    5. What is the child's temperament?

E. Family history

    1. Siblings. Feeding problems, significant illnesses, and deaths during infancy among other children in the family should be noted. If circumstances are suspicious, it may be appropriate to query the local authorities about any prior reports of child abuse or neglect within the family.

    2. Parents. Document the height, body habitus, and head size of each parent.

F. Physical examination

    1. Measurements. The child's height, weight, and head circumference should be noted in the chart.

    2. Vital signs. Worrisome vital signs include low blood pressure, a low pulse rate for age, and hypothermia.

    3. Overall assessment

        a. Note the presence of dysmorphic features, signs of physical abuse or neglect, and signs of neurologic, pulmonary, cardiac, or gastrointestinal disease.

        b. Pay attention to the way the child and caretaker interact. In addition, note the child's response to the examiner (e.g., is the child fearful or withdrawn?).

        c. Ideally, at least one feeding, or meal, should be observed by the physician. If a primary oromotor problem is suspected, additional feedings should be observed by an occupational or physical therapist.

G. Laboratory studies are notoriously low-yield in the evaluation of a patient with failure to thrive, with results contributing to the final diagnosis in approximately 1% of cases. However, some studies may be appropriate, depending on the history and physical examination findings.

    1. Initial tests. The following tests may be helpful initially:

        a. A complete blood count (CBC), to evaluate for anemia

        b. A urinalysis, to evaluate for diabetes or nephropathy

        c. A serum electrolyte panel, to evaluate for metabolic or renal disease

        d. A serum creatinine level, to evaluate for renal disease

      e. A 48- to 72-hour stool analysis for fats, to evaluate for malabsorption

  2. Additional tests. History and physical examination findings may render one or more of the following tests appropriate:

      a. A purified protein derivative (PPD) test

      b. Bone age (chronic disease or an endocrine abnormality is unlikely in light of a normal bone age)

      c. Albumin, alkaline phosphatase, calcium, and phosphorous levels

      d. Sweat test

      e. HIV test

IV TREATMENT

A. Treatment of the underlying causes

  1. Counseling. Because failure to thrive is typically multifactorial, extensive individual and family counseling may be indicated to address underlying psychosocial problems.

  2. Physical therapy. The child may require physical or occupational therapy to improve her feeding skills.

  3. Treatment of medical causes. If a medical cause for the failure to thrive is diagnosed, appropriate therapy should be initiated.

B. Refeeding. All children with failure to thrive require a refeeding plan for catch-up growth.

  1. Nutritional requirements should be estimated at 50% greater than average (i.e., 150 kcal/kg/day). In infants, increased caloric density can be achieved by concentrating or supplementing infant formulas. Toddler diets can be fortified by adding dairy products, margarine, oil, and peanut butter to meals and snacks.

  2. Some children may need short-term nasogastric feedings, and a few eventually require gastrostomy tube placement.

HOT KEY — Children who show signs of abuse, are less than 60% of their ideal weight, or continue to grow poorly despite 1–2 months of intensive outpatient efforts may require hospital admission.

V PROGNOSIS. Given the complexities of diagnosis and treatment of failure to thrive, a long-term and close therapeutic alliance between the medical team and the family of the patient is essential.

A. A child whose standardized weight began to decrease immediately after birth until it was more than two standard deviations below normal may suffer a loss in predicted mental or psycho-motor abilities in the second postnatal year.

B. Children with failure to thrive are at risk for poor cognitive development if they do not receive careful monitoring and treatment.

References

Gahagan S, Holmes R: A stepwise approach to evaluation of undernutrition and failure to thrive. *Pediatr Clin North Am* 45(1):169–187, 1998.

Zenel JA Jr: Failure to thrive: a general pediatrician's perspective. *Pediatr Rev* 18(11):371–378, 1997.

6. Child Abuse and Neglect

I INTRODUCTION

A. Definition. Child abuse and neglect is the physical or mental injury, sexual abuse, or negligent treatment of a child younger than 18 years by a person who is responsible for the child's welfare.

B. Risk factors
  1. **Characteristics of parents**
     a. **Substance abuse** is commonly associated with neglect as well as abuse.
     b. **Psychological disorders** (e.g., antisocial personality disorder, depression) are also associated with abuse.
     c. Parents may have **unrealistic expectations** of a child (e.g., expecting a child to be fully toilet trained by 1 year of age).
     d. **Young parental age** is a risk factor for abuse.
  2. **Characteristics of child**
     a. **Age.** Children younger than 1 year are at a greater risk of death.
     b. **Gender.** Girls are more likely to be victims of abuse.
     c. **Physical health.** Children who are born prematurely or with a low birth weight have a higher risk of being abused.
  3. **Characteristics of family.** Risk factors include poverty, unemployment, unplanned pregnancies, large family size, intergenerational abuse, domestic violence, and poor social supports.

C. Epidemiology
  1. Approximately 1 million children are abused each year in the United States.
  2. About 2000 children die each year as a result of nonaccidental trauma.
  3. Ten percent of injuries to children younger than 5 years of age are caused by abuse.
  4. Abuse by men is more likely to lead to hospitalization, neurologic damage, and death.

II CLINICAL MANIFESTATIONS OF CHILD ABUSE

A. Specific physical injuries
  1. **Bruises**
     a. **Normal bruises** are found on bony prominences (e.g., knees, chin, elbow, or forehead).
     b. **Suspicious bruising** is located on well-padded areas (e.g.,

buttocks, cheeks, thighs, ears, or genitals). **Linear bruising** is suggestive of trauma from cords, belts, or rulers. Bruises in a **child who is not yet cruising** should be a cause for concern and investigation.

c. **Staging of bruise age.** Knowing how to date a bruise by its appearance can help determine the validity of the explanation given for the injury (**Table 6-1**).

TABLE 6-1. Determining Age of Bruise by Color	
Age of Bruise (Days)	**Color**
1–2	Red-blue
3–5	Blue-purple
6–7	Green
8–10	Yellow/brown
13–28	Resolved

2. **Burns**
   a. **Incidence.** Ten to twenty-five percent of childhood burns are caused by abuse.
   b. **Scalds.** Burns resulting from intentional scalding are sharply demarcated and usually are caused by forced immersion in hot liquid. Splash marks are usually missing when the injury is intentional.
   c. **Contact burns.** Burns are suspicious when they appear on parts of the body normally covered with clothing or when they have sharply demarcated patterns that follow the shape of the hot item (e.g., cigarettes, irons, heating grates). Accidental injuries usually have blurred borders.

HOT KEY Patterns such as "doughnut holes" on the buttocks and "stocking" or "glove" burns on the extremities can be seen when restraint is used in scalding water immersions. Full-thickness palmar burns may indicate that the child's hand was forced against a hot surface for a prolonged time.

3. **Head injuries.** Head injuries are the most common cause of fatal or devastating physical abuse. They are seen primarily in children younger than 3 years of age. Injury may occur during shaking (e.g., shaken baby syndrome) or from sudden decelerations when hitting a surface (even if it is padded).
   a. **Symptoms** include lethargy, irritability, seizures, vomiting, apnea, irregular respiration patterns, and changes in neuromuscular tone.

      b. Examination findings include retinal hemorrhages, subdural or subarachnoid bleeding (often associated with bloody cerebrospinal fluid), and skull fractures (most commonly occipital or parieto-occipital fractures).

  4. Abdominal injuries are the second most common cause of death from abuse. These injuries are most commonly caused by a penetrating blow or from the crushing of viscera against the spine.

      a. Characteristics. Injuries to hollow viscera are often caused by abuse. Injuries to the spleen usually are not seen in abuse, but injuries to other solid organs (e.g., the pancreas, kidneys, and liver) are seen in equal numbers in both abusive and unintentional injury.

      b. Symptoms include vomiting (which is not always bilious), peritoneal signs, and abdominal pain and distention.

  5. Skeletal injuries

      a. Incidence. Fractures are found in 10%–20% of abused children. Fractures often are occult (especially in children younger than 1 year) and often are detected during the evaluation of other, more visible injuries.

      b. Fractures of abuse include epiphyseal and metaphyseal chip fractures and rib fractures, which can be caused by shaking or squeezing. Other fractures that are likely to be caused by abuse include midshaft femur and humerus fractures in children younger than 1 year, spinous process fractures, scapular fractures, fractures of the lateral aspect of the scapula, fractures of different ages, complex skull fractures, and sternal fractures.

B. Psychological consequences

  1. Guilt. The child often feels that she is responsible for the abuse.

  2. Anger. Adolescents who are angry may display antisocial behavior.

  3. Fear. The child often fears the consequences of reporting the abuse.

  4. Depression. Child abuse can cause depression and is a significant risk factor for low self-esteem and adolescent suicide attempts.

III APPROACH TO THE PATIENT

A. The interview. Always approach the family in a nonjudgmental fashion. If the injury has no explanation or has an implausible mechanism of action, or there is significant delay in bringing an injured child to medical attention, child abuse should be suspected.

HOT KEY

Be suspicious of stories of self-inflicted injuries that do not match the child's developmental age.

B. Laboratory studies
1. If the bruising is generalized, consider ordering a complete blood cell count (CBC) and prothrombin time (PT) and partial thromboplastin time (PTT) studies to rule out idiopathic thrombocytopenic purpura or a bleeding diathesis.
2. If abdominal trauma is suspected, obtain pancreatic and hepatic enzyme tests and urinalysis.

C. Imaging studies
1. **Radiographs**
   a. **Skeletal survey**
      (1) **A complete survey** includes the following views: anteroposterior (AP) supine chest, lateral chest, AP humeri, AP forearms, posteroanterior hands, AP pelvis, lateral lumbar spine, lateral cervical spine, AP femurs, AP tibias, AP feet, AP skull, and lateral skull.
      (2) **Estimating ages of injuries. Table 6-2** provides guidelines for estimating the age of fractures and soft tissue injuries.
   b. **Abdominal films.** Perforation of a hollow viscus will cause free air or fluid on abdominal plain films.
2. **Computed tomography (CT)**
   a. **Common head CT findings** include subdural and subarachnoid bleeding and hypodensity that spares the basal

TABLE 6-2. Estimating Ages of Fractures and Soft Tissue Injuries

Category	Early	Peak	Late
Resolution of soft tissue swelling	2–5 days	4–10 days	14–21 days
Periosteal new bone definition	4–10 days	10–14 days	14–21 days
Loss of fracture line definition	10–14 days	10–14 days	–
Soft callus	10–14 days	14–21 days	–
Hard callus	14–21 days	21–42 days	41–90 days
Remodeling	3 months	1 year	2 years to physis closure

ganglia and the posterior fossa. Hypodensity may not be present in the initial CT but will appear in the first few days after injury.

b. **Common abdominal CT findings** include duodenal hematoma, pancreatic hemorrhage or pseudocyst formation, liver laceration, and adrenal hemorrhages.

IV MANAGEMENT

A. **Evaluate the child** with a multidisciplinary team, including a pediatrician, a social worker, a psychiatrist, a nurse, and an attorney.

B. **Treat obvious injuries** (e.g., burns, fractures, lacerations, and abdominal injuries).

C. **Order further laboratory and imaging studies** to elucidate any occult injuries.

D. **Take photographs to document any suspicious injuries** such as burns, bruising, bite marks, and other outward signs of physical trauma.

E. **Consider hospitalization** if the diagnosis is unclear or if no alternative for safe custody can be found.

F. **Call Child Protective Services** if social worker has not done this already.

HOT KEY Eighty to ninety percent of families involved in child abuse and neglect can be rehabilitated to provide adequate care for their children.

HOT KEY Medical professionals are mandated by law to report any suspicions of physical or sexual abuse or neglect to the proper authorities. Abused children returned to their homes without intervention have a 25% chance of serious injury and a 5% chance of death.

References

Duhaime AC, Christian CW, Rorke LB, et al: Nonaccidental head injury in infants— the "shaken baby syndrome." *N Engl J Med* 338(25):1822–1829, 1998.

Nimkin K, Kleinman P: Imaging of child abuse. *Pediatr Clin North Am* 44(3):615–635, 1997.

7. Conjunctivitis

I INTRODUCTION

A. Background. The degree of workup and treatment for conjunctivitis depends largely on the age of the patient.

B. Pathogenesis

1. **Neonatal conjunctivitis.** Conjunctival inflammation often is caused by chemical irritation from the routine use of topical antimicrobial prophylaxis agents in the perinatal period. Bacterial conjunctivitis in neonates (ophthalmia neonatorum) can result from inoculation of the conjunctiva during passage through the birth canal. *Chlamydia trachomatis* is the most common cause, followed by *Haemophilus influenzae, Streptococcus pneumoniae,* and *Neisseria gonorrhoeae.* Other gram-negative organisms, such as *Pseudomonas aeruginosa, Escherichia coli,* and *Proteus mirabilis,* also have been implicated.

2. **Childhood conjunctivitis (pinkeye)** occurs in children at any time after the neonatal period and is associated with pathogens that reside in the nasopharynx. It is caused by direct inoculation or local spread through the lacrimal duct. Most cases are caused by bacteria (e.g., *H. influenzae, S. pneumoniae*). *Staphylococcus aureus* often is isolated from both infected and uninfected eyes, and is not likely to be a significant cause of infectious conjunctivitis. Viruses, primarily adenoviruses, cause 20% of cases.

II CLINICAL MANIFESTATIONS

A. History

1. **Neonatal conjunctivitis.** The mother should be asked about any history of sexually transmitted infections, and the results of prenatal screening tests for gonococcus and chlamydia should be obtained. Irritant conjunctivitis usually is seen during the first day of life. Gonococcal infection is seen at 3–5 days of life, and chlamydial infection is seen at 2–4 weeks of life. Symptoms may begin earlier if the membranes ruptured prematurely during labor.

2. **Conjunctivitis in older children.** Older children usually have acute onset of conjunctival erythema and discharge. If allergic conjunctivitis is suspected, the physician should inquire about seasonal recurrences or a history of atopy in either the family or the child. Splash injury from household agents, especially those containing alkali, should be ruled out.

B. Physical examination. Bacterial infection is more likely to be unilateral, with a copious purulent exudate. Viral infection is more likely to be bilateral, with a lower-volume mucoid discharge and associated pharyngitis and preauricular adenopathy. Both types show scleral injection and hyperemia. However, these findings are not pathognomonic.

1. **Gonococcal conjunctivitis** often causes hyperacute onset of strikingly copious purulent discharge and edema of the eyelids.
2. **Chlamydial conjunctivitis** may be associated with a pseudomembrane. It has a more indolent presentation with modest purulence. Pneumonitis may be an accompanying symptom.
3. **Herpes simplex viral conjunctivitis** is characterized by dendritic ulcers and keratitis. It may be accompanied by vesicular eruptions on the skin and mouth.
4. **Allergic conjunctivitis** usually is associated with itchy, red eyes and a small volume of watery exudate.

III APPROACH TO THE PATIENT

HOT
KEY
Neonatal conjunctivitis must be completely investigated.

A. Workup. Swabs of conjunctival membranes should be sent for the following studies.
1. **Gram stain.** Intracellular gram-negative diplococci on Gram stain indicate a gonococcal infection.
2. Culture and direct fluorescent antibody (DFA) testing for *C. trachomatis* should be performed.
3. Herpes culture and DFA or electroimmunoassay (EIA) should be performed if associated vesicular lesions are present or if exposure is suspected.
4. Routine bacterial culture and sensitivity tests should be performed. In older children, culture usually is not necessary unless symptoms persist for longer than 7–10 days.
5. Gonococcal culture should be performed on Thayer-Martin media.
B. Differential diagnosis
1. **Corneal abrasion and trauma** should be considered in any acutely red eye. The eyelid should be everted and the eye examined for foreign bodies. Fluorescein examination should be performed to look for corneal abrasions. If abrasions are found, topical antibiotics are prescribed, and the patient is

HOT KEY

Discovery of a corneal abrasion should always prompt a search for a retained foreign body.

seen in 24 hours to confirm resolution. Patching may provide some relief if tolerated.

2. **Nasolacrimal duct obstruction.** Infants with blocked naso-lacrimal ducts have a history of persistent tearing. Therapy consists of gentle lacrimal sac massage with a cotton-tip swab directed toward the nose. Topical antibiotics are added if purulent discharge is present. Infants whose ducts do not open by 12 months of age may require surgical probing.

3. **Dacryocystitis** is a complication of lacrimal duct obstruction. It presents with swelling, erythema, and tenderness at the nasal corner of the eye. Systemic antibiotics are required.

4. **Systemic illnesses** such as Kawasaki disease, Lyme disease, leptospirosis, juvenile rheumatoid arthritis, and Stevens-Johnson syndrome should also be considered.

5. **Acute glaucoma** presents with perilimbal injection, decreased visual acuity, a poor pupillary response to light, and a mildly dilated pupil. No discharge is present.

6. **Periorbital or orbital cellulitis** (see Chapter 37 V)

C. **Therapy**

1. **Neonatal conjunctivitis.** Neonatal chemical conjunctivitis from topical antibiotic prophylaxis requires no treatment. If the results of a Gram stain suggest gonococcus, treatment with a parenteral third-generation cephalosporin (e.g., cefotaxime, ceftriaxone) is indicated. Conjunctivitis caused by *C. trachomatis* is treated with oral erythromycin for 14 days. Other bacterial infections can be treated topically, but close follow-up is needed.

2. **Topical agents.** Topical antibiotics speed recovery from bacterial infections. Good initial choices include **trimethoprim-polymyxin (Polytrim)** and **erythromycin. Sulfacetamide** is effective, but often causes burning. **Gentamicin** is ineffective for pneumococcal infections, but is helpful for gram-negative infections. Treatment is continued three times daily for 5 days, or until symptoms abate. Because it is difficult to distinguish viral from bacterial causes, all patients who have mucopurulent drainage should receive antibiotic treatment. Cold compresses and lubricants are good adjuvant measures.

3. **Herpes simplex conjunctivitis.** Idoxuridine with or without acyclovir is required. Because of the high incidence of corneal scarring, all suspected cases should be referred to an ophthalmologist immediately.

4. **Allergic conjunctivitis** is treated with topical or systemic antihistamines.
5. **Chemical conjunctivitis.** Chemical splash injuries require aggressive continuous irrigation and ophthalmology consultation.
D. **Ongoing management.** In cases of chlamydia and gonorrhea, the mother and her sexual partner(s) need treatment. All infants with conjunctivitis require isolation; this practice is particularly important in nurseries.

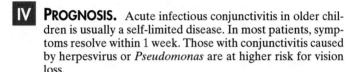 **PROGNOSIS.** Acute infectious conjunctivitis in older children is usually a self-limited disease. In most patients, symptoms resolve within 1 week. Those with conjunctivitis caused by herpesvirus or *Pseudomonas* are at higher risk for vision loss.

References
Gigliotti F: Acute conjunctivitis. *Pediatr Rev* 16(6):203–207, 1995.
King RA: Common ocular signs and symptoms in childhood. *Pediatr Clin North Am* 40(4):753–766, 1993.
Weiss AH: Chronic conjunctivitis in infants and children. *Pediatr Ann* 22(6):366–374, 1993.

8. Varicella (Chickenpox)

▐ INTRODUCTION

A. Epidemiology. Varicella is a herpesvirus that is extremely contagious. Ninety-eight percent of susceptible people who live with a person who has varicella become infected. If not immunized, approximately 90% of people become infected during childhood. The disease can be more serious in the very young (< 3 months old) and in adolescents and adults.

B. Pathogenesis. Person-to-person transmission occurs by direct contact with lesions as well as through exposure to respiratory droplets. Prodromal patients are typically asymptomatic, and the incubation period is 10–21 days after contact.

> **HOT**
> **▶**
> **KEY**
> Patients are most contagious during the period from 2 days before the rash appears to 5 days after the last new lesions appear.

▐ APPROACH TO THE PATIENT

A. History and physical examination

1. **Prodrome.** Mild fever and malaise precede the exanthem. The temperature is less than 38.8°C (102°F), and fever usually lasts less than 1 week.

2. **Exanthem.** The exanthem develops over 3–6 days. Lesions typically evolve as erythematous macules that develop rapidly into vesicles with the characteristic "dewdrops on rose petals" appearance. These lesions collapse, become umbilicated, rupture, and crust over. The presence of crops of lesions at varying stages is common and helps to confirm the diagnosis. Typically, lesions start along the hairline and later emerge in successive crops, first on the trunk and later on the extremities.

3. **Key aspects of the physical examination**
   a. What do the lesions look like?
   b. Are there crops of lesions at different stages?
   c. Do any lesions appear to be superinfected?
      (1) Impetigo and cellulitis often occur, particularly when patients scratch the lesions excessively.

49

(2) Necrotizing fasciitis is increasingly reported as a complication.

HOT KEY

A high fever [temperature > 39.5°C (103°F)] in a patient with varicella should prompt a search for a possible intercurrent infection.

B. Differential diagnosis. Milder or earlier cases may be more difficult to diagnose than more established cases. It is important to consider the following alternate diagnoses:
   1. Coxsackievirus infection (predominance of lesions on the hands, feet, mouth, and buttocks)
   2. *Mycoplasma* infection
   3. Eczema herpeticum
   4. Insect bites
   5. Other viral exanthems
C. Laboratory tests. In uncertain cases, diagnosis can be confirmed by Tzanck preparation or by immunofluorescence of vesicular fluid.
D. Therapy
   1. Acyclovir, if initiated within 24 hours of the appearance of lesions, reduces the severity of varicella and speeds recovery. Acyclovir is not recommended for routine use in healthy children, but its use is considered in the following situations, which can be remembered using the mnemonic ACYC:

"ACYC"

All siblings (of any age) who sequentially contract varicella within the same household, because varicella becomes more severe as it is passed from family member to family member

Comorbid conditions (e.g., asthma, eczema, diabetes, rheumatoid arthritis)

Young (e.g., < 1 year of age) or older (> 12 years of age) patients

Chronic administration of steroid or aspirin therapy

---

   2. Immunocompromised children should receive **varicella zoster immunoglobulin (VZIg)** within 72 hours of exposure. They should be hospitalized and given intravenous acyclovir.
   3. All children with varicella should be kept home from school or daycare until all lesions are crusted over.

HOT KEY **Aspirin** is never given to children with varicella because of the risk of Reye syndrome, which is characterized by irritability or lethargy, intractable vomiting, elevated liver function tests, and elevated serum ammonia levels.

HOT KEY Hospitalized patients require strict isolation in negative-pressure rooms.

E. Prophylaxis

1. **Varicella zoster virus (VZV) vaccine** (see Chapter 2). Routine vaccination is now recommended for all children older than 1 year of age who have a reliable history of never having had varicella. The vaccine has changed the frequency and spectrum of the disease considerably.

2. According to the AAP, varicella vaccine should be given to susceptible children 72 to up to 120 hours after varicella exposure to prevent or modify disease.

3. VZIg must be given within 96 hours of significant exposure. Only select candidates with a significant exposure history qualify for VZIg administration.

   a. **Candidates for VZIg** include:

   (1) Immunocompromised children who have no history of VZV

   (2) Susceptible pregnant women

   (3) Neonates, if the mother had onset of varicella within 5 days before delivery or within 2 days after delivery

   (4) Premature infant (> 28 weeks gestation) whose mother is seronegative or has no history of VZV

   (5) Any infant < 28 weeks of age

   b. **Significant exposure** includes the following:

   (1) Residence in the same house as a person who has varicella

   (2) Sharing a hospital room with a patient who has varicella

   (3) Spending > 5 minutes in face-to-face contact with a person who has varicella

   (4) Hugging or touching a person who is actively infected with herpes zoster

   (5) In neonates, onset of varicella in the mother 5 days or fewer before delivery; however, VZIg is not indicated if the mother has herpes zoster

F. Complications. Most children have no complications. In children who do experience complications, the most common include the following:
   1. Superinfection (e.g., impetigo, cellulitis, necrotizing fasciitis)
   2. Pneumonia (rare)
   3. Neurologic conditions (e.g., aseptic meningitis, Guillain-Barré syndrome, cerebellitis)
   4. Neonatal varicella infections, which include:
      a. Congenital varicella syndrome. This syndrome can result from maternal infection in the first or second trimester. Effects include limb or finger atrophy, central nervous system disease (e.g., cortical atrophy, hydrocephalus, seizures), ocular disease (e.g., chorioretinitis, cataract, anisocoria, nystagmus), and skin scarring, usually in a dermatomal distribution.
      b. Infant varicella. Severe varicella with a 30% mortality rate can occur if varicella develops in the mother fewer than 5 days before delivery. The infant is relatively protected by transplacental maternal antibody if varicella develops in the mother 6–21 days before delivery.

References
Weller TH: Varicella: historical perspective and clinical overview. *J Infect Dis* 174(suppl)3:S306–S309, 1996.
Wharton M: The epidemiology of varicella-zoster virus infections. *Infect Dis Clin North Am* 10(3):571–581, 1996.

9. Pharyngitis

I INTRODUCTION

A. Definition. Pharyngitis is inflammation of the mucous membranes and the underlying structures of the tonsils and pharynx.

B. Causes. Pharyngitis is typically caused by viral or bacterial pathogens.

    1. Bacterial causes. Group A β–hemolytic streptococci are the most common bacterial cause of pharyngitis. Other bacterial causes include **group C or G streptococci** (occasionally), *Mycoplasma* **species,** *Neisseria gonorrhoeae,* and *Treponema pallidum.*

    2. Viral causes include **adenovirus, Epstein–Barr virus (EBV), influenza virus A or B, parainfluenza virus, rhinovirus,** and **respiratory syncytial virus (RSV).**

> **HOT KEY** In making the diagnosis, it is most important to distinguish pharyngitis caused by bacteria (which is treatable) from pharyngitis caused by viruses (which has no specific therapy).

C. Epidemiology. Pharyngitis is one of the most common reasons for visits to the pediatrician for acute illness.

    1. Streptococcal pharyngitis is most common in children between the ages of 5 and 15 years.

    2. Viral pharyngitis is more common in children younger than 5 years.

II APPROACH TO THE PATIENT

> **HOT KEY** Clinical assessment alone is not often diagnostic; a culture or rapid test is frequently required to confirm the diagnosis.

A. Patient history. The patient history is critical to making a correct diagnosis.

    1. Symptoms. A sore throat can exist in isolation or in conjunction with a number of additional symptoms, the presence or absence of which can make streptococcal pharyngitis more or less likely.

   a. The triad of sore throat, headache, and abdominal pain in the absence of other viral symptoms is *extremely* suggestive of streptococcal pharyngitis.

   b. The presence of cough, rhinorrhea, and conjunctivitis makes streptococcal pharyngitis much less likely.

   2. **A history of recent exposure** to a person with known streptococcal infection raises the index of suspicion for this diagnosis.

B. Physical examination

   1. **Head, ears, eyes, nose, and throat (HEENT)**

   a. The appearance of the **tonsils** is generally not helpful in distinguishing between viral and bacterial causes of sore throat.

   b. **Palatal petechiae** are strongly suggestive of Group A Beta Hemolytic Streptococcal Infection **(GABHS) infection.**

   c. **Concomitant conjunctivitis** suggests a viral cause.

   d. **Prominent anterior cervical nodes** are consistent with GABHS infection. **Prominent posterior cervical nodes** suggest EBV.

   2. **Abdomen. Splenomegaly** suggests EBV.

   3. **Skin**

   a. **Scarlatiniform rash** with accentuation in body creases (e.g., in the antecubital fossa) is diagnostic of scarlet fever and should be treated similarly to streptococcal pharyngitis.

   b. **Other rashes** may suggest viral causes.

C. Diagnostic tests

   1. In general, it is appropriate to order a diagnostic test to rule out streptococcal pharyngitis. The risk of other bacterial causes should be assessed by history.

   2. For the diagnosis of GABHS infection, there are three possible tests:

   a. **Latex agglutination rapid test**

   b. **Optical immunoassay (OIA) rapid test**

   c. **Culture (the "gold standard")**

HOT
▶
KEY

Culture confirmation is not required for a positive latex agglutination, a positive OIA, or a negative OIA result. However, because of its poor sensitivity, a negative latex rapid test result should be followed up with a throat culture.

■ III TREATMENT

A. Viral pharyngitis. Most viral infections resolve on their own within 5 days, although symptoms of EBV infection may persist for 1–2 weeks.

B. Streptococcal pharyngitis is treated with antibiotics.
   1. **Penicillin VK** is standard therapy.
   2. **Benzathine penicillin** is administered intramuscularly as a single dose and may be preferable if compliance is a concern.
   3. **Erythromycin** is the drug of choice for children who are allergic to penicillin.
   4. **Azithromycin** is also well tolerated and effective.

IV FOLLOW-UP

A. Complications of streptococcal pharyngitis. Although treatment with antibiotics speeds the resolution of the acute symptoms of GABHS infection somewhat, the principal reason for drug treatment is to avoid the suppurative and nonsuppurative complications of infection.
   1. **Suppurative complications** include peritonsillar abscess in older children and retropharyngeal abscess in younger children.
   2. **Acute rheumatic fever** (Table 9-1)

TABLE 9-1. Jones Criteria (Revised) for Guidance in the Diagnosis of Rheumatic Fever

Major Manifestations	Minor Manifestations
Carditis (myocarditis, pericarditis, or valvular involvement such as mitral or aortic valve involvement)	Clinical
	Previous rheumatic fever or rheumatic heart disease
	Arthralgia
	Fever
Polyarthritis	Laboratory
Chorea	Acute phase reactants
Erythema marginatum	Accelerated erythrocyte sedimentation rate, increased C-reactive protein, leukocytosis
Subcutaneous nodules	Prolonged P-R interval
	Plus

Supporting evidence of preceding streptococcal infections (increased ASO or other streptococcal antibodies, positive throat culture for group A streptococcus, recent scarlet fever)

The presence of two major criteria, or of one major and two minor criteria, indicates a high probability of the presence of rheumatic fever if supported by evidence of a preceding streptococcal infection. The absence of the latter should make the diagnosis doubtful, except in situations in which rheumatic fever is first discovered after a long latent period from the antecedent infection (e.g., Sydenham chorea or low grade carditis.) (From Stollerman GH, Markowitz M, Taranta A, et al: Jones criteria (revised) for guidance in diagnosis of rheumatic fever. *Circulation* 32:664–668, 1965.)

3. Poststreptococcal glomerulonephritis
B. Repeat cultures are not routinely indicated.

References
Gerber MA: Diagnosis of group A streptococcal pharyngitis. *Pediatr Ann* 27(5): 269–277, 1998.
Pichichero ME, Marsocci SM, Murphy ML, et al. Incidence of streptococcal carriers in private pediatric practice. *Arch Pediatr Adolesc Med* 153(6):624–628, 1999.

10. Sinusitis

I INTRODUCTION

A. Background. Sinusitis is a much more common condition in the pediatric population than was previously realized.

B. Definitions

1. **Sinusitis** is characterized by inflammation of the paranasal sinuses.

2. **Acute sinusitis** is defined as symptoms of upper respiratory tract infection that last 10–30 days.

3. The symptoms of **subacute, or chronic sinusitis** last 30 days or longer.

C. Pathogenesis. Episodes of sinusitis are usually preceded by viral upper respiratory tract infections. Mucosal swelling combined with changes in mucous viscosity and ciliary function can lead to ostial obstruction. Bacteria that populate the nasal chamber are drawn into the normally sterile sinus cavity, causing acute sinusitis. The maxillary sinuses are most susceptible to infection.

D. Epidemiology

1. The average child has five to ten upper respiratory tract infections each year; 5%–10% of these are complicated by bacterial sinusitis (see Chapter 12 II A 2).

2. As in otitis media and acute conjunctivitis, *Streptococcus pneumoniae* (30%–40%), *Haemophilus influenzae* (20%), and *Moraxella catarrhalis* (20%) are the most common bacterial pathogens in acute sinusitis. Acute sinusitis can also be caused by viruses, including adenovirus, parainfluenza virus, influenza virus, and rhinovirus.

3. Chronic sinusitis is more likely to be caused by *Staphylococcus aureus* and anaerobes.

II CLINICAL MANIFESTATIONS

A. Acute sinusitis presents in two ways:

1. **Persistent presentation** is the most common and is characterized by relatively mild, localized symptoms (e.g., runny nose, cough, malaise, low-grade fever) that last at least 10 days. Nasal discharge may be of any quality. Cough must be present during the day, but it is often worse at night. Foul-smelling breath may be present. Facial pain or high fever is unusual.

2. **Severe presentation** is characterized by severe "cold" symptoms (e.g., runny nose, sore throat, cough, malaise) coupled

with high fever and purulent nasal discharge. These symptoms usually occur several days after the onset of the upper respiratory tract infection. Affected patients may also have headaches or facial pain.

B. Chronic sinusitis is characterized by symptoms that last longer than 30 days. Nasal congestion and cough are the most common symptoms. Often, sore throat accompanies mouth breathing, which is secondary to nasal congestion. Nasal discharge is not present in all cases. Fever is rare.

HOT **KEY** The persistence or worsening of symptoms over 10 days differentiates bacterial sinusitis from a simple viral upper respiratory tract infection. Most upper respiratory tract infections last 7–9 days; even if symptoms do not completely abate by the 10th day, they are almost always improved.

III ⬛ APPROACH TO THE PATIENT

A. Diagnosis

 1. A **radiograph** of the sinus is considered positive if it shows diffuse opacification, mucosal thickening of more than 4 mm, or an air-fluid level.

HOT ▶ **KEY** In children younger than 6 years of age, sinus films are of little use because many children have abnormal radiographs in conjunction with persistent respiratory symptoms. For these patients, the diagnosis is made based on either the persistence or the severity of symptoms.

---

 2. **Computed tomography scans** are performed when the patient has chronic or recurrent sinusitis or orbital or central nervous system complications.
 3. **Aspiration** of the sinus is useful for patients who do not respond to multiple courses of antibiotics, those who have severe facial pain, and those who have orbital or intracranial complications. Sinus aspirates should always be sent for quantitative culture. A finding of more than 10^4 colony-forming units per milliliter indicates a true infection.

B. Initial antibiotic therapy. A 10-day course of therapy is usually sufficient, and clinical improvement is typically seen within 3–4 days. For patients who respond more slowly, therapy is continued for 7 days after symptoms resolve.

1. **Amoxicillin** (40–60 mg/kg/day) is an effective first-line agent for uncomplicated acute sinusitis.

HOT
KEY

High-dose amoxicillin (80 mg/kg/day) is used if the patient lives in an area with a high prevalence of intermediate-resistant pneumococcus or *H. influenzae*.

---

2. **Amoxicillin-clavulanic acid or a second-generation cephalosporin** is indicated in the following situations:
   a. The patient does not improve while taking amoxicillin.
   b. The patient has had recent (< 30 days) therapy with amoxicillin.
   c. Symptoms are prolonged or sinusitis is complicated.
C. **Adjuvant therapy**
   1. The role of **antihistamines** and **topical or systemic decongestants** in acute sinusitis has been poorly studied. Topical saline sprays may provide some benefit by aiding in the drainage of secretions. Topical corticosteroid sprays may provide a modest benefit during the second week of treatment.
   2. **Surgical therapy** to improve sinus drainage is rarely required and should be limited to patients who do not improve with maximal medical therapy administered for a prolonged period.

References
Bussey MF, Moon RY: Acute sinusitis. *Pediatr Rev* 20(4):142, 1999.
Isaacson G: Sinusitis in childhood. *Pediatr Clin North Am* 43(6):1297–1318, 1996.
Wald ER: Sinusitis. *Pediatr Ann* 27(12):811–818, 1998.

11. Ear Infections (Otitis Media and Otitis Externa)

I DEFINITIONS

A. Otitis externa, sometimes called swimmer's ear, is an infection of the external auditory canal.

B. Serous otitis media is the presence of fluid in the middle ear.

C. Acute otitis media is an infection of the middle ear.

II OTITIS EXTERNA

A. Epidemiology. Because of its association with swimming, otitis externa is most prevalent in the summer months. It typically affects older children and adolescents.

B. Pathophysiology. Protective factors against infections of the outer ear include acidic pH of the cerumen and an intact squamous epithelium. Removal of cerumen or disruption of the skin surface leads to bacterial invasion and inflammation. The two most common risk factors for otitis externa are excess moisture (e.g., swimming) and trauma (e.g., use of cotton swabs). Common pathogens are listed in **Table 11-1.**

TABLE 11-1. Common Pathogens Involved in Otitis Externa

Pathogens	Examples
Bacteria	*Pseudomonas aeruginosa, Staphylococcus aureus,* group A streptococcus
Viruses	Herpes simplex, herpes zoster
Fungi	*Candida* spp., *Aspergillus* spp.

C. History. The physician should ask whether the patient has recently experienced trauma to the ear, been swimming, or been submerged in water.

D. Physical examination

1. Pain is typically elicited when traction is applied to the tragus (i.e., the cartilage below the opening of the ear). Traction usually does **not** cause pain in otitis media, and this maneuver can help to distinguish the two entities.

2. The canal itself may appear red and swollen, and may contain frank pus. The tympanic membrane should appear normal unless there is concomitant otitis media.

HOT **KEY** It is important to distinguish between otitis externa and otitis media with drum rupture. Visualization of the tympanic membrane is important.

E. Tests. Culture of the external canal fluid or debris is **not** routinely indicated because it is not specific and does not guide therapy.

F. Therapy. Analgesics such as Auralgan (antipyrine 5.4% and benzocaine 1.4%) may be instilled in the ear every 2 hours as needed. Topical otic antibiotics (e.g., polymixin, neomycin, hydrocortisone) are helpful. Suspensions are preferred over solutions, especially when the tympanic membrane is perforated.

G. Prevention. Affected children should be advised to avoid trauma to the external canal (no swabbing!) and to dry out their ears after swimming or to wear earplugs. In addition, 2% acetic acid drops may be applied prophylactically to the ear canals after swimming.

III OTITIS MEDIA

A. Epidemiology

1. Otitis media is commonly associated with upper respiratory tract infections. Therefore, it is most prevalent in the winter.
2. Otitis media typically affects children between 6 months and 3 years of age. Approximately 75% of children have at least one episode of otitis media before 18 months of age.
3. Breast-feeding is mildly protective against otitis media.
4. Factors that increase the risk of otitis media include daycare attendance, craniofacial abnormalities, low socioeconomic status, and allergic rhinitis.

B. Pathophysiology

1. The middle ear is normally sterile, air-filled, and ventilated through the eustachian tube.
2. Malfunction of the eustachian tube (either mechanical or as a result of obstruction, often secondary to a viral upper respiratory infection) can lead to the accumulation of fluid. As a result, bacteria and viruses from the nasopharynx can be drawn into the middle ear.
3. In young children, the small caliber and angle of insertion of the eustachian tube predispose it to obstruction.

C. Pathogens. Viruses (e.g., respiratory syncytial virus, adenovirus, influenza virus, rhinovirus, parainfluenza virus) account for approximately 30% of infections. **Table 11-2** shows the bacterial causes of otitis media.

TABLE 11-2. Prevalence of Bacterial Pathogens Involved in Otitis Media and the Percentage of Penicillin Resistance

Bacterial Pathogen	Prevalence	Penicillin Resistance
Streptococcus pneumoniae	40%	Varies greatly, depending on geography
Nontypeable *Haemophilus influenzae*	40%	30% (beta-lactamase)
Moraxella catarrhalis	15%	90% (beta-lactamase)
Streptococcus pyogenes	3%	0%
Others (e.g., *Staphylococcus aureus*, gram-negative bacteria)	2%	90%

HOT KEY Penicillin-resistant pneumococcus is an increasingly recognized problem that varies by geographic region. The resistance is not beta-lactamase–mediated, but is based on the presence of penicillin-binding proteins that may be overcome with high doses of penicillins.

D. History. The classic symptoms of acute otitis media are fever, otalgia, and hearing loss. Many children are irritable; some have associated vomiting. Tugging at the ears is a common nonspecific sign.

E. Physical examination. Otitis media is one of the most common and challenging diagnoses to make. It is critical to learn the range in appearance of normal ears to help define what is abnormal. A normal tympanic membrane is translucent, with a pearly gray appearance. The short process and handle of the malleus should be visible through it. A cone of light should be present, and the membrane should move laterally and medially with negative and positive pressure. Key questions and considerations during physical examination include the following:

1. Are the landmarks visible? Is the tympanic membrane red or yellow? Is it bulging or retracted? Is it mobile?
2. A patient with serous otitis media typically has a dull, retracted, immobile tympanic membrane.

HOT KEY The diagnosis of otitis media should be based on changes in the color, contour, and mobility of the tympanic membrane. It is important to distinguish between serous otitis media (i.e., fluid without superinfection) and acute otitis media (i.e., middle ear infection).

3. A patient with acute otitis media typically has a yellow or red, bulging tympanic membrane.

HOT KEY The tympanic membrane normally turns red with crying. Therefore, a red tympanic membrane is not itself diagnostic of otitis media.

F. Diagnostic tests
  1. Tympanometry uses electroacoustic impedance to establish middle ear compliance. It is highly sensitive and specific for middle ear fluid; however, it does not distinguish between serous and acute otitis media.
  2. Tympanocentesis removes fluid from the middle ear for Gram stain and culture. It is used only in severe, refractory cases of otitis media.
G. Therapy. Acute otitis media can be treated effectively with antibiotics. However, the rate of spontaneous resolution is high, even without therapy. Approximately 90% of treated children and 85% of untreated children are free of pain and fever within 72 hours.
  1. First-line therapy consists of amoxicillin (40 mg/kg/day) to a maximum of 500 mg orally twice daily. For penicillin-sensitive patients, acceptable substitutes include erythromycin plus sulfisoxazole, clarithromycin, and azithromycin. Single-dose ceftriaxone (50 mg/kg intramuscularly) is used as first-line therapy in patients who cannot tolerate oral therapy or who have concomitant vomiting.
  2. Failure of first-line therapy is assumed when patients remain symptomatic (i.e., fever, otalgia) 72 hours after the initiation of therapy. These children are likely to have infection with a beta-lactamase–producing organism or penicillin-resistant pneumococcus. Second-line therapy is indicated.
  3. Second-line therapy may be a second- or third-generation cephalosporin. In areas where penicillin-resistant pneumococcus is common, high-dose amoxicillin-clavulanate (80–90 mg/kg/day) may be used.
  4. Although most practitioners treat otitis media for 7–10 days, 5 days of oral therapy is probably adequate for children older than 2 years of age.

HOT KEY No antibiotic is more effective than amoxicillin as first-line therapy for otitis media.

H. Ongoing management

1. **Antimicrobial prophylaxis** (amoxicillin 20 mg/kg/day given once daily for 3 months, or sulfisoxazole, 75 mg/kg/day in two divided doses) is considered for children who have more than three episodes of otitis media in 6 months or more than four episodes in 1 year.
2. **Tympanostomy tube placement** may be needed if prophylaxis fails.
3. Approximately 50% of children still have an effusion 1 month after an episode of acute otitis media. This finding is expected, and retreatment is not required.

I. Prognosis. Most children do not have complications as a result of otitis media. In those who do, the most common complications include the following:

1. **Mastoiditis** causes swelling and pain over the mastoid process. The earlobe moves superiorly and laterally in infants, and posteriorly and laterally in older patients. Computed tomography (CT) of the mastoid shows coalescence of mastoid air cells and loss of bony trabeculations. Treatment includes myringotomy and intravenous antibiotics (nafcillin plus ceftriaxone) for 21 days. Complications include meningitis, brain abscess, epidural abscess, facial nerve paralysis, jugular venous thrombosis, and internal carotid artery erosion.
2. **Perforation of the tympanic membrane** may occur.
3. **Cholesteatomas** may appear as spherical white oily masses within a perforation. In addition, persistent otorrhea may be present. Retraction pocket deformities may progress to cholesteatomas, which can destroy the delicate structures of the ear. If cholesteatoma is suspected, an otolaryngologist should be consulted.
4. **Hearing loss** is the most common complication. It is usually conductive, but also may be sensorineural. Tympanosclerosis may be an associated finding.

References

Blumer JL: Fundamental basis for rational therapeutics in acute otitis media. *Pediatr Infect Dis J* 18(12):1130–1140, 1999.

Klein JO: Review of consensus reports on management of acute otitis media. *Pediatr Infect Dis J* 18(12):1152–1155, 1999.

McCracken GH Jr: Prescribing antimicrobial agents for treatment of acute otitis media. *Pediatr Infect Dis J* 18(12):1141–1146, 1999.

O'Neill P: Acute otitis media. *BMJ* 319(7213):833–835, 1999.

12. Upper Respiratory Tract Infections (Coryza)

I INTRODUCTION

A. Background. Coryza is the most common reason for outpatient visits to pediatricians. Although coryza typically is not serious, it can be a source of concern to parents and can lead to complications, including lower respiratory tract infection, sinusitis, otitis media, and rarely, bacteremia and meningitis.

B. Pathogenesis

1. More than 200 viruses cause coryza. The most common is rhinovirus. Others include parainfluenza, enterovirus, and influenza.
2. Hand contact is the most important route of transmission. Inhalation of small aerosolized droplets can also lead to spread.
3. The incubation period varies by etiologic agent, but is typically 2–5 days. Viral shedding can precede the development of symptoms by as much as 48 hours.

HOT KEY

Exposure to cold is not a causative agent.

II CLINICAL MANIFESTATIONS

A. History

1. The most important details in the history are those that help to distinguish infectious from allergic causes. Gradual and persistent onset, long-standing duration, exposure to known allergens, seasonal variations, and a history of atopy all point to possible allergic triggers.
2. Sinusitis should be considered in children whose nasal discharge lasts longer than 10–14 days (see Chapter 10).
3. Conjunctivitis, systemic symptoms, and fever all point to infectious causes.

B. Physical examination. The most important aspects of the physical examination are directed at distinguishing infectious from allergic causes as well as ruling out complications or superinfections.

HOT KEY

Cocaine use is a possible cause of chronic rhinitis in adolescents.

1. **Head, ears, eyes, nose, throat (HEENT).** Boggy, pale, or blue turbinates suggest allergy. Unilateral nasal discharge, especially in young children, can be a sign of a foreign body. One should always check for otitis media.

2. **Chest.** Ensure that the lungs are clear and that there is no asymmetry to the examination. Coryza is an infection of the upper respiratory tract and should not involve the lungs. Parents often mistake noisy breathing for wheezing and may worry that a pulmonary process is present.

HOT KEY

Purulent nasal discharge is nonspecific and does not, by itself, suggest a bacterial superinfection.

III APPROACH TO THE PATIENT

A. Workup

1. No routine laboratory tests are indicated.
2. Viral cultures are expensive and unnecessary, and results typically arrive after symptoms resolve.
3. Rapid diagnostic tests are available for respiratory syncytial virus, parainfluenza virus, and influenza virus. However, the results of these tests typically are not helpful in management.
4. A nasal smear for eosinophils may be useful for identifying allergic etiology.

B. Therapy

1. Supportive care, including antipyretics and fluids, is the mainstay of treatment.
2. Nonprescription cold remedies do not speed resolution; however, because they often contain antihistamines, they can be sedating and may help children sleep at night.
3. Topical nasal decongestants (e.g., phenylephrine) can provide symptomatic relief. However, more than 3 days of use can lead to rebound rhinorrhea.
4. Using humidifiers, elevating the head of the bed, and administering vitamin C give concerned parents something to do, but do not affect the course of the disease.
5. Zinc is ineffective in children.

HOT KEY

Systemic cold remedies should not be used in children younger than 6 months of age.

References

Berlin CM Jr: Advances in pediatric pharmacology, toxicology, and therapeutics. *Adv Pediatr* 46:507–538, 1999.

Turner RB: Epidemiology, pathogenesis, and treatment of the common cold. *Ann Allergy Asthma Immunol* 78(6):531–539, 1997.

13. Croup

I INTRODUCTION

A. **Background.** Croup is a common reason for visits to emergency departments. Before the use of glucocorticoids, approximately 5% of all children in the United States required hospitalization for croup, and a substantial proportion of those with croup required intubation. Intubation is now rare, and outpatient management is increasingly common.

B. **Definitions.** Croup is a syndrome characterized by laryngotracheobronchitis, or inflammation of the upper airway. There are two types, infectious and spasmodic, but the treatment and natural history are the same.

C. **Pathogenesis.** Infectious croup is caused by parainfluenza virus, influenza A, adenovirus, respiratory syncytial virus, enterovirus, and possibly *Mycoplasma pneumoniae*. The etiology of spasmodic croup is poorly understood. Patients often have a personal or family history of atopy. Several studies suggest a link between gastroesophageal reflux and recurrent croup. Untreated, croup tends to worsen over the course of 2–3 days.

D. **Epidemiology.** Parainfluenza 1 outbreaks tend to occur in the fall, although croup is seen throughout the winter. Croup presents most commonly at night in children 1–6 years of age.

II CLINICAL MANIFESTATIONS.
Croup is most commonly preceded by coryza and low-grade fever for 12–72 hours. The fever may continue throughout the illness. Symptoms usually are worse at night. In spasmodic croup, the symptoms of coryza may be diminished or absent.

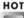

HOT KEY

Croup often presents as a classic triad of barking "seal-like" cough, inspiratory stridor, and hoarseness.

III APPROACH TO THE PATIENT

A. **Diagnosis.** The diagnosis of croup is almost exclusively clinical.
   1. **Respiratory viral direct fluorescent antibody testing or viral culture** can identify the causative agent, although results usually do not affect therapy.

    2. Radiographs. Croup classically presents with a "steeple sign," or narrowing of the tracheal air column to a steep point, on anteroposterior radiographs. This finding is only moderately specific and sensitive for the diagnosis of croup. However, radiographs can be useful for evaluating other possible diagnoses, such as bacterial tracheitis, epiglottitis, and aspirated foreign body.

B. Differential diagnosis

    1. Foreign body aspiration should be suspected in cases of asymmetric wheezing, sudden onset of symptoms, drooling, or differential lung volumes on inspiratory and expiratory films. Bronchoscopy may be needed to remove the object.

    2. Retropharyngeal abscess, peritonsillar abscess, and **epiglottitis** should also be considered (see Chapter 38).

    3. Bacterial tracheitis may be a complication of croup. It can be caused by *Staphylococcus aureus, Haemophilus influenzae, Streptococcus pneumoniae,* or *Moraxella catarrhalis.* It should be considered in children who are recovering from viral croup but then have a sudden decompensation, with fever and prolonged inspiratory stridor. Intubation often is required.

C. Therapy. The classic home management of croup is to provide mist (usually by steaming up the bathroom) or to take the child out into the cool night air. Many children improve by the time they present for medical care because of the effect of cold air augmented by the distraction of the car or ambulance ride to the hospital.

HOT   **KEY**

Distraction and minimal disturbance are keys to preventing hyperventilation and exacerbation of the croup symptoms.

---

    1. Racemic epinephrine is routinely given to all patients who have significant respiratory distress at presentation. Until recently, all children who received racemic epinephrine were hospitalized because of concerns about "rebound" stridor. However, recent studies show that it is safe to discharge a patient home after 3–4 hours of observation if the patient has received dexamethasone and remains symptom-free during this time. Patients should not be treated at home with racemic epinephrine.

    2. Dexamethasone is given as a single oral or intravenous dose (0.6 mg/kg/dose) and should be considered for all children who have significant symptoms, especially those who are seen early in the course of their illness. Clinical improvement occurs approximately 6 hours after administration.

3. **Cool mist** has been a mainstay of hospital treatment of croup for decades. However, little empiric evidence supports this practice. Humidification may be detrimental in children who have concurrent wheezing, and mist tents may exacerbate the stridor by increasing the patient's anxiety. If supplied, mist is best administered by a tube held near the child's face.
4. **Nebulized budesonide** may be a useful adjunct or replacement therapy, but is not yet available in the United States.

D. Adjuvant therapies
   1. In children with poorly responsive, severe croup, helium–oxygen mixtures may reduce viscosity enough to avoid intubation.
   2. Intubation should be performed under controlled circumstances with a tube that is 0.5–1 size smaller than would normally be used.

References

Geelhoed GC: Croup. *Pediatr Pulmonol* 23(5):370–374, 1997.
Kaditis AG, Wald ER: Viral croup: current diagnosis and treatment. *Pediatr Infect Dis J* 17(9):827–834, 1998.
Klassen TP: Croup: a current perspective. *Pediatr Clin North Am* 46(6):1167–1178, 1999.

14. Outpatient Asthma

I INTRODUCTION

A. Definitions
1. **Asthma** is a form of obstructive lung disease that is characterized by **recurrent inflammation and spasm** of small airways. These changes are triggered by **hyperresponsiveness to various stimuli** and are at least partially reversible with appropriate therapy.
2. **Status asthmaticus** (see Chapter 47) describes **progressive respiratory distress and failure** that is **resistant to therapy.**

B. Pathogenesis
1. **Airway inflammation** is caused by CD4+ lymphocytes, neutrophils, eosinophils, and mast cells.
2. Inflammation may be triggered by a variety of **stimuli,** including the following:
   a. **Infections** (e.g., viral upper respiratory infections, sinusitis)
   b. **Smoke** from tobacco products or wood-burning fires
   c. **Chemical irritants,** including perfumes and cleaning agents
   d. **Allergens**
      (1) **Molds** and other **fungi**
      (2) **Pollen** from many sources, especially trees, grasses, and weeds
      (3) **Pets,** especially indoor cats and dogs
      (4) Cockroaches
      (5) Dust mites
   e. **Food or drug sensitivities,** e.g., sulfites, shellfish, dried fruits, processed potatoes, aspirin

C. Epidemiology
1. About 5 million children are affected.
2. Asthma is more prevalent in boys, but the male:female ratio evens out with increased age.
3. Asthma is 2.5 times more common in African Americans than Caucasians.
4. Income is inversely related to asthma incidence.
5. Asthma is 1.5 times more prevalent in inner city than in suburban populations.

II CLINICAL MANIFESTATIONS: SYMPTOMS

A. Asthma has no single pathognomic symptom or sign. However, wheezing, cough, shortness of breath, and chest pain or tightness may be noted. These symptoms may be exacerbated by exercise. A nocturnal cough may be a predominant symptom.

B. The severity of an exacerbation is determined primarily by the patient's mental status and the amount of air movement in the lungs. Severe exacerbations are characterized by marked dyspnea, extensive accessory muscle use, poor air entry, and an inability to speak comfortably.

HOT

KEY

No or mild wheezing may represent states ranging from mild exacerbation to imminent respiratory arrest.

 APPROACH TO THE PATIENT

A. The **history** should include the following:
   1. **Symptoms,** including frequency, duration, intensity, and pattern
   2. **Response to therapy** and an indication of how the response was measured
   3. **Triggers** for asthma attacks
   4. **Burden of illness**
      a. Frequency of clinic visits, emergency department visits, and hospitalizations
      b. Effect on school and other activities
B. **Differential diagnosis** includes the following:
   1. Infections, especially viral
   2. Aspiration of foreign bodies or secretions
   3. Gastroesophageal reflux disease
   4. Pulmonary edema
   5. Cystic fibrosis
   6. Anatomic obstructions such as vascular rings or slings.

HOT

KEY

Not all that wheezes is asthma.

C. **Additional tests to consider**
   1. **Pulse oximetry** or **arterial blood gas** measurement may be useful in severe exacerbations.
   2. **Chest radiographs** may be useful with first exacerbations or unusual presentations to delineate anatomy and rule out concomitant infection or aspiration of foreign bodies.

   3. **Pulmonary function tests** (e.g., spirometry, peak flow measurements) can be used to determine the severity of disease.
   4. Allergy testing, provocational testing, pH probe and swallow studies, and bronchoscopy are of limited usefulness.
   5. Worsening asthma or failure to respond to appropriate medical management demands further workup.

D. Acute management
   1. Initial management of an exacerbation may be guided by the treatment nomogram (see Figure 47-1).
   2. Regardless of the severity of disease, quick relief is accomplished by **short-acting inhaled β_2 agonists.** β_2 agonists also may be given orally in children 5 years of age and younger who are having a mild exacerbation of mild intermittent disease.
   3. **Criteria for hospital admission**
      a. The frequency with which the child requires β_2 agonists dictates the most appropriate setting for treatment.
         (1) **Treatment at home.** Treatment is needed three or four times daily for children up to 5 years of age, or every 4 hours for those older than 5 years of age.
         (2) **Treatment as a hospital inpatient.** Treatment is needed more frequently, but continuous nebulization is not necessary.
         (3) **Treatment in the intensive care unit.** Continuous nebulization is needed.
      b. Any patient who requires supplemental oxygen should be hospitalized.
      c. Patients with peak flows of less than 70% of baseline despite pharmacologic therapy require hospital care. Patients with peak flows of less than 50% of baseline despite aggressive therapy need treatment in the intensive care unit **(Table 14-1).**
      d. Patients who require moderate to severe use of accessory muscles in breathing should receive hospital care.
   4. Those who are discharged may be given a short (3- to 5-day) course of systemic corticosteroids in addition to increased use of β_2 agonist treatments.
   5. Concurrent otitis media, sinusitis, or pneumonia should be treated with appropriate antibiotics. Asthma alone does not require antibiotics.

E. Ongoing management
   1. Scheduled follow-up every 1–6 months (separate from doctor visits because of exacerbations) is necessary to reinforce teaching and to reassess the severity of disease.
   2. Appropriate use of controller medications is an essential component of ongoing management. The use of controller

TABLE 14-1. Predicted Average Peak Expiratory Flow Rates for Normal Children

Height (in)	PEFR (L/min)	Height (in)	PEFR (L/min)
43	147	56	320
44	160	57	334
45	173	58	347
46	187	59	360
47	200	60	373
48	214	61	387
49	227	62	400
50	240	63	413
51	254	64	427
52	267	65	440
53	280	66	454
54	293	67	467
55	307		

Reprinted with permission from Polger G, Promedhat V. Pulmonary function testing in children: techniques and standards. Philadelphia, WB Saunders, 1971, p 530.

medications is based on the severity of disease and the child's age **(Table 14-2).**

3. **Prophylaxis.** No evidence supports the need for special efforts to provide influenza immunizations to children with mild or moderate asthma.

4. Patients with cold-induced and exercise-induced asthma may benefit from the short-acting β_2 agonists cromolyn or nedocromil, used 20 to 30 minutes before exposure. If long-term control is needed, regular use of an inhaled steroid should be considered.

IV PROGNOSIS

A. **Mortality**
   1. **Patient education** helps to decrease the rates of morbidity and mortality through early recognition of triggers and symptoms and early intervention.
   2. **Risk factors for mortality** include previous hospitalizations, especially in the intensive care unit, for asthma; multiple emergency department visits; sudden exacerbations; the presence of other chronic diseases; and low socioeconomic status.

B. **Morbidity**
   1. Asthma is a chronic disease with variable morbidity; thus, many children do not "outgrow" asthma.

TABLE 14-2. Use of Controller Medications in Asthma

Disease Severity	Controller Medications	
	Age ≤ 5 Years	Age > 5 Years
Mild intermittent Symptoms = 2×/week Nighttime symptoms = 2×/month Asymptomatic; normal PEF between exacerbations Exacerbations brief, but variable in intensity PEF or FEV_1 = 80% predicted PEF variability < 20%	None needed	None needed
Mild persistent Symptoms > 2×/week but < 1×/day Nighttime symptoms > 2×/month Exacerbations may affect activity PEF or FEV_1 = 80% predicted PEF variability 20%–30%	Low-dose inhaled corticosteroids or cromolyn or nedocromil	Low-dose inhaled corticosteroids or cromolyn or nedocromil or leukotriene modifiers or sustained-release theophylline
Moderate persistent Daily symptoms Nighttime symptoms > 1×/week Daily use of inhaled, short-acting β_2 agonists Exacerbations affect activity Exacerbations = 2×/week, with exacerbations lasting days PEF or FEV_1 > 60% but < 80% predicted PEF variability > 30%	Medium-dose inhaled corticosteroids or low- or medium-dose inhaled corticosteroids plus long-acting β_2 agonists if needed or medium-high dose inhaled corticosteroid plus long-acting β_2 agonists	Medium-dose inhaled corticosteroids or low- or medium-dose inhaled corticosteroids plus long-acting β_2 agonists or medium- or high-dose inhaled corticosteroid plus long-acting β_2 agonists

(continued)

TABLE 14-2. Use of Controller Medications in Asthma (Continued)		
	Controller Medications	
Disease Severity	**Age ≤ 5 Years**	**Age > 5 Years**
Severe persistent Continual symptoms Frequent nighttime symptoms Limited physical activity Frequent exacerbations PEF or FEV_1 = 60% predicted PEF variability > 30%	High-dose inhaled corticosteroids plus long-term systemic cortico-steroids if needed	High-dose inhaled corticosteroids plus long-acting β_2 agonists plus long-term systemic corticosteroids if needed

PEF, peak expiratory flow; FEV_1 = Forced expiratory volume in one second.

2. Patients with a family history of asthma, eczema, or allergies are at increased risk of more persistent disease.

References

Cates CJ, Jefferson TO, Bara AI, et al: Vaccines for preventing influenza in people with asthma. *Cochrane Database Systemic Reviews* 2:CD000364, 2000.

Mannino DM, Homa DM, Pertowski CA, et al: Surveillance for asthma—United States, 1960–1995. *MMWR* 47(SS-1):1–29, 1998.

National Asthma Education and Prevention Program. *Expert Panel Report: Guidelines for the Diagnosis and Management of Asthma.* Bethesda, MD, NHLBI, May 1997. NIH Publication No. 97–4051A.

15. Colic

I INTRODUCTION

A. Definition. Colic is intractable crying in an otherwise healthy infant. The crying is of the same intensity and character as that of other infants; the only difference is in its duration.

HOT **KEY** Rule of Threes: Colic is three hours of inconsolable crying occurring at least three times per week for at least three weeks. It usually starts at the age of three weeks and resolves by the age of three months.

B. Incidence. Approximately one in four children are affected to varying degrees.

C. Cause. The cause of colic is **not known.** Researchers have speculated that gastroesophageal reflux disease (GERD), a neuro-maturational disorder, the child's temperament, allergies, or the way the parent and child interact may play a role, but none of these factors has been reliably shown to be the cause.

HOT **KEY** Colic does not predict future temperament!

II DIFFERENTIAL DIAGNOSIS

A. Normal crying. Infants normally cry intermittently for as many as three hours per day at the age of 6 weeks, but usually are consolable.

B. Feeding problems. Overfeeding can lead to reflux, particularly in bottle-fed infants. Underfeeding can lead to hunger. Improper burping can lead to gas. All of these problems can lead to crying.

C. Physical problems that can lead to prolonged, inconsolable crying include otitis media, corneal abrasion, hair tourniquet, an incarcerated hernia, and GERD.

D. Breast milk constituents (e.g., caffeine) can affect the baby.

▐ III ▌ APPROACH TO THE PATIENT

A. Patient history

1. **Review the prenatal and perinatal history.** Was the pregnancy complicated? Were there exposures to drugs or alcohol?

2. **Characterize the crying.** Query the caretaker about the frequency and intensity of the crying, what time of day it occurs and how long it lasts, the baby's age at the onset of the problem, and whether or not the crying is associated with feeding.

3. **Ask for a demonstration.** Ask the care giver to tell you about (and to demonstrate) the techniques she is using to soothe the baby.

B. Physical examination. No findings are expected on physical examination.

C. Laboratory studies are not routinely indicated.

▐ IV ▌ TREATMENT. Colic resolves spontaneously by the age of 3–4 months. In the meantime, there is little to do other than to reassure the care giver that the child is healthy and to offer strategies for coping.

A. Advise the caretaker that it is permissible to take breaks, even if doing so means that the child is left to cry for 15 minutes at a time.

B. Offer reassurance and compassion. Make sure parents know that there is a light at the end of the tunnel!

C. Suggest measures that may bring relief (e.g., a change in formula, white noise, avoidance of overstimulation).

Babies "OUTGROW" Colic

Okay for the parent to take breaks
Understand and recognize how stressful colic can be to care givers
Tell care givers that all infants outgrow colic in a few months
Giving a new formula may help
Reassure the caregiver that the child is not sick or abnormal
Overstimulation should be avoided
White noise (e.g., hair dryers, radio static, or a commercial noisemaker) can bring relief

References
Berkowitz CD: Management of the colicky infant. *Compr Ther* 23(4):277–280, 1997.
Lehtonen LA, Rautava PT: Infantile colic: natural history and treatment. *Curr Probl Pediatr* 26(3):79–85, 1996.
Garrison M, Christakis DA: A systematic review of therapies for infantile colic. *Pediatrics* 106(1):184–90, 2000.

16. Constipation

I INTRODUCTION

A. Definition. Constipation is the infrequent passage of hard, often painful stools. There is no readily applicable gold standard for diagnosis, and a provisional definition is fewer than three bowel movements per week. Severe constipation can lead to impaction and overflow incontinence (i.e., encopresis).

HOT **KEY** Normal infants grunt, cry, scream, and draw up their legs with bowel movements because they do not properly relax the pelvic floor with defecation. This behavior is NOT a sign of constipation, as many parents think it is.

B. Epidemiology
1. Approximately 5% of visits to a pediatrician are related to constipation.
2. Approximately 25% of referrals to gastroenterologists involve constipation.
3. Almost 2% of all children have encopresis (repeated bouts of involuntary passage of feces).

C. Causes of constipation are listed in **Table 16-1.**

TABLE 16-1. Secondary Causes of Constipation	
Cause	**Clues**
Neurologic	
Aganglionosis (Hirschsprung disease)	Rare in children older than 4 years of age; seen in fewer than 1:1600 referrals to encopresis clinics
Tethered cord	Look for hair tufts, dimples, signs of lower extremity weakness
Obstructive	
Anal stenosis	Narrow-caliber stools
Meconium ileus or equivalent (cystic fibrosis)	Other signs of cystic fibrosis
Pelvic tumor or mass	Look for lower extremity weakness, progressive incontinence of urine and stool
	(continued)

TABLE 16-1. Secondary Causes of Constipation (*Continued*)

Cause	Clues
Endocrine	
Hypothyroidism	Failure to thrive, low energy level, alopecia
Pharmacologic (**"NAILED"**)	Thorough medical history is required
Narcotics	
Aluminum antacids	
Iron	
Lead	
Elavil and other tricyclic antidepressants	
Diuretics	

The most common causes are idiopathic and behavioral factors.

II APPROACH TO THE PATIENT

A. **Differential diagnosis.** An organic cause is rarely found. In most cases, the cause is either idiopathic and related to genetic predisposition or behavioral (caused by stool withholding or avoidance).

B. **History.** The following questions should be asked.

1. **How much time elapsed before the child passed meconium as an infant?** If it was longer than 48 hours, Hirschsprung disease may be the cause.

2. **How frequent, large, and painful are the child's bowel movements?** Hirschsprung disease typically produces narrow-caliber stools. Decreased motility and active withholding can produce large-caliber stools.

3. **Is the child soiling (i.e., having accidents)?**

4. **Does the child show signs of stooling phobia or avoidance?**

5. **Was toilet training traumatic?**

C. **Physical examination.** Key aspects of the physical examination include:

1. **Skin.** Is it thick, dry, and yellow?

2. **Neck.** Does the patient have thyromegaly?

3. **Abdomen.** Is the abdomen distended or tender? Are there masses or palpable loops of bowel?

4. **Back.** Is a hair tuft or pilonidal dimple present? Is any abnormal pigmentation visible?

5. **Anorectal region.** Does the patient have evidence of sexual abuse? Is there an anal wink? Is the rectal tone normal?

6. **Lower extremities.** Are strength, tone, and reflexes within normal limits?

D. Laboratory studies. Routine laboratory studies are not indicated. Laboratory testing should be based on clues elicited from the history and physical examination.

E. Additional tests that may be useful include:

1. **Abdominal radiographs** can be helpful in assessing the degree of constipation.

2. **Barium enemas** are not routinely helpful, but findings can be abnormal in patients with Hirschsprung disease if the affected area is large. Hirschsprung disease is not likely to be found in older children because most cases are diagnosed during infancy.

3. **Suction rectal biopsy** searches for the presence of ganglion cells to rule out Hirschsprung disease; it is rarely needed.

F. Therapy (Table 16-2) is instituted according to the cause. Encopresis requires a comprehensive approach that may include referral to a specialist.

1. In idiopathic cases without a behavioral component, increased activity, fluids, and fiber can be beneficial. Mild stool softeners (e.g., mineral oil) also may help.

2. Children who withhold stool and have encopresis require a multifaceted approach, including prolonged use of stool softeners, mild stimulants, and a behavioral program.

 HOT KEY Avoid the use of fiber early in the treatment of children with a history of withholding stool. Increased bulk is NOT what they need!

References

Abi-Hanna A, Lake AM: Constipation and encopresis in childhood. *Pediatr Rev* 19: 23–30, 1998.

Nowicki MJ, Bishop PR: Organic causes of constipation in infants and children. *Pediatr Ann* 28:293–300, 1999.

TABLE 16-2. Medications

Class/Generic Name	Trade Name	Action	Dosage	Cautions
Bulk-forming laxatives				
Psyllium preparations	Metamucil; Perdiem	Admixture of plantain, plantago seed, psyllium. Adsorbs water in the intestine to form viscous liquid that promotes peristalsis	< 12 years of age: 0.5–1 packet 1–3 ×/day; Adults: 1–2 packets 1–3 ×/day	Care needed for children with retention who have bulky stools
Hyperosmotic laxatives				
Lactulose	Cephulac	Prevents absorption of ammonia in colon, thereby lowering pH and causing osmotic effect with distension and increased peristalsis	Infants: 3–10 ml divided three times daily; Children: 40–90 ml divided three times daily	Can cause gas

(continued)

TABLE 16-2. Medications (*Continued*)

Class/Generic Name	Trade Name	Action	Dosage	Cautions
Magnesium citrate	Citroma	Leads to osmotic retention of fluid	< 6 years of age: 2–4 ml/kg/day 6–12 years of age: 1/3–1/2 bottle Adults: 1/2–1 bottle	
Magnesium hydroxide	Milk of Magnesia	Leads to osmotic retention of fluid	< 2 years of age: 0.5 ml/kg/dose 2–5 years of age: 5–15 ml/day 6–12 years of age: 15–30 ml/day	
Lubricant laxatives Mineral oil	Fleet	Decreases water resorption, lubricates intestine	5–20 ml/day	Not to be used in children at risk for aspiration

Stimulant laxatives				
Bisacodyl	Dulcolax	Stimulates peristalsis by direct action on intestinal smooth muscle; alters water and electrolyte secretion to increase net water in intestine	< 2 years of age: 5 mg/day 2–11 years of age: 5–10 mg/day >12 years of age: 10 mg/day	May cause abdominal pain if stools are hard
Senna	Senokot, Ex-Lax	Active metabolite stimulates Auerbach plexus to produce peristalsis	Children: 0.5–1 tsp (granules)	Can cause abdominal pain if stools are hard
Stool softeners				
Docusate sodium	Colace	Reduces surface tension in oil–water interface of stool, causing increased water and fat retention in stool, softening them	< 3 years of age: 10–40 mg/day divided 3–6 years of age: 20–60 mg/day 6–12 years of age: 40–120 mg/day	Not to be used concomitantly with mineral oil

17. Atopic Dermatitis (Eczema)

HOT KEY

Eczema is the itch that rashes. Itch is often the first presenting sign.

I INTRODUCTION

A. **Definition.** The term **atopic dermatitis** is used to describe skin that has an unusual response to stimuli and typically is dry, itchy, and prone to inflammation. The term is derived from the Greek word *atopia,* which means "without place." Although the terms *atopic dermatitis* and *eczema* often are used interchangeably, eczema is a general term for a condition that involves redness, itching, scaling, and vesicles.

B. **Epidemiology**
   1. Eczema affects approximately 10%–15% of the pediatric population. It is associated with hay fever and asthma. As many as 50% of children with **eczema** have **hay fever**, **asthma**, or both. Together, the three conditions are often called the **atopic triad.**
   2. Nearly 60% of affected individuals have symptoms in the first year of life. Approximately 85% of affected patients have symptoms in the first 5 years of life.
   3. As many as 40% of affected children are not affected in adulthood.

II APPROACH TO THE PATIENT

A. **Diagnosis.** The diagnosis of eczema is based on the patient's signs, symptoms, and family history as well as the course of the condition. Typically, eczema appears as pruritic, erythematous, papular, and vesicular eruptions with diffuse borders that blend into normal skin. It often includes serous discharge and crusting. When eczema is chronic, scaling, thickening, and fissuring of the skin are common.

B. The **differential diagnosis** includes seborrheic dermatitis, psoriasis, scabies, and contact dermatitis **(Table 17-1).**

C. **Physical examination.** Key aspects of the physical examination include the following:
   1. **Location of the lesions.** During infancy and early childhood, lesions are common on the face and extensor areas. Moist ar-

TABLE 17-1. Differential Diagnosis of Atopic Dermatitis

Clinical Entity	Distinguishing Features
Seborrheic dermatitis	Salmon- or yellow-colored, greasy, nonpruritic, circumscribed lesions
Psoriasis	Rich, red color with silvery scale; predilection for the extensor surfaces of knees and elbows; often involves dimpling of the nail beds
Scabies	Pathognomonic burrows in the skin; predilection for intertriginous areas; other family members affected; itching is worse at night
Contact dermatitis	Location or distinctive patterns of lesions, history of exposure

eas under the diaper are usually spared. During adolescence, lichenifications of the elbows and knees are common.

2. **Appearance of the lesions.** The lesions may be dry or greasy; the skin is usually dry. Periauricular fissures are common, and the lesions may be superinfected.

D. Management

1. Dryness should be reduced.

    a. **Harsh soaps should be limited** (e.g., no bubble baths), and only soaps containing moisturizers should be used. Alternatively, the use of soap can be limited to skin folds only.

    b. **Bath time should be minimized.** Water should be tepid, and bath oils may be helpful.

    c. **Emollients** (e.g., Eucerin, Lubriderm) should be applied liberally within 5 minutes after bathing. In some cases, two applications per day are useful.

2. **Irritants should be avoided.** Some fragrances, perfumes, fabrics (e.g., wool), laundry detergents, and fabric softeners can exacerbate atopic dermatitis.

3. **Allergens should be limited.** House dust mites are the most common allergens associated with atopic exacerbations. Washing sheets regularly in hot ($> 125°F$) water kills dust mites. Impermeable mattress and pillow covers may be necessary.

4. **Anti-inflammatory medications**

    a. Topical corticosteroids should be applied to areas of severe exacerbations.

    b. The strength of the steroid needed is governed by the severity and location of the lesions. For mild exacerbations, 1% hydrocortisone is appropriate. More severely affected areas may require increased potency.

    c. Potent corticosteroids should not be applied to the face or diaper area for prolonged periods (> 1 week). The use of too potent a steroid may cause telangiectasis and skin atrophy. Never use a fluorinated steroid on the face or perineum.

    d. Extreme, generalized cases of atopic dermatitis may require brief systemic administration of steroids (2 mg/kg/day for 5 days).

5. Antipruritic medications

    a. Scratching affected areas exacerbates lesions. Eczema is an "itch that rashes" rather than a "rash that itches"; therefore, controlling itching is paramount.

    b. Nonsedating antihistamines are used to control itch as needed.

    c. Placing cool, moist towels on the itchy area or letting the child "scratch" with an ice cube may be helpful.

6. Antibiotics. If there is suspicion of bacterial superinfection, an oral antistaphylococcic antibiotic should be started. Often recalcitrant cases of atopic dermatitis are dramatically improved after the addition of antibiotics.

E. Complications. The most common complications include superinfection (e.g., impetigo, cellulitis) or eczema herpeticum, which is a widespread varicelliform infection with herpes simplex or varicella virus. Eczema herpeticum can be serious, especially in infants or immunocompromised individuals. Treatment with acyclovir is indicated.

References

Crowson AN, Magro CM: Recent advances in the pathology of cutaneous drug eruptions. *Dermatol Clin* 17:537–560, 1999.

Hanson SG, Nigro JF: Pediatric dermatology. *Med Clin North Am* 82:1381–1403, 1998.

18. Attention Deficit Hyperactivity Disorder

I INTRODUCTION

A. Background. Attention disorders are among the most common chronic behavior problems affecting children and adolescents. Attention problems may occur alone [i.e., attention deficit disorder (ADD)] or in combination with hyperactivity [i.e., attention deficit hyperactivity disorder (ADHD)].

B. Pathogenesis. The pathogenesis of ADD is poorly understood. The results of studies of brain morphology, cerebral glucose metabolism, and catecholamine production have been inconclusive.

C. Epidemiology

1. In the United States, approximately 5% of children are affected by attention disorders.
2. Girls are more likely to have ADD than ADHD.
3. Boys are diagnosed six times more often than girls with ADHD; however, this finding may partly reflect underdiagnosis in girls.
4. Approximately one half of affected children have symptoms that persist in adulthood.
5. Children with ADHD typically are diagnosed at a younger age because of behavioral problems. Children with ADD are identified when they are older, as their school performance deteriorates.

II CLINICAL MANIFESTATIONS

A. The most prominent **symptoms** are inattention, impulsivity, and overactivity that is inappropriate for the child's age.

B. Diagnosis is based on the criteria described in the *Diagnostic and Statistical Manual of Mental Disorders,* 4th edition (DSM-IV) **(Table 18-1).** The most recent criteria define three subtypes of ADD:

1. ADHD primarily of the inattentive type (ADHD/I), in which the patient meets six of nine inattention behaviors
2. ADHD primarily of the hyperactive-impulsive type (ADHD/ HI), in which the patient meets six of nine hyperactive-impulsive behaviors
3. ADHD combined type (ADHD/C), in which the patient has six of nine behaviors in both the inattention and hyperactive-impulsive symptom lists

TABLE 18-1. Diagnostic Criteria for Attention Deficit Hyperactivity Disorder (ADHD)

A. Either 1 or 2
  1. Six (or more) of the following symptoms of inattention have persisted for at least 6 months to an extent that is maladaptive and inconsistent with developmental level:
     a. Inattention
        (1) Often fails to pay close attention to details or makes careless mistakes in schoolwork, work, or other activities
        (2) Often has difficulty with sustaining attention in tasks or play activities
        (3) Often does not seem to listen when spoken to directly
        (4) Often does not follow through on instructions and fails to finish schoolwork, chores, or duties in the workplace (not due to oppositional behavior or failure to understand instructions)
        (5) Often has difficulty organizing tasks and activities
        (6) Often avoids, dislikes, or is reluctant to engage in tasks that require sustained mental effort (e.g., schoolwork or homework)
        (7) Often loses things necessary for tasks or activities (e.g., toys, school assignments, pencils, books, or tools)
        (8) Is often easily distracted by extraneous stimuli
        (9) Is often forgetful in daily activities
  2. Six (or more) of the following symptoms of hyperactivity-impulsivity have persisted for at least 6 months to a degree that is maladaptive and inconsistent with the child's developmental level:
     a. Hyperactivity
        (1) Often fidgets with the hands or feet or squirms in his seat
        (2) Often leaves his seat in the classroom or in other situations in which people are expected to remain seated
        (3) Often runs about or climbs excessively in situations in which these actions are inappropriate (in adolescents or adults, this behavior may be limited to subjective feelings of restlessness)
        (4) Often has difficulty playing or engaging in leisure activities quietly
        (5) Is often "on the go" or behaves as if "driven by a motor"
        (6) Often talks excessively

(continued)

TABLE 18-1. Diagnostic Criteria for Attention Deficit Hyperactivity Disorder (ADHD) (Continued)

    b. Impulsivity
        (1) Often blurts out answers before questions have been completed
        (2) Often has difficulty awaiting his turn
        (3) Often interrupts or intrudes on others (e.g., interrupts conversations or games)
        (4) Some hyperactive-impulsive or inattentive symptoms that caused impairment were present before 7 years of age
B. A degree of impairment from the symptoms is present in two or more settings [e.g., at school (or work) or at home].
C. Clinically significant impairment is clearly evident in social, academic, or occupational functioning.
D. The symptoms do not occur exclusively during the course of a pervasive developmental disorder, schizophrenia, or other psychotic disorder and are not better accounted for by another mental disorder (e.g., mood disorder, anxiety disorder, dissociative disorder, or personality disorder).

Reprinted with permission from the *Diagnostic and Statistical Manual of Mental Disorders*, 4th ed (DSM-IV). Washington, DC, American Psychiatric Association, 1994.

HOT KEY Office visit assessments have poor sensitivity and specificity. As many as 80% of children diagnosed by home and school criteria as having ADHD displayed no symptoms in their physicians' offices.

C. Differential diagnosis includes learning disability, anxiety, depression, and oppositional or conduct disorder.
D. Comorbidities are common among children with attention problems. They include:
  1. Oppositional defiant disorder (35%)
  2. Conduct disorder (25%)
  3. Anxiety disorder (25%)
  4. Depression (15%)

III APPROACH TO THE PATIENT

A. History. Diagnosis requires a comprehensive history. Important questions to ask include the following: When did the problems start? (Problems typically are present before 7 years of age.) How do the problems manifest themselves? Does the child fidget? Is the child unable to wait for things? Can the child focus on particular activities? Is there a family history of learning disabilities or ADD?

B. Diagnosis. The diagnosis should not be made during the child's initial visit and should not be based solely on the parents' input. When possible, multiple sources of information (e.g., questionnaires filled out by parents and teachers) are best.

　　1. Structured rating scales that are specific for ADD (e.g., Conner questionnaire) should be used to make the diagnosis. The rating scales have excellent test characteristics and have > 90% sensitivity and specificity. Parents and teachers should complete the forms and return them at a subsequent visit.

　　2. Neuropsychological testing is indicated for children with poor school performance and a family history of learning disabilities as well as those who do not meet the criteria for ADD.

C. Treatment

　　1. Pharmacotherapy is a mainstay of treatment.

　　　　a. First-line medical therapy consists of stimulants [typically, for children > 6 years of age, methylphenidate (Ritalin) 2.5–5 mg per dose before breakfast or lunch]. Longer-acting stimulants [e.g., amphetamine aspartate (Adderall)] are effective for some children.

　　　　b. Second-line therapy consists of treatment with pemoline. Although it is effective, pemoline is not the drug of choice because of its rare side effect of hepatic failure. Liver function tests should be performed every 3–6 months.

　　　　c. Data on **tricyclic antidepressant drugs and clonidine** have yielded mixed results.

　　2. Behavioral therapy also can be effective for milder cases or for older children. Recent studies have failed to demonstrate an additive benefit of behavioral therapy to medication alone.

HOT KEY Response to stimulant medication is not diagnostic of ADD. Even normal children focus better when they take these medications!

D. Follow-up

　　1. Initially, therapy is monitored monthly and then periodically (i.e., every 3–4 months).

　　2. The child's performance in school is reassessed, and the dose of medication is titrated to achieve the desired results.

　　3. Some physicians discontinue the medication during summer vacation.

　　4. The child is evaluated annually to determine whether medication should be continued.

References

Adesman AR, Morgan AM: Management of stimulant medications in children with attention-deficit/hyperactivity disorder. *Pediatr Clin North Am* 46(5):945–963, vii–viii, 1999.

American Academy of Pediatrics: Clinical practice guideline: diagnosis and evaluation of the child with attention deficit/hyperactivity disorder. *Pediatrics* 105(5):1158–1170, 2000.

NEONATOLOGY

19. Initial Stabilization of the Premature Infant

I **INTRODUCTION.** There are significant stylistic differences in the care of premature infants. The approaches discussed in this chapter are suggested guidelines.

II **APPROACH TO THE PATIENT BY SYSTEMS**

A. Delivery room resuscitation

1. **Anticipation and preparedness** are the keys to avoiding perinatal ischemic injury **(Figure 19-1).** All resuscitation equipment and personnel should be available before delivery.

2. **Resuscitation medications (Table 19-1).** The need for emergent access should be anticipated when the heart rate does not respond to positive pressure ventilation. Obtaining peripheral intravenous access in an emergent situation can be difficult. A catheter placed 3–4 cm into the umbilical vein is an efficient method of access.

3. If resuscitation is going poorly, pneumothorax, diaphragmatic hernia, persistent fetal circulation, and airway obstruction are considered.

B. Environment. A neutral thermal environment is essential because of a newborn's lack of energy reserves and inability to maintain core temperature. Humidity should be kept at 40%–50%. Incubators should be adjusted to maintain core body temperature at 36°C–37°C and skin temperature at 36°C–36.5°C.

C. Fluids and electrolytes

1. **Initial fluids.** All premature infants need intravenous fluids. Initial total fluids vary, depending on the weight of the infant

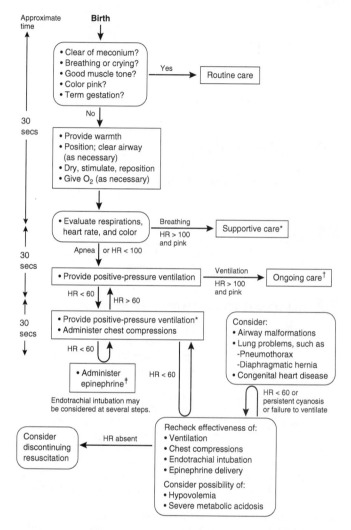

FIGURE 19-1. Overview of resuscitation in the delivery room. ***Supportive care:*** Babies who have prenatal or intrapartum risk factors, have meconium staining of the amniotic fluid or skin, have depressed breathing or activity, and/or are cyanotic will need some degree of resuscitation at birth. These babies are still at risk for developing problems associated with perinatal compromise and should be evaluated frequently during the immediate neonatal period. **†Ongoing care:** Babies who required positive-pressure ventilation or more extensive resuscitation may require ongoing

(*continued*)

(Table 19-2). Micropreemies require more fluid because of their higher insensible fluid losses and immature renal function.

2. **Fluid advancement. Table 19-3** shows the suggested fluid advancement schedule for infants who weigh more than 1000 g.

3. **Modifying factors.** A decrease in weight of approximately 10%–15% is expected in the first week of life. This weight loss is usually caused by the loss of free water. For patients who receive phototherapy, total fluids are increased by 20 ml/kg/day per light to account for increased insensible water losses. Fluid overload should be avoided if there is an associated patent ductus arteriosus (PDA) [150 ml/kg/day may be a prudent limit].

4. **Glucose and electrolytes**

   a. **Hypoglycemia** (glucose level < 40 mg/dl) should be treated initially with a 2–3 ml/kg bolus of $D_{10}W$ (i.e., 10% aqueous dextrose solution). At least 4–6 mg/kg/min of glucose should be delivered in the maintenance intravenous fluid (IVF).

   b. **Hyperglycemia.** Micropreemies may not tolerate $D_{10}W$ as maintenance IVF. Their urine is monitored for significant glucosuria. An insulin drip may be needed if the patient cannot tolerate D_5W.

   c. **Hyponatremia and hypernatremia.** A decrease in the serum sodium level is expected after day of life (DOL) 3. Persistent hypernatremia [sodium (Na) level > 145 mEq/L] may indicate ongoing dehydration; Na level < 133 mEq/L may indicate fluid overload.

   d. **Hyperkalemia.** Premature infants are susceptible to hyperkalemia because of their immature renal function. A decline in serum potassium is expected after DOL 3.

      (1) Infants whose potassium level is higher than 8 mEq/L require electrocardiogram (ECG) monitoring. The physician should look for peaked T waves, wide QRS, a prolonged PR interval, wide and flat P waves, ventricular tachycardia, and ventricular fibrillation. Urine

FIGURE 19-1. (*continued*) support and are at high risk for developing subsequent complications of an abnormal transition. Transfer to an intensive care nursery may be necessary. **‡Heart rate** should increase to more than 60 bpm within 30 seconds. Repeat doses may be given every 3 to 5 minutes. Endotracheal intubation and placement of an umbilical catheter should be strongly considered. (Adapted with permission from Braner DAV, Denson SE, Ibsen LM and the AHA/AAP Neonatal Resuscitation Program Steering Committee: *Textbook of Neonatal Resuscitation.* Elk Grove Village, IL, American Heart Association, 2000, pp 6–14.)

TABLE 19-1. Resuscitation Medications

Drug	Indication	Dose/Route	Administration
Epinephrine	Give if HR = 0 at any time or if HR < 80 after 30 seconds of PPV and chest compressions	0.1–0.3 ml/kg 1:10,000 solution IV/ETT	Bring volume to 1 ml if giving IV; bring volume to 1–2 ml/kg if giving by ETT; consider giving 1–2 ml/kg by ETT or IV only if patient does not respond or if IV is not available; may repeat every 3–5 minutes; HR should increase to > 100 within 30 seconds
Volume expanders	Pallor, weak pulses with a good HR, poor response to resuscitation, suspicion of blood loss (e.g., placental abruption)	10 ml/kg IV; may give lactated Ringer's solution, normal saline, O-negative blood cross-matched to mother, 5% albumin-saline	Give over 5–10 minutes; faster rates may cause intraventricular hemorrhage; may repeat if symptoms persist
Sodium bicarbonate	Use if there is prolonged arrest (> 30 minutes); document that there is no concurrent respiratory acidosis; use only on ventilated patients	2 mEq/kg IV 4.5% (0.5 mEq/ml) solution	Give over at least 2 minutes (1 mEq/kg/min)
Naloxone (Narcan)	Use for severe respiratory depression with a history of maternal use of narcotics within 4 hours of delivery; if mother is addicted to narcotics, use with caution because of the risk of precipitating seizures	0.1 mg/kg ETT, IV, IM SQ	IV push

ETT = endotracheal tube; HR = heart rate; IM = intramuscularly; IV = intravenously; PPV = positive-pressure ventilation; SQ = subcutaneously.

TABLE 19-2. Initial Fluids for Premature Infants

Weight (g)	Dextrose Concentration	Volume (SGA; ml/kg/day)	Volume (AGA; ml/kg/day)
500–599	D_5	140	200
600–699	D_5	120	180
700–799	D_5	100	160
800–899	D_5	80	120
900–999	D_{10}	70	100

Adapted with permission from Gomella TL, Cunningham MD, Eyal FG: *Neonatology: Management, Procedures, On-call Problems, Diseases and Drugs.* Stamford, CT, Appleton & Lange, 1994, p 114.
AGA = appropriate for gestational age; D_5 = 5% dextrose; D_{10} = 10% dextrose; SGA = small for gestational age.

output should also be monitored, and blood urea nitrogen and creatinine levels should be measured.

(2) Infants whose potassium level is higher than 8 mEq/L and those with ECG changes require bicarbonate, calcium, or glucose and insulin infusions (250–500 mg/kg dextrose followed by 0.2 U/kg/dose insulin over 1 hour). The physician should rule out acidosis, hypocalcemia, and necrotizing enterocolitis.

e. **Hypocalcemia.** The iCa level is maintained at > 1.0 mmol/L, and serum calcium levels are maintained at > 7.5 mg/dl with calcium gluconate supplements.

D. **Nutrition.** All premature infants initially have an NPO order (i.e., nothing orally). However, 100–120 kcal/kg/day is needed for growth.

1. **Hyperalimentation with intralipids** is started when electrolytes have stabilized by DOL 3–5. Hyperalimentation is

TABLE 19-3. Suggested Fluid Advancement Schedule for Infants Weighing > 1000 g

DOL 1	80 ml/kg/day D_{10}W
DOL 2	100 ml/kg/day D_{10}W with 3 mEq NaCl/100 ml
DOL 3	120 ml/kg/day D_{10}W with 3 mEq NaCl and 2 mEq KCl/100 ml
DOL 4	140–160 ml/kg/day D_{10}W with 3 mEq NaCl and 2 mEq KCl/100 ml

DOL = day of life.

discontinued when more than 75% of calories are received from enteral feedings.

    a. Amino acids are started at 0.5 g/kg/day and advanced by 0.25–0.5 g/kg/day, as tolerated, to a maximum of 3–4 g/kg/day. Metabolic acidosis can occur secondary to protein overload.

    b. Intralipids are begun at 0.5 g/kg/day and advanced by 0.5 g/kg/day to a maximum of 3 g/kg/day. Intralipids are discontinued when more than 50% of calories are received from enteral feedings.

  2. Enteral feedings. Continuous drip feedings administered through a nasogastric or orogastric tube are usually started within 5 days. Typically, feedings are begun at 8–10 cc/kg/day (trophic feeds) and gradually increased to full over 5–7 days. Bolus or nipple feedings are started at 34–35 weeks gestational age. Initiation of enteral feedings is delayed and advancement schedules are lengthened if there is extreme prematurity, significant birth asphyxia, or other evidence of end-organ compromise. Many clinicians delay enteral feedings while umbilical artery catheters are in place because of the theoretical risk of necrotizing enterocolitis.

E. Cardiovascular

  1. Hypotension may be related to cardiogenic shock (e.g., tension pneumothorax, arrhythmia, asphyxia, metabolic disease), distributive shock (e.g., sepsis), neurogenic shock (e.g., intracranial hemorrhage), or hypovolemic shock (e.g., abruption, fetomaternal hemorrhage, twin–twin transfusion).

    a. Workup. A chest radiograph is obtained. A small cardiac silhouette may indicate hypovolemia, cardiomegaly may indicate congenital heart disease, and pneumothoraces may be identified. In addition, a complete blood count is obtained, and arterial blood gases are measured. Arrhythmia is ruled out, and a cranial ultrasound is considered. Urine output is noted. A Kleihauer-Betke test is considered if fetomaternal transfusion is suspected.

    b. Management. In general, patients who are in cardiogenic shock need inotropic agents (e.g., dopamine, dobutamine) rather than fluid boluses. Patients who are in distributive, neurogenic, or hypovolemic shock require volume expansion (10 ml/kg normal saline, lactated Ringer's solution, or 5% albumin). Inotropes are added if the response to initial volume expansion is poor. Shock-dose hydrocortisone (1–2 mg/kg bolus followed by 25–150 mg/kg/day in 3–4 divided doses) is considered for extremely premature infants who may have adrenal insufficiency.

  2. PDA prophylaxis. Recommendations for PDA vary according to the institution. Indomethacin prophylaxis is considered if the infant weighs less than 1000 g and is younger than

12 hours old. Symptomatic PDAs are characterized by hyper-carbia, metabolic acidosis, left-sided cardiomegaly, increased pulmonary vasculature, hyperdynamic precordium, palmar pulses, and a characteristic murmur.

F. Pulmonary (see Chapter 21)

1. Infants who weigh less than 750 g usually require intubation. To reduce barotrauma, the lowest possible ventilator settings are used.

2. Failure to maintain oxygenation may indicate cyanotic heart disease, persistent pulmonary hypertension of the newborn, pulmonary hemorrhage, or pneumothorax.

3. Any abrupt change in arterial blood gases requires chest wall illumination, auscultation, and an immediate chest radiograph to rule out tube displacement or pneumothorax. A patient who has a pneumothorax requires immediate evacuation with a needle or chest tube. This procedure should not be delayed if the need is clear on clinical grounds alone (i.e., absence of breath sounds combined with a chest wall that becomes brightly lit during illumination).

4. Blood suctioned from the endotracheal tube or patchy densities seen on the chest radiograph may indicate pulmonary hemorrhage. If pulmonary hemorrhage is present, positive end-expiratory pressure is increased (4–8 cm H_2O), and coagulation studies, hematocrit, and platelet count are checked. Further doses of surfactant are contraindicated.

G. Unconjugated hyperbilirubinemia

1. Thresholds for phototherapy and exchange transfusion are lower for premature or ill infants and those with hemolytic disease.

2. General recommendations for premature infants

a. Adequate hydration should be ensured. Total fluid is increased by 0.5–1.0 ml/kg/h.

b. Phototherapy (DOL 1) begins when the bilirubin level is greater than 0.5% of the patient's weight in grams (e.g., if the infant weighs 1100 g, phototherapy starts at 5.5 mg/dl) **(Table 19-4).** Intensive phototherapy with multiple lights and a phototherapy blanket is required if bilirubin levels do not decrease. Intensive phototherapy should decrease serum bilirubin by 1–2 mg/dl every 4–6 hours.

c. Exchange transfusion is required (DOL 1) at 10–15 mg/dl if the infant is well and at 10–12 mg/dl if the infant is ill, if there is evidence of hemolysis, if the rate of increase is higher than 1 mg/dl/h, or if the hemoglobin level is < 10 g/dl.

d. Phototherapy is discontinued when the bilirubin level decreases to 2 points below the level at which phototherapy was begun. A rebound bilirubin level is obtained in 48 hours.

TABLE 19-4. Phototherapy and Exchange Transfusion Thresholds

Age	Weight (g)		
	< 1500	1500–2000	> 2000
Phototherapy thresholds (mg/dl)			
< 24 h	> 4	> 4	> 5
24–48 h	> 5	> 7	> 8
49–72 h	> 7	> 9	> 12
>72 h	> 8	> 10	> 14
Exchange transfusion thresholds			
< 24 h	> 10–15	> 15	> 16–18
24–48 h	> 10–15	> 15	> 16–18
49–72 h	> 10–15	> 16	> 17–19
> 72 h	> 15	> 17	> 18–20

H. Neurologic
  1. Retinopathy of prematurity (ROP) is characterized by neo-vascularization and fibrosis. Retinal detachment may occur. The pathogenesis is controversial; oxygen exposure may not be the only causative factor. In managing ROP, PaO_2 is maintained at < 90 mm Hg. All oxygen-exposed infants who weigh less than 1800 g or are younger than 35 weeks gestational age require ophthalmologic evaluation at hospital discharge. Infants who weigh less than 1300 g or are younger than 30 weeks gestational age require ophthalmologic evaluation, regardless of oxygen exposure.
  2. Intraventricular hemorrhage. The germinal matrix and periventricular regions are delicate and susceptible to hemorrhage.
    a. Risk factors. Prematurity, asphyxia, respiratory distress syndrome, mechanical ventilation, acidosis, and pneumothorax are risk factors. Patients may be asymptomatic or may have catastrophic bleeding, with seizures, hypotension, flaccid quadriparesis, and fixed and dilated pupils.
    b. Management. Meticulous care is required to avoid intraventricular hemorrhage. Wide swings in mean arterial pressure (MAP) and bicarbonate boluses are avoided. Good fluid and acid–base balance is maintained; fluid boluses should run over at least 30 minutes. A screening cranial ultrasound is required at 4–7 days for all infants who weigh less than 1500 g.
I. Infectious disease (see Chapter 23). Because of their immuno-suppressed state, many premature infants require initial antibiotics. Ampicillin and gentamicin or ampicillin and cefotaxime are used if meningitis is suspected.

III PROGNOSIS

A. **Limits of viability.** Survival of premature infants depends on both gestational age and birth weight. Most consider 23 weeks and 500 g to be the lower limits of viability.

B. **Hyaline membrane disease.** Patients who have hyaline membrane disease and weigh less than 750 g are at significant risk for bronchopulmonary dysplasia.

C. **Intraventricular hemorrhage.** Approximately 35% of patients who have stage III hemorrhage and approximately 90% of patients who have stage IV hemorrhage have significant sequelae. Posthemorrhagic obstructive hydrocephalus develops in nearly 10%–15% of all groups with these hemorrhages. Stage I or II hemorrhage does not increase the morbidity or mortality rate. Periventricular leukomalacia is a poor prognostic finding.

D. **ROP.** Approximately 90% of patients who have stage I and II ROP and approximately 50% of those who have stage III ROP experience spontaneous regression. At preschool age, 20% of all cases of blindness are attributed to ROP.

References

American Academy of Pediatrics: Clinical considerations in the use of oxygen. In *Guidelines for Perinatal Care,* 3rd ed. Elk Grove Village, IL, American Academy of Pediatrics and American College of Obstetricians and Gynecologists, 1992.

American Heart Association: *Textbook of Neonatal Resuscitation.* Elk Grove Village, IL, American Academy of Pediatrics, 1990.

Cashore WJ: The neurotoxicity of bilirubin. *Clin Perinatol* 17(2):437–47, 1990.

Dietch JS: Periventricular-intraventricular hemorrhage in the very low birth weight infant. *Neonatal Network* 12(1):7–16, 1993.

Gomella TL, Cunningham MD, Eyal FG: *Neonatology: Management, Procedures, On-call Problems, Diseases and Drugs.* Stamford, CT, Appleton & Lange, 1994.

20. Hyaline Membrane Disease

I INTRODUCTION

A. **Background.** Hyaline membrane disease [HMD; also referred to as respiratory distress syndrome (RDS)] affects premature newborns. Until the recent advent of surfactant replacement therapy, HMD was the major cause of mortality and morbidity in premature infants.

B. **Surfactant** is a lipoprotein produced by type II alveolar cells. It forms a surface monolayer at the air–fluid interface of the alveoli. Surfactant decreases surface tension, enabling the alveoli to remain open.

C. **Etiology and epidemiology**

1. **Pathogenesis.** The combination of an inadequate surfactant system (i.e., decreased surfactant synthesis, secretion, or function; surfactant inactivation) and the poor chest wall compliance found in premature infants results in alveolar collapse (atelectasis). As a result, hypoxemia and acidosis occur and increase pulmonary vascular resistance, causing shunting of blood (through a patent ductus foramen or patent foramen ovale) away from the lungs, exacerbating the hypoxemia and acidosis.

2. **Histologic examination** shows diffuse alveolar atelectasis, pancellular damage of alveolar epithelia, proteinaceous fluid in the alveoli, edema of the alveolar septum, and overdistended alveolar ducts.

3. **Risk factors**

a. The risk of HMD is **increased** by prematurity, male gender, maternal diabetes, cesarean delivery without labor, birth asphyxia, maternofetal hemorrhage, chorioamnionitis, a family history of infants with RDS, and hydrops fetalis. It is also increased in second-born twins.

b. The risk of HMD is **decreased** by antenatal steroids (approximately a 50% reduction), premature rupture of the membranes (2 days to 1 week), maternal hypertension with decreased fetal growth, maternal heroin or alcohol addiction, female gender, and an African-American racial background.

4. **Epidemiology**

a. **Occurrence.** HMD occurs in approximately 0.5% of all

deliveries. In the United States, approximately 40,000 neonates are affected annually.

    b. Incidence. The incidence of HMD is 90% at 26 weeks gestation, 80% at 28 weeks, 70% at 30 weeks, 55% at 32 weeks, 25% at 34 weeks, 3% at 35 weeks, and less than 1% at 40 weeks.

II CLINICAL MANIFESTATIONS

A. Natural history. The onset of symptoms is usually within the first hour of life; peak respiratory distress occurs between 24 and 48 hours. Resolution of the disease usually begins after 72 hours; however, patients can remain symptomatic for as long as 2 weeks.

B. Symptoms include tachypnea, increased work of breathing (e.g., retractions, grunting, nasal flaring), cyanosis, and apnea.

III APPROACH TO THE PATIENT

A. Diagnosis is based on the presence of specific symptoms (see II B) in combination with the infant's history (i.e., gestational age, presence of risk factors), findings of hypoxemia ($PaO_2 < 50$ on room air, or decreased SaO_2), and characteristic findings on chest radiograph (i.e., granular lung fields with air bronchograms, small lung volumes).

    1. Essential laboratory tests include an arterial blood gas measurement to determine the degree of respiratory compromise, complete blood cell count with differential and blood culture to assess for pneumonia or sepsis, hematocrit to assess for anemia or polycythemia, and glucose level measurement.

    2. Additional tests to consider. Prenatally, amniotic fluid can be tested for lecithin, sphingomyelin, and phosphatidylglycerol to assess the risk for HMD. HMD is associated with a lecithin:sphingomyelin ratio of less than 2 or an absence of phosphatidylglycerol.

B. Differential diagnosis. Many diseases cause similar symptoms; they must be considered when evaluating an infant in respiratory distress.

    1. Pneumonia. It is difficult to differentiate pneumonia from HMD in premature infants. Unlike adults, newborn pneumonia is nonfocal because the infectious agent diffuses through the fluid-filled lung in utero. Often, pneumonia is not associated with positive blood culture results.

    2. Sepsis. Neutropenia, or a left shift of the white blood cell differential, suggests infection; however, the absence of this finding does not rule out infection.

   3. Transient tachypnea of the newborn can occur in full-term infants and those delivered by cesarean section.
   4. Aspiration may cause symptoms similar to those of HMD. A history of thick meconium or a finding of patchy fluffy infiltrates on chest radiograph suggests aspiration of amniotic fluid before birth.
   5. Pneumothorax is diagnosed with a chest radiograph, physical examination, or needle aspiration.
   6. Congenital heart disease may be present if there is cyanosis despite oxygen delivery or if there is tachypnea without distress.

C. Therapy
   1. General management (see Chapter 19)
      a. Stress on the infant should be minimized. The infant should be kept in a thermoneutral environment, and the serum glucose level should be maintained. Stimulation should be minimized, and enteral feedings avoided initially. Sedation may be required, and adequate blood pressure should be maintained.
      b. Fluid restriction is associated with decreased severity of HMD.
      c. In patients with severe HMD, arterial access is required for frequent blood draws.
   2. Respiratory support (see Chapter 21)
      a. Continuous positive airway pressure (CPAP) often is appropriate as a starting measure.
      b. Mechanical ventilation is required if FiO_2 on CPAP > 60% or PCO_2 > 60.
      c. Surfactant replacement is most effective if given within 2 hours of delivery. Surfactant rapidly increases lung compliance; expect the need for rapid lowering of ventilator settings.
   3. Antibiotics. Because clinical distinction between infection and HMD is difficult, infants should receive antibiotics empirically. Consider discontinuing antibiotics in the following situations: respiratory distress and chest radiograph findings resolve after surfactant replacement; blood cultures are negative; white blood cell count and differential remain reassuring.

D. Prevention
   1. Premature delivery should be avoided, if possible, through the use of bed rest, tocolysis, and antibiotics.
   2. Administration of steroids decreases the incidence of HMD by approximately 50% if given 24 hours before delivery and within 7 days after delivery. Steroids are not beneficial after 31 weeks gestation.

E. Ongoing management. Infants with respiratory distress require frequent assessment. Associated complications include pulmonary hypertension, pneumothorax, pneumomediastinum, hypotension, pulmonary hemorrhage, patent ductus arteriosus, and intracranial hemorrhage.

 IV PROGNOSIS. Accurate estimates of morbidity and mortality are difficult to make. The advent of surfactant therapy has dramatically changed the initial management of premature infants and lowered the gestational age of infants considered viable. Although surfactant therapy has decreased the overall mortality rate as well as HMD-associated complications (e.g., pneumothorax), it has not decreased the rate of chronic lung disease.

References
Haas M, Rice WR: Respiratory distress syndrome for the practicing pediatrician. *Pediatr Ann* 24(11):572–580, 1995.
Merenstein GB, Gardner SL, Halliday HL (eds): *Handbook of Neonatal Intensive Care,* 4th ed. Philadelphia, WB Saunders, 1998, pp 143–155.
Rennie JM, Roberton NRC (eds): *Textbook of Neonatology,* 3rd ed. Philadelphia, Churchill Livingstone, 1999, pp 481–514.

21. Ventilator Management

....

I INTRODUCTION

A. Background

1. **Goals of mechanical ventilation (MV)**
   a. To facilitate alveolar ventilation (i.e., maintain an adequate $PaCO_2$)
   b. To reduce ventilation-perfusion mismatch (maintain an adequate PaO_2 or SaO_2)
   c. To reduce the work of breathing, and to re-expand regions of atelectatic lung
2. While pursuing these goals, it is critical to minimize ventilator-related lung injury.

B. Definitions

1. **Conventional mechanical ventilation (CMV)** is designed to deliver breaths to a patient with a positive pressure applied to the lungs for inspiration (expiration is passive) (Figure 21-1). This differs from normal breathing, in which a negative pressure is generated to initiate inspiration, and also from high-frequency oscillatory ventilation (HFOV), in which a constant positive pressure is applied to the lungs.
2. **Peak inspiratory pressure (PIP)** is the maximum pressure applied to the lung during inspiration (see Figure 21-1).
3. **Positive end-expiratory pressure (PEEP)** is the pressure maintained on the lung at the end of expiration (see Figure 21-1).

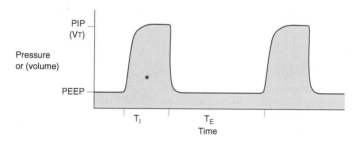

FIGURE 21-1. Basic ventilator cycle. *Area under the curve represents the mean airway pressure. PIP = peak inspiratory pressure; VT = tidal volume; PEEP = positive end-expiratory pressure; T_I = inspiratory time; T_E = expiratory time. (Adapted with permission from Tarczy-Hornoch P, Jones D, Zerom B, et al: *Primer on Mechanical Ventilation*. 1998. Available at http:/neonatal.peds.Washington.edu/NICU-WEB/vents.stm.)

4. **Tidal volume (V_T)** is the volume delivered to the lung during an inspiratory cycle (see Figure 21-1).

5. **Inspiratory time (T_I)** is the amount of time during a single respiratory cycle spent in inspiration (see Figure 21-1), expressed either in seconds or as a percentage of a single respiratory cycle.

6. **Expiratory time (T_E)** is the period of time during a single respiratory cycle spent in expiration (see Figure 21-1), expressed either in seconds or as a percentage of a single respiratory cycle.

7. **Mean airway pressure (MAP)** is a calculated value used to describe the average pressure applied to the lung by the ventilator. In Figure 21-1, the MAP is represented as the area under the curve.

8. **Minute ventilation (V_A) = rate $\times$ V_T** is the total volume of air delivered to the lung over 1 minute.

9. **Fraction of inspiratory oxygen (FIO_2)** of room air is 21% O_2, or an FIO_2 of 0.21.

C. **Potential indications for intubation and MV**
   1. Respiratory failure (i.e., failure to oxygenate or ventilate)
   2. Need for heavy sedation and paralysis
   3. $PaCO_2 > 60$ mm Hg, $PaO_2 < 60$ mm Hg despite supplemental O_2, or severe respiratory distress

D. **Complications of mechanical ventilation**
   1. **Barotrauma** is injury to the lungs due to excessive pressure. Pressure itself is not thought to be as injurious to the lungs as is the stretch on the lungs caused by excessive volume.
   2. **Volutrauma** is injury to the lungs due to excessive volume. Forms of injury include pulmonary edema, epithelial injury, hyaline membrane formation, and air leak syndromes (e.g., pneumothorax, interstitial emphysema).
   3. **Hyperventilation.** Low $PaCO_2$ (caused by excessive ventilation) causes cerebral vasoconstriction with consequent decreased cerebral perfusion.
   4. **Oxygen toxicity.** Exposure to high oxygen tension can lead to the formation of oxygen free radicals and oxidant injury to tissues.
   5. **Impaired cardiac output.** Overexpansion of the lungs with high MAP, inadequate T_E, or high PEEP can compress the pulmonary vasculature. This can impair venous return to the heart and, consequently, decrease cardiac output.
   6. **Pain and agitation.** Endotracheal intubation and lack of control of respiration is distressing. Sedation and analgesia often are required to keep patients comfortable.
   7. **Anatomic deformities.** Endotracheal tubes can cause nose deformities, palatal grooves, subglottic stenosis, vocal cord injury, tracheal ulceration, and mucosal injury (due to suc-

tioning). In addition, damage caused by mechanical ventilation and oxygen can alter the cellular organization of vascular and airway structures.

II MODES OF VENTILATION. **Figure 21-2** shows the modes
of ventilation described in this section.

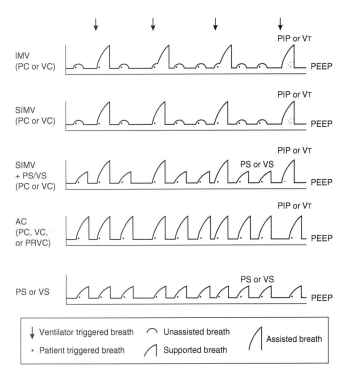

FIGURE 21-2. Modes of ventilation, showing the action of ventilators in
different modes of operation. Although a rate pressure, or volume, is set in
each mode, the response of the ventilator to the patient's effort to breathe
differs among the various modes. Note the difference in mean airway
pressure between the modes. IMV = intermittent mandatory ventilation;
PC = pressure control; VC = volume control; PIP = peak inspiratory
pressure; VT = tidal volume; PEEP = positive end-expiratory pressure;
SIMV = synchronized intermittent mandatory ventilation; PS = pressure
support; VS = volume support; AC = assist control; PRVC = pressure-
regulated volume control. (Adapted with permission from Tarczy-Hornoch
P, Jones D, Zerom B, et al: *Primer on Mechanical Ventilation.* 1998.
Available at http:/neonatal.peds.Washington.edu/NICU-WEB/vents.stm.)

A. **Continuous positive airway pressure (CPAP)** is supplied to the lungs via nasal prongs or a nasopharyngeal tube. CPAP helps stabilize the upper airway and helps prevent atelectasis; its effect is similar to that of PEEP. Pressures usually range from 3 to 8 cm H_2O. CPAP is useful in respiratory distress syndrome (RDS), in apnea, or as a support measure after extubation. However, excessive CPAP can cause CO_2 retention as a result of overdistension and air-trapping. A nasogastric tube can be used in conjunction with CPAP to prevent gastric distension.

B. **Intermittent mandatory ventilation (IMV)** describes intermittent breaths delivered to a set pressure or tidal volume, at a fixed rate. These breaths are not synchronized to the patient's effort to breathe, nor are the patient's efforts to breathe recognized or assisted by the ventilator. Because of this lack of synchronization, the patient may "fight" the ventilator.

   1. **Pressure control (IMV-PC).** The lungs are inflated to a set pressure (i.e., PIP) with each breath given to the patient via the ventilator.

   2. **Volume control (IMV-VC).** The ventilator delivers a set tidal volume (VT) for each ventilator breath.

C. **Synchronized intermittent mandatory ventilation (SIMV) with volume or pressure support.** Intermittent breaths are delivered to a set pressure or tidal volume, at a fixed rate. These breaths are synchronized to the patient's efforts to breathe. The patient can take extra breaths between the scheduled breaths given by the ventilator, either independently or with ventilator support (pressure support or volume support).

   1. **Pressure control (SIMV-PC).** The lungs are inflated to a set PIP at a set rate, but the breaths are synchronized with the patient's respiratory efforts.

   2. **Volume control (SIMV-VC)** is similar to SIMV-PC, except that the lungs are inflated to a set VT.

   3. **Pressure control with pressure support (SIMV-PC/PS)** is the same as SIMV-PC; however, breaths initiated by the patient, over the set ventilator rate, are supported by a set amount of pressure (often set to one-half the PIP or twice the PEEP). At high rates [i.e., > 40 breaths per minute (bpm)], the ventilator cannot synchronize the SIMV breaths effectively with the additional patient-initiated breaths and provide adequate time for expiration. The result may be "breath stacking" (i.e., trapping of air because of inadequate time for expiration).

   4. **Volume control with volume support (SIMV-VC/VS)** is the same as SIMV-VC; however, breaths initiated by the patient, over the set ventilator rate, are supported by a set amount of volume (usually 50%–75% of VT). SIMV-VC/VS has the same limitation as SIMV-PC/PS at high rates.

5. **Pressure support (PS)** does not involve a set ventilator rate or mandatory breaths. All breaths are initiated by the patient and supported by a set amount of pressure. The patient can inhale air beyond that generated by the pressure support. Pressure support guarantees the delivery of a minimal volume of air to the lungs. It also helps the patient to overcome the resistance of pulling air through the endotracheal tube (ETT).

6. **Volume support (VS)** is similar to PS, except that all breaths are supported by a set amount of volume.

D. **Assist control (AC).** Intermittent breaths are delivered to a set pressure or tidal volume at a set rate. All patient-initiated breaths above the set rate are supported with the same amount of pressure or volume as the scheduled breaths. The addition of fully supported patient-initiated breaths provides significantly more support than SIMV-PC/PS or SIMV-VC/VS for both MAP and minute ventilation. Because the patient initiates every breath, this mode can be useful for the patient who needs significant support, but is "fighting" the ventilator. The ventilator recognizes breaths initiated by the patient only when adequate time for expiration is possible, thus preventing "breath stacking." Therefore, these modes are useful when high rates are needed.

1. **Pressure control (PC).** The lungs are inflated to a set pressure.

2. **Volume control (VC).** The ventilator delivers a set volume of air to the lungs.

3. **Pressure-regulated volume control (PRVC).** The ventilator delivers a set volume, but does not push that volume of gas above a set pressure. Pressure-regulated volume control is useful when major changes in lung compliance over brief periods are anticipated (e.g., after the administration of surfactant). Each breath delivers the same degree of lung expansion; however, as compliance improves, less pressure is required to deliver that volume. In PC mode, pressure would be maintained at a constant level while lung compliance improves, thus leading to a situation in which the lungs would become overdistended and at risk for volutrauma.

E. **HFOV** often is used as a rescue mode when conventional ventilation fails. Some physicians use HFOV as a first line of ventilatory support, however. The lungs are kept inflated at a set MAP. Ventilation occurs by the rapid exchange of extremely small volumes, substantially less than the dead space. The rate of ventilation, which is expressed in cycles per second or hertz (Hz), ranges from 480 to 900 breaths/min (about 8–15 Hz). The amplitude of the "puffs" is manipulated to control PCO_2, whereas the MAP and FIO_2 are manipulated to control oxygenation **(Table 21-1).**

TABLE 21-1. Guidelines for Initial Ventilator Settings	
Parameter	**Initial Setting Guidelines**
CMV	
PEEP	3–8 cm H_2O, with higher values for larger patients, airway malacia, pulmonary edema, or significant pulmonary disease
Rate	20–60 breaths per minute depending on severity of pulmonary disease, degree of sedation, age, and PCO_2 value
T_I	0.3–0.6 seconds, with lower values for less compliant lungs, and high rates (need to maintain adequate expiratory time)
PIP	18–26 cm H_2O, or whatever pressure moves the chest
PS	Twice the PEEP or half of the PIP
V_T	4–8 ml/kg, although the accuracy of volume measurement by ventilators is variable, especially in neonates, due to the dead space of the tubing
VS	50%–75% of V_T
HFOV	
MAP	10% higher than MAP on CMV
AMP	Increase until perceptible chest wall motion noted
Hz	8–15 Hz

CMV = conventional mechanical ventilation; PEEP = positive end-expiratory pressure; T_I = inspiratory time; PIP = peak inspiratory pressure; PS = pressure support; VS = volume support; V_T = tidal volume; HFOV = high-frequency oscillating ventilation; MAP = mean airway pressure; AMP = amplitude; Hz = Hertz.

1. **Advantages**
   a. HFOV may cause less injury to the patient because ventilator-induced cycles of expansion and collapse are avoided.
   b. HFOV often is preferred for air-leak syndrome, pulmonary hemorrhage, and pulmonary interstitial emphysema.
2. **Disadvantages**
   a. Logistic limitations include the use of stiff ventilation tubing that requires minimal patient movement and activity.
   b. An unstable patient may have difficulty making the transition to HFOV.
   c. Cardiac output may be impaired as a result of the lack of phasic respirations and the corresponding venous return to the heart.

III GOALS OF MECHANICAL VENTILATION

A. **Appropriate goals** for oxygenation, ventilation, and acid–base balance are dictated primarily by the disease process and can vary among institutions.

1. **Premature infant with RDS.** Ventilator-induced lung injury must be minimized. Permissive hypercapnia often is the goal: pH > 7.25, $PaCO_2$ 45–60 mm Hg, and PaO_2 > 50 mm Hg or SaO_2 > 90%.

2. **Congenital heart disease.** The goal may be to minimize oxygen-induced pulmonary vasodilation. An FIO_2 that is capable of maintaining PaO_2 > 25 mm Hg may be acceptable.

3. **Pulmonary hypertension.** The goal is to optimize oxygenation and acid–base balance while minimizing ventilator-induced lung injury and avoiding hypocarbia.

4. **Otherwise-healthy infant with normal lungs after surgery.** The goals are relatively normal values.

B. **Complications**

1. **Acidosis (pH < 7.25) should be avoided** because it can impair protein function and myocardial contractility.

2. **Wide swings in CO_2 level must be avoided** because they cause wide variations in cerebral perfusion.

IV MONITORING

A. **Blood gases.** Arterial blood samples give reliable estimates of all parameters. Capillary and venous specimens are useful for determining pH, PCO_2, and base excess or deficit values; however, the values will be different than for arterial specimens (higher PCO_2, lower pH).

B. **Transcutaneous CO_2 monitoring (TCM).** Accuracy of TCMs can vary with skin perfusion, subcutaneous fat, and time. In addition, its use is limited by the need for frequent calibration with blood gases and the propensity to damage the skin of premature infants.

C. **End-tidal CO_2 monitoring** is reliable, but requires calibration with blood gases. It is inaccurate in disease states associated with high ventilation-perfusion mismatch and in small premature infants.

D. **Pulse oximetry (SaO_2).** Oxygen saturation reflects the oxygen content of arterial blood. An SaO_2 of 88%–93% corresponds to a PaO_2 of 50–80 mm Hg. SaO_2 is a useful indicator of oxygenation (assuming an adequate hematocrit), right-to-left shunting of blood, and potential oxygen toxicity.

V ADJUSTMENT OF VENTILATOR SETTINGS

A. **Considerations.** A common mistake is to adjust ventilator settings based solely on blood gas information. The following information should be taken into consideration before settings are adjusted.

1. **Physical examination**
   a. **Air entry** is assessed. Is it bilaterally equal? Is there a long expiratory phase? Does the chest rise adequately?
   b. The **patient's comfort level** is determined. Would the patient benefit from sedation? Is the patient breathing out of "sync" with the ventilator?
   c. The **ETT** is checked to ensure that it is not obstructed with mucus.
   d. The physician should also look for evidence of **bronchoconstriction or air trapping** (e.g., high inspiration–expiration ratio, hyperinflated lungs). If air trapping is detected, it may be appropriate to decrease the inspiratory time, PEEP, or IMV rate.

2. A **chest radiograph** can be useful when an acute change in the patient's condition or blood gas value is noted. The physician should assess the position of the ETT and look for signs of atelectasis, air trapping, pulmonary edema, or air leak. In premature infants, chest illumination with a fiberoptic device should be considered if a pneumothorax is suspected. If the patient's condition deteriorates rapidly, emergent needle aspiration may be necessary.

3. **Laboratory tests** usually include a blood gas measurement (arterial or capillary), and, when appropriate, a hematocrit.

4. The nature of the **patient's disease process** is an important consideration in making ventilator adjustments. For example, decreasing support prior to anticipated postoperative edema may be inappropriate, as might increasing ventilatory support as diuresis begins.

B. **Conventional mechanical ventilator adjustments**
   1. **Oxygenation** is monitored by measurements of arterial PO_2 measurement and FIO_2, and pulse oximetry. Oxygenation improves with maneuvers that increase MAP or FIO_2 **(Figure 21-3).**
   2. **Ventilation (PCO_2)** is monitored by PCO_2 measurement. Ventilation improves with maneuvers that increase alveolar minute ventilation (V_A = rate × VT). VT usually is adjusted by changing either PIP or VT. If air exchange is adequate, the rate usually is adjusted.

C. **High-frequency oscillating ventilator adjustments.** The HFOV settings that usually are adjusted include the MAP and FIO_2, both of which affect oxygenation, and the amplitude (AMP), which affects ventilation (CO_2). Serial chest radiographs often are required when assessing MAP because it is difficult to assess lung inflation by physical examination on the HFOV. In addition, as the patient's condition changes, it is critical to monitor

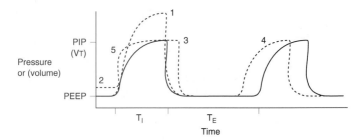

FIGURE 21-3. Ventilator changes that increase mean airway pressure. PIP = peak inspiratory pressure; V$_T$ = tidal volume; PEEP = positive end-expiratory pressure; T$_I$ = inspiratory time; T$_E$ = expiratory time. (Adapted with permission from Tarczy-Hornoch P, Jones D, Zerom B, et al: *Primer on Mechanical Ventilation.* 1998. Available at http:/neonatal.peds. Washington.edu/NICU-WEB/vents.stm.)

for both overdistension (which can impair cardiac output) and atelectasis. When the MAP is adequate, lungs are inflated to the eighth or ninth rib. Changes in both MAP and AMP are not immediate. With changes in MAP, this delay occurs because alveolar recruitment takes time. With changes in AMP, the delay is due to the HFOV mechanics of exchanging extremely small breaths and obtaining equilibrium within the alveolar environment.

VI SUGGESTED MANAGEMENT STRATEGIES (Tables 21-2 and 21-3)

VII WEANING FROM A VENTILATOR

A. **Conventional mechanical ventilation**
   1. The PIP is decreased as soon as possible to minimize lung injury from overdistension, while at the same time providing adequate support to avoid atelectasis. When air exchange is considered adequate, FIO_2 is decreased.
   2. Rates can be decreased progressively while the patient is monitored for hypercarbia.
   3. Extubation often is considered in neonates, when the ventilator settings are around 10–15 breaths/min, PIP is decreased (16–18 cm H$_2$O), and FIO_2 is relatively low ($< 35\%$).
   4. The patient also should be breathing spontaneously and

TABLE 21-2. Problem Solving for the Ventilated Patient

Compartment	Examples	Ventilator Strategies
Mechanical		
ETT	Displaced ETT	Reposition/replace ETT
	Obstructed ETT	Suction or replace ETT
	Air leak around ETT	Reposition or up-size ETT
Equipment	Disconnection, malfunction	Reconnect, check air supply, replace vent
Airway		
Obstruction	Mucus, blood, gastric contents, meconium	Suction, replace ETT, consider lavage
Collapse	Malacia	Increase PEEP
	Bronchospasm	Bronchodilator
	Compression	Increase PEEP
Alveoli		
Congestion	Edema, pulmonary hemorrhage	Increase PEEP to tamponade bleed/edema
	Pneumonia	Treat and support pneumonia
Overdistension	Airway collapse	Increase PEEP
	High PEEP, low T_E, high MAP	Decrease PEEP or T_I Decrease MAP
Atelectasis	Airway obstruction	Suction
	Inadequate support	Increase MAP (PIP/rate)
	ETT malposition	Reposition ETT
Compression	Pneumothorax, pleural effusion	Aspirate air or fluid, or increase support if needed; consider HFOV
Decreased number	Pulmonary hypoplasia (multiple causes)	Support in least injurious manner
Vasculature		
Excess flow	Heart disease	Minimize oxygen
	Heart failure, fluid overload, PDA	Increase PEEP to help tamponade edema
Decreased flow	Heart disease	Increase oxygen
	Pulmonary hypertension	Increase FIO_2, MAP, consider HFOV and nitric oxide therapy

(continued)

TABLE 21-2. Problem Solving for the Ventilated Patient (*Continued*)

Compartment	Examples	Ventilator Strategies
Thoracic cage		
Too compliant	Sedation, paralysis, neuromuscular disease, trauma	Decrease drugs, or increase support (PIP or V_T and rate)
	Prematurity	Maintain PEEP
Too restrictive	Agitation	Sedation
	Seizure	Anticonvulsant therapy
	Thoracic dystrophy or scoliosis	Support in least injurious manner

ETT = endotracheal tube; PEEP = positive end-expiratory pressure; T_E = expiratory time; MAP = mean airway pressure; T_I = inspiratory time; PIP = peak inspiratory pressure; HFOV = high-frequency oscillating ventilation; PDA = patent ductus arteriosus; FIO_2 = fraction of inspiratory oxygen; V_T = Tidal volume.

TABLE 21-3. Potential Responses to Blood Gas Values

Most common ventilator adjustments:
To increase MAP
CMV: Increase PIP or V_T (common), PEEP or T_I (rare), or rate
HFOV: Increase MAP on HFOV
To increase V_A
CMV: Increase rate, PIP, or V_T
HFOV: Increase the AMP

$PaCO_2$	PaO_2	Suggested response (always consider *why* a change is needed: ETT position or obstruction, pneumothorax, heart disease, pulmonary hypertension, agitation)
Low	Low	Decrease V_A, increase FIO_2 and MAP
		Consider sedation
		Consider HFOV to improve oxygenation
Low	Normal	Decrease V_A
		Recheck gas—a low CO_2 decreases cerebral perfusion
		Consider changing to mode with less support
Low	High	Decrease V_A and decrease MAP
		Recheck gas—a low CO_2 decreases cerebral perfusion
		Consider changing to a mode with less support
		(*continued*)

TABLE 21-3. Potential Responses to Blood Gas Values (*Continued*)

$Paco_2$	Pao_2	Suggested response (always consider *why* a change is needed: ETT position or obstruction, pneumothorax, heart disease, pulmonary hypertension, agitation)
Normal	Low	Increase Fio_2 or MAP
		Consider sedation for low Pao_2
		Consider HFOV to improve oxygenation
Normal	Normal	Do not change (consider weaning support)
Normal	High	Decrease MAP or Fio_2
High	Low	Increase V_A and MAP
		Consider sedation
		Consider changing to a mode with more support
High	Normal	Increase V_A
		Consider sedation
		Consider changing to a mode with more support
High	High	Increase V_A and decrease Fio_2
		Consider sedation
		Consider changing to a mode with more support

MAP = mean airway pressure; CMV = conventional mechanical ventilation; PIP = peak inspiratory pressure; VT = tidal volume; PEEP = positive end-expiratory pressure; T_I = inspiratory time; HFOV = high-frequency oscillating ventilation; V_A = minute ventilation; AMP = amplitude; ETT = endotracheal tube; Fio_2 = fraction of inspiratory oxygen.

comfortably above the ventilator rate and have normal respiratory drive.

5. Infants can be extubated to CPAP or nasal prongs; some physicians use a trial of PS before the patient is extubated.

B. High-frequency oscillating ventilation

1. Usually Fio_2 (rather than MAP) is decreased if lung inflation on chest radiograph is appropriate.

2. Mean airway pressure usually is decreased slowly to prevent atelectasis. However, it may be necessary to decrease MAP aggressively if signs of overdistension are present (e.g., overexpansion on radiograph, tachycardia, decreased blood pressure, urine output, or perfusion).

3. AMP is adjusted to maintain adequate Pco_2 levels.

4. CMV can be reinstituted, or the infant can be extubated directly from HFOV.

References
Ambalavanan N, Carlo WA: Current approaches to mechanical ventilation. *Neonatal Respiratory Diseases* 8:1, 1998
Carlo WA, Ambalavanan N: Conventional mechanical ventilation: traditional and new strategies. *Pediatr Rev* 20:e117, 1999.
Eichenwald EC, Stark AR: High-frequency ventilation: current status. *Pediatr Rev* 20: e126, 1999.
Tarczy-Hornoch P, Jones D, Zerom B, et al: Primer on Mechanical Ventilation. 1998. Available at http:/neonatal.peds.Washington.edu/NICU-WEB/vents.stm

22. Neonatal Jaundice (Unconjugated Hyperbilirubinemia)

I INTRODUCTION

A. Background. Almost all newborns have hyperbilirubinemia relative to adult normal values. It is important to differentiate physiologic jaundice from pathologic jaundice and to identify which infants require intervention and which need only observation.

B. Bilirubin physiology. The toxic insoluble form of bilirubin (unconjugated bilirubin) is transported in the circulation bound to albumin until it is taken up by the liver for conjugation. Unconjugated bilirubin is conjugated by glucuronyl transferase, and is secreted into bile. In enterohepatic circulation, the intestines hydrolyze conjugated bilirubin back to unconjugated bilirubin, which is then either reabsorbed into the circulation or converted by the intestinal flora into urobilinogen or stercobilin. The neonatal intestine reabsorbs bilirubin, thus contributing to physiologic jaundice.

C. Definitions and pathogenesis

    1. Jaundice is clinically evident yellowing of the skin or sclera.

> **HOT KEY**
>
> Jaundice usually is not apparent until the serum bilirubin level exceeds 5 mg/dl.

    2. Physiologic jaundice is caused by decreased bilirubin conjugation, increased enterohepatic circulation, and increased heme degradation, which results in an increase in unconjugated bilirubin. The bilirubin level peaks between day of life (DOL) 3 and day 6.

    3. Pathologic jaundice is defined as a serum bilirubin > 5 mg/dl in the first day of life or an increase in serum bilirubin at a rate greater than 0.5 mg/dl/h; such a rate of increase suggests hemolysis. After the first day, jaundice is defined as pathologic if the infant requires phototherapy. **Table 22-1** lists the risk factors for pathologic jaundice.

TABLE 22-1. Risk Factors for Pathologic Jaundice

Jaundice in the first 24 hours of life
Rate of bilirubin rise > 0.5 mg/dl/h
History of hemolytic disease
Hemolysis (Rh or ABO incompatibility)
Polycythemia
Bleeding (e.g., hematoma, gastrointestinal bleeding)
Prematurity
Suboptimal breast-feeding
Ethnicity (Near and Middle East, Asia)
Swallowed maternal blood
Maternal diabetes
Evidence of bowel obstruction
Evidence of sepsis
Evidence of hypothyroidism
Evidence of galactosemia

---

4. **Breast-feeding jaundice** occurs in the first week of life in breast-fed infants. It is caused by physiologic jaundice combined with a relatively low oral intake. Optimal breast-feeding does not result in more jaundice than formula feeding.

5. **Breast milk jaundice** is a normal extension of physiologic jaundice in breast-fed infants. It is thought to occur when fatty acids in breast milk interfere with the uptake and conjugation of bilirubin. It occurs in 10%–30% of breast-fed infants and starts later than breast-feeding jaundice. Breast milk jaundice may persist for up to 3 months, but rarely requires intervention. It resolves when breast-feeding is discontinued.

6. **Bilirubin encephalopathy** results from the toxicity of bilirubin to the central nervous system. Early clinical manifestations include lethargy, change in muscle tone, abnormal hearing, opisthotonus, and seizures. Later clinical manifestations include choreoathetoid cerebral palsy, high-frequency hearing loss, and upward gaze palsy.

7. **Kernicterus** is characterized by neuronal death and pigment deposition in specific regions of the brain (i.e., basal ganglia, cerebellum).

8. **Phototherapy** is the use of fluorescent or halogen lighting at a wavelength of 425–475 nm to convert bilirubin in the skin into water-soluble photoisomers.

9. **Exchange transfusion** is the transfusion of whole blood into an infant while simultaneously removing an equal volume of blood. The goals are to lower the serum bilirubin concentra-

tion and to remove sensitized erythrocytes (if hemolysis is present).

D. Epidemiology

    1. Approximately 60% of neonates have jaundice; 30% of healthy term infants remain jaundiced after 2 weeks of age.

    2. Physiologic jaundice causes a higher peak bilirubin level in Asian and Native American infants than in African American or Caucasian infants.

II   **CLINICAL MANIFESTATIONS.** Except for yellowing of the skin and sclera, jaundice usually is asymptomatic. Pathologic jaundice can lead to feeding problems because of decreased alertness.

III   **APPROACH TO THE PATIENT**

A. Physical examination should be performed in sunlight. Jaundice is detected by gently blanching the skin to reveal its underlying color. Jaundice progresses steadily from the face down to the lower extremities in approximate proportion with increasing serum bilirubin levels. Face-only jaundice is associated with bilirubin levels of 5–8 mg/dl; face and trunk (above the umbilicus) jaundice is associated with bilirubin levels of 12–15 mg/dl; jaundice of the face, trunk, hands, and feet is associated with a bilirubin level of greater than 15 mg/dl.

B. Evaluation should focus on identifying the risk factors for pathologic jaundice (see Table 22-1). If the physical examination and the infant's risk factors suggest pathologic jaundice, laboratory investigation should be considered. Initial laboratory tests for detection of pathologic jaundice include direct and indirect bilirubin levels, infant and maternal blood types, direct Coombs test on the infant's blood (to look for isoimmune hemolysis), and complete blood cell count (CBC) with smear.

C. Differential diagnosis (Table 22-2)

D. Initial therapy. Therapy is initiated to prevent the devastating morbidity and mortality associated with bilirubin encephalopathy and kernicterus.

    1. The threshold for therapy is lower in premature or sick infants (**Table 22-3** and see Table 19-4) and those with hemolysis.

    2. The risk of kernicterus or bilirubin encephalopathy is much higher in infants with hemolysis (50% of infants with a bilirubin level > 31 mg/dl; 18% of infants with a bilirubin level of 16–30 mg/dl). The current standard is to maintain bilirubin levels of less than 20 mg/dl in infants with hemolysis. Bilirubin encephalopathy also occurs in healthy, breast-fed term infants without hemolysis; however, the threshold of serum

TABLE 22-2. Differential Diagnosis of Unconjugated
Hyperbilirubinemia

Increased bilirubin production from the degradation of heme
  Hemolytic disease (hereditary or acquired)
    Isoimmune hemolysis
      Rh or ABO incompatibility, transfusion reaction, auto-
      immune disease
    Membrane defects
      Spherocytosis, elliptocytosis, infantile pyknocytosis
    Erythrocyte enzyme deficiencies
      Glucose-6-phosphate dehydrogenase, pyruvate kinase,
      hexokinase
    Hemoglobinopathy
      Sickle cell disease, thalassemia
    Sepsis or infection
    Microangiopathy
      Hemolytic-uremic syndrome, hemangioma, mechanical trauma
    Ineffective erythropoiesis
    Drugs
      Vitamin K, maternal oxytocin, phenol disinfectants
    Bleeding
      Enclosed hematoma, swallowed maternal blood
    Polycythemia
      Maternal diabetes, fetal transfusion recipient, delayed cord
      clamp
Decreased delivery of unconjugated bilirubin to hepatocyte
  Right-sided congestive heart failure, portacaval shunt
Decreased bilirubin uptake across hepatocyte membrane
  Presumed enzyme deficiency (i.e., Gilbert syndrome)
  Competitive inhibition
    Breast milk, Lucey-Driscoll syndrome, drug inhibition
  Miscellaneous
    Hypothyroidism, galactosemia, hypoxia, acidosis
Decreased storage in cytosol (decreased Y and Z proteins)
  Competitive inhibition, fever
Decreased conjugation
  Neonatal jaundice, drugs, Crigler-Najjar syndrome, hepato-
  cellular dysfunction
Enterohepatic recirculation
  Intestinal obstruction
    Ileal atresia, Hirschsprung disease, cystic fibrosis, pyloric
    stenosis
  Antibiotic administration
Breast-milk jaundice

TABLE 22-3. Management of Hyperbilirubinemia in Full-Term Infants

| Age (hours) | Healthy Infant | | Sick Infant | |
	Phototherapy (mg/dl)	Exchange Transfusion (mg/dl)	Phototherapy	Exchange Transfusion (mg/dl)
< 24	10–12	20	7–10	18
25–48	12–15	20–25	10–12	20
49–72	15–18	25–30	12–15	20
> 72	18–20	25–30	12–15	20

bilirubin required is higher (the range for six reported cases was 39–47 mg/dl).

E. Ongoing management

1. **Prevention.** Frequent feeding is encouraged to decrease enterohepatic recirculation.

2. **Hydration** with intravenous fluids is provided only if signs or symptoms of dehydration are evident. Intravenous fluids should also be considered for patients with polycythemia.

3. **Treatable risk factors (e.g., infection) should be addressed.**

4. **Total bilirubin levels should be followed.** The frequency of monitoring is dictated by the risk of needing an exchange transfusion or expected resolution of pathologic jaundice.

5. **The hematocrit is followed** if there is ABO or Rh incompatibility.

IV PROGNOSIS: MORBIDITY AND MORTALITY

A. **Physiologic jaundice** is not associated with morbidity or mortality.

B. **Pathologic jaundice—morbidity and mortality** are associated with the degree and duration of hyperbilirubinemia, the etiology, and the therapies used to lower the serum bilirubin level.

C. **Risks of phototherapy** include retinal damage, bronze baby syndrome (in infants with conjugated hyperbilirubinemia), thermal stress (especially in premature infants), skin rash (due to histamine release), dehydration, diarrhea, and oxidant stress (in sick premature infants or patients with glucose-6-phosphate dehydrogenase deficiency).

D. Complications of exchange transfusions are significantly greater than those of phototherapy. They include anemia, apnea, bradycardia, thrombocytopenia, hypothermia, sepsis, transmission of infection in blood products (e.g., HIV, hepatitis B and C), necrotizing enterocolitis, thromboembolic phenomena, graft-versus-host disease, transient metabolic abnormalities, and death (rate is approximately 0.5%).

References

Alkalay AL, Sola A: Neonatal jaundice guidelines. *Neonatal Intensive Care* 13(3): 15–24, 2000.

Hammerman C, Kaplan M: Recent developments in the management of neonatal hyperbilirubinemia. *Neoreviews* 1(2):e19–e24, 2000.

23. Neonatal Sepsis

I INTRODUCTION

A. Background

1. **Trends in responsible pathogens.** In the 1930s, group A streptococci predominated; in the 1950s, staphylococci were common; in the 1960s and 1970s, group B streptococci (GBS) and *Escherichia coli* emerged; and the 1980s saw an emergence of *Staphylococcus epidermidis*.

2. **Onset** may be early (first 5–7 days of life) or late (> 7 days of life).

    a. **Early-onset disease** usually is a systemic fulminant process with prominent respiratory symptoms.

    b. **Late-onset disease** may be the result of a nosocomial infection. Meningitis is a more common finding in late-onset disease.

3. **Intrapartum antibiotic prophylaxis (IAP)** often is given to mothers who are known to be colonized with GBS, are in preterm labor, or are at risk for chorioamnionitis (e.g., maternal fever, premature rupture of membranes). Administration of IAP provides protection to the fetus. However, failure to continue antibiotic treatment after delivery may result in a partially treated infection. In addition, IAP may complicate the evaluation of culture studies obtained after birth as well as decisions about the length of empiric therapy.

B. Pathogenesis. Neonatal infections occur by four routes:

1. **Bloodborne transmission.** Infections occur in utero via the maternal bloodstream [e.g., *Listeria monocytogenes*, STORCH (see Chapter 24), and tuberculosis].

2. **Vertical transmission.** Infections can occur as a result of the ascent of bacteria into the amniotic cavity from the vagina or cervix (e.g., GBS, *E. coli*, and *L. monocytogenes*).

3. **During passage through the birth canal.** The neonate may acquire gonococcal ophthalmia, *E. coli* infection, or late-onset GBS sepsis.

4. **Environmental transmission.** Infections may be acquired from the home environment or in a nosocomial setting (e.g., *Pseudomonas, Klebsiella, S. epidermidis*).

C. Risk factors. The most important risk factors for neonatal sepsis include the degree of prematurity (i.e., a greater degree of prematurity is correlated with a higher risk of infection) and

certain maternal conditions. Risk factors for systemic infection in the first 7 days of life include the following:

1. **Maternal conditions:** GBS colonization, chorioamnionitis, premature rupture of the membranes (> 18 hours), maternal temperature greater than 38°C, urinary tract infection, preterm labor, and cerclage.

2. **Infant characteristics:** prematurity, Apgar score less than 6 at 5 minutes, meconium-stained amniotic fluid, persistent respiratory distress or oxygen requirement, fever, neutropenia, male gender, skin wounds, polymorphonuclear cells and organisms in a gastric aspirate, and sustained fetal tachycardia of greater than 160 beats/min prior to delivery.

3. **Systemic bacterial disease in a sibling before 3 months of age** is an additional risk factor.

D. Epidemiology

1. The incidence of neonatal sepsis in full-term infants is 1–4:1000 live births.

2. The incidence of neonatal sepsis in very-low-birthweight infants (< 1000 g) is 300:1000.

3. *E. coli* and GBS account for 70% of cases of systemic neonatal disease.

4. The colonization rate for GBS in pregnant women and newborns is 5%–35%.

5. The incidence of neonatal GBS disease is 1–4:1000 live births.

6. The prognosis is worse in boys.

7. The mortality rate for African American infants is twice that for Caucasian infants.

II **CLINICAL MANIFESTATIONS.** **Signs and symptoms** often are nonspecific, but are not necessarily subtle. Longitudinal evaluation in the first day of life is critical because any infant whose condition deteriorates should undergo a workup for sepsis **(Table 23-1).**

III **APPROACH TO THE PATIENT**

A. Identifying affected patients. Determining which infants should be evaluated for sepsis is not a straightforward process. Gestational age, signs, symptoms, and significant risk factors should be considered.

HOT
KEY

Symptomatic infants of any gestational age should receive a full evaluation and empiric therapy.

TABLE 23-1. Clinical Manifestations of Sepsis/Meningitis

System	Clinical Manifestation
Constitutional	Temperature instability manifests either as hyperthermia (> 99.6°F [37.5°C]) or hypothermia (< 97°F [36°C])
Respiratory	Oxygen requirement, grunting, flaring, retractions, tachypnea, increased ventilator settings; the combination of respiratory distress and an oxygen requirement strongly suggests sepsis
Cardiovascular	Hypotension, shock, metabolic acidosis, poor perfusion, mottled appearance
Gastrointestinal	Abdominal distension, ileus, diarrhea, vomiting, poor feeding, hepatomegaly, conjugated hyperbilirubinemia
Hematologic	Petechiae, purpura, abnormal coagulation study findings
Endocrine	Glucose instability
Neurologic	Seizures; change in level of consciousness; apnea; lethargy; bulging, full fontanel; nuchal rigidity; seizures in newborns should be considered to have an infectious cause until proven otherwise

Adapted with permission from Cole FS: Bacterial infections of the newborn. In *Avery's Diseases of the Newborn*, 7th ed. Edited by Taeusch HW, Ballard RA. Philadelphia, W.B. Saunders, 1999, p 493.

1. **Neonates older than 34 weeks gestational age or weighing more than 2000 g at birth.** An initial workup should be considered for asymptomatic infants who have significant risk factors. Workup should include a complete blood cell (CBC) count with differential and a band:total neutrophil (I:T) ratio, and blood culture. Some physicians also advocate a C-reactive protein (CRP) or gastric aspirate examination as part of the initial workup. If the results of the initial workup suggest infection, empiric antibiotics should be strongly considered.
2. **Neonates younger than 34 weeks gestational age or weighing less than 2000 g at birth.** All asymptomatic preterm infants who weigh less than 1250 g at birth or are younger than 30 weeks gestational age should receive a full workup and empiric treatment. Workup and empiric treatment also should be considered for any asymptomatic infant who is younger

than 34 weeks gestational age or who has a birthweight less than 2000 g if the mother received IAP more than 4 hours before delivery.

B. Treatment
1. Antimicrobial therapy
a. Ampicillin and gentamicin provide adequate coverage in most patients.
b. Cefotaxime should be substituted for ampicillin if the patient has clinical or laboratory evidence of meningitis.
c. Nafcillin or vancomycin plus cefotaxime can be used in patients who are suspected of having a nosocomial infection.
2. Duration of therapy
a. Patients who have a **positive blood culture result** should receive 10–14 days of treatment with intravenous antibiotics.
b. Documented meningitis usually necessitates at least 21 days of treatment with intravenous antibiotics.
c. When **culture findings remain negative,** antibiotics typically can be discontinued in 2–3 days if the patient's symptoms can be attributed to another process. However, longer courses of antibiotics may be required for infants who are premature or symptomatic as well as for those who have persistently worrisome laboratory values or whose mothers received IAP.

C. Diagnostic tools
1. Blood culture. A minimum of 0.5–1 ml blood should be obtained, preferably from an umbilical artery or a peripheral vein. The femoral artery or vein should be avoided because of the risk of joint capsule perforation and contamination by perineal organisms.
2. CBC. A total white blood cell count of less than 5000 cells/mm^3 or an I:T ratio greater than 0.2–0.3 suggests infection. The CBC is most predictive of infection if it is obtained after 12 hours of age because maternal hypertension, asphyxia, and intraventricular hemorrhage can cause leukopenia and abnormal I:T ratios. Serial CBC counts may be helpful in these situations.
3. Gastric aspirate. A positive gastric aspirate culture or Gram stain result or the presence of white blood cells may indicate infection. In a full-term infant, a positive culture result increases the risk of sepsis from approximately 1:1000 to 5:100.
4. Cerebrospinal fluid (CSF). Some institutions perform a lumbar puncture on all newborns who are evaluated for sepsis; others perform this test only if the results of primary blood cultures are positive. However, as many as 15% of cases of meningitis occur without a positive finding on blood culture.

   5. **Urine.** A bladder tap is the preferred method of obtaining a sample in infants younger than 6 weeks of age. A urine specimen is usually not necessary in infants younger than 24 hours of age because the risk of urinary tract infection in this population is low.
   6. **Arterial blood gas** measurements may show metabolic acidosis or respiratory failure.
   7. **Chest radiographs** may show diffuse pulmonary infiltrates similar to those seen in respiratory distress syndrome.
   8. **Abdominal radiographs** should be considered for patients who have gastrointestinal symptoms (e.g., abdominal distension, vomiting).
   9. **CRP** level greater than 1 suggests infection. Longitudinal evaluation of CRP may be helpful; some centers state that three normal CRP values taken 12 hours apart is a reassuring sign.
   10. **Latex agglutination.** Antigen detection tests on CSF and urine can be helpful in detecting GBS, *Neisseria meningitidis, Haemophilus influenzae* type B (HIB), and *Streptococcus pneumoniae,* especially if the mother received IAP. Significant cross-reactivity occurs between *E. coli* and the HIB capsular antigen, so a positive HIB titer may indicate infection with *E. coli.*

References

Singhal KK, La Gamma EF: Management of 168 neonates weighing more than 2000 g receiving intrapartum chemoprophylaxis for chorioamnionitis. Evaluation of an early discharge strategy. *Arch Pediatr Adolesc Med* 150(2):158–163, 1996.

Yancey MK, Duff P, Kubilis P, et al: Risk factors for neonatal sepsis. *Obstet Gynecol* 87(2):188–194, 1996.

24. STORCH Infections

....

I **INTRODUCTION.** STORCH infections are a collection of congenital infections that share a constellation of manifestations.

"STORCH"

Syphilis
Toxoplasmosis
Other (e.g., hepatitis, parvovirus, varicella zoster virus)
Rubella
Cytomegalovirus
Herpes

II **CLINICAL MANIFESTATIONS.** Table 24-1 shows the major clinical manifestations shared by STORCH infections. **Table 24-2** lists findings that suggest a specific diagnosis.

III **APPROACH TO THE PATIENT.** The clinical findings, maternal history, and prepartum screening studies should be considered, and the diagnostic workup should be focused ac-

---

TABLE 24-1. Clinical Features Associated with Congenital Infection

Intrauterine growth retardation
Hydrops
Hepatosplenomegaly
Microcephaly, intracranial calcifications, hydrocephalus
Anemia, thrombocytopenia, petechiae
Jaundice (especially conjugated hyperbilirubinemia)
Pneumonitis
Cardiac malformations, myocarditis
Eye abnormalities (chorioretinitis, cataracts)
Bone abnormalities (osteochondritis, periostitis)

Reprinted with permission from Schwartz MW, Bell LM, Bingham PM: *The 5-Minute Pediatric Consult*, 2nd ed. Baltimore: Lippincott Williams & Wilkins, 2000.

TABLE 24-2. Clinical Findings in Congenitally Infected Infants That Suggest a Specific Diagnosis

Infection	Suggestive Findings
Syphilis	Osteochondritis and periostitis
	Eczematoid skin rash
	Hemorrhagic rhinitis ("snuffles")
Toxoplasmosis	Hydrocephalus with generalized calcifications
	Chorioretinitis
Rubella	Cataracts, cloudy cornea, pigmented retina
	"Blueberry muffin" syndrome
	Vertical striation
	Malformation (PDA, pulmonary artery stenosis)
	Sensorineural hearing loss
CMV	Microcephaly with periventricular calcifications
	Inguinal hernias in boys
	Petechiae with thrombocytopenia
Herpes	Skin vesicles
	Keratoconjunctivitis
	Acute CNS findings

Adapted with permission from Stagno S, Pass RF, Alford CA: Perinatal infections and maldevelopment. In *The Fetus and the Newborn*, vol 17, series 1. Edited by Bloom AD, James LS. New York: Wiley-Liss, 1981. CMV = cytomegalovirus; CNS = central nervous system; PDA = patent ductus arteriosus.

cordingly. Because many infants are asymptomatic at birth, the diagnosis may depend on findings outside of the immediate neonatal period.

IV SPECIFIC INFECTIONS

A. Syphilis

1. **Pathogenesis.** Congenital syphilis is still seen in large urban areas and in rural areas of the southern United States. Transmission of syphilis can occur at any time during pregnancy or at birth. The rate of vertical transmission is almost 100% during the primary or secondary stage of the illness, 40% during the latent phase, and 6%–14% in the late latent stage. Infants who acquire syphilis earlier in gestation have a more severe form of the disease. The overall mortality rate from congenital syphilis in infants is 54%.

2. **Incidence.** Approximately two to five infants contract congenital syphilis for every 100 infected women.

    3. Clinical manifestations. The symptoms resemble those of secondary syphilis, but no primary chancre is present. As many as 50% of infants are asymptomatic at birth.

      a. Early congenital syphilis (< 2 years of age). Periostitis is the most common finding. In periostitis, the metaphysis and diaphysis of the long bones have multiple lines of periosteum that are visible on a radiograph. Hemorrhagic rhinitis ("snuffles") is also common.

      b. Late congenital syphilis (> 2 years of age). Noninfectious sequelae include eighth cranial nerve damage (deafness), gummas, Hutchinson teeth, and keratitis of the cornea. Hutchinson teeth, deafness, and keratitis compose Hutchinson's classic triad.

    4. Diagnosis. Transfer of maternal nontreponemal and treponemal antibodies confounds testing of the child. The following criteria are used to help confirm the diagnosis:

      a. Long bone findings combined with a positive result on a nontreponemal or treponemal test

      b. Venereal Disease Research Laboratory (VDRL) level four times the mother's level

      c. Positive VDRL finding on cerebrospinal fluid (CSF) tests

      d. Positive serum test results for antitreponemal immunoglobulin M (IgM)

      e. Evidence of treponemes on antibody staining of the placenta or umbilical cord

    5. Treatment. Aqueous crystalline penicillin G is the drug of choice for infected infants. Postpartum management involves treating any infant of a mother who was inadequately treated, whose treatment cannot be confirmed, who received a drug other than penicillin G, or who was treated in the last 4 weeks of pregnancy.

B. Toxoplasmosis

    1. Pathogenesis. Toxoplasmosis is acquired by handling infected cat feces or by eating raw meat or eggs. Most maternal infections are subclinical, but some women may have mononucleosis-like symptoms. Congenital toxoplasmosis may occur when there is a primary infection acquired during pregnancy. The rate of transmission is directly related to gestational age at the time of infection. The degree of fetal damage has an inverse relationship.

      a. First trimester: 17% rate of infection; spontaneous abortion

      b. Second trimester: 25% rate of infection; spontaneous abortion or severe disease

      c. Third trimester: 65% rate of infection; subclinical disease

    2. The **incidence** has been estimated to be between 1:1000 and 1:10,000 live births.

3. **Clinical manifestations** include obstructive hydrocephalus, chorioretinitis, and intracranial calcifications (the classic triad of toxoplasmosis).

4. **Diagnosis.** An elevated level of toxoplasmosis IgM in the serum or CSF implies disease in the infant. A positive maternal skin test result indicates chronic infection and almost no risk of transmission to the fetus.

5. **Treatment.** The effectiveness of therapy for infected infants is unclear; however, most regimens use a combination of pyrimethamine and sulfadiazine. Spiramycin can prevent congenital infection if it is given to pregnant mothers with primary infections.

C. Rubella

1. **Pathogenesis.** Despite vaccination, congenital rubella still occurs. Approximately 5%–20% of young adults are susceptible to rubella. The maternal illness is mild and is characterized by low-grade fever, generalized lymphadenopathy, and faint erythematous rash. The rate of transmission varies with gestational age: 1–12 weeks, 81%; 13–16 weeks, 54%; 17–22 weeks, 36%; 23–30 weeks, 30%; 31–36 weeks, 60%; 36–40 weeks, 100%.

2. **Clinical manifestations.** At birth, 50% of neonates are normal; the presentation may be acute or chronic.

3. **Diagnosis.** Cultures from the pharynx, conjunctiva, urine, and CSF are useful. Measuring the serum level of IgM also may be helpful; however, the disease may suppress immune function, reducing the effectiveness of this test.

4. **Treatment** is supportive. Vaccination is the main mode of prevention.

D. Cytomegalovirus

1. **Pathogenesis.** Cytomegalovirus (CMV) is a ubiquitous pathogen that may cause an upper respiratory tract infection or mononucleosis-like symptoms in adults. Although most congenital infections occur during primary maternal infections (50% transmission rate), they also can occur during recurrences (1% transmission rate). Infection also can occur through infected vaginal secretions or breast milk. Although gestational age does not influence the rate of vertical transmission, an infant who acquires CMV early in gestation has a more severe form of the disease.

2. **Incidence.** CMV affects 1%–2% of live births.

3. **Clinical manifestations.** Only 5%–10% of all patients are symptomatic within the first few weeks of life. Symptomatic patients have a 20%–30% mortality rate. Classic multisystemic CMV inclusion disease is rare.

4. **Diagnosis.** Isolation of the virus from urine is the gold standard. Urine shell vial assays are also helpful. Beyond the first

3 weeks of life, the diagnosis of CMV infection is difficult because of its ubiquitous nature.

5. **Treatment.** Ganciclovir is useful in the treatment of CMV retinitis; however, this drug is not routinely used because of insufficient data on its efficacy and its inherent toxicity.

E. **Herpes simplex virus (HSV I/HSV II)**

1. **Pathogenesis.** Direct exposure during delivery is the major mode of infection. Infection can be caused by HSV I or HSV II. Infants born to women with primary infection near the time of delivery have a 50% risk of acquiring HSV. Infants born to mothers with a first episode of nonprimary infection (antibody to type 1, new acquisition type 2 disease, and vice versa) have a 30% risk of acquiring HSV. Infants born to mothers with recurrent infection have a 1%–3% risk. Additional neonatal risk factors include membranes ruptured for more than 6 hours, scalp electrode or other internal monitoring, chorioamnionitis, cervicitis, and vaginal delivery.

2. **Incidence.** The incidence is 1:2000–5000 live births. Fifty percent to seventy percent of affected infants are born to women who are asymptomatic at delivery.

HOT KEY Always consider herpes when evaluating an infant for sepsis, even if the mother was asymptomatic at the time of delivery or has no clinical history of herpes.

3. **Treatment.** All regimens use acyclovir. Consultation with an infectious disease specialist is required because dosages and duration of therapy often change.

4. **Clinical manifestations.** Unlike other congenital infections, asymptomatic presentation is rare.

a. **Disseminated herpes infection** represents 50% of all cases of neonatal herpes. It is a particularly vicious illness.

(1) **Presentation.** Disseminated herpes infection usually occurs by day of life (DOL) 9–11, but may occur as late as DOL 28. The symptoms are dramatic, with involvement of multiple organ systems—e.g., pneumonitis, hepatitis with jaundice, disseminated intravascular coagulation, encephalitis, seizures, keratoconjunctivitis. A characteristic vesicular rash often is present.

(2) **Diagnosis.** Tests include surface culture and fluorescent antibody test of skin lesions, conjunctiva, and oropharynx after 24 hours of life. A rectal swab for culture also is obtained. Blood and CSF samples are

sent to the laboratory for culture and polymerase chain reaction (PCR) studies.

(3) **Prognosis.** The infant mortality rate without treatment is higher than 80%; with treatment, it is 57%. Most infants have significant neurologic sequelae.

b. **Central nervous system (CNS) herpes**

(1) **Epidemiology.** Approximately 70% of infants with neonatal herpes, including those with disseminated herpes infection, have CNS disease.

(2) **Symptoms** are nonspecific and include seizures, irritability, poor feeding, a bulging fontanel, and temperature instability.

(3) **Diagnosis.** CSF findings include an increased white blood cell count and increased protein levels. PCR and culture results are positive for HSV.

(4) **Prognosis.** Approximately 50% of untreated infants with localized CNS disease die; with treatment, the mortality rate decreases to 10%. Nearly 75% of survivors have psychomotor retardation. Associated microcephaly, hydranencephaly, porencephalic cysts, blindness, spasticity, or learning disabilities also may be present.

c. **Skin, eye, and mouth herpes**

(1) **Epidemiology.** Skin, eye, and mouth herpes (SEM) represents 30%–40% of cases of neonatal herpes.

(2) **Presentation.** Affected infants are usually 15–17 days of age. Symptoms may occur as late as 28 days of age.

(a) **Cutaneous.** Classically, herpes appears as clusters of vesicles on an erythematous base. Almost all infants have a recurrence during the first 6 months of life. Many have recurrences after 1 year of age.

(b) **Oral herpes.** These lesions have a similar appearance to cutaneous lesions.

(c) **Ocular herpes** may lead to corneal ulcers, cataracts, optic atrophy, or blindness. Dendritic keratitis is pathognomonic. Referral to an ophthalmologist is required.

(3) **Prognosis.** Without intravenous Acyclovir, 70% of skin lesions progress to CNS involvement or disseminated disease. However, with early treatment, only 5%–20% of skin lesions progress.

(4) **Diagnosis** is made by a positive surface culture or fluorescent antibody test result.

References
Behrman RE, Kliegman R, Jenson HB (eds): *Nelson Textbook of Pediatrics,* 16th ed. Philadelphia, WB Saunders, 2000, pp 514–527.

Bloom AD, James LS: *The Fetus and the Newborn,* vol 17, series 1. New York, Wiley-Liss, 1981.

Committee on Infectious Disease, American Academy of Pediatrics, Pickering LK (ed): *2000 Red Book Report of the Committee on Infectious Diseases,* 25th ed. Elk Grove Village, IL, American Academy of Pediatrics, 2000.

Gomella TL, Cunningham MD, Eyal FG: *Neonatology: Management, Procedures, On-Call Problems, Diseases and Drugs.* Stamford, CT, Appleton and Lange, 1994, pp 345–365.

Zenker PN, Berman SM: Congenital syphilis: trends and recommendations for evaluation and management. *Pediatr Infect Dis J* 10(7):516-522, 1991.

25. Persistent Pulmonary Hypertension of the Newborn

I INTRODUCTION

A. Definitions

1. **Persistent pulmonary hypertension of the newborn (PPHN),** or persistent fetal circulation (PFC), is a physiologic condition characterized by suprasystemic pulmonary vascular resistance. It results in right-to-left flow through the ductus arteriosus, hypoxemia, cyanosis, and poor left ventricular filling. No structural heart defect is present.

2. **Oxygenation index = (OI)**
$$\text{Oxygenation index (OI)} = \frac{\text{mean airway pressure (MAP)} \times \text{F}_{\text{IO}_2}}{\text{postductal Pa}_{\text{O}_2}}$$

3. **Extracorporeal membrane oxygenation (ECMO)** is a continuous mechanized process through which blood is removed from the venous system, oxygenated using an artificial membrane outside of the body, and then pumped back into the arterial circulation.

B. Pathogenesis. The transition from fetal to adult circulation begins soon after birth. It is initiated by increased oxygen tension in the alveoli and a corresponding decrease in pulmonary vascular resistance. Any insult that impairs pulmonary oxygen tension and vascular tone can prevent this transition and may lead to PPHN.

C. Epidemiology

1. PPHN occurs in approximately 1:1000 live births.

2. The most common initiating event is meconium aspiration. Other common triggers are sepsis, pneumonia, perinatal ischemic insult, and respiratory distress syndrome.

3. The incidence is increased in infants of mothers who have diabetes mellitus.

4. PPHN most commonly affects full-term infants.

5. Maternal use of nonsteroidal anti-inflammatory drugs may increase the risk of PPHN.

II CLINICAL MANIFESTATIONS. Signs and symptoms include cyanosis with a structurally normal heart, a significant

oxygen requirement that may not resolve even with 100% oxygen, tachypnea and respiratory distress, hypotension, acidosis, and poor distal perfusion.

III APPROACH TO THE PATIENT

A. Diagnosis. Initial steps in the diagnosis and management of an infant with cyanosis include a thorough cardiac and pulmonary examination, oximetry, blood gas analysis, and chest radiograph.

    1. An **echocardiogram** helps to rule out a structural lesion and may show right-to-left shunting through the foramen or ductus.

    2. Blood cultures are obtained to rule out bacterial sepsis.

    3. Preductal oxygen saturation is measured by placing a lead on the right upper extremity. **Postductal oxygen saturation** is determined by placing a lead on any other extremity. If preductal oxygen saturation is significantly greater than postductal oxygen saturation, then a right-to-left shunt is present through the ductus arteriosus. Right-to-left flow across the ductus arteriosus indicates suprasystemic pulmonary blood pressure, which is the hallmark of PPHN.

B. Additional tests to consider. A complete blood cell count with differential, coagulation studies, electrolytes, and cranial ultrasound may not alter the initial stages of management. However, these tests are an important supplement to ongoing care and may provide clues to the triggering event. Baseline studies should be obtained early in the course of illness.

C. Initial therapy

    1. Oxygen. Liberal use of oxygen, especially in full-term infants, is necessary to maximize oxygen tension and reduce pulmonary vascular resistance.

    2. Mechanical ventilation. The MAP may need to be increased to maximize alveolar oxygen tension. High-frequency oscillatory ventilation (HFOV) can achieve a high MAP while minimizing the risk of corresponding lung trauma.

    3. Inotropics. Catecholamines (e.g., dopamine) function in two ways. First, they increase systemic vascular resistance, encouraging left-to-right flow across the ductus. Second, they enhance cardiac output. This helps to overcome the increased pulmonary vascular resistance, which, in turn, improves lung perfusion and filling of the left ventricle.

    4. Volume expansion. Several boluses of crystalloid, colloid, and blood products may be necessary to maximize preload. Hematocrit should be kept within a normal range to maximize oxygen-carrying capacity.

5. **Alkalinization** is desirable because it reduces pulmonary vascular resistance. Alkalinization may be achieved with an intravenous infusion of sodium bicarbonate or sodium acetate, or through hyperventilation. There is controversy as to whether alkali infusion or hyperventilation is more effective. Recent studies suggest that there is a lower morbidity rate in full-term infants with PPHN if hyperventilation is used to keep the pH above 7.5.

D. Ongoing management

1. **Treating the trigger.** When meconium aspiration or perinatal ischemia is involved, PPHN usually resolves over time. In the case of overwhelming sepsis or pneumonia, the physiologic derangement will not resolve until the infection is successfully treated with antibiotic or antiviral agents.

2. **Nitric oxide (NO).** Inhaled nitric oxide is a potent pulmonary vasodilator, which usually is administered in concentrations ranging from 5 to 40 parts per million (ppm), and typically 20 ppm. The use of NO has been reported to reduce the number of infants requiring ECMO. Appropriate dosage ranges are still the subject of controversy. Escalating dosages and prolonged therapy may cause methemoglobinemia and platelet dysfunction. Doses < 20 ppm have not been associated with toxicity.

3. **ECMO** is indicated for patients who have severe pulmonary hypertension and cannot be stabilized with conventional therapies or nitric oxide.

   a. **Indication.** A numeric indication for ECMO is an **OI > 0.4** on two successive measurements while on maximal support, or an A-a gradient > 620 mm Hg. When the OI exceeds 0.4 on repeated measurements, the mortality rate without ECMO is more than 90%.

   b. **Risks** include those associated with surgery, prolonged anticoagulation (including intraventricular hemorrhage or other acute hemorrhage), organ or vascular injury, and infectious complications. Preexisting intraventricular hemorrhage substantially increases the risks of a major complication. Preexisting structural abnormalities, including major cardiac or central nervous system malformations, decrease the likelihood of successful weaning from the ECMO circuit, resulting in a prolonged indefinite state of cardiopulmonary bypass.

IV PROGNOSIS

A. Mortality. With the advent of new technologies, such as HFOV and ECMO, the mortality rate has been reduced to 10%–15%.

B. Morbidity. Chronic lung disease and central nervous system injury are the most common forms of long-term morbidity.

References

Davidson D, Barefield ES, Kattwinkel J, et al: Inhaled nitric oxide for the early treatment of persistent pulmonary hypertension of the term newborn: a randomized, double-masked, placebo-controlled, dose-response, multicenter study. *Pediatrics* 101(3):325–334, 1998.

Van Marter LJ, Leviton A, Allred EN, et al: Persistent pulmonary hypertension of the newborn and smoking, aspirin, and nonsteroidal antiinflammatory drug consumption during pregnancy. *Pediatrics* 97(5):658–663, 1996.

Walsh-Sukys MC, Tyson JE, Wright LL, et al: Persistent pulmonary hypertension in the era before nitric oxide: practice variation and outcomes. *Pediatrics* 105(1): 14–20, 2000.

26. Neonatal Cholestasis (Conjugated Hyperbilirubinemia)

I INTRODUCTION

A. Background. Conjugated hyperbilirubinemia in the neonate is a potentially serious condition that requires an immediate, thorough evaluation. It is almost always a sign of an underlying disease process. The differential diagnosis is vast, and includes infection, metabolic abnormalities, drugs and toxins, inherited syndromes, and hepatic structural disease.

> **HOT** **KEY**
>
> True conjugated hyperbilirubinemia is rare, with an approximate total frequency of 2.5 per 10,000 live births. In contrast, unconjugated neonatal hyperbilirubinemia is very common and occurs in as many as 50% of term newborns. The cause usually is benign.

B. Definitions
   1. **Cholestasis** is the decreased flow of bile from the liver.
   2. **Jaundice** is a yellow discoloration of the skin. It is clinically apparent when total serum bilirubin levels reach 5–7 mg/dl.
C. A **workup** should be done if the direct (conjugated) bilirubin is greater than 2 mg/dl or greater than 15% of total serum bilirubin.

II CLINICAL MANIFESTATIONS: SYMPTOMS

A. Infants who have cholestatic liver disease typically have jaundice, hepatomegaly, a history of dark urine, and acholic (pale) stools.
B. Cholestatic jaundice often has a distinct green-yellow appearance. In contrast, jaundice caused by increased unconjugated bilirubin has an orange-yellow appearance.
C. Splenomegaly occurs in approximately 50% of cases.
D. Patients who have severe liver disease may have bleeding diatheses [e.g., central nervous system (CNS) or gastrointestinal bleeding] because of malabsorption of fat-soluble vitamins (e.g., vitamin K).

E. Ascites and edema may be present because of decreased synthesis of albumin.

 III **SPECIFIC CAUSES.** Common causes of neonatal cholestasis can be remembered using the mnemonic CHOLESTATIC.

CHOLESTATIC

Cytomegalovirus
Herpes simplex virus, **H**epatitis B, or **H**yperalimentation (> 2 weeks)
Other metabolic causes (e.g., galactosemia, glycogen storage diseases, fructose intolerance, tyrosinemia)
Low α_1-antitrypsin levels
Extrahepatic biliary atresia
Sepsis (bacterial)
Toxoplasmosis
Alagille syndrome and other inherited syndromes
Thyroid disease and other metabolic causes
Idiopathic neonatal hepatitis
Congenital syphilis or **C**ongenital rubella

A. Infection accounts for 3%–5% of all cases. Both perinatal (STORCH) and postnatal (bacterial sepsis) infections can cause neonatal cholestasis (see Chapters 23 and 24).

B. α_1**-Antitrypsin deficiency** causes 7%–10% of all cases of neonatal cholestasis. α_1-Antitrypsin protects cells from damage by trypsin or other proteolytic enzymes. Only a deficiency of protease inhibitor type Z (PiZ) is associated with liver disease. This deficiency is the most common inherited metabolic liver disease.

  1. Clinical presentation. Only 20% of homozygotes have neonatal cholestasis, but as many as 60% have abnormal transaminase levels by 6 months of age. A subset of these patients may have either asymptomatic hepatomegaly or cryptogenic cirrhosis later in childhood. Often, presentation is delayed until adulthood, after the development of pulmonary emphysema. Fulminant liver failure is rare.

  2. Testing. Diagnosis requires liver biopsy and determination of serum Pi type. The biopsy findings overlap with those of biliary atresia and idiopathic neonatal hepatitis.

  3. Treatment is supportive, with an emphasis on good pulmonary hygiene later in life (e.g., avoidance of cigarette smoke).

C. Extrahepatic biliary atresia is responsible for 25%–30% of all cases of neonatal cholestasis. Biliary atresia is caused by the destruction or absence of the extrahepatic biliary tree and is the leading indication for pediatric liver transplantation. In acquired cases (80%–90%), the defect is isolated to the liver and biliary tree. The cause is believed to be viral. The remaining 10%–20% of patients may have other associated anomalies, including polysplenia syndrome, a preduodenal portal vein, intestinal malrotation, an interrupted inferior vena cava, and congenital cyanotic heart disease.

1. **Clinical presentation.** These infants usually are born full term and do well until the insidious onset of jaundice at 2–6 weeks of life.

2. **Testing.** A di-isopropyl iminodiacetic acid (DISIDA) scan shows no excretion from the biliary tree into the intestine. Liver biopsy results show interlobular bile duct proliferation. If biliary atresia is suspected, exploratory laparotomy and intraoperative cholangiogram are indicated.

3. **Treatment.** If a cholangiogram does not show extrahepatic biliary ducts, hepatoportoenterostomy (Kasai procedure) is performed. Remnants of the extrahepatic ducts are dissected up to the hilum of the liver. A jejunojejunostomy (Roux-en-Y anastomosis) is constructed, and the free limb is sutured to the distal biliary tree. Cholangitis is a universal complication that requires aggressive therapy with intravenous antibiotics.

4. **Prognosis.** Before the Kasai procedure was introduced, the mortality rate was 100% by 2 years of age. When the defect is repaired by 70 days of life, 60% of patients establish biliary flow. After 70 days of life, the success rate drops to less than 20%. Long-term survival has been documented into the third decade of life, and the 2-year posttransplantation survival rate approaches 80%. The overall prognosis is better in the acquired form of the disease. Patients who have associated congenital anomalies have a poorer prognosis.

D. **Alagille syndrome,** or arteriohepatic dysplasia, is the fourth most common cause of neonatal cholestasis. It accounts for 5%–6% of all cases. It is an inherited disorder that is characterized by a paucity of interlobular bile ducts, cardiac anomalies (right-sided outflow tract anomalies, such as pulmonic stenosis), and "elfin" facies. Additional features include butterfly vertebrae and ocular anomalies. The inheritance pattern is autosomal dominant, with variable penetrance.

1. **Clinical presentation.** Presentation ranges from very mild liver disease to profound hepatic failure.

2. **Testing.** Diagnosis is based on the clinical features. A DISIDA scan shows poor uptake and delayed excretion. Findings of liver biopsy show fewer than 0.5 ducts per portal triad.

3. **Treatment** is supportive and includes proper nutrition, fat-soluble vitamins, and choleretic or antipruritic agents. To avoid unnecessary operative intervention, it is important to distinguish Alagille syndrome from extrahepatic biliary atresia.

4. The **prognosis** is usually good, although cirrhosis develops in up to 10% of patients and liver transplantation is required.

E. **Metabolic disorders (see also Chapter 95)**

1. **Congenital hypothyroidism** is suggested by a large anterior fontanel, constipation, and somnolence or sluggishness. Newborn screens for thyroid-stimulating hormone and thyroxin should be repeated in the patient with prolonged jaundice. With early clinical detection and treatment (within the first few weeks of life), the prognosis is usually good.

2. **Galactosemia.** Tests for urine-reducing substances and an assay for galactose-1-phosphate uridyltransferase are performed. Neonatal *Escherichia coli* sepsis should prompt a workup for this disorder, regardless of whether jaundice is present.

3. **Glycogen storage disease type IV** is caused by a deficiency of the brancher enzyme in glycogen synthesis. It occurs in older infants and causes a gradual onset of growth failure, hepatomegaly, and liver failure. A liver biopsy is needed for diagnosis.

4. **Hereditary fructose intolerance** occurs after the introduction of fructose or sucrose into the diet, common in citrus fruits and sweetened food. Symptoms occur soon after ingestion and include emesis, seizures, shock, and coma. Laboratory studies reveal non–glucose reducing substances in the urine, hypoglycemia, and lactic acidosis.

5. **Tyrosinemia** occurs in the first 6 months of life. It causes jaundice, hepatomegaly, failure to thrive, developmental delay, and a cabbage-like odor. The presence of succinylacetoacetate and succinylacetone in the serum and urine is diagnostic.

F. **Idiopathic neonatal hepatitis** accounts for 30%–40% of all cases of neonatal cholestasis. It is a diagnosis of exclusion. Undetected viruses or metabolic processes are believed to be responsible.

1. **Clinical presentation.** Idiopathic neonatal hepatitis is more common in low-birthweight male infants. Jaundice and acholic stools begin in the first week of life.

2. **Testing.** Liver biopsy shows multinucleated giant cells without bile duct proliferation.

3. **Treatment** is supportive and includes nutrition, fat-soluble vitamins, and choleretic or antipruritic medications.

4. The **prognosis** is fair: 75% of patients recover without

chronic liver disease; 20% die of progressive liver disease; and 5% have chronic liver disease.

IV APPROACH TO THE PATIENT

A. History. A thorough history should be obtained, including the prenatal history (e.g., unexplained maternal illness or fever), maternal exposures (e.g., exposure to raw meat or cat litter suggests toxoplasmosis), and family history (e.g., metabolic disease, liver disease, inherited clinical syndromes).

B. Physical examination

1. **Head, eyes, ears, nose, and throat (HEENT).** The occipitofrontal circumference is measured to check for microcephaly. Large fontanels may occur with hypothyroidism. Patients should also be checked for dysmorphic features (e.g., classic elfin facies of Alagille syndrome) and cataracts (e.g., in TORCH infections).

2. **Chest.** The physician should listen for murmurs (e.g., pulmonic stenosis in Alagille syndrome).

3. **Abdomen.** The size and consistency of the liver and spleen should be noted.

C. Laboratory studies

HOT KEY Avoid the "shotgun" approach to diagnostic tests; rather, let a good history and physical examination guide the choice of studies.

---

1. **General tests** include a complete blood count with differential, platelet count, blood culture, and glucose.

2. **Liver-specific tests** include prothrombin time, fibrinogen, total protein and albumin, bilirubin (total and conjugated), serum cholesterol, and bile acids.

3. **Tests for hepatobiliary damage include** γ-glutamyltransferase, aspartate aminotransferase, alanine aminotransferase, and alkaline phosphatase.

4. **Urine tests** include urinalysis, urine culture, urine cytomegalovirus (CMV) shell vial, and urine-reducing substances.

5. **Maternal tests** include rubella titers, screening for HIV, toxoplasmosis serology, hepatitis B studies, and Veneral Disease Research Laboratory/Rapid plasma reagin (VDRL/RPR).

6. **Other tests** to consider are thyroid function tests, α_1-antitrypsis Pi type, Herpes Simplex Virus (HSV) polymerase chain reaction, sweat chloride, urine galactose-1-phosphate uridyltransferase, urine organic acids, and serum amino acids.

D. Additional tests
  1. **Abdominal ultrasound** can be used as an initial screening tool to assess the size of the gallbladder (i.e., absence of the gallbladder suggests biliary atresia), ductal dilation, and other obstructive anomalies (e.g., choledochal cysts).
  2. **Ophthalmologic evaluation** is done to look for cataracts (e.g., STORCH) or Axenfeld anomaly (e.g., Alagille syndrome).
  3. **A DISIDA scan** is performed to evaluate the patency of the extrahepatic biliary tree. The sensitivity of this scan is maximized by administering phenobarbital (5 mg/kg/d in 2 doses) 3–5 days before the study. The study is based on hepatic uptake and intestinal excretion of ^{99m}Tc-labeled DISIDA. Biliary obstruction is suggested by uptake of DISIDA in the liver without excretion into the duodenum.
  4. **Percutaneous liver biopsy** is indicated in almost all cases of neonatal cholestasis, unless extrahepatic biliary obstruction is certain.

References

Maller ES: Jaundice. In *Clinical Pediatric Gastroenterology.* Edited by Altschuler SM, Liacouras CA. Philadelphia, Churchill Livingstone, 1998, pp 49–61.

Committee on Infectious Disease, American Academy of Pediatrics, Pickering LK (ed): *2000 Red Book Report of the Committee on Infectious Diseases,* 25th ed. Elk Grove Village, IL, American Academy of Pediatrics, 2000.

27. Necrotizing Enterocolitis

I INTRODUCTION

A. **Background.** Necrotizing enterocolitis (NEC) is one of the most severe problems faced by premature infants.

B. **Pathogenesis.** Ischemic coagulative necrosis is the major finding. The exact pathogenesis is unknown, but it appears that bacterial invasion or colonization needs to take place before NEC occurs.

C. **Epidemiology.** The typical patient with NEC is a premature infant who has been receiving enteral feeding for 7–14 days.
   1. NEC can occur as early as the first day or as late as the 99th day of life. Fetuses are not affected.
   2. NEC occurs in 2% of patients in neonatal intensive care units.
   3. Approximately 90% of affected infants are younger than 36 weeks gestation, and almost all have been fed enterally.
   4. Other risk factors include polycythemia, congenital heart disease, asphyxia, presence of a catheter in the umbilical artery or vein, hyperosmolar feedings, and rapid feed advances.

II CLINICAL MANIFESTATIONS

A. **Symptoms.** Onset is usually acute. It rarely progresses in a stepwise or gradual pattern.
   1. **Abdominal symptoms.** Abdominal distension is a predominant finding. Associated symptoms include vomiting, bilious or bloody gastric aspirates, bloody stool, abdominal tenderness, and abdominal wall redness. A mass may be found in the right lower quadrant. (The ileum is most commonly affected.)
   2. **Systemic symptoms.** The patient may be inactive, hypotonic, and pale, with recurrent episodes of apnea, bradycardia, and cyanosis, increasing oxygen requirements, metabolic acidosis, oliguria, hypotension, poor perfusion, or a bleeding diathesis.

B. **The differential diagnosis** includes feeding intolerance, sepsis, bowel perforation, volvulus, intussusception, appendicitis, mesenteric thrombosis, and spontaneous bowel perforation.

III APPROACH TO THE PATIENT

A. **Initial workup.** Three-way abdominal films should be obtained. Pneumatosis intestinalis is the hallmark finding on abdominal

radiographs. It appears as tiny bubbles that appear to be em-
bedded within the intestinal wall. Other findings include portal
venous air, peritoneal air, hepatic portal gas, asymmetric bowel
loop distension, and free air. The following is the **modified
Bell's staging criteria** for NEC.
1. **Stage I:** intestinal dilation
2. **Stage II:** intestinal distension, pneumatosis intestinalis, and
   portal venous air
3. **Stage III:** perforation of the gut wall with free air or free peritoneal fluid

---

HOT The radiographic triad of distension, gastric retention, and dilation without perforation is usually the result of feeding intolerance. Generalized or abdominal signs suggest NEC.
KEY

B. Laboratory tests
   1. **Complete blood count.** A white blood cell count < 5000
      cells/mm^3 or $> 25,000$ cells/mm^3 is expected. A left shift may
      be present.
   2. **Platelet count** may reveal thrombocytopenia.
   3. **Hyperglycemia** may be present.
   4. **C-reactive protein level** increases as NEC progresses.
   5. **Coagulation studies.** Prothrombin time, partial thrombo-
      plastin time, and fibrinogen level should be evaluated to as-
      sess for disseminated intravascular coagulation (DIC).
   6. **Acidosis** is often present secondary to bowel injury. There
      may be a significant base deficit.
   7. **Blood culture and culture of cerebrospinal fluid and urine.**
      The likelihood of positive blood cultures increases as NEC
      becomes more severe.
   8. **Electrolytes** may indicate severe hyponatremia or dehydra-
      tion.
C. Initial therapy
   1. **Stage I.** Enteral feedings are stopped, and adequate intra-
      vascular volume is ensured. A nasogastric tube should be
      placed on low intermittent continuous suction. Antibiotics
      (vancomycin and cefotaxime or ampicillin and gentamicin)
      are administered (clindamycin is added later if perforation
      occurs). If improvement is seen, feeding may be restarted in
      1–3 days.
   2. **Stage II.** Treatment as described for stage I continues. In ad-
      dition, mechanical ventilation may be required, especially if
      there is significant acidosis or shock. Acidosis is corrected
      with bicarbonate. Removal of any umbilical artery catheter
      should be considered. Correct any anemia, thrombocyto-

penia, DIC (cryoprecipitate is preferred if the fibrinogen level is low), and hypotension. Enteral feedings are withheld for at least 10 days.

3. **Stage III.** Treatment as described for stages I and II continues. Surgery is indicated whenever the bowel has become perforated. Other indications for surgery include persistent focal distension, persistent or worsening acidosis, worsening respiratory status, and unremitting neutropenia or thrombocytopenia. Venous portal air is a cause for concern; the threshold for surgery may be lower in these patients. Emergency external peritoneal drainage may precede laparotomy.

D. **Ongoing management** includes serial abdominal radiographs obtained every 8 hours. In addition, electrolytes, blood urea nitrogen (BUN), creatinine, complete blood count, coagulation studies, creatine phosphate (CRP), and arterial blood gases are followed. Because of the high incidence of fungal infection, some physicians recommend administration of an oral antifungal agent postoperatively. A barium gastrointestinal study should be considered before feedings are restarted to rule out a stricture, especially if the patient required surgery.

IV PROGNOSIS

A. **Morbidity.** Approximately 10% of patients will develop a postnecrotic stricture. For those requiring surgery, the overall prognosis depends on the amount of bowel remaining. Short-bowel syndrome may occur if significant amounts of the bowel are resected.

B. **Mortality.** Approximately 20% of infants with pneumatosis intestinalis die. The mortality rate is higher if perforation occurs.

References

Kennedy J, Holt CL, Ricketts RR: The significance of portal vein gas in necrotizing enterocolitis. *Am Surg* 53(4):231–234, 1987.

Kliegman RM, Walsh MC: Neonatal necrotizing enterocolitis: pathogenesis, classification, and spectrum of illness. *Curr Probl Pediatr* 17(4):213–288, 1987.

Sheldon B, Korones MD, Henrietta S, et al: *Neonatal Decision Making.* Philadelphia, Mosby-Year Book, 1993, pp 168–171.

PART IV

INFECTIOUS DISEASE

28. Fever Without Focus

I INTRODUCTION

A. Background. The neonate, infant, or young child who has a fever without an apparent source presents a common challenge in pediatrics. It is convenient to classify pediatric patients with fever into one of four groups, each of which has unique etiologic, diagnostic, and therapeutic considerations:

1. The infant younger than 1 month of age with fever
2. The infant 1–3 months of age with fever
3. The young child (3–36 months of age) with fever
4. The infant or child with fever of unknown origin (see Chapter 30)

B. Definitions

1. **Fever** is abnormal elevation of temperature [38°C (100.4°F)]. Rectal temperature (or sublingual temperature in children older than 3–4 years of age), measured with a glass mercury thermometer, is the most accurate method of determining core temperature. Tympanic and axillary measurements are not sufficiently accurate; both methods tend to underestimate core temperature. Although some attribute fevers to bundling, bundling alone should not cause temperatures > 38°C.

2. **Occult bacteremia** is the finding of a positive blood culture in a non–toxic-appearing febrile patient without a focus of infection.

3. **Serious bacterial illness** is a result of occult bacteremia. This category includes meningitis, sepsis, bone and joint infections, urinary tract infections, pneumonia, and enteritis.

C. Pathogenesis. Fever is caused by a resetting of the hypothalamic thermoregulatory center by cytokines. These cytokines are released in response to viral or bacterial pathogens, circulating immune complexes, or tumor cell pyrogens. Central nervous system lesions may also affect the thermoregulatory center. Once it is reset, the thermoregulatory center maintains a higher body temperature through physiologic mechanisms (e.g., shivering, cutaneous vasoconstriction). The febrile response is unreliable and less mature in infants.

D. Epidemiology

1. Fifteen percent of visits to pediatricians are for acute episodes of fever.

2. Bacteremia is present in 42% of patients whose white blood cell (WBC) count is higher than 30,000 cells/mm^3, 17% of patients whose WBC count is 15,000–30,000 cells/mm^3, and 3% of patients whose WBC count is 10,000–15,000 cells/mm^3.

3. Other indicators, such as C-reactive protein, erythrocyte sedimentation rate, band form count, and vacuolization, have been used to identify serious illness, but they do not show a clear advantage over the WBC count.

4. The height of fever is associated with an increased risk of bacteremia ($<$ 1% risk if fever $<$ 40°C; 8% risk if fever $>$ 40°C; 11% risk if fever $>$ 40.5°C).

5. **History and physical examination** are not as sensitive in detecting serious illness in infants younger than 3 months of age (78% sensitivity) as they are among children 3–36 months of age (89%–92% sensitivity).

E. Microbiology and etiology

1. Among **infants younger than 3 months of age,** serious bacterial illnesses are most often caused by group B streptococcus, gram-negative organisms (e.g., *Escherichia coli*), *Listeria monocytogenes,* and enterococci.

2. Organisms that commonly are seen in **older children** include *Streptococcus pneumoniae, Haemophilus influenzae* type b, group A streptococcus, and *Neisseria meningitidis.*

HOT KEY In infants and children 3–36 months of age, *S. pneumoniae* is the etiologic agent of occult bacteremia in approximately 90% of cases. In children, bacteria may circulate in the blood without apparent sepsis or focal infection.

II **CLINICAL MANIFESTATIONS.** Identifying children with serious illness in the setting of fever without focus is a difficult task, even for experienced pediatricians. The Acute Illness Observation Scale **(Table 28-1)** is a useful tool. A score $>$ 10 has a sensitivity of 88% and a specificity of 77% for serious illness. However, its utility in patients younger than 8 weeks of age is limited (22% with a score $<$ 10 may have a serious illness; 45% with a score $>$ 16 have a serious illness).

TABLE 28-1. Predictive Model: Six Observation Items and Their Scales			
Observation Item	1 Normal	3 Moderate Impairment	5 Severe Impairment
Quality of cry	Strong with normal tone OR Content and not crying	Whimpering OR Sobbing	Weak OR Moaning OR High-pitched
Reaction to parent stimulation	Cries briefly then stops OR Content and not crying	Cries off and on	Continual cry OR Hardly responds
State variation	If awake → stays awake OR If asleep and stimulated → wakes up quickly	Eyes close briefly → awake OR Awakes with prolonged stimulation	Falls to sleep OR Will not rouse
Color	Pink	Pale extremities OR Acrocyanosis	Pale OR Cyanotic OR Mottled OR Ashen
Hydration	Skin normal, eyes normal, AND Mucous membranes moist	Skin, eyes-normal AND Mouth slightly dry	Skin doughy OR Tented AND Dry mucous membranes AND/OR Sunken eyes
Response (talk, smile) to social overtures	Smiles OR Alerts (≤2 months)	Brief smile OR Alerts briefly (≤2 months)	No smile Face anxious, dull, expressionless OR No alerting (≤2 months)

Reprinted with permission from McCarthy PL, Sharpe MR, Spiesel SZ, et al: Observation scales to identify serious illness in febrile children. *Pediatrics* 70(5):802–809, 1982.

III APPROACH TO THE PATIENT

A. **Laboratory evaluation.** There is no consensus about the most appropriate laboratory evaluation of febrile infants and young children. In general, febrile infants who are younger than 3 months of age require a full sepsis workup (including complete blood count with differential, blood and urine culture, and cerebrospinal fluid analysis and culture). Chest radiograph and stool studies (e.g., culture, Gram stain, and examination for leukocytes) are ordered if appropriate symptoms are present.

B. **Management**

1. **Patients younger than 1 month of age.** Because the findings of clinical examination are unreliable in neonates, all febrile infants younger than 30 days of age should be admitted to the hospital, undergo a full workup, and receive treatment with intravenous antibiotics. Antibiotics are continued until cultures remain negative for 48–72 hours. In febrile neonates, the most appropriate choice of empiric antibiotics may be a combination of ampicillin and gentamicin. Alternatively, ampicillin and a third-generation cephalosporin (e.g., cefotaxime) may be used if meningitis is considered.

2. **Patients 1–3 months of age.** Although febrile infants sometimes are admitted to the hospital and treated empirically, some clinicians opt for outpatient management if "low-risk criteria" (see III B 2 b) are met, the patient is clinically well, and follow-up within 24 hours is assured.

   a. Most pediatricians recommend using ceftriaxone (50 mg/kg intramuscularly) in infants 31–90 days old who are managed as outpatients.

   b. **Low-risk criteria include the following:**

      (1) No history of prematurity, perinatal complications, or recent antibiotic use

      (2) Normal findings on physical examination

      (3) WBC count 5000–15,000 cells/mm^3, with an absolute band count < 1500, and urinalysis < 10 WBC/high-power field

      (4) No cerebrospinal fluid abnormalities

3. **Patients 3–36 months of age.** If the child looks well and the temperature is < 39°C, no further workup is required. If the fever is > 39°C, WBC count, urinalysis, urine culture (for boys younger than 6 months of age and for girls younger than 2 years of age), and blood culture are obtained. Some experts advocate the use of intramuscular ceftriaxone for all patients; other experts advocate ceftriaxone only for patients whose WBC count is higher than 15,000 cells/mm^3. All patients should be re-examined in 24 hours.

HOT

KEY

Any toxic-appearing infant or child requires inpatient admission, a full workup, and intravenous antibiotics, regardless of laboratory values.

References

Baraff LJ, Bass JW, Fleisher GR: Practice guideline for the management of infants and children 0–36 months of age with fever without focus. *Pediatrics* 82(1), 1–12, 1993.

Jaffe DM, Fleisher GR: Temperature and total white blood cell count as indicators of bacteremia. *Pediatrics* 87(5):670–674, 1991.

McCarthy PL: Fever. *Pediatr Rev* 19(12):401–407, 1998.

McCarthy PL, Sharpe MR, Spiesel SZ, et al: Observation scales to identify serious illness in febrile children. *Pediatrics* 70(5):802–809, 1982.

29. Empiric Antibiotic Therapy by Clinical Scenario

....

I **INTRODUCTION.** **Table 29-1** lists recommendations for empiric therapy in specific clinical scenarios.

II **ADDITIONAL RECOMMENDATIONS**

A. The antibiotic should provide adequate coverage for the organism that is most likely to be the causative agent.
B. Antibiotic therapy should be tailored to provide the most specific coverage once the organism is identified.
C. Always inquire about the patient's drug allergies before initiating therapy.
D. A patient may not respond to therapy because of resistance to the drug, inadequate dosing, or fungal infection. The physician should reconsider the original diagnosis if the patient's condition does not improve.

References
Long SS, Pickering LK, Prober CG: *Principles and Practice of Pediatric Infectious Diseases.* New York, Churchill Livingstone, 2002, pp 1643–1646.

TABLE 29-1. Antimicrobial Therapy for Clinical Syndromes

	Drug(s)	Alternative(s)	Comments
Upper respiratory tract infections			
AOME	Amoxicillin; amoxicillin-clavulanate; erythromycin-sulfisoxazole; TMP-SMX	Cefprozil; loracarbef; cefpodoxime; ceftibuten; cefuroxime axetil; cefixime; cefaclor; clarithromycin	Amoxicillin is therapy of choice for first or sporadic episode unless clinical experience portends high failure rate
Chemoprophylaxis for recurrent AOME	Amoxicillin; sulfisoxazole	TMP-SMX	TMP-SMX is not approved for chemoprophylaxis
Sinusitis, acute	As AOME		As AOME
Mastoiditis			
Acute	Cefuroxime; cefotaxime; ceftriaxone	Oral β-lactamase-resistant agent for mild disease or continuation after parenteral therapy	Consider adding nafcillin if third-generation cephalosporin used for severe cases
Chronic	As acute mastoiditis		As acute mastoiditis
Recurrent, sporadic Pseudomonas	Ceftazidime; piperacillin; aztreonam; ticarcillin plus aminoglycoside	Mezlocillin; piperacillin-tazobactam; ticarcillin-clavulanate; imipenem	Choice based on local pattern of susceptibility
Tonsillopharyngitis			
Group A Streptococcus	Penicillin V; benzathine penicillin	Penicillin-allergic: erythromycin or clindamycin; cephalosporins (oral)	Inconsistent superiority of other agent(s) to supplant penicillin as the drug of choice

(continued)

TABLE 29-1. Antimicrobial Therapy for Clinical Syndromes (Continued)

	Drug(s)	Alternative(s)	Comments
Upper respiratory tract infections (continued)			
Peritonsillar abscess	Penicillin V; benzathine penicillin	As tonsillopharyngitis	
Epiglottitis or bacterial tracheitis	Cefuroxime; nafcillin *plus* cefotaxime or ceftriaxone or chloramphenicol		Hib is infrequent pathogen; add antistaphylococcal coverage (nafcillin, vancomycin) to third-generation cephalosporin or chloramphenicol
Parapharyngeal or retro-pharyngeal cellulitis/abscess	Clindamycin	Chloramphenicol	
Diphtheria	Penicillin G (IV); erythromycin		Antitoxin
Lower respiratory tract infections			
Lobar pneumonia, mild to moderate	Penicillin; ampicillin; cephalo-sporins (second- or third-generation); amoxicillin-clavulanate; erythromycin-sulfisoxazole	Erythromycin; clarithromycin	Age-dependent selection; local incidence of penicillin-resistant, cephalosporin-resistant *Streptococcus pneumoniae* is important; oral cefixime and ceftibuten have poor *S. pneumoniae* coverage

Lobar pneumonia, moderate to severe	Cefuroxime; cefotaxime; ceftriaxone	Nafcillin; erythromycin; clarithromycin	Consider adding vancomycin if severe disease and penicillin and cephalosporin resistance in area; consider adding or substituting a macrolide in specific cases
			Consider cefuroxime alone if milder disease pending culture/susceptibility testing
Empyema	Nafcillin, clindamycin, or vancomycin *plus* cefotaxime or ceftriaxone		Clindamycin alone if community-associated, history or risk of aspiration
Necrotizing pneumonia or lung abscess	Clindamycin *plus* cefotaxime or ceftriaxone		
Immunocompromised host	Nafcillin or vancomycin *plus* ceftazidime or imipenem	Broad-spectrum penicillin *plus* aminoglycoside	Consider vancomycin depending on presence of methicillin-resistant staphylococci; choose gram-negative coverage based on local pattern or patient's susceptibility tests; consider TMP-SMX for *Pneumocystis carinii* or erythromycin for *Legionella*
Acute pulmonary exacerbation of cystic fibrosis	Ticarcillin *plus* tobramycin	Antipseudomonal aminoglycosides; cephalosporins; monobactams; carbapenems; other broad-spectrum penicillins based on susceptibilities	Choose agents based on patient's susceptibility tests; tobramycin can be given as aerosol

(continued)

TABLE 29-1. Antimicrobial Therapy for Clinical Syndromes (Continued)

	Drug(s)	Alternative(s)	Comments
Lower respiratory tract infections (continued)			
Pneumonia unresponsive to β-lactam antibiotics	Add erythromycin; consider other etiologies and agents: tuberculosis, fungus, tularemia	Tetracycline; clarithromycin; azithromycin	Epidemiology, regional location, and exposure history are important
Afebrile pneumonia of infancy	Erythromycin	TMP-SMX	
Pertussis	Erythromycin		See Chapter 7
Eye infections			
Conjunctivitis, acute	Polymyxin B-bacitracin, topically; sulfacetamide, topically		
Periorbital or orbital cellulitis Associated with ethmoid sinusitis or idiopathic	Cefuroxime; or nafcillin plus cefotaxime or ceftriaxone	Nafcillin plus chloramphenicol	Avoid cefuroxime unless meningitis excluded; limited data on oral therapy
Associated with peri-orbital skin lesion	Nafcillin	Clindamycin (plus cephalosporin)	Consider nafcillin plus third-generation cephalosporin, if severe
Endophthalmitis	Clindamycin plus third-generation cephalosporin	Vancomycin	Assess need for intravitreal antibiotic(s)
Skin and soft tissue infections			
Impetigo	Cloxacillin; dicloxacillin; clindamycin; erythromycin; mupirocin topically (mild, single lesion)	Cephalexin; cefadroxil	Use cephalosporin only if compliance at issue

Condition		Alternative	Comments
Cellulitis			
Mild to moderate	As impetigo	As impetigo	
Severe	Nafcillin	Clindamycin	
Scalded skin syndrome	Nafcillin	Clindamycin	
Lymphangitis or lymph-adenitis	As impetigo or severe cellulitis		
Buccal cellulitis	Cefuroxime; cefotaxime; ceftriaxone	Chloramphenicol	Avoid cefuroxime unless meningitis excluded
Ludwig angina	Clindamycin; cephalexin; cefadroxil; cloxacillin		
Necrotizing fasciitis	Nafcillin *plus* aminoglycoside or ceftazidime	Clindamycin; ticarcillin-clavulanate	Clindamycin may be superior for high inoculum *S. pyogenes*; consider need for anaerobic coverage; include penicillin if clostridial
Suppurative myositis	Nafcillin	Anti-staphylococcal β-lactams	
Gas gangrene (*Clostridia*)	Penicillin G (IV)		
Animal bites			
Outpatient	Amoxicillin-clavulanate		
Inpatient	Ticarcillin-clavulanate; ampicillin sulbactam		Ampicillin-sulbactam is not approved in children

(continued)

TABLE 29-1. Antimicrobial Therapy for Clinical Syndromes *(Continued)*

	Drug(s)	Alternative(s)	Comments
Skeletal infections			
Pyogenic arthritis			
Neonates	Methicillin *plus* gentamicin		
Infants and children (< 6 y)	Cefuroxime; nafcillin	Cefotaxime	Avoid cefuroxime unless meningitis excluded; occasional non-Hib occurs
Children (≥ 6 y)	Nafcillin; cefazolin	Clindamycin; vancomycin (MRSA)	
Osteomyelitis			
Neonates	Methicillin *plus* gentamicin	Cefotaxime	Add nafcillin to cefotaxime based on Gram stain results
Infants (< 6 y, Hib vaccine incomplete)	Cefuroxime; cefotaxime		
Children (Hib vaccine complete or age ≥ 6 y)	Nafcillin; cefazolin	Clindamycin	
Osteochondritis (foot wound)	Ceftazidime; broad-spectrum penicillin *plus* antipseudomonal aminoglycoside	Ticarcillin-clavulanate	Surgery required for short-duration therapy; consider use of quinolones for patients ≥ 18 y
Chronic osteomyelitis	Antistaphylococcal β-lactam initially; continuation therapy: dicloxacillin or cloxacillin or cefadroxil or cephalexin	Clindamycin	Consider use of quinolones for patients ≥ 18 y depending on pathogen

Cardiac infections		
Purulent pericarditis	Nafcilin *plus* cefotaxime or cefotriaxone	Vancomycin	Consider substitution vancomycin, or adding aminoglycoside or both if nosocomial infection
Endocarditis			
Native valve	Penicillin *plus* gentamicin	Nafcillin *plus* gentamicin	Nosocomial or line-related infection requires special choices
Prosthetic valve	Vancomycin *plus* gentamicin		
SBE prophylaxis	See Chapter 52		
Gastrointestinal infections			
Travelers' diarrhea	TMP-SMX	Ciprofloxacin	Age-dependent selection; quinolones not approved if age < 18 y
Bacterial enteritis			
Shigella species	Ampicillin; TMP-SMX	Tetracycline	Many geographic areas have limited ampicillin susceptibility
Salmonella species (invasive)	Cefotaxime; ceftriaxone	TMP-SMX	Consider use of quinolones
Escherichia coli	TMP-SMX		Antibiotics should be withheld in patients with bloody diarrhea; antibiotics are not indicated for *E. coli* 0.157:H7 infections due to the risk of hemolytic uremic syndrome

(continued)

TABLE 29-1. Antimicrobial Therapy for Clinical Syndromes (Continued)

	Drug(s)	Alternative(s)	Comments
Gastrointestinal infections (continued)			
Yersinia enterocolitica	No therapy	Gentamicin (invasive)	Therapy indicated in children with iron overload states
Campylobacter jejuni	Erythromycin	Gentamicin	
Antibiotic-associated colitis	Metronidazole orally; vancomycin orally		*Clostridium difficile* toxin-mediated disease
Perirectal abscess	Clindamycin *plus* aminoglycoside or third-generation cephalosporin		
Peritonitis			
Primary	Cefotaxime; ceftriaxone		Consider vancomycin (penicillin- and cephalosporin-resistant *Pneumococcus*)
Secondary	Ampicillin *plus* clindamycin *plus* gentamicin		Can substitute metronidazole for clindamycin, broad spectrum β-lactam for gentamicin, or consider monotherapy using cefoxitin
Peritoneal dialysis	Vancomycin parenterally plus gentamicin in dialysate		Intraperitoneal therapy alone can be considered for mild infection

Genitourinary tract infections

Cystitis			
Acute	Amoxicillin	Sulfisoxazole; TMP-SMX; cefpodoxime; cefixime	
Recurrent	TMP-SMX	Cephalosporin	
Prophylaxis	TMP-SMX; nitrofurantoin	TMP-SMX	
Acute pyelonephritis	Ampicillin *plus* gentamicin or cefotaxime or ceftriaxone		
Renal or perinephric abscess	Nafcillin *plus* gentamicin or third-generation cephalosporin		
Epididymitis	Cefuroxime; cefotaxime		
Sexually transmitted diseases	See Chapter 41		

Central nervous system infections

Bacterial meningitis			
Neonates	Ampicillin *plus* gentamicin or cefotaxime		
Infants < 3 months	Ampicillin *plus* cefotaxime or ceftriaxone		Consider pneumococcal resistance (below)
Children > 3 months	Cefotaxime; ceftriaxone	Ampicillin *plus* chloramphenicol	Consider pneumococcal resistance (below)

(continued)

TABLE 29-1. Antimicrobial Therapy for Clinical Syndromes (Continued)

	Drug(s)	Alternative(s)	Comments
Central nervous system infections (continued)			
Pneumococcus (penicillin/cephalosporin-resistant)	Vancomycin *plus* cefotaxime; ceftriaxone		Consider adding rifampin to vancomycin therapy; use of dexamethasone is controversial
Ventriculoperitoneal shunt infection	Vancomycin *plus* aminoglycoside; cefotaxime *plus* aminoglycoside		Consider vancomycin plus rifampin for coagulase-negative staphylococci
Suspect coliforms	Third-generation cephalosporin *plus* aminoglycoside		
Brain abscess	Nafcillin *plus* cefotaxime and metronidazole	Vancomycin for nafcillin; chloramphenicol	

Adapted with permission from Long SS, Pickering LK, Prober CG: *Principles and Practice of Pediatric Infectious Diseases.* New York, Churchill Livingstone, 2002, pp 1643–1646.

AOME = acute otitis media with effusion; TMP-SMX = trimethoprim-sulfamethoxazole; Hib = *Haemophilus influenzae* type b; MRSA = Methicillin resistant Staph Aureus; SBE = Subacute bacterial endocarditis.

30. Fever of Unknown Origin

I **INTRODUCTION**

A. Definition. Fever of unknown origin (FUO) is defined as fever (temperature > 38.5°C) without a known source that lasts longer than 10 days. The fever may wax and wane during that period.

> **HOT**
> ▶
> **KEY**
>
> FUO is most often a manifestation of a common diagnosis presenting in an uncommon way.

B. Epidemiology. Causes include infection (> 50%), connective tissue disorder (15%), neoplasm (7%), and inflammatory bowel disease (IBD) [4%]. The origin remains undetermined in 20% of cases.

II **APPROACH TO THE PATIENT.** Evaluation of a patient with FUO requires a systematic approach that is based on history and physical examination. Involvement of multiple organ systems is more likely to indicate a connective tissue, hematologic, or oncologic disorder.

> **HOT**
> ▶
> **KEY**
>
> FUO is not without clues. Approximately two-thirds of patients with FUO have significant signs or symptoms at presentation; the remaining one third have them at some point.

A. History
1. **Fever pattern** (i.e., sustained, relapsing, spiking). Daily high spikes may indicate bacteremia or juvenile rheumatoid arthritis. Although the absolute peak of a fever has no prognostic value, the higher the fever, the greater the chance of a positive blood culture. A sustained fever may indicate tularemia, Rocky Mountain spotted fever, typhus, or typhoid. A relapsing fever may indicate malaria, brucellosis, subacute bacterial endocarditis, borreliosis, rat-bite fever, or lymphoma.
2. **Pertinent historical factors (Table 30-1)**

TABLE 30-1. Pertinent Historical Factors for FUO	
History	**Associations**
Chills	Bacterial or viral infection
Decreased growth (weight or height)	Chronic condition, e.g., Inflammatory Bowel Disease (IBD)
Recurrent infections	Immunodeficiency
History of transfusion	Possible human immunodeficiency virus (HIV) or hepatitis C as cause of the fever
Medications	Possibility of drug fever
Family and contact history	Possibility of IBD or tuberculosis (TB)
Daycare attendance	Possibility of exposure to Epstein–Barr virus, cytomegalovirus, hepatitis, and salmonella
Contact with animals	Dogs: leptospirosis Cats: toxoplasmosis Rats: rat-bite fever Birds: psittacosis Amphibians: salmonella Rodents: hantavirus
Travel to endemic areas	Exposure to diseases such as malaria, enteric fever, TB, histoplasmosis, and coccidioidomycosis. Time spent in wooded areas may lead to tick bites (Lyme disease), Rocky Mountain spotted fever, relapsing fever, and arboviruses.
Consumption of unusual foods	Eating raw meat can lead to brucellosis or toxoplasmosis. Eating game meat may lead to exposure to tularemia. Raw fish can harbor pathogens that cause hepatitis and salmonella. Unpasteurized milk can harbor pathogens that cause brucellosis and salmonella.
Pica	Visceral larva migrans or toxoplasmosis

B. Physical examination

   1. HEENT. Conjunctivitis may indicate Kawasaki disease, leptospirosis, tularemia, or systemic lupus erythematosus. Uveitis may be a symptom of Kawasaki disease, juvenile rheumatoid arthritis, IBD, or toxoplasmosis. Transilluminate and palpate the sinuses and examine the nasal mucosa for evidence of sinusitis. Check dentition for the presence of dental abscesses.

2. Reticuloendothelial system

  a. Hepatosplenomegaly or generalized adenopathy may indicate mononucleosis, connective tissue disease, leukemia, or HIV.

  b. Localized adenopathy may indicate abscess, cat-scratch disease, or neoplasm.

3. Musculoskeletal system

  a. Joint swelling or pain can be a symptom of a connective tissue disorder, brucellosis, shigellosis, or hepatitis, or an infectious arthritis.

  b. Bone tenderness can be present in osteomyelitis, neoplasm, sinusitis, or mastoiditis.

  c. Muscle tenderness may be related to an abscess.

4. Cardiovascular system. The physician should listen for murmurs, which can indicate endocarditis. Friction rubs indicate pericarditis.

5. Genitourinary system

  a. Perianal tenderness can indicate abdominal or pelvic abscess.

  b. Pelvic examination is considered for sexually active girls, especially if there is a history of vaginal discharge or lower abdominal pain.

6. Integumentary system

  a. A **perineal rash** may be a clue to Kawasaki syndrome.

  b. An **evanescent rash** at the time of fever can indicate juvenile rheumatoid arthritis.

  c. A **seborrheic rash** may signify histiocytosis.

  d. Petechiae or purpura may indicate subacute bacterial endocarditis or vasculitis.

  e. Eczema can be associated with Wiskott-Aldrich syndrome or HIV.

C. Initial workup

  1. Initial workup includes a complete blood count with differential, blood cultures (i.e., aerobic, anaerobic, fungal), urinalysis and urine culture, liver function tests, albumin, blood urea nitrogen (BUN), creatinine and PPD with controls. In older children, tests for heterophil antibodies, an erythrocyte sedimentation rate, and antinuclear antibodies are included. Further workup is dictated by clues in the initial workup (e.g., sterile pyuria is seen in TB, Kawasaki disease, and Reiter syndrome).

  2. A chest radiograph and sinus radiographs should be obtained.

  3. The erythrocyte sedimentation rate and the C-reactive protein level do not have great diagnostic value, but they allow the patient's course to be followed up over time.

4. In cases of prolonged FUO, consider further imaging studies [gallium white blood cell (WBC) scan, bone scan, or CT scan] to rule out infection or neoplasm. A bone marrow biopsy should also be considered.

D. Therapy

1. Fever. The fever itself usually is not treated; it is more important to identify the cause. Fever is treated only if the patient is uncomfortable or if the absolute temperature is higher than 41°C. In these cases, nonsteroidal anti-inflammatory drugs or acetaminophen is given every 6 hours for 2–3 days.

HOT

    Antipyretics may obscure the only clinical clue.

KEY

---

2. Empiric antibiotics have **no** role in the management of FUO.

3. Most patients are managed on an outpatient basis, but hospital admission for serial examinations may be helpful.

4. Good hydration should be maintained. There is an increased evaporative loss of 10% for each degree of fever higher than 37°C.

E. Morbidity and mortality. Approximately 40% of children with FUO have serious or lethal diseases. The overall mortality rate is 9%–17%.

References

Committee on Infectious Disease, American Academy of Pediatrics, Pickering LK (ed): *2000 Red Book Report of the Committee on Infectious Diseases,* 25th ed. Elk Grove Village, IL, American Academy of Pediatrics, 2000.

Nizet V, Vinci RJ, Lovejoy FH Jr: Fever in children. *Pediatr Rev* 15(4):127–135, 1994.

31. Meningitis

I INTRODUCTION

A. Background. Few pediatric diseases are as important as meningitis. It is especially important to rule out meningitis when evaluating febrile children younger than 3 months of age. Because meningitis can have devastating medical and social effects, prompt evaluation and treatment are vital.

B. Definitions

1. **Meningitis** is inflammation of the meninges in the dura, arachnoid space, or pia mater.
2. **Encephalitis** is inflammation of the cerebral cortex. Symptoms include confusion, hallucinations, memory loss, combativeness, seizures, coma, or unprovoked emotional outbursts.
3. **Meningoencephalitis** is inflammation of both the meninges and the cortex.
4. **Relapse** from the same organism occurs on days 3–14, often secondary to parameningeal foci.
5. **Recrudescence** is continued infection secondary to inadequate therapy.
6. **Recurrence** from the same organism or a different organism suggests an underlying anatomic abnormality.

C. Pathogenesis. Central nervous system (CNS) invasion into the meninges occurs by hematogenous spread or by direct invasion. Bacterial cell wall and membrane elements (e.g., phosphorylcholine endotoxin) incite inflammation, which results in capillary leak and diffusion of low-molecular-weight proteins into the CNS. This diffusion leads to increased intracranial pressure (ICP). Antibiotics cause lysis of the bacterial cell wall, which may exacerbate this inflammation and further increase ICP.

D. Epidemiology (Table 31-1)

II CLINICAL MANIFESTATIONS

A. Presentation of meningitis according to age

1. **Infants** may exhibit nonspecific symptoms, including somnolence, a full fontanel, anorexia, vomiting, and low-grade fever.

HOT KEY Meningitis must always be considered in infants who have a fever and no clear source of infection, especially those < 3 months of age.

TABLE 31-1. Epidemiology of Meningitis

Age/Condition	Organisms	Comments
Preterm infant	Consider less common pathogens (e.g., viruses, *Mycoplasma*, ureaplasma, and fungi)	Treat as an immuno-compromised host; all organisms isolated should be considered pathologic
Neonate (0–3 months)	Group B streptococcus, *Escherichia coli*, *Listeria*, Enterococcus, gram-negative enteric bacilli (other than *E. coli*)	See **Chapter 23**
Infant/Toddler (3 months–3 years)	*Neisseria meningitidis*, pneumococcus, *Haemophilus influenzae*, and viral infections, including enteroviruses and herpes simplex virus	The incidence of *H. influenzae* has decreased by more than 98% since the introduction of HIB vaccine
Child (3–21 years)	*N. meningitidis, H. influenzae, S. pneumoniae*	Signs of meningeal irritation are more reliable in this age group
Ventriculo-peritoneal shunts	Consider *S. epidermidis, Corynebacterium*	Obtain a neurosurgical consultation

HIB = *Haemophilus influenzae* type B.

2. **Younger children** characteristically exhibit fever, vomiting, and irritability. They may not show signs of meningeal irritation, but they may show signs of increased ICP. Evidence of meningeal irritation often is a late sign.
3. **Older children and adults** characteristically exhibit a profound change in level of consciousness, positive Kernig and Brudzinski signs, seizures, coma, back pain, and headache.

B. **Specific signs and symptoms**
   1. **Brudzinski sign.** Flexion of the neck with the patient supine causes involuntary flexion of the hips.
   2. **Kernig sign.** Passive extension of the knees with the hips fully flexed while the patient is supine causes pain and spasm in the hamstrings.
   3. **Neurologic manifestations** occur in 20%–30% of patients in

the first 3 days of illness. Herpesvirus encephalitis characteristically manifests as temporal lobe seizures. Cranial nerve
dysfunction is common (deafness, disturbances in vestibular
function, paralysis of extraocular or facial nerves).

4. **Syndrome of inappropriate secretion of antidiuretic hormone (SIADH)** occurs in 30%–60% of patients. Concurrent
dehydration may cause appropriately high ADH levels.

C. Organisms and their characteristics

1. *Haemophilus influenzae* may cause a subdural effusion that
usually does not require drainage. The incidence of *H. influenzae* meningitis has decreased drastically since the introduction of the *Haemophilus influenzae* type B (HIB) vaccine.

2. *Neisseria meningitidis* causes endemic meningitis in people
living in college dormitories and army barracks. Death may
occur in as little as 15 hours. All people who have been in
contact with the index case should be treated prophylactically. (See also Chapter 32.)

3. *Streptococcus pneumoniae* causes a purulent exudate that can
accumulate in the cerebral convexities. The incidence of infection with penicillin-resistant *S. pneumoniae* is increasing.

4. **HSV-1 and HSV-2** are important causes of neonatal sepsis.
In addition, they may cause meningoencephalitis in older
children or adults. HSV is the most common cause of sporadic fatal encephalitis in the United States.

III APPROACH TO THE PATIENT

A. Diagnosis (Table 31-2)

1. **Lumbar puncture (LP)** is the critical test and should be performed on most febrile neonates.

   a. Early therapy may be guided by cerebrospinal fluid (CSF)
   cell count and differential.

   b. CSF culture is the gold standard for diagnosis.

2. **Computed tomography (CT) scan and funduscopic examination** (papilledema) should be done before performing the
lumbar puncture to rule out increased ICP caused by a
space-occupying lesion (e.g., brain abscess, tumor). Patients
with focal neurologic findings should also be imaged prior to
lumbar puncture. A head CT is not a necessary prerequisite
for lumbar puncture in infants who have an open fontanel
and open sutures.

HOT KEY The most important step when approaching a patient with possible meningitis is to consider the diagnosis early in the evaluation stage.

TABLE 31-2. Cerebrospinal Fluid Findings				
Condition	Pressure (mm H$_2$0)	Leukocytes (per mm^3)	Protein (mg/dl)	Glucose (mg/dl)
Normal newborn	80–110	0–30	19–149	32–121
Normal child	< 200	0–6	20–30	40–80
Bacterial	Elevated, often > 300	100–60,000	100–500	Decreased compared with blood
Partially treated bacterial	Slightly elevated	1–10,000 monocytes	100+	Slightly decreased
Tuberculosis	Increased or decreased if the flow of cerebrospinal fluid is blocked	10–500 polymorphonuclear leukocytes early; lymphocytes late	100–500	< 50
Viral	Slightly elevated	Rarely > 1000	50–100	Normal
Herpes	Slightly elevated	10–1000	> 75	> 30
Fungal	Elevated	25–500, polymorphonuclear cells early; monocytes late	20–500	< 50

3. Additional tests

   a. Peripheral blood cultures, complete blood cell count (CBC), platelets, urine electrolytes, and serum electrolytes and osmolality (to screen for SIADH) should be obtained.

   b. If a viral cause is suspected, enteroviral throat swabs, CSF polymerase chain reaction (PCR) for enterovirus and herpesvirus, viral cultures of CSF, and peripheral buffy coat cultures should be considered.

   c. For patients with significant encephalopathy, workup for mycoplasma, rabies, arboviruses, and *Leptospiros* species should be considered. The differential diagnosis also should include toxic ingestion and metabolic disease.

   d. If the patient is immunocompromised, a cryptococcal antigen or an India ink smear should be considered.

   e. Results of liver function tests may be significantly elevated in herpetic infection.

B. Initial antibiotic therapy. Empiric therapy begins immediately pending culture results. Ideally, all patients should undergo LP before the administration of antibiotics.

   1. Preterm, low-birthweight infants who have late-onset meningitis while in the nursery are given an antistaphylococcal agent (e.g., methicillin, vancomycin) plus gentamicin.

   2. Term infants younger than 1 month old are treated with ampicillin plus gentamicin or ampicillin plus cefotaxime.

   3. Term infants 1–2 months old are given ampicillin plus cefotaxime or ampicillin plus ceftriaxone.

   4. Children older than 2–3 months of age are treated with vancomycin plus cefotaxime or ceftriaxone. Vancomycin is added to treat possible resistant strains of pneumococcus.

   5. Acyclovir should be added if there is suspicion of neonatal transmission of HSV from the mother, temporal lobe seizures, unexplained encephalopathy, or CT/MRI or electroencephalogram (EEG) evidence of temporal lobe involvement.

C. Adjuvant therapy: Dexamethasone reduces complications in *H. influenzae* meningitis; its benefit in pneumococcal or meningococcal meningitis is uncertain. The dose is 0.6 mg/kg/day given twice daily to four times daily for 2–4 days. Dexamethasone should be administered 30 minutes before antibiotics to quell the meningeal inflammatory response.

D. Prophylaxis. Rifampin is administered to contacts of patients who have *N. meningitidis* or *H. influenzae* meningitis.

E. Fluid and electrolyte management. Patients should be monitored for SIADH, but fluids should not be restricted initially because cerebral autoregulation may be lost in meningitis. Lowering vascular volume and blood pressure may adversely affect

HOT
KEY

Consider intensive care unit admission for all patients with bacterial meningitis or any patient with suspected increased intracranial pressure.

cerebral perfusion. Systolic blood pressure should be maintained at normal to high-normal levels.

F. Ongoing management
   1. Indications for a repeat LP at 24–36 hours
      a. All neonates
      b. Meningitis caused by resistant strains of *S. pneumoniae*
      c. Meningitis caused by gram-negative enteric bacilli
      d. Lack of clinical improvement in 24–36 hours after the start of therapy
      e. Prolonged or second fever. Fever may not be due to continued CNS disease, but often is the result of nosocomial or iatrogenic infections, or drug fever from either β-lactam or anticonvulsant medications.
      f. Recurrent meningitis
      g. Immunocompromised host
   2. Indications for CT or MRI in patients with meningitis. The primary goal of imaging is to monitor for abscess, hydrocephalus, subdural effusion, subdural empyema, hemorrhage, or infarction. MRI is more sensitive than CT, but also is more expensive and should be used judiciously. Imaging is considered in the following cases:
      a. Meningitis in a newborn (except for *Listeria,* and in most cases of *N. meningitidis,* because these organisms are killed quickly)
      b. Prolonged obtundation
      c. Seizures 72 hours after the start of treatment
      d. Continued excessive irritability
      e. Focal neurologic findings
      f. Persistently abnormal CSF indices
      g. Relapse or recurrence

IV PROGNOSIS

A. Mortality
   1. In neonates: 15%–20%
   2. *Pneumococcus* species: 10%
   3. *Meningococcus* species, *H. influenzae:* 3%–5%
B. Morbidity
   1. Sequelae (in order of prevalence) may include deafness, seizures, learning difficulties, blindness, paresis, ataxia, and hydrocephalus.

2. **Incidence of morbidity by organism**
   a. Pneumococcus (25%–30%)
   b. Enterococcus or *Escherichia coli* (15%–30%)
   c. *H. influenzae* (15%)
   d. Meningococcus (10%)

HOT KEY Children who have meningitis should have a complete developmental follow-up, including a hearing evaluation, at the end of therapy.

References
Committee on Infectious Disease, American Academy of Pediatrics, Pickering LK (ed): *2000 Red Book Report of the Committee on Infectious Diseases,* 25th ed. Elk Grove Village, IL, American Academy of Pediatrics, 2000.
Wubbel L, McCracken GH Jr: Management of bacterial meningitis. *Pediatr Rev* 19(3):78–84, 1998.

32. Meningococcemia

I INTRODUCTION

A. Background. *Neisseria meningitidis* is an encapsulated, gram-negative diplococcus. Meningococcal disease can range from a benign, self-limited condition to fulminant septic shock. A good outcome often depends on rapid diagnosis and immediate institution of antibiotics and supportive measures.

B. Pathogenesis. *N. meningitidis* colonizes the nasopharynx of 5%–15% of the population. Humans are the only known reservoir. Acute disease often is preceded by a mycoplasmal or viral upper respiratory infection. *N. meningitidis* infection is transmitted through respiratory droplets, saliva, and nasopharyngeal secretions. Endotoxins and lipopolysaccharides are released and activate cytokines and anaphylatoxins, causing endothelial cell injury. Major pathogenetic mechanisms include:

1. Severe capillary leak, volume loss, and hypotension
2. Vasodilation of some vascular beds coexisting with vasoconstriction of others
3. Intravascular thrombosis, or disseminated intravascular coagulation (DIC)
4. Multisystem organ failure

C. Risk factors in the host include terminal complement deficiency (C5–C9), properdin deficiency, functional or anatomic asplenia, and immunoglobulin deficiency.

D. Epidemiology
1. The annual incidence of invasive meningococcal disease is 1:100,000 population per year. Meningococcemia is most common in children younger than 4 years of age (8:100,000).
2. Meningococcemia is most common in late winter and early spring. Most cases are sporadic and are not associated with outbreaks (< 1% of reported cases).
3. There are 13 different serogroups. The incidence by serogroup is B (32%), C (35%), and Y (26%).
4. Meningococcemia is associated with exposure to passive tobacco smoke or crowded living conditions (e.g., military barracks, dormitories).

II CLINICAL MANIFESTATIONS.
Meningitis and meningococcal sepsis are the most common clinical presentations. Severe meningococcal sepsis may be rapidly progressive; the time from onset of fever to death can be as short as 12 hours.

Early symptoms include fever, chills, malaise, vomiting, irritability, prostration, rash, myalgias, and arthralgias.

A. **Shock, or hemodynamic instability,** manifests as tachycardia, cool extremities, prolonged capillary refill, and depressed mental status. Hypotension is a late sign of shock. Waterhouse–Friderichsen syndrome (i.e., massive adrenal hemorrhage) also may be a source of shock.

B. **Central nervous system.** Between 50% and 70% of all patients have meningitis.

C. **Skin**
   1. **Purpura.** Purpuric or ecchymotic lesions are more specific than are petechiae for fulminant meningococcemia. Lesions may be extensive and may progress to digital and limb ischemia, which requires amputation or orthopedic and plastic repair.
   2. **Petechiae** occur in 50%–60% of patients. Petechiae often start on the ankles, wrists, or axillae, and usually spare the palms, soles, and head.
   3. A maculopapular rash occurs in 10%–15% of patients.

D. **Pulmonary:** manifestations include pulmonary edema, acute respiratory distress syndrome (ARDS), and pneumonia

E. **Cardiac:** myocarditis, pericarditis, pancarditis, and myocardial infarction

F. **Renal:** acute renal failure

G. **Hematologic:** DIC

H. **Endocrine:** adrenal hemorrhage and adrenal insufficiency

I. **Ophthalmologic:** endophthalmitis and conjunctivitis

> **HOT** ▶ **KEY** Meningococcal disease must be considered in any patient who has fever and petechiae. As many as 5% may have meningococcemia. Such patients may appear remarkably stable just before sudden deterioration occurs.

III APPROACH TO THE PATIENT

A. The **diagnosis** of invasive meningococcal disease requires bacteriologic isolation of *N. meningitidis* from a sterile site, such as blood, cerebrospinal fluid (CSF), or synovial, pericardial, or pleural fluid, or from petechial or purpuric lesions. Samples should be sent for culture and Gram stain.
   1. **Lumbar puncture (LP)** is performed only if the patient is hemodynamically stable. The procedure is deferred if there are signs of DIC or increased intracranial pressure.
   2. A presumptive diagnosis is based on the presence of gram-negative diplococci in any normally sterile fluid or aspirate.

The Gram stain from the buffy coat of a blood sample may be particularly useful.

3. A polymerase chain reaction (PCR) study of blood or cerebrospinal fluid is especially useful in patients who have previously been treated with antibiotics.

4. *N. meningitidis* normally colonizes the nasopharynx. Therefore, isolation of the organism from a nasopharyngeal or conjunctival site is not diagnostic.

5. All cases of meningococcemia must be reported to the Department of Public Health.

B. Initial therapy (Figure 32-1)

1. **Antibiotics.** Fluid samples should be drawn before antibiotics are administered, but the procedure should not delay treatment. Ceftriaxone is the typical first-line therapy; chloramphenicol is considered for patients who are allergic to cephalosporins.

2. **Intensive care management.** Early admission to a pediatric intensive care unit is prudent. Patients with evidence of hemodynamic instability require immediate and aggressive fluid resuscitation. Severely ill patients may require mechanical ventilation or inotropic support.

3. **Adjuvant therapies**

   a. **Respiratory isolation** is recommended for at least 24 hours after the first dose of antibiotics.

   b. **The use of corticosteroid therapy** for meningitis is controversial.

      (1) Data on the effect of steroids in meningococcal meningitis are not available. Consultation with an infectious disease expert is advised.

      (2) No evidence supports the routine use of adrenal replacement with corticosteroids. Steroids may be added for patients who have hypotension that persists despite aggressive volume resuscitation and inotropic support.

   c. **DIC** can progress rapidly in the first 24–48 hours.

      (1) Platelets, prothrombin time (PT), partial thromboplastin time (PTT), d-dimers, and fibrinogen should be evaluated.

      (2) Fresh frozen plasma (FFP) is considered if PT or PTT is two to three times the normal value, if d-dimer level is elevated, or if the patient is actively bleeding. Cryoprecipitate also may be given, especially if the fibrinogen level is low.

      (3) Vitamin K is given if PT level is elevated.

      (4) Platelets are given if the patient's count is lower than 20,000 μl, if there is active bleeding, or if platelet counts are rapidly decreasing.

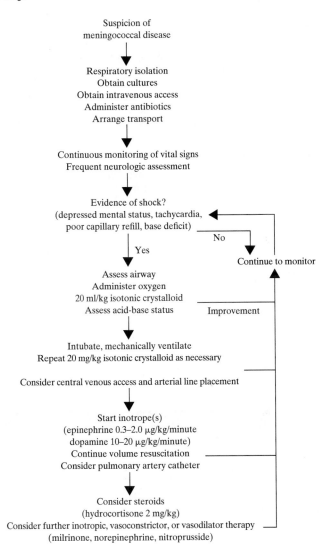

FIGURE 32-1. Management scheme for meningococcemia. (Adapted with permission from Kirsch EA, Barton RP, Kitchen L, et al: Pathophysiology, treatment and outcome of meningococcemia: a review and recent experience. *Pediatr Infect Dis J* 15:967–78, 1996.)

IV PROGNOSIS

A. The Glasgow Meningococcal Septicemia Prognostic Score **(Table 32-1)** can be used to assess the patient's prognosis.

B. The **overall mortality rate** is 10%–20%.

C. **Morbidity.** Serious sequelae of meningococcal disease include neurologic problems (e.g., seizures, cerebral infarcts, subdural hematoma, atrophy, hearing loss), amputation, and skin grafting.

V PREVENTION

A. Chemoprophylaxis and immunization are available to help prevent meningococcal infections (see Chapter 2).

B. Patients with documented immunodeficiencies should receive the meningococcal vaccine.

References

American Academy of Pediatrics: Meningococcal disease prevention and control strategies for practice-based physicians. *Pediatrics* 97(3):404–412, 1996.

Committee on Infectious Disease, American Academy of Pediatrics, Pickering LK (ed): *2000 Red Book Report of the Committee on Infectious Diseases,* 25th ed. Elk Grove Village, IL, American Academy of Pediatrics, 2000.

Rosenstein NE, Perkins BA, Stephens DS, et al: The changing epidemiology of meningococcal disease in the United States, 1992–1996. *J Infect Dis* 180(6):1894–1901, 1999.

Salzman MB, Rubin LG: Meningococcemia. *Infect Dis Clin North Am* 10(4):709–725, 1996.

TABLE 32-1. Glasgow Meningococcal Septicemia Prognostic Score	
Blood pressure < 75 mm Hg systolic in child younger than age 4 years, or < 85 mm Hg systolic in child age 4 years or older	3
Skin/rectal temperature difference > 3°C	3
Modified coma scale score < 8, or deterioration of 3 or more points in 1 hour	3
Deterioration in the hour before scoring	2
Absence of meningismus	2
Extending purpura or widespread ecchymoses	1
Base deficit > 8 mEq/L	1
Maximum score	15

In a study of 123 children with meningococcemia, 100% of the 104 with a score of 7 or less survived, whereas only 26% of the 19 with a score of 8 or greater survived.

33. Bronchiolitis

I INTRODUCTION

A. Definition. Bronchiolitis is a type of lower respiratory tract infection. It typically affects infants and young children and is a clinical diagnosis.

B. Pathogenesis. Damage to the bronchial epithelium results in inflammation of small airways (i.e., bronchioles), leading to expiratory wheezes and crackles. Bronchiolitis is most commonly caused by respiratory syncytial virus (RSV), but other agents are also responsible. These agents include RSV, parainfluenza viruses (especially types I and III), influenza A, adenoviruses, rhinoviruses, and *Mycoplasma pneumoniae.*

HOT

KEY
Bronchiolitis + severe conjunctivitis = adenovirus

C. Epidemiology
1. Approximately 80% of cases occur in the first year of life. By age 5, nearly all children will have had RSV at least once.
2. Approximately 1% of infected children are hospitalized.
3. Marked seasonal variation occurs, with peaks in the winter and early spring.
4. Bronchiolitis is especially serious for infants younger than 6 months of age and for children with underlying chronic disease, including bronchopulmonary dysplasia, congenital heart disease, cystic fibrosis, and immunodeficiency.

II CLINICAL MANIFESTATIONS

A. Symptoms
1. Fever
2. Tachypnea
3. Use of accessory muscles during breathing (i.e., suprasternal or subcostal retractions)
4. High-pitched wheezing
5. Fine inspiratory crackles

B. Differential diagnosis
1. Pneumonia
2. Asthma

3. Gastroesophageal reflux
4. Inhalation injury

> **HOT KEY** ▶ Infants < 1 month of age may have minimal respiratory signs. These patients may present with lethargy, irritability, poor feeding, or apnea.

III APPROACH TO THE PATIENT

A. History
  1. Wheezing, typically preceded by profuse rhinorrhea
  2. Clinical course (Is the patient getting better or worse?)
  3. Feeding and hydration
  4. Apnea or color changes
B. Physical examination
  1. General appearance (Does the child appear fatigued or toxic?)
  2. Work of breathing (What is the child's respiratory rate? Is he or she using accessory muscles?)
  3. Air exchange (How well are breath sounds heard?)
  4. Mental status (Does the child engage the parents or smile?)
C. Laboratory tests
  1. Pulse oximetry to assess oxygenation
  2. Enzyme-linked immunosorbent assay (ELISA) from a nasal wash for rapid identification of viral pathogens
  3. Chest radiograph (typical findings include atelectasis, hyperinflation, diffuse infiltrates); chest radiograph is not routinely indicated
  4. Arterial blood gas level, if the patient appears severely ill or fatigued
D. Hospitalization should be considered for a child with bronchiolitis who has one or more of the following characteristics (remembered with the mnemonic MONITOR):

"MONITOR"

Medical conditions in addition to bronchiolitis (e.g., chronic lung disease, congenital heart disease)
Oxygen requirement
No reliable caregiver
Infant, especially if younger than 3 months of age
Toxic appearance
Oral intake diminished or evidence of dehydration
Respiratory rate > 60 breaths/minute *or* evidence of **Res**piratory failure on arterial blood gas measurements

In addition, any patient with a history of apnea should be admitted to the hospital.

HOT KEY

> Premature infants with bronchiolitis are at high risk for apnea; therefore, the admission threshold should be very low.

E. Therapy
1. **Bronchodilators** are not uniformly helpful, but may improve symptoms in 25% of children. A trial of bronchodilators is usually warranted. Typically, nebulized albuterol is tried first. Some patients may have a greater response to nebulized racemic epinephrine.
2. **Supplemental oxygen** can be administered as needed.
3. **Corticosteroid** use remains controversial. Use of these agents is more accepted in a patient with underlying chronic lung disease. There has been recent evidence that steroids may be helpful in reducing the length of stay in hospitalized patients.
4. **Antibiotics** are not routinely indicated. Chest films show areas of atelectasis, which are often mistakenly interpreted as bacterial pneumonia.
5. **Ribavirin** therapy is considered only in infants who have severe underlying chronic cardiopulmonary disease or are otherwise immunocompromised.

F. Prophylaxis. Palivizumab (Synagis), a recombinant monoclonal antibody, is indicated in certain situations. Synagis has been proven to reduce the hospitalization rate by 55% in randomized controlled trials. Candidates for palivizumab therapy include:
1. Children with respiratory illnesses requiring daily medications or treatments (e.g., oxygen, diuretics, corticosteroids, bronchodilators) within the last 6 months and who are < 2 years of age at the onset of RSV season
2. Infants born at < 32 weeks gestation who are < 6 months old at the onset of RSV season
3. Infants born at > 33–35 weeks gestation who are < 6 months old at the onset of RSV season and have at least one environmental risk factor (e.g., passive tobacco smoke exposure, daycare, siblings, persistent hospitalization)
4. Palivizumab may also be indicated for patients < 2 years of age at the onset of RSV season who are symptomatic from or who require daily medications for congenital heart disease. Use of palivizumab should be done in concert with a cardiologist for infants with cyanotic heart disease.

PROGNOSIS. Most uncomplicated cases resolve within 3–5 days. However, morbidity can be considerable in patients with underlying chronic lung disease.

References

Shaw KN, Bell LM, Sherman NH: Outpatient assessment of infants with bronchiolitis. *Am J Dis Child* 145(2):151–155, 1991.

Welliver JR, Welliver RC: Bronchiolitis. *Pediatr Rev* 14(4):134–139, 1993.

34. Tuberculosis

I INTRODUCTION

A. **Background.** Worldwide, nearly 500 children die each day of tuberculosis (TB). The occurrence of TB in children implies recent transmission and reflects the effectiveness of adult TB control programs.

B. **Definitions.** Tuberculosis is caused by *Mycobacterium tuberculosis,* an acid-fast bacillus. Disease is differentiated from infection by the presence of clinical symptoms or a positive finding on chest radiograph. The risk of disease is highest in the first 2 years of life, but disease does not develop in most healthy children.

C. **Pathogenesis.** Tuberculosis is transmitted by aerosolized droplets. Because young children cannot expectorate with sufficient force to expel the droplets, children usually are infected by adults rather than by other children. A peripheral lesion begins in any lobe of the lung and is accompanied by alveolitis. The infection spreads through the lymphatic system to regional hilar lymph nodes. Approximately 95% of cases heal spontaneously, and the site calcifies in 6–12 months, producing the **Ghon complex** (i.e., a primary focus of inflammation plus involvement of draining lymph nodes). However, lymphohematogenous spread may occur to extrapulmonary sites (e.g., apical pleura of the lungs, bone, brain, kidneys).

D. **Epidemiology.** Pediatric cases have increased by 33% since 1990. Risk factors include household exposure, foreign birthplace (especially Asia, the Middle East, Africa, and Latin America), travel to endemic countries, low socioeconomic status, immunosuppression, homelessness, and exposure to high-risk individuals (e.g., people infected with HIV, homeless people, illicit drug users, incarcerated people, migrant farm workers).

II CLINICAL MANIFESTATIONS.

A. The **initial infection** often is detected when the patient is asymptomatic; the primary complex often is not seen on a chest radiograph. Some patients experience an initial febrile illness that lasts for 1–3 weeks, with erythema nodosum and phlyctenular conjunctivitis (i.e., small yellow nodules at the corneal limbus). It may take weeks to years for the disease to appear.

B. **Early manifestations** of TB disease (1–6 months after initial infection) include fever, weight loss, cough, night sweats, chills,

189

lymphadenopathy, pleural effusion (as a result of rupture of a subpleural focus), meningitis, or miliary TB.

C. **Late manifestations** of TB disease are primarily extrapulmonary and include middle ear, bone, skin, or joint lesions that may occur within 3 years after infection. Renal lesions occur after 5 years or more. Renal TB and pulmonary reactivation in the apices of the lung (i.e., adult-type TB) can occur in adolescents, but rarely are found in children.

HOT

 Extrapulmonary disease occurs in 25% of children younger than 15 years of age.

KEY

III APPROACH TO THE PATIENT

A. **Tuberculin skin test.** Targeted skin testing is used only in high-risk populations. Skin testing is the best method for identifying TB infection. In a child with a normal immune system, tuberculin sensitivity develops in 3–12 weeks. In the **purified protein derivative (PPD) skin test,** five tuberculin units of PPD are administered intradermally on the volar surface of the arm. The induration, not the erythema, is then measured 48–72 hours later.

1. An **area of induration larger than 5 mm** is considered a positive result in the following settings:
   a. If the child's **contacts** include people at home who have active cases of TB, people in whom treatment cannot be verified as adequate or was started after contact, or those in whom reactivation is suspected
   b. If the chest radiograph is consistent with TB (active or previously active) or if there is clinical evidence of extrapulmonary TB
   c. If the child is **immunosuppressed** because of oncologic drugs, high-dose steroids, or HIV infection

2. An **area of induration larger than 10 mm** is considered positive in the following settings:
   a. If the child is younger than 4 years of age or has Hodgkin's disease, lymphoma, diabetes, chronic renal failure, or malnutrition
   b. If the child has any **environmental exposures.** These include time spent in an endemic area and exposure to people with the following risk factors: HIV-positive status; homelessness; intravenous drug abuse; low socioeconomic status, especially in an urban setting; living or working in a

nursing home, prison, or other institution; and employment as a migrant farm worker.

3. An **area of induration larger than 15 mm** in a child older than 4 years of age who has no risk factors is considered a positive result.

4. False-negative results can occur during the incubation period (in which case the test is repeated in 2–3 months) or during severe systemic illness (e.g., meningeal or miliary disease). Malnutrition, use of steroids, viral infections, or infection with *Mycoplasma pneumoniae* also may cause false-negative results.

HOT

KEY
Previous vaccination with bacille Calmette-Guérin (BCG) is not a contraindication to skin testing. Interpretation of the PPD result is the same, regardless of previous BCG vaccination. BCG status has no effect on management or therapy!

B. **Additional tests**
1. A **chest radiograph** is performed if the PPD result is positive.
2. **Culture.** A positive culture from any fluid (e.g., gastric aspirate, sputum, pleural fluid, cerebrospinal fluid, urine, tissue biopsy) is helpful in establishing a diagnosis; however, this takes weeks to determine, and is only 50% sensitive.
3. **Acid-fast bacillus stain (Ziehl-Nelson test).** An acid-fast stain should be performed on all fluids. However, this test has a low sensitivity. Fluorescence microscopy with auramine-rhodamine staining is a helpful adjunctive test.
4. **Gastric lavage** is performed in children younger than age 12 years because they do not produce sputum easily. On three consecutive early mornings, the stomach contents should be aspirated and then washed with 50 ml of sterile distilled water. The sample should be neutralized to a pH of 7 with a 10% sodium bicarbonate solution and sent immediately for smear and culture.

HOT

KEY
HIV testing should be considered in any patient who has TB disease.

C. **Therapy**
1. **Management of contacts.** All patients who are immunosuppressed and those younger than 4 years of age who were exposed within the previous 3 months to a potentially contagious case of TB should undergo PPD and chest radiograph,

and begin treatment with isoniazid, even if the result of the PPD is negative. The patient should be retested 12 weeks after contact has been broken. All patients with a positive PPD result should receive 9 months of isoniazid therapy.

2. **Management of infection** [with infection defined as a positive PPD test result without disease, or latent tuberculosis infection (LTBI)]. The efficacy of isoniazid in preventing disease in children is nearly 100%. Treatment duration ranges from 9 months for a healthy child to 1 year in children who have an underlying immunodeficiency. The dose is 10 mg/kg orally once daily (maximum dose, 300 mg). If resistance to isoniazid is suspected, rifampin (10 mg/kg once daily) should be added, and an infectious disease expert should be consulted.

3. **Management of disease.** Proper treatment is difficult because of low compliance, slow growth of the organism, and spontaneous resistance of the organism to drug therapy.

   a. **Pulmonary disease.** Patients are treated for a total of 6 months. Therapy includes rifampin, isoniazid, and pyrazinamide for the first 2 months, followed by isoniazid and rifampin for the remaining 4 months.

   b. **Extrapulmonary disease.** Treatment is the same as for pulmonary disease (see III C 3 a). Patients with miliary, meningeal, bone, or joint disease also receive streptomycin for the first 2 months. Steroids are indicated in patients with tuberculous meningitis.

   c. **If drug resistance is suspected,** either ethambutol or streptomycin is added, and treatment is continued for a total of 18 months.

   d. **If pleural or pericardial effusions** are present, steroids are considered.

D. **Ongoing management**

   1. The health department should be notified to ensure that all contacts are identified and tested.

   2. If compliance with therapy is in doubt, directly observed therapy should be ensured.

   3. Drug sensitivity testing should be performed on all isolates from the patient and from adult contacts. Drug resistance can be as high as 30% in some populations, including the foreign-born, homeless, and patients previously treated for TB. Drug resistance also should be suspected in patients whose source case has ongoing evidence of active TB after 2 months of appropriate therapy.

   4. Children with TB are not contagious if the results of sputum smears are negative.

   5. The treatment standards for TB change frequently. Therefore, consultation with infectious disease specialists is essen-

tial, especially in cases involving immunodeficiency states, pregnancy, and newborns.

References

Nobert E, Chernick V: Tuberculosis: pediatric disease. *CMAJ* 160(10):1479–1482, 1999.

Committee on Infectious Disease, American Academy of Pediatrics, Pickering LK (ed): *2000 Red Book Report of the Committee on Infectious Diseases,* 25th ed. Elk Grove Village, IL, American Academy of Pediatrics, 2000, pp 593–613.

35. Pneumonia

I INTRODUCTION

A. **Definition.** Pneumonia is inflammation of the pulmonary paren-chyma caused by bacterial or viral pathogens. It often is classi-fied according to pulmonary anatomy (e.g., lobar, interstitial, bronchopneumonia).

B. **Epidemiology.** Pneumonia can affect all children, although those younger than 2 years of age and those with underlying immuno-suppression are more commonly infected. It often occurs as a su-perinfection after a viral illness. There are mild seasonal predilec-tions; pneumonia occurs more often in the winter and spring.

II APPROACH TO THE PATIENT

A. **History.** Pneumonia is often preceded by a viral illness and of-ten causes systemic signs of toxicity. The physician should ask about recent fever, cough, malaise, anorexia, and respiratory distress. The character of the cough (e.g., "deep," "rattling") has no clinical significance, although it may be a source of con-cern to parents.

B. **Physical examination**

1. **Vital signs,** especially body temperature, oxygen saturation, and resting respiratory rate, are crucial.

2. **Head, ears, eyes, nose, throat (HEENT).** The physician should check for tonsillitis, pharyngitis, and ulcerative stom-atitis, which are more common with viral or mycoplasmic disease. Severe conjunctivitis suggests adenoviral infection.

3. **Chest.** Auscultation of the chest is crucial, but does not reli-ably distinguish between types of pneumonia. Crackles may be heard with viral or bacterial pneumonia. Wheezing is of-ten heard in cases of bronchiolitis or in children with an un-derlying diagnosis of asthma. Decreased breath sounds may be present secondary to atelectasis, consolidation, or asthma. Therefore, the findings on clinical examination must be considered in the larger context of the patient's history and laboratory findings.

> **HOT KEY**
> The absence of fever and tachypnea makes pneumonia un-likely.

C. Admission criteria. The presence of any of the following criteria should cause the physician to strongly consider hospital admission:

ADMIT

Age younger than 6 months
Dehydration requiring vigorous rehydration
Medications that need to be given intravenously, or the need for supplemental oxygen
Immunocompromised condition (e.g., AIDS, cancer)
Toxic appearance

D. Follow-up. In uncomplicated cases, improvement can be expected in 1–5 days. A chest radiograph should appear normal within 6 weeks. A repeat chest radiograph is not indicated unless a large effusion or severe atelectasis was noted initially.

III CLINICAL TYPES OF PNEUMONIA

A. Bacterial pneumonia
1. **Pathogenesis.** In children younger than 2 months of age, the most common organism is group B streptococcus. Afterward, the most common bacterial pathogen is pneumococcus, although mycoplasma infection (discussed later) increases in frequency in children older than age 5 years. Other causes include *Haemophilus influenzae,* which is nontypeable now that *H. influenzae* type B vaccine is widespread, and *Staphylococcus aureus,* which is rare but serious.
2. **Symptoms.** Bacterial pneumonia can have an acute onset accompanied by fever and chills. Grunting respirations are also common.
3. **Additional tests to consider**
   a. **Chest radiograph.** Lobar consolidation suggests bacterial origin, whereas diffuse interstitial distribution suggests mycoplasma or a viral etiology.
   b. **Complete blood cell count.** A white blood cell count lower than 15,000/mm^3 suggests viral pneumonia. Blood cultures should be obtained from children who appear moderately ill. As many as 30% of children with bacterial pneumonia and toxicity have bacteremia.
   c. **Pulse oximetry** should be obtained on children who appear to be in moderate to severe respiratory distress.
4. **Therapy.** Oral or parenteral antibiotics are the mainstays of therapy. Cefuroxime is usually indicated as first-line intra-

Chapter 35

venous therapy; amoxicillin is appropriate for outpatient treatment. Macrolide therapy (e.g., clarithromycin, erythromycin) is appropriate in older children and adolescents, in penicillin-allergic patients, and when mycoplasma is suspected.

> **HOT KEY** In a dehydrated child, a chest radiograph may not show lobar infiltrates early in the course of illness. In toxic-appearing children with fever and tachypnea, presumptive antibiotic therapy may be indicated, even with nonspecific findings on chest radiograph.

B. Viral pneumonia
  1. **Pathogenesis.** The most common viral pathogens that cause pneumonia include respiratory syncytial virus and parainfluenza.
  2. **Symptoms.** Viral pneumonia typically has a more indolent onset than does bacterial pneumonia, with symptoms developing over 3–4 days. Fever is typically lower than in bacterial pneumonia.
  3. **Additional tests to consider.** A chest radiograph may show peribronchial thickening, air trapping, or diffuse interstitial infiltrates. Rapid virologic tests can be performed on nasopharyngeal specimens to look for viral causes of illness; although these tests typically have little clinical value, they can be useful for epidemiologic or infection control purposes.
  4. **Therapy.** No specific therapies other than supportive care (i.e., antipyretics, oral hydration) are necessary.
C. Mycoplasma pneumonia
  1. **Pathogenesis.** Mycoplasma pneumonia is one of the most common types of pneumonia in school-age children.
  2. **Symptoms.** Onset typically is insidious, with fever and malaise. Children may have a nonproductive cough, hoarseness, a sore throat, and, occasionally, chest pain. Respiratory symptoms typically are mild. Occasionally, associated otitis media, especially bullous myringitis, is seen.
  3. **Additional tests to consider.** Chest radiographs vary greatly and typically "look worse than the patient does." Scattered segmental infiltrates, interstitial disease, or even lobar infiltrates may be seen. Cold agglutinins suggest mycoplasma, but they are neither sensitive nor specific.
  4. **Therapy.** Macrolide therapy is indicated in suspected cases.

References

Margolis P, Gadomski A: Does this infant have pneumonia? *JAMA* 279(4):308–313, 1998.

Nelson JD: Community-acquired pneumonia in children: guidelines for treatment. *Pediatr Infect Dis J* 19(3):251–253, 2000.

36. Hepatitis

I INTRODUCTION. Hepatitis has a variety of etiologies, from viral to metabolic.

A. Pathogenesis. Hepatitis leads to hepatocellular destruction, leakage of cellular enzymes [glutamate oxaloacetate transaminase (AST), glutamate pyruvate transaminase (ALT), lactate dehydrogenase (LDH), glutamyl transpeptidase (GGT), alkaline phosphatase], and decreased liver function (e.g., increase in indirect or direct bilirubin, decrease in albumin, abnormal coagulation).

B. Fulminant hepatic failure (FHF) is characterized by sudden impairment of all hepatic function—synthetic, excretory, and detoxifying—within 8 weeks of the onset of liver disease. For this diagnosis to be made, associated hepatic encephalopathy and coagulopathy must be present. The condition often is fatal.

C. Differential diagnosis
1. **Infectious causes**
   a. **Viral.** Hepatitis A, B, and C; Epstein-Barr virus (EBV); and cytomegalovirus (CMV)
   b. **Bacterial.** Leptospirosis, syphilis, gonorrhea, and chlamydia
   c. **Parasitic.** Malarial and amebic infections
2. **Drug-related causes.** Acetaminophen, phenothiazines, valproate, isoniazid, methyldopa, intravenous tetracycline, erythromycin, indomethacin, oral contraceptives, gold, and ethanol
3. **Toxic causes.** Mushroom (*Amanita phalloides*) ingestion
4. **Metabolic causes.** Alpha-1-antitrypsin deficiency, Wilson disease (hepatolenticular degeneration), tyrosinemia, urea cycle defect, and disorder of carbohydrate metabolism
5. **Systemic disorders.** Hypoxemia and hypotension
6. **Other causes.** Reye syndrome, chronic autoimmune hepatitis, and infiltrative disease (e.g., lymphohistiocytosis, leukemia, choledocholithiasis, cholecystitis, cholangitis)

II CLINICAL PRESENTATION

A. Symptoms
1. Most **acute forms** are accompanied by fever, malaise, nausea and vomiting, and abdominal pain. Later, patients may have jaundice, dark urine, and light stools. Viral hepatitides often

improve after the onset of jaundice, whereas other hepatitides often do not.

   2. **Chronic forms** may occur more insidiously. For example, Wilson disease may cause psychiatric disturbances, dysarthria, diminished work or school performance, or dystonias.

B. Physical examination
   1. The patient is examined for signs of hyperbilirubinemia (e.g., jaundice, scleral icterus).
   2. The abdomen is examined closely, with particular attention given to the size of the liver and to the consistency of the liver and spleen.
   3. Kayser-Fleischer rings may indicate Wilson disease.
   4. Severe myositis, conjunctival suffusion, photophobia, ocular pain, and meningismus may indicate leptospirosis. Jaundice is not always present.
   5. If the patient has acute encephalopathy, then Reye syndrome, FHF, and leptospirosis should be considered.
   6. The presence of cirrhosis, acne, ascites, edema, spider hemangioma, asterixis, palmar erythema, clubbing, gynecomastia, or amenorrhea suggests chronic liver disease.

III APPROACH TO THE PATIENT

A. Basic workup
   1. Complete blood cell count (CBC) with differential
   2. Urinalysis, bilirubin, blood urea nitrogen (BUN), and creatinine
   3. Liver-specific tests (albumin, AST, ALT, GGT, LDH, and alkaline phosphatase)
      a. A hepatocellular pattern of injury is characterized by alterations in AST, ALT, and LDH.
      b. A cholestatic pattern of injury is characterized by elevations in alkaline phosphatase and GGT. AST and ALT are only mildly elevated.
   4. Coagulation studies (prothrombin time and partial thromboplastin time). Prothrombin time is a sensitive indicator of the liver's synthetic function.
   5. Hepatitis serologic studies [IgG anti-HAV, IgM anti-HAV, HBS Ag, HBC Ag, HBe Ag, anti-HBS, anti-HBc, anti-HBe, IgM anti HCV]
   6. EBV and CMV serologies

B. Additional tests to consider
   1. Wilson disease must be ruled out in patients who are older than age 5 years. The workup includes a serum ceruloplasmin and copper level as well as a thorough slit-lamp examination to detect Kayser-Fleischer rings.

2. Alpha-1-antitryspin deficiency is considered, especially if the patient has a history of neonatal cholestasis.

3. Autoimmune hepatitis is considered if the patient has relapsing or chronic hepatitis, or if there is an associated Coombs-positive hemolytic anemia or thyroiditis. The workup includes tests for anti-nuclear antibodies (ANA), anti–smooth muscle antibodies, and quantitative gammaglobulin level.

4. Reye syndrome, metabolic disease, or drug-induced disease is considered if the patient has hyperammonemia.

5. A microscopic agglutination titer for **leptospirosis** may be performed, especially if the patient has unexplained azotemia or the characteristic constellation of symptoms.

6. The possibility of an undiagnosed **inborn error of metabolism** also must be considered (see Chapter 95).

C. Initial management

1. All potentially hepatotoxic drugs are discontinued.

HOT KEY
If the results of liver function tests are elevated for longer than 3 months, a chronic cause may be responsible. Chronic causes include systemic lupus erythematosus, autoimmune chronic hepatitis, Wilson disease, and alpha-1-antitrypsin deficiency. In this situation, a liver biopsy may be required.

---

2. Vitamin K is indicated if the patient has an associated coagulopathy.

3. Chronic hepatitis requires management by a pediatric gastroenterologist.

4. FHF requires care in the intensive care unit and may necessitate liver transplantation.

IV VIRAL HEPATITIS

A. Hepatitis A Virus (HAV) (Figure 36-1)

1. Pathogenesis

a. The main **mode of transmission** is via the fecal–oral route. Transmission also may occur by person-to-person contact, sexual intercourse, and intravenous drug abuse.

b. The **incubation time** is approximately 3–4 weeks. The virus is believed to replicate in the gastrointestinal tract and then spread hematogenously to the liver.

2. Epidemiology

a. Epidemics can occur in crowded conditions, such as classrooms and boarding schools.

b. In the United States, 50% of the population will show IgG to HAV by 50 years of age.

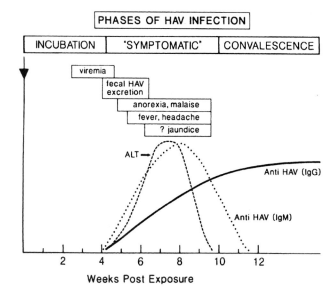

FIGURE 36-1. Phases of hepatitis A infection. (Reprinted with permission from Balistreri WF: Viral hepatitis. *Pediatr Clin North Am* 1988;35:640.)

    c. Hepatitis A is more prevalent in developing countries.
3. Symptoms
    a. Fever, anorexia, vomiting, dark urine, light stools, and jaundice are the classic symptoms of HAV and other hepatitis viruses.
    b. Many patients have a prodrome (fever, HA, fatigue, vomiting, and right upper quadrant pain).
    c. Symptoms last 2–4 weeks; however, most infections in children are asymptomatic.
4. Diagnosis
    a. IgM anti-HAV indicates an **acute** infection.
    b. IgG anti-HAV implies **prior** infection, with protection from subsequent infection.
5. Treatment is supportive. No specific therapy is available. A vaccine is available.
6. Prognosis. There are usually no long-term sequelae, FHF is rare, and chronic infection does not occur.
B. Hepatitis B virus (HBV) (Figure 36-2)
    1. Pathogenesis. Transmission occurs through body fluids (e.g., blood, wound exudates, semen, cervical secretions, saliva).

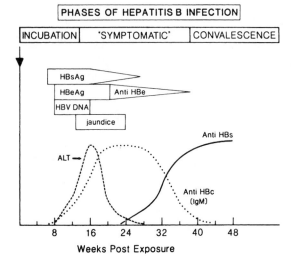

FIGURE 36-2. Phases of hepatitis B virus infection. (Reprinted with permission from Balistreri WF: Viral hepatitis. *Pediatr Clin North Am* 1988;35:647.)

Transmission by **transfusion** is rare. The **incubation** period is 45–160 days (average, 120 days).

2. Epidemiology

    a. Groups at high risk include intravenous drug abusers, heterosexuals with multiple partners, homosexual men, health care workers, hemodialysis patients, and sexual or household contacts of people with acute or chronic infections.

    b. One third of cases have no identifiable risk factor.

3. Symptoms

    a. Symptoms range from asymptomatic seroconversion to classic clinical hepatitis to FHF.

    b. Early symptoms include arthralgia, arthritis, and macular rash.

    c. Most children with HBV infection are **asymptomatic.**

4. Diagnosis

    a. Surface antigen (HBsAg) is the first marker to appear, it occurs late in the incubation period, 2–5 weeks before the onset of symptoms. It persists for 1–4 months and then disappears. Patients with chronic infection continue to have this marker; it does not distinguish between chronic and acute infection.

   b. Antibody to s-antigen (anti-HBs) appears after HBsAg
      clears. It indicates previous infection and protection from
      chronic disease, and also indicates immunity after immu-
      nization.
   c. Antibody to c-antigen (anti-HBc). IgM HBc antibody is
      the best marker for active HBV infection, except in cases
      of perinatal transmission, in which it often is negative. It
      appears before the onset of symptoms. This marker helps
      to distinguish a vaccinated patient from one with a pre-
      vious viral infection. This marker is present during the
      window period when HBsAg and anti-HBs are negative.
      IgG anti-HBc persists for life.
   d. The **e antigen (HBeAg)** indicates a high level of virus. The
      patient is at increased risk for transmitting HBV. This
      marker is shorter-lived than HBsAg.
   e. Antibody to e-antigen (anti-HBe) appears soon after the
      antigen disappears. This marker is a good prognostic sign,
      because resolution coincides with conversion. The patient
      is at low risk for transmitting HBV.
   f. Summary of serology results
      (1) Previous vaccination: (+) anti-HBs
      (2) Acute infection: (+) IgM anti-HBc
      (3) Resolved infection: (+) anti-HBs, (+) anti-HBc
      (4) Chronic healthy: (+) HBsAg, (+) anti-HBc, (+) anti-
          HBe
      (5) Chronic active: (+) HBsAg, (+) HBeAg
 5. Treatment. No specific therapy is available. Alpha-interferon
    may have limited effectiveness for those with chronic infec-
    tions.
 6. Prognosis
   a. The risk of chronic infection is inversely related to the age
      of the patient at the time of primary infection.
   b. Chronic carriers are at increased risk for HCC and chronic
      liver disease. Most do not go on to have cirrhosis, but those
      with cirrhosis are at greatest risk for hepatocellular carci-
      noma.
   c. The risk of transmission for infants born to mothers who
      are HBeAg-positive is 70%–90%.
C. Hepatitis C Virus (HCV)
 1. Pathogenesis. HCV is a major cause of posttransfusion
    hepatitis. HCV accounts for 50% of sporadic or community-
    acquired cases of hepatitis (i.e., cases without obvious sexual
    contact or intravenous inoculation). The **incubation time** is 2
    weeks to 2 months.
 2. Epidemiology. HCV is uncommon in children younger than
    age 15 years.
 3. Symptoms. Infection with HCV usually causes chronic asymp-

tomatic elevation of transaminase levels. Symptoms are similar to those of other hepatitis viruses and usually are mild. Infection often is asymptomatic. Cirrhosis develops in 10%–25% of patients.

  4. Diagnosis
   a. Diagnosis is made by **antibody titer.** However, anti-HCV may be absent during acute infection.
   b. No antigen test is available, and it may be necessary to wait for 6–12 months before the antibody (Ab) test result becomes positive.
   c. Polymerase chain reaction (PCR) is available, but its use is not standardized.
   d. Transaminase levels can vary from normal to 10 times the normal level. Usually, they are lower than in patients infected with HBV or HAV.

  5. Treatment
   a. Alpha-interferon may be of some benefit for patients with chronic hepatitis.
   b. Patients should be vaccinated against HAV and HBV.

  6. Prognosis. If hepatitis progresses to chronic infection, the patient is at risk for HCC and chronic liver disease. Between 50% and 70% of patients go on to have chronic disease, and cirrhosis develops in 20% of those patients.

D. Hepatitis D virus (HDV)
  1. Pathogenesis. The HBsAg serves as the coat of HDV; therefore, infection with HDV requires pre-existing active HBV infection (co-infection) or chronic HBV infection (superinfection). HDV infection cannot outlast HBV infection.

  2. Epidemiology
   a. Hepatitis D is sexually transmitted in endemic areas and percutaneously and parenterally transmitted in nonendemic areas.
   b. Any HBsAg carrier is at risk for HDV infection.
   c. In the United States, patients with hemophilia and those who abuse intravenous drugs are at greatest risk.

  3. Symptoms
   a. Co-infection may result in FHF. Superinfection may result in chronic active hepatitis and increases the risk of cirrhosis.
   b. Serologic findings
    (1) Co-infection. IgM anti-HBc (+) and IgM anti-HD (+)
    (2) Superinfection. HBsAg (+), IgM anti-HBc (-), and IgG anti-HD (+)

  4. Treatment is supportive. Vaccination against HBV also provides protection against HDV.

References

American Academy of Pediatrics: *2000 Red Book: Report of the Committee on Infectious Diseases,* 25th ed. Elk Grove Village, IL, American Academy of Pediatrics, 280–309, 2000.

Balistreri WF: Viral hepatitis. *Pediatr Clin North Am* 35:638, 1988.

Bhaduri BR, Mieli-Vergani G: Fulminant hepatic failure: pediatric aspects. *Semin Liver Dis* 16:349, 1996.

Brewer GJ, Yuzbasiyan-Gurkan V: Wilson's disease. *Medicine* 71:139, 1992.

Czaja AJ: Autoimmune hepatitis: evolving concepts and treatment strategies. *Dig Dis Sci* 40:435, 1995.

Norman MR, Mowat AP, Hutchison DC: Molecular basis, clinical consequences and diagnosis of alpha-1 antitrypsin deficiency. *Ann Clin Biochem* 34:230, 1997.

37. Soft Tissue Infections and Toxic Shock Syndrome

I **INTRODUCTION.** Soft tissue infections are common in children. They range in severity from simple annoyances to life-threatening systemic processes.

II **DERMATOPHYTE INFECTIONS**

A. **Pathogenesis.** Dermatophyte infections (tinea, or ringworm) are fungal infections (e.g., *Trichophyton*) of the skin. They are spread by person-to-person contact.

B. **Symptoms**
1. **Tinea corporis (ringworm)** is a superficial dermatophyte infection. Its manifestations vary greatly. A minimally inflamed annular plaque is most common, but nonannular, erythematous, and indurated lesions also occur. Severe forms with perifollicular granulomas are rare. If there is widespread neck, face, and chest involvement, **tinea capitis** may be serving as a nidus for spread.
2. **Tinea pedis (athlete's foot)** consists of erythema, burning, itching, and scaling on the sole and dorsal surfaces of the foot, most often in the interdigital webs. It often serves as a port of entry for bacterial infection or cellulitis (tinea pedis complex).
3. **Tinea unguium (onychomycosis)** is often associated with tinea pedis. There are three types:
   a. **Distal,** which causes yellow-brown discoloration of the nail plate
   b. **Proximal,** which causes white discoloration and debris under the nail fold
   c. **White superficial onychomycosis,** which causes a white, plaque-like layer on top of the nail that easily scrapes off.
4. **Tinea capitis** may cause scaling, alopecia, and cervical lymphadenopathy. Impetigo-like crusting may occur as well. In severe forms, a kerion (erythema, induration, crusting) may develop. Classic black-dot tinea is rare.

C. **Diagnosis.** The edge of the lesion is scraped with a glass slide; 20% potassium hydroxide (KOH) and a coverglass are added; and the slide is examined under a microscope. Arthrospores and hyphae are diagnostic. In questionable cases, the scraping should be cultured to confirm the diagnosis.

D. Therapy

    1. Topical (tinea corporis or tinea pedis). Clotrimazole or miconazole is applied to the lesions twice daily for 2–3 weeks. Terbinafine, which is applied for 4 weeks, is a second-line therapy. Topical steroids should be avoided. Selenium shampoo helps to prevent the spread of tinea capitis.

    2. Systemic (tinea capitis, tinea unguium, failed topical therapy for tinea corporis or tinea pedis, and all immunocompromised hosts). Itraconazole or griseofulvin is commonly used. Tinea capitis and tinea unguium require 3–12 months of treatment. Kerions often respond to treatment with an antifungal agent plus a 2-week tapering course of prednisone. Treatment-resistant tinea corporis or tinea pedis requires 2–3 weeks of therapy. An infectious disease expert should be consulted when the patient is immunocompromised.

E. Morbidity and mortality rates usually are low unless the patient has an associated immunodeficiency.

III IMPETIGO

A. Pathogenesis. Impetigo is a superficial skin infection that is usually caused by *Staphylococcus aureus* or *group A streptococcus*. *S. aureus* is the most common agent in both the crusted and bullous varieties of impetigo.

B. Epidemiology. Impetigo is most common in the summer and among those living in crowded conditions with poor hygiene.

C. Symptoms. Classically, the lesion may be crusted and golden or bullous. Local adenopathy is common. Any part of the body may be involved.

D. Therapy. Systemic therapy is needed if the lesions are widespread. Topical therapy with mupirocin is adequate if the infection is localized. If the lesions are resistant to treatment, culture is indicated.

IV CERVICAL LYMPHADENITIS

A. Pathogenesis. Cervical lymphadenitis is often a bacterial complication of tonsillitis or tooth infection. It may also occur by direct extension from skin trauma. However, a clinically recognizable source of infection is not a prerequisite for diagnosis. Adenitis may be acute (< 2 weeks) or subacute.

    1. Causes of acute adenitis include *S. aureus, group A streptococcus, Haemophilus influenzae, actinomyces, herpes simplex virus, Epstein-Barr virus* (EBV), *adenovirus*, and *cytomegalovirus*.

    2. Causes of subacute adenitis include *Bartonella henselae*, atypical mycobacteria, tuberculosis, HIV, fungus (*Histoplasma* species, *Coccidioides* species), and *Toxoplasma gondii*.

B. Symptoms. Nodes are erythematous, indurated, and often tender to palpation.

C. Therapy

1. For **suppurative adenitis,** antibiotics that cover streptococci and staphylococci (e.g., cephalexin, dicloxacillin) are given. Anaerobic coverage should be provided if a dental focus is suspected (e.g., clindamycin, trimethoprim-sulfamethoxazole). Treatment-resistant cases require intravenous antibiotics (e.g., nafcillin, cefazolin) and surgical drainage.

2. If adenopathy is **chronic,** or if antibiotic therapy does not ameliorate the condition, consider the causes of subacute adenitis (see IV A 2). Malignancy should also be considered.

V PERIORBITAL OR ORBITAL CELLULITIS

A. Pathogenesis. Periorbital and orbital cellulitis may be a complication of sinusitis, conjunctivitis, tooth abscess, or cellulitis. Periorbital cellulitis involves the tissues in front of the orbital septum, whereas orbital cellulitis involves the structures of the orbit, including the extraocular muscles and cranial nerves. Causative organisms include *S. aureus, Streptococcus pyogenes, Peptostreptococcus* species, *Bacteroides* species, or *H. influenzae.*

B. Symptoms. Although both conditions may cause fever as well as swelling and erythema of the eyelid and preseptal tissues, orbital cellulitis is distinguished by proptosis, extraocular motor palsies, and pain with eye movement.

C. Diagnosis. Computed tomography scan is indicated if orbital cellulitis is suspected.

D. Therapy. Intravenous antibiotics are needed for both periorbital and orbital cellulitis. Cefuroxime is the drug of choice. Periorbital cellulitis requires intravenous antibiotics until the induration subsides. Orbital cellulitis is a medical emergency that requires prompt consultation with an ophthalmologist. Orbital cellulitis requires at least 2 weeks of therapy; surgical debridement is often required.

E. Morbidity and mortality. In patients with orbital cellulitis, morbidity is greatly reduced with early diagnosis and treatment.

VI TOXIC SHOCK SYNDROME (TSS)

A. Pathogenesis. Toxic shock syndrome is caused by a bacterial toxin from *S. aureus* or *group A streptococcus*. It is a multisystemic disease process that is associated with tampon use, surgical wound infections, septic abortions, cutaneous lesions (e.g., varicella zoster virus), sinusitis, and pneumonia.

B. Clinical case definitions of staphylococcal and streptococcal TSS are presented in **Tables 37-1** and **37-2,** respectively.

TABLE 37-1. Staphylococcal Toxic Shock Syndrome: Clinical Case Definition

- Fever: temperature $\geq$ 38.9°C (102.0°F)
- Rash: diffuse macular erythroderma
- Desquamation: 1–2 weeks after onset, particularly palms and soles
- Hypotension: systolic blood pressure $\leq$ 90 mm Hg for adults; lower than fifth percentile by age for children younger than 16 years of age; orthostatic decrease in diastolic blood pressure of $\geq$ 15 mm Hg from lying to sitting; orthostatic syncope or orthostatic dizziness
- Multisystem involvement: three or more of the following:
  - Gastrointestinal: vomiting or diarrhea at onset of illness
  - Muscular: severe myalgia or creatinine phosphokinase level greater than twice the upper limit of normal
  - Mucous membrane: vaginal, oropharyngeal, or conjunctival hyperemia
  - Renal: serum urea nitrogen or serum creatinine level greater than twice the upper limit of normal or urinary sediment with $\geq$ five white blood cells per high-power field in the absence of a urinary tract infection
  - Hepatic: total bilirubin, aspartate aminotransferase, or alanine aminotransferase level greater than twice the upper limit of normal
  - Hematologic: platelet count, $< 100 \times 10^9$/L ($< 100 \times 10^3$/µl)
  - Central nervous system: disorientation or alterations in consciousness without focal neurologic signs when fever and hypotension are absent
- Negative results on the following tests, if obtained:
  - Blood, throat, or cerebrospinal fluid cultures; blood culture may be positive for *Staphylococcus aureus*
  - Serologic tests for Rocky Mountain spotted fever, leptospirosis, or measles

Case Classification

Probable: A case with five of the six aforementioned clinical findings

Confirmed: A case with all six of the clinical findings, including desquamation
If the patient dies before desquamation could have occurred, the other five criteria constitute a definitive case

Adapted with permission from Wharton M, Chorba TL, Vogt RL, et al: Case definitions for public health surveillance. *MMWR Morb Mortal Wkly Rep* 39(RR-13):1–43, 1990.

TABLE 37-2. Streptococcal Toxic Shock Syndrome: Clinical Case Definition

I. Isolation of group A β-hemolytic streptococci
   A. From a normally sterile site (e.g., blood, cerebrospinal fluid, peritoneal fluid, tissue biopsy specimen)
   B. From a nonsterile site (e.g., throat, sputum, vagina)
II. Clinical signs of severity
   A. Hypotension: systolic blood pressure ≤ 90 mm Hg in adults or lower than the fifth percentile for age in children

   AND

   B. Two or more of the following signs:
   - Renal impairment: creatinine level, ≥ 177 μmol/L (≥ 2 mg/dl) for adults or two times or more the upper limit of normal for age
   - Coagulopathy: platelet count, $\leq 100 \times 10^9$/L ($\leq 100 \times 10^3$/μl) or disseminated intravascular coagulation
   - Hepatic involvement: alanine aminotransferase, aspartate aminotransferase, or total bilirubin levels two times or more the upper limit of normal for age
   - Adult respiratory distress syndrome
   - A generalized erythematous macular rash that may desquamate
   - Soft tissue necrosis, including necrotizing fasciitis or myositis, or gangrene

An illness fulfilling criteria IA and II A and II B can be defined as a *definite* case. An illness fulfilling criteria IB and IIA and IIB can be defined as a *probable* case if no other cause for the illness is identified. (Adapted with permission from The Working Group on Severe Streptococcal Infections: Defining the group A streptococcal toxic shock syndrome: rationale and consensus definition. *JAMA* 269:390–391, 1993.)

C. The **differential diagnosis** of TSS includes Rocky Mountain spotted fever, leptospirosis, measles, and ehrlichiosis.
D. Therapy. Aggressive intravenous fluid administration is needed for all patients. Antibiotics are given to eliminate the toxin-producing bacterial focus. Nafcillin and clindamycin (to disable protein synthesis) should be started empirically. Intravenous immunoglobulin is reserved for patients who do not respond to conventional treatment or for those with an infection in a site that cannot be drained. A pelvic examination should be performed to look for a retained tampon, diaphragm, or contraceptive sponge. Patients with hypotension need aggressive fluid resuscitation and admission to an intensive care unit.

VII NECROTIZING FASCIITIS

A. Pathogenesis. Necrotizing fasciitis (NF) may be a complication of omphalitis, late-onset group B *Streptococcus,* sepsis, circumcision, necrotizing enterocolitis, appendicitis, impetigo, varicella zoster virus, or Hirschsprung disease. The hallmark of NF is rapid extension of infection within the fascial planes. It is usually caused by staphylococci or streptococci, but may be polymicrobial if the source of infection is abdominal. Toxic shock syndrome may accompany NF.

B. Epidemiology. Between 10% and 16% of patients with omphalitis progress to necrotizing fasciitis.

C. Signs and symptoms include tachycardia, fever, white blood cell count greater than 20,000 cells/mm^3, peau d'orange (tough skin resembling an orange), and violaceous skin. Leukopenia is a worrisome finding.

HOT

Pain is often out of proportion to physical findings.

KEY

D. Diagnosis is made by clinical criteria. Patients with suspected necrotizing fasciitis need frequent assessments to monitor for rapidly spreading infection.

E. Therapy. Antibiotic regimens should cover staphylococci, gram-negative organisms, and anaerobes. Surgical debridement is the cornerstone of therapy. Hyperbaric oxygen therapy should be considered as an adjunctive measure.

F. Morbidity and mortality. A good outcome depends on prompt surgical intervention.

References

Herold BC, Immergluck LC, Maranan MC, et al: Community-acquired methicillin-resistant *Staphylococcus aureus* in children with no identified predisposing risk. *JAMA* 279(8):593–598, 1998.

Howard RM, Frieden IJ: Dermatophyte infections in children. *Adv Pediatr Infect Dis* 14:73–107, 1999.

38. Epiglottitis, Retropharyngeal Abscess, and Peritonsillar Abscess

I INTRODUCTION

A. Background
1. Retropharyngeal abscess, peritonsillar abscess, and epiglottitis are major pediatric otolaryngologic emergencies.
2. The incidence of epiglottitis has decreased dramatically since the introduction of the *Haemophilus influenzae* type B (HIB) vaccine.

B. Pathogenesis (Table 38-1)
1. **Retropharyngeal abscess** occurs as a result of necrosis of the retropharyngeal nodes. This type of abscess is also seen in the setting of a perforated pharynx. Purulent material collects between the retropharyngeal and prevertebral layers of the cervical fascia, which is normally a potential space that extends from the mediastinum to the base of the skull.
2. **Peritonsillar abscess** results from an accumulation of purulent material in the tonsillar fossa. This abscess typically produces a bulge in the posterior aspect of the soft palate, which causes uvular deviation.
3. **Epiglottitis** results from infection and swelling of the epiglottis and arytenoepiglottic folds. Epiglottitis is characterized by sudden, severe compromise of the airway.

C. Epidemiology (see Table 38-1)
D. Etiology (see Table 38-1)

II CLINICAL MANIFESTATIONS (see Table 38-1)

> **HOT** **KEY**
> All can present with fever, sore throat, and dysphagia. Children with epiglottis or retropharyngeal abscess appear more toxic and have associated stridor and drooling. Those with peritonsillar abscesses may have the classic triad of trismus, muffled ("hot potato") voice, and uvular deviation.

III APPROACH TO THE PATIENT

A. History. Typically, retropharyngeal and peritonsillar abscesses

TABLE 38-1. Comparison of Features of Retropharyngeal Abscess, Peritonsillar Abscess, and Epiglottitis

Feature	Retropharyngeal Abscess	Peritonsillar Abscess	Epiglottitis
Pathogenesis	Necrosis of retropharyngeal nodes, perforated pharynx, collection of purulent material between layers of cervical fascia	Accumulation of purulent material in the tonsillar fossa	Infection and swelling of the epiglottis and arytenoepiglottic folds
Epidemiology	Children < 4 years of age	Older children, adolescents	Children 3–6 years of age, second peak at 15–30 years of age
Etiology	Streptococcus (e.g., group A), Staphylococcus aureus, anaerobic species, usually mixed flora	Streptococcus (e.g., group A), S. aureus, anaerobic species	Haemophilus influenzae type B, group A streptococcus, Epstein-Barr virus
Symptoms	Fever, sore throat, dysphagia, cervical lymphadenopathy, neck pain, toxic appearance, stridor, drooling	Fever, sore throat, dysphagia, cervical lymphadenopathy, neck pain, trismus muffled ("hot potato") voice, uvular deviation	Fever (sudden onset, often > 39°C in the first 24 hours), sore throat, dysphagia, cervical lymphadenopathy, neck pain, toxic or anxious appearance, inspiratory stridor, respiratory distress, tripoding or sniffing position (sitting forward with the neck extended and the chin thrust out), drooling, hoarse cough, tachypnea, cyanosis

first appear as routine pharyngitis; these abscesses represent severe suppurative complications. Epiglottitis begins more acutely, with sudden onset of severe symptoms. Usually there have been no preceding symptoms of an upper respiratory infection or pharyngitis.

B. Workup and treatment. Retropharyngeal abscesses and epiglottitis are true emergencies because the airway may become compromised. If the security of the airway is in question, the patient must be kept calm. The patient should be allowed to assume a comfortable position and should not be restrained or forced to lie down. In addition, procedures or examinations that might agitate the patient (e.g., placement of peripheral intravenous lines, blood tests, examination using a tongue depressor) should be avoided.

 1. **Retropharyngeal abscess**
    a. If the airway is secure, a lateral neck film is obtained. Widening of the retropharyngeal space (more than one half of the width of the adjacent cervical vertebrae) or the finding of an air–fluid level is diagnostic of this type of abscess. A computed tomography (CT) scan can also be used as a more sensitive and specific test.
    b. An otolaryngologist should be consulted immediately because surgical drainage may be required. Mild cases may respond to antibiotic therapy alone, but most patients require surgery. Spontaneous drainage of a retropharyngeal abscess may lead to life-threatening aspiration.
    c. **Broad-spectrum antibiotics** (e.g., clindamycin or ampicillin-sulbactam) are started empirically and modified pending culture results.
 2. **Epiglottitis.** A patient with epiglottitis is at great risk of having a sudden, fatal airway obstruction.
    a. **If the patient is unstable or if the diagnosis of epiglottitis is clear on clinical grounds alone,** the child is immediately anesthetized and intubated in the operating room. Intravenous access, a complete blood cell (CBC) count with differential, blood cultures, and culture swabs are obtained only after the airway is secured. Ceftriaxone is the treatment of choice.
    b. **If the patient is stable and the diagnosis is unclear clinically,** lateral and anteroposterior neck films are obtained with the patient's chin extended in the sniffing position. An enlarged epiglottis "thumb sign" or blurred folds may be visible. Because emergent intubation may be required, intubation equipment and rapid sequence intubation medications should accompany the patient to the radiography suite.

3. Peritonsillar abscesses

   a. If the patient's airway is secure, examination with a tongue depressor is allowed. A classic finding is a bulge in the posterior aspect of the soft palate, with uvular deviation.
   b. Fluctuant masses should be aspirated and drained.
   c. Intravenous antibiotic therapy (e.g., clindamycin or a first-generation cephalosporin) is started empirically pending the results of a culture of tonsillar aspirate.
   d. Tonsillectomy may be required if the patient does not respond to therapy within 48–72 hours.

References

Friedman NR, Mitchell RB, Pereira KD, et al: Peritonsillar abscess in early childhood: presentation and management. *Arch Otolaryngol Head Neck Surg* 123(6):630–632, 1997.

Lalakea ML, Messner AH: Retropharyngeal abscess management in children: current practices. *Otolaryngol Head Neck Surg* 121(4):398–405, 1999.

39. Osteomyelitis

I INTRODUCTION

A. Background. Osteomyelitis is an infection of bone that affects 1:5000 children in the United States each year. It is difficult to treat and is most common between 3 and 12 years of age.

B. Pathogenesis occurs by three different mechanisms.

1. **Hematogenous seeding during bacteremia** is the most common mechanism. In children with hematogenously disseminated disease, seeding most often occurs in the metaphyses of long bones, usually as a single focus. The femur and tibia are the most commonly affected bones, followed by the humerus, calcaneus, and pelvis. Forty percent of affected neonates have multiple infected bone sites.

2. **Local invasion from contiguous infected structures** can occur with cellulitis, decubitus ulcer, or periodontal disease.

3. **Direct inoculation** of bone, surgically or from trauma.

II CLINICAL MANIFESTATIONS.

A broad range of symptoms occur, including fever, discrete pain and swelling, persistent limp, and refusal to use a limb. Joint movement may be limited because of local muscle spasm. In older children, symptoms tend to localize to the affected bone.

HOT KEY

The clinical presentation can be similar to that of septic arthritis. However, in older children, palpation of the affected portion of bone is more painful than isolated movement of the affected joint.

III APPROACH TO THE PATIENT

A. Diagnosis. Any two of the following findings satisfy the diagnostic criteria for osteomyelitis. These criteria can be remembered using the mnemonic "PIPE"

PIPE

Purulence of bone (white blood cells, organisms, pus)
Imaging study results (e.g., radiograph, bone scan, magnetic resonance imaging) consistent with osteomyelitis
Positive culture of bone or blood
Erythema or edema in the area overlying the presumed site of infection

B. Differential diagnosis includes fracture, rheumatic fever, septic arthritis, toxic synovitis, cellulitis, bone infarction secondary to hemoglobinopathy, leukemia, and bone neoplasms (particularly Ewing sarcoma or metastatic neuroblastoma).

C. If the **initial workup** suggests osteomyelitis, an orthopedic surgeon should be consulted and a bone aspirate obtained.

1. Laboratory tests

    a. A **complete blood count (CBC) with differential** should be obtained. Leukocytosis with a left shift and thrombocytosis may be present.

    b. The **erythrocyte sedimentation rate (ESR)** is often elevated. The ESR is also helpful in determining the length of therapy (see III E 2).

    c. The **C-reactive protein (CRP)** level is useful in evaluating the early response to therapy.

2. Imaging studies

    a. Standard radiographs may not show bony changes associated with osteomyelitis for 7–10 days. However, many of the diseases included in the differential diagnosis can be excluded by standard radiographs.

    b. A **bone scan** is highly sensitive (80%–100% in older children). It can define multiple foci of infection and is helpful if the radiograph is negative because it shows changes in the first 24–48 hours of infection. However, a bone scan is less sensitive in neonates (30%–100% sensitivity) and in patients with sickle cell disease.

    c. Magnetic resonance imaging (MRI) scans are useful for delineating the extent of infection in complex cases. They also are used when infection occurs as a complication of trauma, surgery, or sickle cell anemia. MRI is 92%–100% sensitive, but somewhat less specific.

HOT KEY Identification of the causative microorganism is essential for treatment. Bone aspirates (80% are positive) and blood cultures (60% are positive) must be obtained.

D. Initial antibiotic therapy

1. Parenteral antibiotics are required to guarantee rapid peak serum concentrations and limit local and disseminated spread of infection. Therapy is continued for 4–6 weeks.

2. Empiric therapy is guided by the child's age and clinical history **(Table 39-1).** Tissue samples (e.g., blood, bone biopsy specimen) are obtained before therapy is initiated.

    a. In a fully immunized child beyond the newborn period, the most likely pathogens are *Staphylococcus aureus*

TABLE 39-1. Etiology of Acute Hematogenous Osteomyelitis in Infants and Children

Organism	Infants (%)	Children > 5 Years of Age (%)	Special Clinical Associations
Staphylococcus aureus	50	80	—
Group A streptococci	10	5	—
Haemophilus influenzae	10	2	Unimmunized children < 4 years of age
Atypical agents	15	13	—
Salmonella species	1	4	Patients with hemoglobinopathy
Escherichia coli	1	2	Patients with hemoglobinopathy
Pseudomonas aeruginosa	1	3	Foot puncture wound in sneaker wearers
Klebsiella species	1	1	—
Streptococcus pneumoniae	4	1	—
Anaerobes	1	1	Bite wounds, dental procedures
Candida species	1	1	Immunocompromised patients

Adapted with permission from Sonnen G, Henry N: Pediatric bone and joint infections: diagnosis and antimicrobial management. *Pediatr Clin North Am* 43(4):933–943, 1996.

and *Streptococcus pyogenes.* Therefore, a β-lactamase–resistant penicillin (e.g., nafcillin, oxacillin) or first-generation cephalosporin (e.g., cefazolin) is a good choice.

b. Children younger than 4 years of age who have not been fully immunized against *Haemophilus influenzae* should be given cefuroxime.

c. Vancomycin may be used if infection with methicillin-resistant *S. aureus* is suspected or if the patient is allergic to penicillin or cephalosporins.

d. Gonococcal osteomyelitis should be considered in adolescent patients who have concurrent pustular or hemorrhagic distal skin lesions. Ceftriaxone is the drug of choice.

e. Once a specific organism is isolated and the results of antimicrobial susceptibility tests are available, therapy is tailored accordingly.

E. Ongoing management

1. Surgical drainage is required if a subperiosteal or bone abscess is present on radiographs or if pus is found on bone aspiration.

2. Switching to **oral therapy** may be considered in patients who show improvement clinically and based on laboratory values (e.g., CRP = 2 mg/dl, ESR decreased 10–20 mm/hr from initial value).

a. Therapeutic levels of an oral agent (e.g., cephalexin) are assessed by an oral dosing trial while the patient continues to receive parenteral therapy. After a therapeutic drug level of the oral agent is documented, further assessment of therapeutic levels is not necessary if compliance is not in question.

b. The reliability of the family and patient as well as their ability to administer the therapy on an outpatient basis must be considered before discharge.

c. A CBC with differential is performed weekly for patients who are receiving β-lactam therapy because of the potential for bone marrow suppression.

HOT

KEY
Consider tuberculosis in patients who show a poor response to treatment or who have negative culture results.

 PROGNOSIS. Prompt recognition and appropriate treatment are essential to prevent serious complications. Inadequate or delayed antibiotic therapy often leads to chronic

abscess formation, draining sinus tracts, pathologic fractures, and orthopedic deformity.

References
Lew D, Waldvogel F: Osteomyelitis. *N Engl J Med* 336(14):999–1007, 1997.
Sonnen G, Henry N: Pediatric bone and joint infections: diagnosis and antimicrobial
    management. *Pediatr Clin North Am* 43(4):933–943, 1996.

40. Septic Arthritis

I INTRODUCTION

A. Background. Septic arthritis, a bacterial infection within the joint space, is one of the rare infectious disease emergencies in pediatrics. Failure to initiate therapy at an early stage can have devastating effects on the affected limb.

B. Pathogenesis

1. There are three general modes of bacterial entry into the joint space:
   a. Hematogenous spread (the synovial membrane receives a high amount of blood flow)
   b. Direct inoculation (usually from a puncture wound)
   c. Contiguous extension from osteomyelitis (this is relatively rare)

2. **Sequence of events.** Bacteria enter the joint space, forming a pannus. Polymorphonuclear cells release granules that degrade cartilage. This degradation increases vascular permeability and fluid production, ultimately increasing pressure within the joint space. The increased pressure causes compression and thrombosis of intra-articular vessels, which leads to further joint destruction.

3. **Joint pain** is caused by stretching of the fibrous joint capsule. Inflammation within the joint cavity elicits an axon reflex that causes vasodilation and warmth over the affected joint.

C. Epidemiology. Septic arthritis is more common in children than in adults. Among children, there is a 2:1 male:female predominance. The relationship between trauma and septic arthritis is unknown, although a history of trauma often is sought as a predisposing determinant.

D. Microbiology

1. The most common pathogen routinely isolated is *Staphylococcus aureus* (60%), followed by group A streptococcus (26%), *Enterobacter* species (7%), and *Streptococcus pneumoniae* (6%).

2. *Haemophilus influenzae,* once a common culprit, has almost disappeared since the advent of routine vaccination.

3. *Salmonella* should be considered in patients who have sickle cell disease or other hemoglobinopathies.

4. *Neisseria gonorrhoeae* should be considered in newborns and sexually active adolescents. Septic arthritis due to *N. gonorrhoeae* almost always occurs in association with infection in the genitourinary tract, rectum, or pharynx.

5. In one third of cases, no specific type of bacteria is identified. In such cases, the causative organism may be *Kingella* species, which is notoriously difficult to culture.
6. Other rare causes include rat-bite fever, *Borrelia burgdorferi,* and *Corynebacterium diphtheriae.*

II **CLINICAL MANIFESTATIONS.** Most patients have fever and constitutional symptoms. Focal findings (e.g., erythema, effusion, tenderness) are almost always present. The most commonly affected joints are the knees (38%) and hips (32%). Less commonly affected are the ankles (11%), elbows (8%), shoulders (5%), wrists (4%), and small diarthrodial joints (2%).

A. **Single joint involvement.** Only 5% of patients with septic arthritis have more than one involved joint. Multiple joint involvement suggests a rheumatologic cause.
B. **Tenderness with movement.** Any movement that increases intracapsular pressure causes pain. This pain causes muscle spasm, which places the joint in a position that maximizes articular volume and minimizes intra-articular pressure and pain (i.e., antalgic position). Hips are held in abduction, flexion, and external rotation. Knees are held in partial flexion, shoulders are held in adduction and internal rotation, and elbows are held in midflexion.

HOT **KEY** A septic hip should be suspected in infants or young children with thigh or buttock swelling or in those presenting in an antalgic position, even in the absence of systemic symptoms or leukocytosis.

III **APPROACH TO THE PATIENT**

A. **Diagnosis.** Plain films usually are of little use in making the initial diagnosis, unless the joint in question is the hip.
1. **Hip films** should be obtained in the frog leg position and with the legs extended at the knee and slightly rotated internally. When swelling is present in the hip joint capsule, the gluteal fat lines are laterally displaced. As the hip joint capsule continues to swell, the femoral head is displaced laterally and upward.
2. **Aspiration of joint fluid.** Because of the potential risk of missing a diagnosis, the threshold for tapping a joint should be low. The gold standard for diagnosis is joint fluid culture. Fluid should be sent for Gram stain and cell count. The joint fluid should be sent in a heparinized syringe **(Table 40-1).**
a. Because noninfectious causes of arthritis also may present

TABLE 40-1. Characteristic Synovial Fluid Findings

Diagnosis	WBC/μL		% PMNs (typical)
	Typical	Range	
Normal	< 150	—	< 25
Bacterial arthritis	> 50,000	2,000–300,000	> 90
Tuberculosis arthritis	10,000–20,000	40–136,000	> 50 (10–99)
Lyme arthritis	40,000	180–100,000	> 75
Candida arthritis	—	7,500–150,000	> 90
Viral arthritis	15,000	3,000–50,000	< 50 (variable)
Reiter syndrome	15,000	10,000–22,000	> 70 (37–98)
Rheumatoid arthritis	—	2,000–50,000	> 70
Rheumatic fever	25,000	2,000–50,000	> 70

Reprinted with permission from Long SS, Pickering LK, Prober CG: *Principles and Practice of Pediatric Infectious Diseases.* Philadelphia, WB Saunders, 1997, p 538.
PMNs = polymorphonuclear cells; WBC = white blood cells.

with leukocytes in the synovial fluid, fluid should always be cultured.

   b. Synovial fluid is bacteriostatic; therefore, organisms seen on Gram stain may not grow from synovial fluid. Synovial culture results are positive in 50% to 60% of cases.

   c. Latex agglutination may be helpful for identifying *H. influenzae* or *S. pneumoniae.*

  3. A **blood culture** should always be obtained because it may provide another means to identify the pathogen. Blood culture results are positive in 40% of cases.

B. The differential diagnosis includes toxic synovitis, osteomyelitis, Henoch-Schönlein purpura, viral arthritis, mycobacterial and fungal arthritis, traumatic arthritis, leukemia, serum sickness, and inflammatory bowel disease.

C. Additional tests to consider. The white blood cell count, erythrocyte sedimentation rate, and C-reactive protein level are usually elevated.

HOT **KEY**   The most common laboratory abnormalities in septic arthritis are an elevated C-reactive protein (mean, 9 mg/dl) and erythrocyte sedimentation rate (usually > 20 mm/h).

D. Antibiotic therapy. Empiric therapy is started with nafcillin or cefazolin.

  1. Therapy may be modified based on the results of Gram stain.

   a. Gram-negative cocci. Ceftriaxone therapy should be started to cover *Neisseria gonorrhoeae.*

   b. Gram-negative bacilli. Aminoglycoside and third-generation cephalosporin therapy should be started.

  2. The joint fluid concentration of antibiotics is high (approximately 30% of the serum level). Moreover, efflux is slow, so antibiotic levels in the joint space become cumulative. Antibiotic levels within the joint space actually may exceed levels in blood.

  3. Length of antibiotic therapy

   a. Gonococcus: 2 weeks

   b. Other bacteria: at least 3–4 weeks

   c. Once defervescence occurs, joint swelling decreases, and inflammatory markers (erythrocyte sedimentation rate and C-reactive protein level) return to normal, switching to oral antibiotics (e.g., high-dose cephalexin, dicloxacillin) is acceptable. Strict compliance with the oral medication regimen is essential. Most patients require serial synovial fluid analysis. Bactericidal concentrations in the serum and synovial fluid should be verified if the patient's condition is not improving.

E. Surgical management. Septic hips and shoulders require immediate open surgical debridement in the operating room. For
other joints, repeat aspirations may be as effective as open surgical drainage; however, tissue debris and loculations eventually may make surgical drainage necessary. Surgical drainage is
also necessary for recurrent culture-positive effusions.

F. Ongoing management includes immobilization of the joint in a
neutral functional position. Passive range-of-motion devices
help maintain circulation of synovial fluid and prevent contractures. Active range-of-motion and weight bearing are restricted
until pain and inflammation resolve.

IV PROGNOSIS

A. Morbidity. Complications include abscess, osteomyelitis, early
degenerative changes, and limited range of motion. The duration of symptoms before the initiation of specific therapy seems
to be the most important prognostic factor. *S. aureus* and
Enterobacteriaceae are associated with more sequelae than *H.
influenzae.*

B. Poor prognostic factors include age younger than 6 months, delayed therapy (> 5 days after the onset of symptoms), hip or
shoulder involvement, *S. aureus* infection, infection with gram-
negative organisms, and fungal infection.

References
Feigin RD, Cherry JD: *Textbook of Pediatric Infectious Disease,* 3rd ed. Philadelphia,
    WB Saunders, 1992, pp 739–745.
Dagan R: Management of acute hematogenous osteomyelitis and septic arthritis in the
    pediatric patient. *Pediatr Infect Dis J* 12:90, 1993.
Nade SML: Acute septic arthritis in infancy and childhood. *J Bone Joint Surg* [Br]
    65:234, 1983.

41. Sexually Transmitted Infections

....

I INTRODUCTION. Background:

A. Sexually transmitted infections (STIs) are a major cause of morbidity and mortality among adolescents.

B. Risk-taking behaviors put adolescents at greater risk for acquiring STIs.

II HISTORY AND PHYSICAL EXAMINATION

A. **History.** Inquire about sexual activity, sexual orientation, the number of sexual partners, the history of prior STIs, urethral or vaginal discharge, last menstrual period, dysuria, dyspareunia, genital lesions, fever, rashes, scrotal pain, and joint or abdominal pain.

B. **Physical examination**
   1. **Routine screening** for gonorrhea and chlamydia is recommended for all asymptomatic sexually active adolescents.
   2. All sexually active female adolescents should undergo an **annual pelvic examination** that includes the following components:
      a. Assessment for adnexal tenderness, adnexal masses, or cervical motion tenderness; note the appearance of the vaginal mucosa and cervical epithelium
      b. Cultures from the cervical os for chlamydia and gonococcus
      c. Additional viral cultures of suspicious lesions
      d. Wet mount, Gram stain, potassium hydroxide preparation, and pH of vaginal pool secretions
      e. Papanicolaou (Pap) smear annually to screen for cervical dysplasia and cancer

II CLINICAL SCENARIOS (Table 41-1)

A. **Pelvic inflammatory disease (PID)**
   1. **Introduction**
      a. **Description.** PID is an infection of the female upper genital tract that can include endometritis, salpingitis, or tubo-ovarian abscess. Unrecognized recurrent PID is a major cause of infertility.

TABLE 41-1. Overview of Sexually Transmitted Diseases

	Chlamydia (*Chlamydia trachomatis*)	Gonorrhea (*Neisseria gonorrhoeae*)	Herpes (HSV types I and II)	Syphilis (*Treponema pallidum*)	Candida (*Candida albicans*)	Genital Warts (*Human papilloma virus*)	Trichimonas (*Trichomonas vaginalis*)	Bacterial Vaginosis (*G. vaginalis, M. hominis, Anaerobes*)
General	Cervicitis, PID, urethritis Most common STI in adolescents 40% progress to upper tract infections if untreated	A gram-negative diplococcus cervicitis, PID, urethritis Chlamydia co-infection in 50% patients	HSV II is usually a genital pathogen; HSV I can also cause genital disease Primary and recurrent infections	Systemic disease Higher prevalence in HIV-positive people, IVDA, sex workers	Vulvovaginitis	Warts in genital region	Vulvovaginitis, urethritis	Vaginitis

(continued)

TABLE 41-1. Overview of Sexually Transmitted Diseases (Continued)

	Chlamydia (*Chlamydia trachomatis*)	Gonorrhea (*Neisseria gonorrhoeae*)	Herpes (HSV types I and II)	Syphilis (*Treponema pallidum*)	Candida (*Candida albicans*)	Genital Warts (*Human papilloma virus*)	Trichomonas (*Trichomonas vaginalis*)	Bacterial Vaginosis (*G. vaginalis, M. hominis*, Anaerobes)
Symptoms	General: 75% of cases are asymptomatic Females: lower abdominal pain, dysuria, fever, mucopurulent discharge, dyspareunia Males: asymptomatic (25%) dysuria, penile discharge	Females: 80% are asymptomatic. Lower abdominal pain, purulent vaginal discharge, dyspareunia Males: penile discharge, dysuria Both: rectal symptoms, pharyngitis	Primary outbreak: fever, malaise, lymphadenopathy, genital dysesthesia, burning followed by vesicles and painful ulcers Recurrent: dysesthesias, painful ulcers, usually no systemic symptoms	Primary: painless chancre or ulcers at infection site Secondary: rash, mucocutaneous lesions, adenopathy Tertiary: aortitis, iritis, gummas, Argyl-Robertson pupils, tabes dorsalis	Thick, white vaginal discharge, vaginal pruritus, burning, erythema	Warts grow on the perineum, vulva, and anus Itching, vaginal discharge	Females: copious frothy vaginal discharge; vulvar irritation ± pruritus dyspareunia, dysuria Males: asymptomatic, occasionally urethritis	Females: thin, malodorous, fishy-smelling discharge, vulvar itching or burning

Diagnosis	Gold standard: endocervical or urethral culture Sensitivity, 70%–90%; Specificity, 100% Cervicitis: friable erythematous cervix and vaginal discharge Urethritis: Gram stain of urethral secretions with > 5 WBCs per HPF or LE+	Gold standard: endocervical or urethral culture Sensitivity, 80%–95% Cervicitis: pelvic exam findings are the same as for chlamydia Urethritis: same diagnostic criteria as for chlamydia	Gold standard: viral culture within 72 hours Sensitivity varies: vesicles, 93%; ulcers, 72%; crusted lesions, 27% Lesion appearance: shallow painful ulcers, clustered, linear, or serpiginous, erythematous borders, may be crusted	Darkfield examinations and DFA tests of lesion exudate = definitive diagnosis OR serologies (nontreponemal: VDRL and RPR, or treponemal: FTA-ABS or MHA-TP) Nontreponemal tests correlate with disease activity	Vaginal erythema: vaginal pH < 4.5 KOH preparation: buds, pseudohyphae; these may also be seen on wet mount	Verrucous-appearing lesions, weak (3%) acetic acid may help the diagnosis	Cervicitis: vaginal erythema, "strawberry" appearance of cervix Vaginal pH > 4.5 Wet mount: WBCs, trichomonads	Vaginal erythema "whiff test": fishy odor after the addition of KOH solution Vaginal pH > 4.5 Wet mount: clue cells

(continued)

TABLE 41-1. Overview of Sexually Transmitted Diseases (Continued)

	Chlamydia (Chlamydia trachomatis)	Gonorrhea (Neisseria gonorrhoeae)	Herpes (HSV types I and II)	Syphilis (Treponema pallidum)	Candida (Candida albicans)	Genital Warts (Human papilloma virus)	Trichimonas (Trichomonas vaginalis)	Bacterial Vaginosis (G. vaginalis, M. hominis, Anaerobes)
Additional tests to consider	Endocervical or urethral sample for EIA or DFA Sensitivity, 70%–90%; Specificity, 97%–99% First-void urine for LCR, sensitivity/ specificity > 95%	Gram stain: consider when culture is not available Symptomatic males: sensitivity 90%–95% Asymptomatic males: sensitivity, 70% Symptomatic females: sensitivity 30%–65% First-void urine for LCR, sensitivity/ specificity > 95%	HSV PCR Tzanck stain Pap may also be diagnostic Serum antibodies: not specific, titers are 10–100 times lower in asymptomatic patients	Sensitivity of tests increases in secondary syphilis (62%–76% to 100%) Always investigate for HIV co-infection	Vaginal culture	Pathology specimen	Pap may also be diagnostic	Vaginal culture

Therapy	Azithromycin (1 g orally once) OR doxycycline (100 mg twice daily for 7 days) Alternative antibiotic therapies: erythromycin (500 mg four times daily for 7 days) or emycin (250 mg four times daily for 14 days) or ofloxacin (300 mg twice daily for 7 days)	Cefixime (400 mg orally one time) or ceftriaxone (125 mg intramuscularly once) or ciprofloxacin (500 mg orally once) or ofloxacin (400 mg orally once) plus chlamydia treatment	First episode/primary infection: acyclovir (400 mg orally twice daily or 200 mg 5 times per day for 7 days) or famciclovir (250 mg three times daily for 7-10 days) or valacyclovir (1 g twice daily for 7-10 days)	Primary and secondary: benzathine penicillin G (50,000 units/kg intramuscularly up to the adult dose of 2.4 million units in a single dose) Tertiary: benzathine penicillin G 2.4 units intramuscularly weekly for 3 doses	Patient applied: podofilox × 0.5% solution or gel (apply twice daily for 3 days, then off for 4 days; may repeat for 4 cycles) or imiquimod 5% cream (apply once daily three times per week; wash after 6-10 hours; may use for up to 16 weeks)	Clotrimazole (1% cream (5 g) intravaginal application once daily for 7 days) Miconazole (2% vaginal cream once daily for 7 days or 200-mg vaginal suppository hourly for 3 days) Diflucan (150 mg orally for 1 dose)	Metronidazole (2 g orally once or 500 mg twice daily for 7 days)	Metronidazole (500 mg orally twice daily for 7 days) or clindamycin cream 2% (one application) or 5 mg (once daily for 7 days); or metronidazole gel 0.75% (1 application once daily for 7 days)

(continued)

TABLE 41-1. Overview of Sexually Transmitted Diseases (Continued)

	Chlamydia (Chlamydia trachomatis)	Gonorrhea (Neisseria gonorrhoeae)	Herpes (HSV types I and II)	Syphilis (Treponema pallidum)	Candida (Candida albicans)	Genital Warts (Human papilloma virus)	Trichimonas (Trichomonas vaginalis)	Bacterial Vaginosis (G. vaginalis, M. hominis, Anaerobes)
Therapy (continued)								Alternative therapies: metronidazole (2 g orally once) or clindamycin (300 mg orally twice daily for 7 days)
Ongoing management	Treat partners Abstinence during treatment or for 7 days if single dose	Treat for co-infection with chlamydia Abstinence with therapy Report to	Recurrent infections: acyclovir (400 mg orally three times daily or 200 mg	Test for cure is required: titers (RPR or VDRL) should decrease fourfold at	If recurrences: consider diabetes and HIV, extend treatment Do not need	Provider applied: cryotherapy, laser surgery, podophyllin 10%–25%	Treatment failure: metronidazole (500 mg twice daily for	Do not need to treat partners

(continued)

is used
Check health
department
for reporting
regulations
Test of cure
only if
persistent
symptoms

health
department
Test of cure
only if
persistent
symptoms

5 times daily
or 800 mg
twice daily
for 5 days)
or famciclo-
vir (125 mg
twice daily
for 5 days)
or valacyclo-
vir (500 mg
twice daily
for 5 days)
Suppression
(> 6 epi-
sodes per
year)
Acyclovir
(400 mg
twice daily)
or famciclo-
vir (250 mg
twice daily)
or valacyclo-
vir (250 mg
twice daily)

6 months
to undetect-
able at
12 months
Seek infectious
disease
specialist
consultation
for treatment
failures

to treat
partners

or trichloro-
acetic acid
8%–90%,
apply
weekly as
needed

7 days
or 2 g
orally for
5 days)
Discourage
alcohol use
when on
metro-
nidazole
Treat partners

TABLE 41-1. Overview of Sexually Transmitted Diseases (*Continued*)

	Chlamydia (*Chlamydia trachomatis*)	Gonorrhea (*Neisseria gonorrhoeae*)	Herpes (HSV types I and II)	Syphilis (*Treponema pallidum*)	Candida (*Candida albicans*)	Genital Warts (*Human papilloma virus*)	Trichimonas (*Trichomonas vaginalis*)	Bacterial Vaginosis (*G. vaginalis, M. hominis, Anaerobes*)
Prognosis	Cured with treatment Untreated chlamydia can cause PID, ectopic pregnancy, and infertility In males: epididymitis and Reiter syndrome	Cured with treatment Can become disseminated with arthralgias, skin lesions, endocarditis, and meningitis	Potential perinatal transmission, neonatal HSV	Variable based on stage	Cured with treatment	HPV 16 and 18 association with cervical dysplasia	Cured with treatment	Curable Associated with endometritis, PID

PID = pelvic inflammatory disease; STI = sexually transmitted infection; HSV = herpes simplex virus; IVDA = intravenous drug abuse; WBC = white blood count; HPF = high-power field; LE+ = leukocyte esterase-positive; DFA = direct fluorescent antibody; VDRL = Venereal Disease Research Laboratory; RPR = rapid plasmin reagin; FTA-ABS = fluorescent treponemal antibody; MHA-TP = microhemagglutination-*Treponema pallidum*; KOH = potassium hydroxide; EIA = enzyme immunoassay; LCR = ligase chain reaction; PCR = polymerase chain reaction; Pap = Papanicolaou.

*All dosages are for adult-sized patients.

      b. Causative agents include *Neisseria gonorrhoeae* and *Chlamydia trachomatis.* Gram-negative rods and anaerobes may co-infect to produce a polymicrobial infection.

2. Diagnosis

      a. Minimal criteria include lower abdominal tenderness, adnexal tenderness, and cervical motion tenderness.

      b. Definitive criteria include endometrial biopsy showing endometritis, transvaginal ultrasound showing a thickened tube or free fluid, or positive laparoscopic findings.

      c. Additional criteria that increase the likelihood of PID include an oral temperature higher than 101°F (38.3°C), abnormal cervical or vaginal discharge, elevated erythrocyte sedimentation rate or C-reactive protein, or a cervical culture that is positive for chlamydia or gonorrhea.

3. Treatment

      a. Hospitalization is appropriate in the following circumstances: failure to respond to 72 hours of oral therapy, tubo-ovarian abscess, immunodeficiency, severe illness, or noncompliance.

      b. Outpatient antibiotic regimens commonly include ofloxacin (400 mg orally twice daily for 14 days) plus metronidazole (500 mg orally twice daily for 14 days). Alternatively, ceftriaxone (250 mg intramuscularly) or another third-generation cephalosporin, such as cefixime, plus doxycycline (100 mg orally twice daily for 14 days) may be used.

      c. Parenteral antibiotic regimens include cefotetan (2 g every 12 hours) or cefoxitin (2 g every 6 hours) plus doxycycline (100 mg every 12 hours) or clindamycin (900 mg every 8 hours) plus gentamicin (2 mg/kg load, then 1.5 mg/kg every 8 hours; or a single daily dose).

B. Sexual assault

  1. Introduction. Sexual assault is the most rapidly growing violent crime in the United States. More than 700,000 women are sexually assaulted each year. Approximately 54% of the college women surveyed had been the victims of some form of sexual abuse; more than 25% of college-age women have been the victim of rape or attempted rape.

  2. Workup. Consultation should be sought for forensic sampling as well as counseling services.

      a. Sexual assault in children. A child abuse team should be consulted, a report should be made to Child Protection Services, and the child should be admitted to the hospital for protection if necessary.

      b. Laboratory studies. Samples are taken for chlamydia and gonococcus culture at any site of penetration. A wet mount is performed, and serum is tested for HIV, hepatitis B, and syphilis.

    c. Preventive antibiotics. Three antibiotics are administered:
    ceftriaxone (125 mg intramuscularly), metronidazole (2 g
    orally, in a single dose), and azithromycin (1 g orally, in a
    single dose).

    d. Hepatitis B prophylaxis. Vaccination (without hepatitis B
    immunoglobulin) at the time of the initial examination is
    sufficient. Follow-up vaccines are administered at 1–2 and
    4–6 months after the first dose.

    e. HIV prophylaxis is considered on a patient-by-patient
    basis.

    f. Emergency contraception should be considered within 72
    hours of assault (e.g., Ovral, two white pills for the first
    dose, repeated in 12 hours). Benadryl may be adminis-
    tered as required for nausea.

3. Ongoing management. A follow-up examination should be
performed at 2 weeks; at this time, the cultures and wet
mount should be repeated. Serologic tests are repeated at 6,
12, and 24 weeks. The need for ongoing psychological support should be assessed.

References
Biro FM: New developments in diagnosis and management of adolescents with sexu-
    ally transmitted disease. *Curr Opin Obstet Gynecol* 11(5):451–455, 1999.
Centers for Disease Control and Prevention: 1998 Guidelines for treatment of sexu-
    ally transmitted diseases. *MMWR Morb Mortal Wkly Rep* 47(RR-1):1–118, 1998.
United States Preventive Services Task Force: *Guide to Clinical Preventive Services,*
    2nd ed. Alexandria, VA, International Medical Publishers, 1996.

42. Human Immunodeficiency Virus

··

I **INTRODUCTION.** AIDS is caused by infection with HIV-1 or HIV-2. Pediatric patients with AIDS account for about 2% of known cases in the United States.

A. **Risk factors.** Birth to an HIV-infected mother and breast-feeding are the main risk factors for children. Because of blood bank screening, the risk of blood product–associated transmission is less than 1:200,000.

B. **Transmission.** Only blood, semen, cervical secretions, and breast milk are implicated in transmission. Most cases of pediatric HIV infection result from vertical transmission.

   1. Pediatric HIV infection mirrors HIV infection in women of childbearing age. Therefore, any reduction in the number of infected children depends on the activities of women of childbearing age and their sexual partners.

   2. With perinatal antiretroviral therapy, the rate of vertical infection has decreased from 25% to less than 8%. Despite this reduction, 93% of new cases in children are the result of perinatal infection.

II **CLINICAL MANIFESTATIONS**

A. **Symptoms**

   1. Most perinatally infected infants are asymptomatic for the first few months of life. Once symptoms appear, the disease progresses more rapidly than in adults.

      a. **Rapid progressors.** In approximately 10% of infected children, AIDS develops in less than 5 years. These children present most often with *Pneumocystis carinii* pneumonia (PCP), failure to thrive, hepatitis, diarrhea, and neurocognitive deterioration.

      b. **Slow progressors.** The remaining 90% of children have no uniform clinical presentation and appear much less sick. Most have at least one of the following conditions: generalized lymphadenopathy, hepatosplenomegaly, failure to thrive, thrush, chronic eczema, onychomycosis, idiopathic thrombocytopenic purpura, recurrent diarrhea, parotitis, cardiomyopathy, hepatitis, nephropathy, central nervous system disease, lymphoid interstitial pneumonia, or recurrent invasive bacterial infections.

2. Opportunistic infections and malignancies are less common in children than in adults.

III APPROACH TO THE PATIENT

A. Diagnosis in infants born to HIV-positive mothers is confounded by the presence of passively acquired maternal antibodies.

1. Criteria for infection

   a. Age younger than 18 months. The most sensitive and specific test for detection of HIV is polymerase chain reaction (PCR) done on DNA extracted from peripheral blood mononuclear cells. The first test should be done in the first 48 hours of life. The test should be repeated at 1 to 2 months of age. A positive result confirms the diagnosis. For patients older than 1 month of age, infection is confirmed by positive results on two separate studies, one of which must be done after 4 months of age.

   b. Age older than 18 months. A positive enzyme-linked immunosorbent assay (ELISA) antibody screening test result followed by a positive confirmatory Western blot for antibodies to HIV is diagnostic.

   c. Any AIDS-defining condition (**Tables 42–1, 42–2, and 42–3**), even if laboratory criteria are not met, is proof of infection with HIV.

2. Infection is excluded when two PCR assay results performed in an infant older than 1 month of age are negative. One of these assays must be performed after 4 months of age. For patients older than 6 months of age, infection is excluded by two blood samples, taken at least 1 month apart, that are negative for HIV antibody.

B. Initial therapy

1. An infectious disease specialist should always be consulted because information in this field changes rapidly.

2. Initiation of therapy does not depend on clinical or immunologic criteria. Therapy should be started at the time of diagnosis. In general, children have a higher baseline viral load than do adults, and they need more aggressive treatment. After obtaining a baseline viral load and resistance testing, a regimen of at least three agents (including at least one protease inhibitor) should be initiated.

HOT

KEY

Adherence to therapy is difficult in children. Gastric tubes may be necessary in young children.

TABLE 42-1. 1993 Revised Case Definition of AIDS-Defining Conditions for Adults and Adolescents 13 Years of Age and Older

Candidiasis of bronchi, trachea, or lungs
Candidiasis, esophageal
Cervical cancer, invasive
Coccidioidomycosis, disseminated or extrapulmonary
Cryptococcosis, extrapulmonary
Cryptosporidiosis, chronic intestinal (> 1 month duration)
Cytomegalovirus disease (other than liver, spleen, or nodes)
Cytomegalovirus retinitis (with loss of vision)
Encephalopathy, HIV-related
Herpes simplex: chronic ulcer(s) (> 1 month duration); or bronchitis, pneumonitis, or esophagitis
Histoplasmosis, disseminated or extrapulmonary
Isosporiasis, chronic intestinal (> 1 month duration)
Kaposi sarcoma
Lymphoma, Burkitt (or equivalent term)
Lymphoma, immunoblastic (or equivalent term)
Lymphoma, primary or brain
Mycobacterium avium complex or *Mycobacterium kansaii,* disseminated or extrapulmonary
Mycobacterium tuberculosis, any site, pulmonary or extrapulmonary
Mycobacterium, other species or unidentified species, disseminated or extrapulmonary
Pneumocystis carinii pneumonia
Pneumonia, recurrent
Progressive multifocal leukoencephalopathy
Salmonella septicemia, recurrent
Toxoplasmosis of brain
Wasting syndrome due to HIV
CD4+ T-lymphocyte count less than 200/µl (0.20 × 10⁹/L) or CD4+ percentage less than 15%

Adapted with permission from Centers for Disease Control and Prevention: 1993 Revised Classification System for HIV Infection and Expanded Case Surveillance Definition for AIDS Among Adolescents and Adults. *MMWR Morb Mortal Wkly Rep* 41(RR-17):1–19, 1992.

C. **Prophylaxis**
　　1. **Reduction of perinatal HIV transmission.** Zidovudine is given orally to pregnant women starting at 14 weeks gestation, intravenously during labor and delivery, and to the newborn from 8–12 hours after birth until 6 weeks of age (2 mg/kg orally four times daily).

TABLE 42-2. Clinical Categories for Children Younger Than 13 Years of Age with HIV Infection

Category N: not symptomatic

Children who have no signs or symptoms considered to be the result of HIV infection or have only one of the conditions listed in category A

Category A: mildly symptomatic

Children with two or more of the conditions listed but none of the conditions listed in categories B and C

Lymphadenopathy ($\geq$ 0.5 cm at more than two sites; bilateral at one site)

Hepatomegaly

Splenomegaly

Dermatitis

Parotitis

Recurrent or persistent upper respiratory tract infection, sinusitis, or otitis media

Category B: moderately symptomatic

Children who have symptomatic conditions other than those listed for category A or C that are attributed to HIV infection

Anemia (hemoglobin < 8 g/dl [< 80 g/l]), neutropenia (white blood cell count < 1000/μl [< 1.0 × 10^9/l]), and/or thrombocytopenia (platelet count < 100 × 10^3/μl [< 100 × 10^9/l]) persisting for $\geq$ 30 days

Bacterial meningitis, pneumonia, or sepsis (single episode)

Candidiasis, oropharyngeal (thrush), persisting (> 2 months) in children older than 6 months of age

Cardiomyopathy

Cytomegalovirus infection, with onset before 1 month of age

Diarrhea, recurrent or chronic

Hepatitis

HSV stomatitis, recurrent (> two episodes within 1 year)

HSV bronchitis, pneumonitis, or esophagitis with onset before 1 month of age

Herpes zoster (shingles) involving at least two distinct episodes or more than one dermatome

Leiomyosarcoma

Lymphoid interstitial pneumonia or pulmonary lymphoid hyperplasia complex

Nephropathy

Nocardiosis

Persistent fever (lasting > 1 month)

Toxoplasmosis, onset before 1 month of age

Varicella, disseminated (complicated chickenpox)

Category C: severely symptomatic

Serious bacterial infections, multiple or recurrent (any combination of at least 2 culture-confirmed infections within a 2-year period), of the following types: septicemia, pneumonia, meningitis, bone or joint infection, or abscess of an internal organ or body cavity (excluding otitis media, superficial skin or mucosal abscesses, and indwelling catheter–related infections)

Candidiasis, esophageal or pulmonary (bronchi, trachea, lungs)

Coccidioidomycosis, disseminated (at site other than or in addition to lungs or cervical or hilar lymph nodes)

Cryptococcosis, extrapulmonary

Cryptosporidiosis or isosporiasis with diarrhea persisting > 1 month

Lymphoma, primary, in brain

Lymphoma, small, noncleaved cell (Burkitt), or immunoblastic; or large-cell lymphoma of B-cell or unknown immunologic phenotype

Mycobacterium tuberculosis, disseminated or extrapulmonary

Mycobacterium, other species or unidentified species, disseminated (at a site other than or in addition to lungs, skin, or cervical or hilar lymph nodes)

Pneumocystis carinii pneumonia

Progressive multifocal leukoencephalopathy

Salmonella (nontyphoid) septicemia, recurrent

Toxoplasmosis of the brain with onset at or after 1 month of age

(continued)

TABLE 42-2. Clinical Categories for Children Younger Than 13 Years of Age with HIV Infection *(Continued)*

Category C: severely symptomatic *(Continued)*

Wasting syndrome in the absence of a concurrent illness other than HIV infection that could explain the following findings: (1) persistent weight loss > 10% of baseline, OR (2) downward crossing of at least two of the following percentile lines on the weight-for-age chart (e.g., 95th, 75th, 50th, 25th, 5th) in a child 1 year of age or older, OR (3) < 5th percentile on weight-for-height chart on two consecutive measurements, ≥ 30 days apart PLUS (1) chronic diarrhea (i.e., at least two loose stools per day for > 30 days) OR (2) documented fever (for > 30 days, intermittent or constant)

Cytomegalovirus disease with onset of symptoms after 1 month of age (at a site other than liver, spleen, or lymph nodes)

Encephalopathy (at least one of the following progressive findings present for at least 2 months in the absence of a concurrent illness other than HIV infection that could explain the findings): (1) failure to attain or loss of developmental milestones or loss of intellectual ability, verified by standard developmental scale or neuropsychological tests; (2) impaired brain growth or acquired microcephaly demonstrated by head circumference measurements or brain atrophy demonstrated by computed tomography or magnetic resonance imaging (serial imaging required for children younger than 2 years of age); (3) acquired symmetric motor deficit manifested by two or more of the following: paresis, pathologic reflexes, ataxia, or gait disturbance

HSV infection causing a mucocutaneous ulcer that persists for more than 1 month; or bronchitis, pneumonitis, or esophagitis for any duration affecting a child older than 1 month of age

Histoplasmosis, disseminated (at a site other than or in addition to lungs or cervical or hilar lymph nodes)

Kaposi sarcoma

Adapted with permission from Centers for Disease Control and Prevention: 1994 Revised Classification System for Human Immunodeficiency Virus Infection in Children Less Than 13 Years of Age: Official Authorized Addenda: Human Immunodeficiency Virus Infection Codes and Official Guidelines for Coding and Reporting ICD-9-CM. *MMWR Morb Mortal Wkly Rep* 43(RR-12):1–19, 1994.

HSV = herpes simplex virus.

TABLE 42-3. Pediatric HIV Classification for Children Younger Than 13 Years of Age

Immunologic Definitions	Clinical Classifications*			Immunologic Categories					
	N: No Signs or Symptoms	A: Mild Signs and Symptoms	B: Moderate Signs and Symptoms[‡]	C: Severe Signs and Symptoms[‡]	Age-Specific CD4+ T-Lymphocyte Count and Percentage of Total Lymphocytes[†]					
					< 12 months		1–5 years		6–12 years	
					µl	%	µl	%	µl	%
1: no evidence of suppression	N1	A1	B1	C1	≥ 1500	≥ 25	≥ 1000	≥ 25	≥ 500	≥ 25
2: evidence of moderate suppression	N2	A2	B2	C2	750–1499	15–24	500–999	15–24	200–499	15–24
3: severe suppression	N3	A3	B3	C3	< 750	< 15	< 500	< 15	< 200	< 15

Modified from Centers for Disease Control and Prevention: 1994 Revised Classification System for Human Immunodeficiency Virus Infection in Children Less Than 13 Years of Age: Official Authorized Addenda: Human Immunodeficiency Virus Infection Codes and Official Guidelines for Coding and Reporting ICD-9-CM. *MMWR Morb Mortal Wkly Rep* 43(RR-12):1–19, 1994.

*Children whose HIV infection status is not confirmed are classified by using this grid with a letter E (for perinatally exposed) placed before the appropriate classification code (e.g., EN2).

[†]To convert values in microliters to Système International units ($\times 10^9$/L), multiply by 0.001.

[‡]lymphoid interstitial pneumonitis in category B or category C is reportable to state and local health departments as AIDS (See Table 42-2 for further definition of clinical categories).

   2. PCP prophylaxis. HIV-exposed infants should receive trimethoprim-sulfamethoxazole (Bactrim) prophylaxis starting at 4–6 weeks of age. Prophylaxis is continued if there is severe suppression of the CD4 count (see Table 42-3). Lifelong chemoprophylaxis is required if the patient has had a previous episode of PCP.

D. Primary care issues

   1. Immunizations. In general, live virus vaccines (e.g., oral polio virus, varicella zoster virus) are not administered. The measles-mumps-rubella vaccination series may be administered if the child is not severely immunocompromised. The pneumococcal vaccine should be given at 2 months of age, with a booster 3–5 years later. An influenza vaccine should be administered annually. Hepatitis A vaccination is recommended if the patient lives in a community with elevated rates of hepatitis A. Antibody titers should be checked to ensure a proper response to vaccines.

   2. Breast-feeding is contraindicated if the mother is HIV-positive.

   3. Contact prevention. Regular bleach (1:10 diluted in water) should be used to clean surfaces that come in contact with emesis, urine, feces, or blood. Universal precautions should always be followed.

E. Prognosis. Rapid progressors have a 5-year survival rate of less than 50%. Slow progressors have a 5-year survival rate higher than 70%.

References

Committee on Infectious Disease, American Academy of Pediatrics, Pickering LK (ed): *2000 Red Book Report of the Committee on Infectious Diseases,* 25th ed. Elk Grove Village, IL, American Academy of Pediatrics, 2000.

Wiznia AA, Lambert G, Pavlakis S: Pediatric HIV infection. *Med Clin North Am* 80(6):1309–1336, 1996.

PART V

CRITICAL CARE AND EMERGENCY MEDICINE

43. Dehydration

I INTRODUCTION

A. Background. The management of dehydrated patients is one of the most common tasks in pediatrics. Management is stepwise, logical, and simple.

B. Definitions

1. **Hyponatremic dehydration** is dehydration in a patient whose serum sodium level is < 130 mEq/L. It may be caused by vomiting, diarrhea, diuretics, burns, pancreatitis, intestinal fistula, mineralocorticoid deficiency, sodium-losing nephropathy, or adrenal insufficiency. It is likely that the patient's losses are mainly of sodium rather than water and that the replacement fluids needed should be relatively devoid of electrolytes.

2. **Hypernatremic dehydration** is dehydration in a patient whose serum sodium level is > 150 mEq/L. The patient's losses are mainly of water rather than electrolytes. Hypernatremic dehydration is caused by severe water depletion and diarrhea or diabetes insipidus. In rare cases, hypertonic breast milk is a factor.

3. **Isotonic fluids** have a tonicity equivalent to that of blood (i.e., 154 mEq/L). Examples include 0.9% normal saline (NS) and lactated Ringer's solution.

II CLINICAL MANIFESTATIONS

A. Symptoms of hypernatremic dehydration. Circulatory volume may be maintained because the tonicity of the blood draws extracellular fluid into the intravascular space; therefore, tachycardia may not be present. The skin is doughy, and the patient often is thirsty, crampy, and irritable. Encephalopathy may occur if the sodium level is > 160 mEq/L or if the total osmolarity is > 340 mOsm/kg. Brain shrinkage predisposes to hemorrhage; venous thrombosis and cerebral infarction also may occur.

B. Clinical symptoms of isotonic or hyponatremic dehydration usually are more prominent than in hypernatremic dehydration. The heart rate usually is higher because the degree of intravascular depletion is greater.

III INITIAL STEPS

A. The fluid deficit is calculated. This calculation may be done by three different methods:

1. **Clinical picture**
   a. **Fluid deficit of 5% (50 ml/kg):** slightly dry mucous membranes, heart rate is increased by 10%, concentrated urine, and poor tear production
   b. **Fluid deficit of 10% (100 ml/kg):** oliguria, decreased skin turgor, severe thirst, or sunken fontanel
   c. **Fluid deficit of 15% (150 ml/kg):** shock, hypotension, Kussmaul breathing, change in mental status, and anuria

2. **Calculations based on weight loss** are made according to the following formula:

$$\% \text{ Dehydration} = \frac{\text{Premorbid} - \text{morbid}}{\text{Premorbid}} \times 100$$

3. As in hypernatremic dehydration (see IV B 2)

B. The total body water (TBW) is calculated as follows:
TBW (L) = 0.6 × weight (kg).

C. Laboratory tests include measuring electrolytes with serum bicarbonate. Substantially low bicarbonate levels (i.e., < 16 mEq/L) usually mandate intravenous fluid therapy.

D. Ongoing management. The patient is monitored carefully during each stage of fluid resuscitation. If mental status does not improve or adequate urine output is not re-established, the initial deficit may have been underestimated. Patients with severe dehydration may require multiple fluid boluses.

IV APPROACH TO THE PATIENT

A. Isotonic or hyponatremic (serum Na < 130) dehydration

1. **Initial intravenous fluid resuscitation** with a 20 ml/kg bolus of NS or lactated Ringer's solution restores circulation to the vital organs and improves cardiac output.

2. **Replacement fluids**
   a. **Replacement of fluid deficit**
      (1) Half of the deficit is replaced during the first 8 hours.
      (2) The remainder of the deficit is replaced during the next 16 hours.

(3) It is important to include maintenance fluids, initial resuscitation fluids, and ongoing losses in the fluid rate calculation.
b. Replacement of sodium deficit

Na deficit = [Na (desired) − Na (actual)] × TBW

If Na > 105 mEq/L, 130 mEq/L is used as desired; if Na < 105 mEq/L, correct deficit by maximum of 20 mEq/L in 24 hours.
(1) Half of the sodium deficit is replaced during the first 8 hours.
(2) The remainder is replaced during the next 16 hours.
(3) After calculation, the fluid is usually D5 ½ NS. Be sure to take into account maintenance Na requirements (3 meq/kg/day).
(4) Potassium is added to the maintenance fluids (20–40 mEq KCl/L) after urine output is restored.
(5) The rate of Na increase should not exceed 2 mEq/L/h because of the risk of central pontine myelinolysis. If the rate of increase is too great, the tonicity of fluids is decreased.

HOT

KEY

In patients with severe hyponatremic dehydration, rapid correction risks central pontine myelinolysis.

HOT

KEY

Consider adrenal insufficiency in patients with low serum sodium and elevated serum potassium.

---

3. Symptomatic hyponatremic dehydration. If a seizure or coma occurs, the focus is on quick restoration of the serum Na by infusing hypertonic saline. Serum sodium should be corrected to 125 mEq/L over a period of 30 minutes to 4 hours using the following formula:

$$\frac{\text{Amount of 3\%}}{\text{NaCl (ml)}} = \frac{[X\text{ mEq/L} \times \text{body weight (kg)}] \times 0.6\text{ L/kg}}{0.513\text{ mEq Na/ml 3\% NaCl}}$$

where X = (125 mEq/L − actual serum [Na]) to initially increase the serum Na^+ rapidly to 125 mEq/L. Alternatively, as an initial estimate, give 10–12 ml/kg of 3% saline over 1 hour.

B. Hypernatremic dehydration (serum Na > 150 mEq/L)

  1. Initial resuscitation: 20 ml/kg NS, D_5 NS, or lactated Ringer's solution as an intravenous bolus

  2. Replacement fluids. The water deficit is calculated as follows:

$$\text{Total Body Water Deficit (L)} = \left[\frac{[\text{Na (actual)} - \text{Na (desired)}]}{\text{Na (desired)}]}\right] \times \text{TBW}$$

  a. The Na (actual) level is adjusted if the glucose level is high:

$$\text{Corrected Serum Sodium} =$$
$$\text{Na (measured)} + \left[1.6 \times \frac{(\text{Glucose (mg/dl)} - 100)}{100}\right]$$

  b. Deficits should be corrected evenly over 48 hours. Initial resuscitation fluids are subtracted. Maintenance fluids and ongoing losses must be taken into account.

  c. The Na level should be decreased no more than 10–12 mEq/L/day (0.5 mEq/L/h). The general rule is that 4 ml/kg free water lowers serum Na by 1 mEq/L. The following equation is helpful in calculating the rate of decline. If the rate of decrease is too great, the tonicity of the fluids should be increased:

$$\text{Free water (L)} = 1 - \left[\frac{\text{Na (IVF)}}{\text{Na (serum)}}\right] \times \text{IVF (L) administered}$$

  where IVF = intravenous fluid.

  d. Usually, the starting resuscitation fluid is D_5 ½ NS. Higher tonicities are used initially if serum osmolarity is very high (> 340) or if the calculated rate of decline is too great.

  e. Potassium is added to maintenance fluids (20–40 mEq KCl/L) after urine output is restored.

  f. The patient is evaluated for hypocalcemia.

HOT **KEY** Rapid correction risks cerebral edema. Free water is replaced slowly to prevent cerebral edema, and the Na level is decreased no more than 10–12 mEq/L/day (0.5 mEq/L/h). If seizures occur, treat with hypertonic saline (see section IV A3).

V ORAL REHYDRATION

A. Limitations

  1. Oral rehydration cannot be used for patients who have > 10% dehydration, stool losses in excess of 10 ml/kg/h, or intractable vomiting.

   2. The rehydration fluid cannot be hyperosmolar because such
   fluid would worsen fluid losses. Recommended concentrations contain 90 mEq/L Na, 20 mEq/L K, and 20 g/L glucose.
   3. In some patients who have carbohydrate malabsorption, diarrhea worsens if the oral rehydration fluid contains glucose.
   These children require intravenous fluid therapy.
B. Rehydration phase. The total fluid deficit is replaced over a period of 4 hours. The goal is 60–80 ml/kg for mild to moderate dehydration. The fluid is given orally in small, frequent amounts.
C. Maintenance phase. Infants may breast-feed on demand. Ongoing stool losses should be replaced 1:1 with oral rehydration
   fluid, not fruit juices. The BRAT diet (i.e., bananas, rice, apple-
   sauce, and toast) can be introduced slowly as tolerated.
D. Ongoing management. Continuing enteral feeding helps cell re-
   newal in the gut. The use of soy-based milk is controversial.
   There are few clear contraindications to breast-feeding; it may
   even speed resolution of acute gastroenteritis.

References

Choukair MK: Fluids and electrolytes. In *The Harriet Lane Handbook: A Manual for
   Pediatric House Officers,* 15th ed. Edited by Barone MA. Philadelphia, Mosby-
   Year Book, 1996, pp 119–130, 229–240.
Edwards WH: Fluids and electrolytes. In *The HSC Handbook of Pediatrics,* 9th ed.
   Edited by Shefler AG, Parkin PC. Philadelphia, Mosby-Year Book, 1997, pp
   87–102.

44. Apparent Life-Threatening Events and Apnea

I. INTRODUCTION

A. Definitions

1. An **apparent life-threatening event (ALTE)** is an episode that is frightening to the observer and is characterized by some combination of apnea (central or occasionally obstructive), color change (usually cyanotic or pallid, but occasionally erythematous or plethoric), marked change in muscle tone (usually marked limpness), choking, or gagging. In some cases, the observer fears that the infant has died. Previously used terminology [e.g., aborted crib death or near-miss sudden infant death syndrome (SIDS)] should be abandoned because it implies a possibly misleading association between this type of episode and SIDS.

2. **High-risk ALTE** is defined by occurrence during sleep, perceived to require cardiopulmonary resuscitation (CPR) or vigorous stimulation.

3. **Apnea of infancy (AOI),** or **idiopathic ALTE,** is an unexplained episode of cessation of breathing for 20 seconds or longer. There may also be a shorter respiratory pause associated with bradycardia, cyanosis, pallor, or marked hypotonia. AOI usually occurs in infants who are older than 37 weeks gestational age. The diagnosis of AOI should be reserved for infants for whom no specific cause of ALTE can be identified.

B. Pathogenesis

1. The pathogenesis of **ALTE** is unclear. Most patients have increased respiratory pauses, normal baseline oxygenation, and normal responses to hypercapnia, but abnormal arousal responses to hypoxia.

2. **Gastroesophageal reflux disorder (GERD)–associated apnea.** When chemoreceptors around the larynx are stimulated by acid, central apnea, bradycardia, and pallor occur as a result of central pooling of blood. These effects are more pronounced in infancy than later in life. GERD can also cause obstructive apnea as a result of laryngospasm.

C. Epidemiology

1. The mean age at presentation is 8–14 weeks; it is more common in boys than in girls.

2. After evaluation, a cause is identified in 45%–60% of patients with ALTE.

3. The incidence of ALTE in all infants is 1%–3%.

4. The prevalence of a previous ALTE in SIDS victims is approximately 5%–6%.

5. Approximately 11% of patients with ALTE have relatives who died of SIDS.

6. Causes include:

   a. GERD and other causes of laryngeal stimulation: 47%

   b. Seizures and other neurologic disorders: 29%

   c. Respiratory disorders: 15%

   d. Infection [e.g., sepsis, respiratory syncytial virus (RSV), pertussis, meningitis]: 5%–40%

   e. Miscellaneous (e.g., postanesthetic effect, vocal cord paralysis, tracheomalacia, vascular ring, child abuse, Munchausen syndrome by proxy, breath-holding spells): 3%

   f. Endocrine or metabolic disorders: 2.5%

   g. Cardiovascular disorders: 2.5%

II APPROACH TO THE PATIENT

A. Initial workup

1. The patient is admitted to the hospital and placed on a cardiac rhythm monitor. A 2-day stay is recommended.

2. The patient is observed for recurrence, which is important because ALTEs tend to occur in clusters.

3. A **detailed history** is crucial and should include the following:

   a. The infant's state of consciousness before, during, and after the event

   b. Whether the infant was asleep or awake

   c. The position of the infant (supine or prone)

   d. The surface of the bedding (e.g., was there potential for microenvironments, such as loose blankets or pillows near the patient's head?)

   e. Duration of the event

   f. Changes in color (being very specific): cyanosis, pallor, plethoral?

   g. Changes in muscle tone

   h. Eye and extremity movements; seizure-like activity

   i. Respiratory efforts

   j. Temporal relationship between the ALTE and feeding

   k. Any previous episodes of choking with feeding or of snoring at night

   l. Any previous episodes of ALTE, feeding problems, seizures, perinatal injuries, or family history of SIDS, apnea, or cardiovascular problems

4. **Physical examination.** Special emphasis is placed on the neurologic, cardiac, and upper airway examinations. Attention should be focused on the patient's respiratory patterns during feeding and sleep. The primary goal of the examination is to search for a cause of the ALTE; however, the physician must also determine whether the episode was a true ALTE or simply parental overreaction.

B. **Laboratory tests** initially are minimal if the findings of the physical examination are normal.

1. **A complete blood count (CBC) with differential** is done to assess for anemia and occult infection (pertussis may cause lymphocytosis).

2. **Electrolyte levels with serum bicarbonate and glucose** should be obtained as soon as possible. This information is helpful in determining whether a significant metabolic acidosis (characterized by low serum bicarbonate) or hypoglycemia was associated with the ALTE.

3. **Urine toxicology screen.** Between 10% and 15% of screen results are positive for over-the-counter medications given by well-meaning but overzealous parents.

HOT KEY A broader workup should be considered if there is a high-risk ALTE, if there is evidence of acidosis, if episodes recur, or if there is a positive family history of SIDS.

---

4. **Additional testing** is pursued if the history or physical examination suggests an identifiable cause, if a severe episode is suspected, or if the episodes recur. Additional tests may include:

a. RSV fluorescent antibody assay, pertussis culture swabs and lumbar puncture to rule out meningitis

b. Electroencephalogram (EEG), electrocardiogram (ECG) or echocardiogram, chest radiograph, and polysomnography (PSG)

(1) PSG measures the heart rate, respiratory effort (chest wall muscle activity), airflow through the mouth, oxygenation, and end-tidal CO_2 ($ETCO_2$). Optional channels are available for a pH probe, an EEG, and an ECG.

(2) PSG is indicated when obstructive symptoms are suspected. This test can diagnose obstructive apnea, apneic seizures, and sleep hypoventilation.

c. Pneumograms show abnormalities in approximately 50% of patients with AOI; however, they cannot identify patients who are at risk for SIDS.

    d. A pH probe or an upper gastrointestinal barium study is considered for patients who may have GERD-associated apnea.

C. Differential diagnosis

  1. Causes of ALTE in relation to sleep state

    a. Asleep. Obstructive sleep apnea, AOI, alveolar hypoventilation, suffocation

    b. Awake. GERD, breath-holding spells, and airway obstruction

    c. No relation. Neurologic dysfunction, infection, cardiac disturbance, inborn error of metabolism, poisoning, autonomic dysfunction, and Munchausen syndrome by proxy

  2. Congenital central hypoventilation syndrome is the most severe hypoventilation syndrome. The brain stem cannot sustain adequate spontaneous ventilation due to inadequate sensitivity to hypercarbia and hypoxia. The major long-term risk is cor pulmonale. Patients who have this condition require long-term mechanical ventilatory support, usually with a tracheostomy.

  3. Apnea of prematurity usually occurs in infants younger than 37 weeks gestation and can persist until 42 weeks.

  4. Obstructive sleep apnea syndrome can be caused by obesity, tonsillar hypertrophy, Pierre Robin syndrome, Down syndrome, cerebral palsy, or myotonic dystrophies.

  5. Breath-holding spells (prolonged expiratory apnea or infantile syncope) are usually preceded by vagal stimulation. The infant does a Valsalva maneuver in response to pain or fright, vigorous activity, coughing, crying, or defecation. This condition is self-limited, but a seizure disorder must be ruled out.

  6. Munchausen syndrome by proxy must be considered when the patient is older than 6 months of age, when a sibling has a similar history, when multiple episodes occur, when the events are seen only by the mother (it is almost always the mother who is involved).

D. Ongoing management

  1. Documentation of a seizure disorder does not indicate whether the seizure caused or was caused by ALTE. Regardless, seizures should be treated appropriately.

  2. Most patients with GERD do not have ALTEs; therefore, the finding of GERD does not unequivocally explain the cause.

  3. If the PSG shows hypoventilation, a trial of methylxanthines is indicated.

  4. ALTEs are clearly stressful for families, so adequate social support should be provided.

  5. Neurodevelopmental follow-up should be considered at age 1–3 years.

6. An event recorder may be the best way to distinguish true events from false alarms.
7. Home monitoring is indicated if the ALTE was severe enough to require mouth-to-mouth resuscitation or vigorous stimulation, if the patient is a sibling in a family with two or more cases of SIDS, if the patient is a premature infant, or if the patient has central hypoventilation or a tracheotomy.
   a. Patients who have less severe episodes may require home monitoring, especially if there is a family history of SIDS, if a sibling has severe ALTE, if the patient has recurrent ALTEs that require intervention, or if there is a history of prolonged apnea with associated definite changes in color or tone.
   b. Home monitoring should be continued until there are no significant episodes of apnea or bradycardia for 2 months or until the child reaches 6 months of age.
8. Parents and care givers should be trained in basic techniques of cardiac life support.

III PROGNOSIS

A. Mortality
1. The combined mortality rate from eight studies of ALTE populations is 1%. The predominant cause of death is SIDS.
2. The combined mortality rate from six studies of AOI populations is 3%.
3. The mortality rate is higher when the ALTE occurs during sleep, when the patient requires resuscitation or vigorous stimulation, and when the patient has recurrent ALTEs that are concurrent with a seizure disorder.
4. The risk of death for patients with high-risk ALTE (i.e., occurrence during sleep, perceived to require CPR or vigorous stimulation) is 8%–10%.

HOT **KEY**   The risk of death for patients with more than one serious episode is 28%.

B. Morbidity
1. Infants who experienced an ALTE show a slight increase in abnormal neurodevelopmental function (i.e., muscle hypotonia), gross motor impairment, and lower mental and psychomotor scores according to Bailey scales.
2. Marked hypoxic-ischemic encephalopathy is rare in patients with ALTE.

References

Brooks JG: Apparent life-threatening events and apnea of infancy. *Clin Perinatol* 19(4):809–838, 1992.

Carroll JL, Marcus CL, Loughlin GM, et al: Disordered control of breathing in infants and children. *Pediatr Rev* 14(2):51–66, 1993.

Brooks JG: Consultation with the specialist: apparent life-threatening events. *Pediatr Rev* 17(7):257–259, 1996.

45. Toxic Ingestions

I BACKGROUND

A. Two thirds of all toxic ingestions occur in children. Toxic ingestions typically fall into one of two categories: the toddler with an accidental ingestion, or the adolescent with an intentional ingestion representing a suicide attempt or gesture.

B. The type and amount of substance ingested may not be known. Therefore, a high index of suspicion is warranted, and the physician needs to cast a wide diagnostic net.

C. Death due to ingestion is unusual. If death occurs, it is most likely to be from ingestion of iron or hydrocarbons.

II APPROACH TO THE PATIENT

A. History. Obtaining a complete history is essential.

1. When did the ingestion occur?
2. What substance or substances did the patient ingest? Co-ingestions should always be considered.
3. What other substances or medications (e.g., parent's medications, grandparent's medications) are available in the household?
4. How much of the substance was ingested? Often, the amount must be estimated by counting the pills that remain in the bottle.
5. Has the patient vomited?
6. Was the substance in its original container?

HOT KEY

There may be no early symptoms of ingestion of certain "time bombs": acetaminophen, iron, monoamine oxidase inhibitors, toxic mushrooms, or slow-release preparations.

B. Initial management. The local poison control center should be contacted early in the course of evaluation and management. A specific diagnosis usually comes late in the course of treatment. The general treatment protocol includes:

1. Evaluating and securing the "ABCs" (airway, breathing, and circulation). Patients who are comatose or who cannot protect their airway should be intubated. Comatose patients should be given intravenous glucose, 0.5 g/kg, followed by naloxone, 0.1 mg/kg. Central nervous system (CNS) injury,

CNS infection, or hypoglycemia should be considered as either a primary or secondary cause in patients with neurologic impairment.

2. Reducing toxin absorption with charcoal, emesis, lavage, or whole-bowel irrigation

3. Identifying the agent

4. Providing a specific antidote

C. **Decontamination**

1. **Activated charcoal** is becoming the sole recommended agent for gastric decontamination. It is most effective if given within 4 hours of ingestion. It is not useful for patients who have ingested iron, heavy metals, volatile hydrocarbons, simple alcohols, or strong acid or alkali. Activated charcoal is contraindicated in patients with airway compromise, gastrointestinal bleeding, or intestinal obstruction. One g/kg (minimum dose, 15 g) is mixed with cold water or fruit juice. Doses of 15–30 g (child) and 30–100 g (adolescent) can be given every 2–6 hours until the first charcoal stool is passed. A cathartic (e.g., sorbitol, magnesium citrate, or magnesium sulfate) can be administered with the initial dose to counteract the constipating effects of charcoal. The cathartic dose is not repeated because fluid shifts may occur. Repeat dosing of activated charcoal is controversial.

2. **Gastric lavage** is becoming less frequently recommended. It must be performed within 30–60 minutes of ingestion. It is contraindicated for patients who ingested acid or alkali and for patients who cannot protect their airway. Gastric lavage probably should not be performed in children because cuffed endotracheal tubes cannot be used to protect the airway. It may be useful for substances that have a low affinity for charcoal (e.g., metals, glycols) or those that decrease gastric motility (e.g., aspirin, opiates). The patient should be placed in the Trendelenburg position, lying on the left side of the body. A large-bore (22–36 French) nasogastric tube is necessary. Lavage should be continued until the solution is clear and free of pill fragments. Activated charcoal administration should follow gastric lavage.

3. **Ipecac** has been virtually abandoned except in rare circumstances. It must be given within 60 minutes of ingestion. It is contraindicated in cases of caustic (e.g., lye, acid) or hydrocarbon ingestions, Nissen fundoplication, recent abdominal surgery, neurologic symptoms, or airway compromise. Ipecac is contraindicated in children younger than 6 months of age. Doses by age group are as follows: 6–9 months, 5 ml; 9–12 months, 10 ml; 1–12 years, 15 ml; and 12 or more years, 20 ml. The dose may be repeated once if there is no vomiting within 20 minutes after the first dose.

4. **Whole-bowel irrigation** is most useful with slow-release preparations, iron, or lithium. The airway must be protected. The dose is 20–40 ml/kg by nasogastric tube with polyethylene glycol solution (e.g., GoLYTELY, Colyte) until rectal effluent is clear.

D. Ongoing management. Tests to consider include serum acetaminophen level, glucose, electrocardiogram (ECG), arterial blood gas, electrolytes with anion gap, urine toxicology screen, serum toxicology screen (may allow quantitation of substance; more specific for sedative/hypnotic drugs), ethanol level, serum aspirin level, complete blood cell (CBC) count, and liver function tests (LFTs). A chest radiograph in patients who have respiratory symptoms or a history of hydrocarbon ingestion is useful.

HOT KEY   Always check the acetaminophen level in a patient with suspected ingestion. All symptomatic patients, all patients with a suicide attempt or gesture, and all patients with potential acetaminophen toxicity should be admitted to the hospital.

III SPECIFIC INGESTIONS

A. Acetaminophen. It is important to have a high clinical suspicion because toxicity is delayed, and the patient may be initially asymptomatic.

1. **Symptoms.** Toxicity occurs in four phases:
   a. In the first 24 hours, there are nonspecific gastrointestinal complaints, nausea, vomiting, malaise, and diaphoresis.
   b. At 24–48 hours, the patient's symptoms mostly abate, although there may be right upper quadrant pain. Laboratory tests reveal elevated liver enzymes and prothrombin time (PT).
   c. At 3–4 days, jaundice and hepatic failure may ensue. LFTs may be very high (approaching 10,000 IU/L), which reflects severe hepatocellular necrosis.
   d. In the terminal stage, only supportive treatment is given. For those who recover, laboratory indices return to normal. Liver transplantation is required for those who progress to hepatic failure.

2. **Diagnosis.** A serum level may be obtained at a minimum of 4 hours after ingestion. Toxicity occurs at doses greater than 150 mg/kg. If the level is in the toxic range or if the ingested amount is high, the following tests should be performed: CBC, LFTs, electrolytes, glucose, and PT (Figure 45-1).

3. **Treatment** is with N-acetylcysteine (Mucomyst). The oral loading dose is 140 mg/kg, followed by 70 mg/kg every 4 hours for 17 more doses. Treatment is most effective if

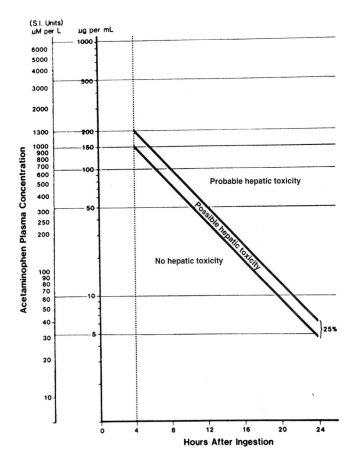

FIGURE 45-1. Semilogarithmic plot of plasma acetaminophen levels over time. Levels drawn fewer than 4 hours after ingestion may not represent peak levels. The lower solid line 25% below the standard nomogram is included to allow for possible errors in acetaminophen plasma assays and estimated time from ingestion of an overdose. (Reprinted with permission from Rumack BH, Matthew H: Acetaminophen poisoning and toxicity. *Pediatrics* 55:871, 1975.)

started within 8 hours of ingestion, but may be useful as late as 36 hours after ingestion. Patients who take medications that induce hepatic microsomal enzymes (e.g., barbiturates, carbamazepine, phenytoin, primidone, and rifampin) have a lower threshold for treatment. If the time of ingestion is unknown, therapy should be started if the serum level is higher than 20 μg/ml. If the patient cannot tolerate oral dosing, a nasogastric or orogastric tube may be used. Intravenous dosing of N-acetylcysteine is an acceptable alterative if oral dosing is not possible; the dose is 100 mg/kg every 8 hours for 3 doses.

B. Salicylates
  1. Symptoms. Lower doses of salicylates cause tinnitus, abdominal pain, vomiting, and tachypnea. Higher doses cause more dramatic tachypnea, respiratory alkalosis, hypoglycemia, or hyperglycemia. Severe poisoning can lead to lethargy, polyuria, metabolic acidosis, hypotension, coma, pulmonary edema, and death. The clinical signs and symptoms often are confused with diabetic ketoacidosis.
  2. Diagnosis. A toxic dose is 100 mg/kg; chronic use can lead to toxicity at lower levels. Serum salicylate level should be tested 6 hours after ingestion (Figure 45-2). Early on, blood gases tend to show respiratory alkalosis. Later, an anion gap metabolic acidosis predominates; some patients will have a mixed metabolic acidosis and respiratory alkalosis.
  3. Treatment should begin before the results of the 6-hour salicylate test are obtained in patients suspected of having a toxic ingestion. Aggressive hydration with glucose-containing isotonic fluids should begin immediately if the patient is hypotensive. Activated charcoal is given and gastric lavage should be considered if the patient comes to medical attention within 12 hours of ingestion. Some clinicians use repeat doses of charcoal for levels > 50 mg/dl. Urine should be alkalinized to enhance excretion and lessen systemic acidosis by giving an intravenous bolus of sodium bicarbonate (2–3 mEq/kg) followed by a glucose-containing intravenous infusion with sodium bicarbonate (20–40 mEq/L) and potassium. Ideally, urine pH should reach 8.0–8.5. Alkalinization can lower potassium levels, so losses must be followed and corrected. Dialysis should be considered for severe acidosis, intractable seizures, or progressive deterioration despite maximum alkalinization.

C. Ibuprofen
  1. Symptoms. Gastrointestinal symptoms (e.g., nausea, epigastric pain, upper gastrointestinal bleeding) predominate. CNS effects (e.g., coma, seizures, apnea) are the most serious. Renal failure also has been reported.
  2. Treatment is mainly supportive. Activated charcoal can be given, and alkaline diuresis should be considered.

D. Beta-blockers
  1. Symptoms. The most common symptoms of beta-blocker toxicity are bradycardia and hypotension. Beta-blockers also

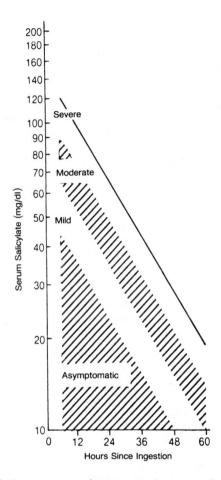

FIGURE 45-2. Done nomogram for estimating the severity of acute, single ingestion of non–enteric-coated aspirin. (Reprinted with permission from Temple AR: Acute and chronic effects of aspirin toxicity and their treatment. *Arch Intern Med* 141:364, 1981.)

may cause delirium, CNS depression, hypoglycemia, and bronchospasm in patients with asthma.
2. **Diagnosis.** An ECG may show a widened QRS and bundle branch block, ventricular tachycardia, or torsades de pointes. The differential diagnosis includes ingestion of digoxin and calcium channel blockers.

   3. Treatment. Hypotension is treated with intravenous fluid
      boluses. If hypotension persists, an isoproterenol drip begin-
      ning at 0.1 μg/kg/min should be considered, followed by
      glucagon infusion, 0.025–0.1 mg/kg bolus followed by con-
      tinuous infusion at 1–5 mg/h, if needed.
E. Calcium channel blockers
   1. Symptoms. Toxicity caused by cardiovascular involvement is
      manifested by hypotension, atrioventricular block, and brady-
      cardia. CNS depression, hyperglycemia, and lactic acidosis
      are also possible.
   2. Treatment. Hypotension is treated with intravenous fluids. If
      hypotension persists, the patient should receive a dopamine
      drip (2–20 μg/kg/min). Glucagon infusion should be consid-
      ered. Pacing may be required if all pharmacologic manage-
      ment fails.
F. Clonidine is very toxic to children, even in small quantities.
   1. Symptoms. Patients have central sympathetic inhibition.
      Symptoms may be similar to those of opiate overdose (e.g.,
      respiratory depression, coma, miosis). Hypotension or hyper-
      tension, bradycardia, and hypothermia also may occur. A
      patient who is asymptomatic initially and is still asympto-
      matic after 4 hours of observation may be sent home.
   2. Treatment for symptomatic bradycardia is atropine, 0.01–
      0.02 mg/kg, with a minimum dose of 0.1 mg. Hypertension
      often is followed by hypotension; therefore, antihyperten-
      sive medications should be avoided. Hypotension is treated
      with fluid boluses and, if needed, a dopamine drip. Naloxone
      (0.1 mg/kg) may be useful to block the endogenous effects of
      opioids, which are primary mediators of clonidine toxicity.
      Therefore, naloxone is helpful for severe respiratory depres-
      sion. Naloxone may block only the central effects of cloni-
      dine, thus allowing the peripheral, vasodilatory effects to
      predominate. Therefore, the patient's blood pressure should
      be monitored closely.
G. Button battery ingestion causes injury only if the battery becomes lodged in the esophagus. The injury is caused by leakage of alkali and generation of current. Chest and abdominal
   radiographs should be obtained. A child with a battery distal
   to the esophagus may be sent home; the parents are instructed
   to screen the child's stool for the battery. The patient should
   return for a repeat radiograph if symptoms develop or if the
   child has not passed the battery in the stool in 1 week. Batteries lodged in the esophagus require immediate endoscopic
   removal.
H. Carbon monoxide poisoning usually is associated with incomplete combustion reactions in closed spaces (e.g., structure fires,
   kerosene heater use, suicide attempts using automobile ex-

haust). A carboxyhemoglobin (COHb) level measurement should be obtained if the history suggests carbon monoxide poisoning.

1. **Symptoms.** There often is a poor correlation between the COHb level and symptoms, especially if the patient has been treated with oxygen or if a prolonged period has passed since the exposure. In such cases, the level may underestimate the degree of toxicity. Symptoms and accompanying COHb levels include:

   a. Headache (20%)

   b. Nausea and vomiting (30%)

   c. Lethargy, tachypnea, and tachycardia (40%)

   d. Coma and possible death (50%–60%)

2. **Treatment.** All patients suspected of having carbon monoxide poisoning should be treated with 100% oxygen via a nonrebreather mask. If the COHb level is greater than 20%, hyperbaric oxygen therapy should be considered. Patients are observed until symptoms have ceased and the COHb level has decreased to less than 5%.

I. Hydrocarbons

1. **Symptoms.** The respiratory system is most affected, especially with rapidly evaporating, low-viscosity substances (e.g., paint thinner, lamp oil, furniture polish, gasoline, lighter fluid). Respiratory symptoms occur within 4–6 hours of ingestion. Fever often accompanies pneumonitis without bacterial infection.

2. **Diagnosis.** Because of the potential for aspiration pneumonitis, a chest radiograph is indicated for any child with respiratory symptoms.

3. **Treatment.** Gastric decontamination usually is contraindicated with hydrocarbon ingestions. The exceptions are ingestions of hydrocarbons with a high likelihood of systemic toxicity: for example, camphor (CNS toxicity), carbon tetrachloride (hepatotoxicity), benzene, heavy metals, or pesticides. Admission to the intensive care unit should be considered for any patient with respiratory symptoms because rapid deterioration can occur. Asymptomatic patients are monitored for at least 4 hours.

J. Acids and alkali

1. **Symptoms.** Alkaline burns are notorious for their ability to cause liquefaction necrosis. Expected symptoms include excessive drooling or visible burns around the lips or in the mouth. Strictures and perforations are late findings.

2. **Treatment.** If the patient can swallow safely, he or she should be given 1–2 cups of milk or water and should be allowed nothing else by mouth. Endoscopy should be performed at 12–24 hours.

K. Iron
  1. Symptoms. Iron poisoning progresses through five stages:
    a. Stage I occurs during the first 6 hours after ingestion and includes gastrointestinal symptoms such as vomiting, abdominal pain, and diarrhea, which may contain blood.
    b. Stage II is an asymptomatic period that may last anywhere from 6 to 72 hours.
    c. Stage III. Some patients may progress to a third stage, in which gastrointestinal symptoms return. Hypotension, shock, seizures, metabolic acidosis, hyperglycemia, and coma occur in this stage.
    d. Stage IV is characterized by severe hepatotoxicity and coagulation abnormalities.
    e. Stage V includes gastric or intestinal stricture, which may occur 4–6 weeks after ingestion.
  2. Diagnosis. A serum iron level measurement should be obtained 2–6 hours after ingestion of more than 20 mg/kg of iron. Abdominal radiographs can show iron tablets; liquid iron preparations may not be visible. The **deferoxamine challenge test** can detect iron poisoning: 50 mg/kg deferoxamine (maximum dose 1 g) is administered intramuscularly, and a rusty orange color to the urine is considered a positive result.
  3. Treatment. Whole-bowel irrigation should be considered for significant ingestions with radiographic evidence of tablets. Deferoxamine (15 mg/kg/h intravenously) is indicated for iron levels greater than 350 μg/dl. Acid–base status measurement, coagulation studies, CBC, electrolyte level measurement, blood urea nitrogen testing, creatinine level measurement, and LFTs should be done.
L. Tricyclic antidepressants include imipramine (Tofranil), amitriptyline (Elavil), clomipramine (Anafranil), desipramine (Norpramin), doxepin (Adapin, Sinequan), and nortriptyline (Aventyl, Pamelor).
  1. Symptoms. Ventricular tachyarrhythmias are the main cause of death. Altered mental status (e.g., delirium, coma), seizures, and unstable blood pressure also may be present. Hypotension is an ominous sign. Anticholinergic symptoms (e.g., hallucinations, dryness of mucous membranes, flushing, urinary retention, arrhythmias, mydriasis) may predominate in the clinical picture—"Mad as a hatter, dry as a bone, red as a beet." These patients may seem well, but their condition may deteriorate abruptly.
  2. Diagnosis. A tricyclic antidepressant overdose should be suspected in any patient with mental status change and arrhythmia, particularly if the QRS is widened. Serum tricyclic levels do not predict the degree of toxicity.

3. **Treatment.** There is a low threshold for hospital admission due to the risk of sudden deterioration. Activated charcoal should be administered, and the patient should be given 1–2 mEq/kg sodium bicarbonate if there is evidence of QRS prolongation. The blood pH should be maintained above 7.45. Seizures should be controlled with benzodiazepines (lorazepam, 0.05–0.25 mg/kg intravenously, or diazepam, 0.1–0.3 mg/kg intravenously). Norepinephrine (0.1–0.2 μg/kg/ min) or dopamine (5–20 μg/kg/min) drips should be considered for hypotension that is unresponsive to fluid boluses. Physostigmine should be considered if the patient's condition is unresponsive to these measures.

M. **Organophosphates (cholinergic)** commonly are found in insecticides and carbamates and may be absorbed through the skin.
   1. **Symptoms** include excessive salivation, urination, or lacrimation; diarrhea; sweating; and miosis.
   2. **Treatment** includes atropine, 0.05 mg/kg, to a maximum of 2–5 mg. The patient should be decontaminated with soap and water. Pralidoxime, a cholinesterase regenerator, may be given for patients with recalcitrant symptoms.

N. **Opiates**
   1. **Symptoms** of opiate overdose include CNS depression, apnea, and miosis.
   2. **Treatment.** Narcan is administered at 0.2 mg/kg/dose every 2–3 minutes for patients 0–5 years of age and 2 mg/kg/dose if the patient is older than 5 years of age.

O. **Ethanol**
   1. **Symptoms.** Respiratory depression is the predominant symptom. Blood alcohol level should decrease from 400 mg/dl to 0 in 20 hours.
   2. **Diagnosis.** There is a risk of death at levels higher than 200 mg/dl. A urine toxicology screen and a head computed tomography (CT) scan should be performed if symptoms do not correlate with the ethanol level.
   3. **Treatment.** Supportive intubation may be required if significant respiratory depression occurs. Dialysis may be needed at levels greater than 350 mg/dl.

P. **Cyanide.** Cyanide may be found in apricot or peach kernels and in apple seeds. Cyanide poisoning may occur by inhalation of certain combustible materials.
   1. **Symptoms.** Symptoms may include a characteristic odor of bitter almonds or peach pits. Coma, seizures, and apnea are the predominant clinical manifestations.
   2. **Diagnosis.** A plasma lactate concentration greater than 10 mmol/L in smoke inhalation or greater than 6 mmol/L after suspected pure cyanide ingestion suggests cyanide poisoning.
   3. **Treatment** is 100% O_2; sodium nitrite, 0.33 ml/kg of a 3%

solution via slow intravenous push; hydroxocobalamin (Vitamin B12), 70 mg/kg intravenously over 30 minutes; and 25% sodium thiosulfate solution (1.65 ml/kg infused 3–5 ml/min).

Q. Plants
1. **Anticholinergics** include jimsonweed, nightshade, and potato. Physostigmine may be used if the reaction is severe.
2. **Foxglove** contains digitalis. Treatment involves the use of Fab fragments, phenytoin, and charcoal.
3. **Oleander** is similar to foxglove. It is unclear whether Fab fragments are effective; thus, phenytoin and charcoal should be used.
4. **Hemlock.** The effects are similar to those of nicotine (i.e., hyperactivity followed by CNS depression). There is no specific treatment.
5. **Arum** (dieffenbachia, caladium, philodendron). Irritation of the oropharynx occurs. If the reaction is severe, steroid administration should be considered.
6. **Castor beans** cause gastrointestinal symptoms, hemolytic anemia, and renal failure. There is no specific treatment.
7. **Amanita (mushroom).** Cells with the most turnover are most affected because the toxin inhibits mRNA formation.
   a. **Symptoms** include watery diarrhea, liver failure, and renal failure.
   b. **Treatment** involves aspiration of duodenal contents and repeated administration of activated charcoal. High-dose penicillin, cimetidine, silibinin, or N-acetylcysteine are controversial therapies.

References
Lovejoy FH Jr, Nizet V, Priebe CJ: Common etiologies and new approaches to management of poisoning in pediatric patients. *Curr Opin Pediatr* 5(5):524–530, 1993.
Vernon DD, Gleich MC: Poisoning and drug overdose. *Crit Care Clin* 13(3):647–667, 1997.
Woolf AD: Poisoning by unknown agents. *Pediatr Rev* 20(5):166–170, 1999.

46. Anaphylaxis

I INTRODUCTION

A. Pathophysiology

1. **Anaphylaxis** is a type I hypersensitivity reaction and is a form of distributive shock. Exposure to the sensitizing antigen leads to an immunoglobulin E (IgE) response, which sensitizes mast cells and basophils. Re-exposure to the antigen leads to mast cell degranulation, which causes increased permeability of postcapillary venules.

2. Manifestations occur when a hypersensitive subject is re-exposed to a sensitizing antigen. Two or more systems (e.g., cutaneous, respiratory, cardiovascular, gastrointestinal) must be involved to make the diagnosis of anaphylaxis.

B. Etiologic agents

1. **Drugs.** The most common cause of drug-related anaphylaxis is penicillin; serious reactions usually occur after intravenous administration. Trimethoprim-sulfamethoxazole and vancomycin are other common offenders. Nearly all antibiotics have been associated with anaphylaxis.

HOT **KEY**

Approximately 5% of patients with penicillin allergy have cross-reactivity with cephalosporins.

---

2. **Foods**
   a. **More common food allergens** include shellfish, fish, nuts, peas, beans, milk, egg white, and seeds (e.g., cottonseed, flaxseed, sesame seed, sunflower seed).
   b. **Less common food allergens** include potato, mango, chamomile tea, corn, grains, bananas, melons, and citrus fruits.

3. **Other offenders** include anesthetics, nonsteroidal anti-inflammatory drugs, narcotics, mannitol, intravenous contrast, and wasp, bee, or yellow jacket venom.

C. Less common types of anaphylaxis

1. **Exercise-induced anaphylaxis** requires both exercise and ingestion of a particular food within 2–6 hours of exercise.

2. **Cold anaphylaxis.** People with cold urticaria can have an anaphylactic reaction to sudden cold exposure (e.g., jumping into a cold lake).

II **CLINICAL MANIFESTATIONS.** **Symptoms** usually start within 30 minutes of contact with the offending agent. The most rapidly evolving reactions usually are the most severe. Symptoms may evolve in the following manner: flushing, sensations of warmth, tingling, pruritus of the skin, and a feeling of impending doom. Physical examination findings can be highly variable due to the multiple systems involved.

A. **Cardiovascular system.** Cardiovascular collapse can occur because of distributive shock. Tachycardia, hypotension, and syncope may occur. Dysrhythmias occasionally occur secondary to hypotension.

B. **Respiratory system.** Airway obstruction may occur in the upper or lower airways. Upper airway effects can cause hoarseness, dysphagia, and stridor. Lower airway obstruction can lead to cough, wheezing, and shortness of breath.

C. **Gastrointestinal system.** Gastrointestinal symptoms are prominent in children and include nausea, vomiting, cramping, tenesmus, and diarrhea.

D. **Skin.** Flushing, urticaria, hives, and facial swelling are common manifestations.

III **APPROACH TO THE PATIENT**

A. **Initial management.** Managing the ABCs (airway, breathing, and circulation) is always paramount. In more severe cases of anaphylaxis, symptoms can worsen despite epinephrine administration, especially if the first dose is delayed. Airway patency then becomes a particular problem due to laryngeal edema and laryngospasm. A suggested treatment scheme is as follows:

1. **Epinephrine** is the first-line therapy. The 1:1000 concentration is used. The subcutaneous dose is 0.01 ml/kg (minimum 0.1 ml, maximum 0.5–1.0 ml) and may be repeated every 15 minutes for a total of three doses. Intravenous epinephrine boluses are not indicated unless full arrest occurs. Although beta-blocker use is not common in children, the physician should keep in mind that beta-blockers may counteract the effectiveness of epinephrine and prolong or exacerbate the anaphylactic response. Atropine (0.05–0.075 mg/kg every 4 hours) or glucagon (1–5 mg intravenously) should be considered for patients who take beta-blockers.

2. To maintain saturations, **100% O_2** is given.

3. **Albuterol** (0.1–0.3 mg/kg) is administered to patients who are wheezing. For persistent wheezing, aminophylline (5–6 mg/kg over 20 minutes as a loading dose, then 0.7–0.9 mg/kg/h infusion) should be considered.

4. Distributive shock should be treated with rapid intravenous

fluid boluses (20 ml/kg) of **normal saline** or **lactated Ringer's solution**. Multiple boluses may be required.

5. If necessary, an **epinephrine drip** (0.1–1.5 μg/kg/min), or **dopamine drip** (2–25 μg/kg/min) can be started for patients with recalcitrant hypotension.

6. A **systemic steroid** (hydrocortisone, methylprednisolone, or prednisone) should be administered to ameliorate the late-phase response.

7. **Cimetidine,** 5–10 mg/kg given intravenously, can be considered in refractory cases.

8. **Diphenhydramine** may be given in less severe cases to treat urticaria, itching, and angioedema.

HOT

 Always be prepared for emergent intubation.

KEY

B. Ongoing management of insect stings

1. To promote local vasoconstriction, a second epinephrine injection directly into the site of the insect sting may be given.

2. A loose tourniquet should be applied proximal to the site of the sting to decrease systemic absorption. If possible, the affected body part should be kept below the heart.

C. Disposition

1. Future episodes should be anticipated, although the cause often cannot be found. It is vital to give family members Epi-Pens (Dey Laboratories, Napa, CA) and instruct them in their use. This simple maneuver can save a child's life.

2. **Skin testing** is performed on an outpatient basis. Only 40% of reactors have positive skin test results.

3. The patient should always wear a **MedicAlert bracelet** that indicates the specific allergy.

4. **Severe reactions.** Because of the risk of recurrent reactions, patients should be admitted to the hospital and observed for 24 hours. Patients should be discharged on a 3-day course of oral steroids and diphenhydramine.

5. Patients with **mild reactions** may be observed for 2–4 hours and discharged on diphenhydramine for 1–2 days.

6. **Immunotherapy** should be considered for patients who have severe reactions to insect venom or for patients who require certain antibiotics.

References

Fisher M: Treatment of acute anaphylaxis. *BMJ* 311:731–733, 1995.
Friday GA, Fireman P: Anaphylaxis. *Ear Nose Throat J* 75:21–24, 1996.

47. Status Asthmaticus

I INTRODUCTION

A. Definitions
1. **Asthma** is an obstructive pulmonary disease of recurrent and reversible airway narrowing.
2. **Status asthmaticus** is progressive respiratory distress and failure that is refractory to usual therapy.

B. Pathogenesis
1. Asthma is characterized by airflow obstruction as a result of bronchial inflammation, airway smooth muscle bronchospasm, and increased mucus production.
2. Allergens, upper respiratory infections, and irritants (e.g., smoke) are the most common triggers of asthma exacerbations.

C. Epidemiology
1. Asthma is a leading cause of admission to children's hospitals.
2. The incidence of fatal asthma attacks has increased in the past decade.
3. Asthma is 2.5 times more common in African Americans than in whites.
4. Income is inversely related to asthma incidence, and asthma is 1.5 times more prevalent in inner city populations.
5. Asthma is a leading cause of missed school days and an increasing cause of hospitalization and emergency treatment.

II CLINICAL MANIFESTATIONS.
Symptoms of asthma include cough, dyspnea, wheezing, prolonged expiration, chest tightness, accessory muscle use, inability to speak in complete sentences, suprasternal retractions, cyanosis, and hyperinflation.

HOT KEY

In extreme respiratory distress, wheezing may be absent until therapy is administered and airflow increases.

III APPROACH TO THE PATIENT

A. Diagnosis
1. The diagnosis is clinical. The patient's history usually in-

cludes episodes of coughing and wheezing. The severity of previous episodes is a risk factor for the current illness. Additionally, the patient's history typically includes a trigger.

2. The differential diagnosis includes infection (e.g., bronchiolitis, pneumonia), anatomical or congenital anomalies, and foreign body aspiration.

HOT
KEY   Not all that wheezes is asthma!

B. Tests

1. **Pulse oximetry** is always obtained.
2. A **chest radiograph** can be useful for evaluation of other causes of symptoms and for pneumothorax and atelectasis associated with status asthmaticus.
3. **Arterial blood gas measurements** should be obtained on patients in extremis (indicated by marked accessory muscle use, poor or diminished inspiratory breath sounds, marked expiratory wheezing, or change in level of consciousness). A child who is well compensated should be able to blow off carbon dioxide. Patients with normal or elevated carbon dioxide levels need aggressive therapy.
4. Handheld **peak expiratory flow** (PEF) meters provide a useful assessment of the degree of airway obstruction, but should not be used in severely dyspneic patients.

HOT   Be wary of the "paradoxically normal" carbon dioxide values
       on arterial blood gas measurements. Children who are not in
       respiratory failure should have low carbon dioxide values; nor-
KEY   mal values may mean that they are tiring.

C. Initial therapy (Figure 47–1)

1. **Oxygen** should be administered as needed to keep the saturation above 95%.
2. The initial therapy for status asthmaticus is a **nebulized selective beta$_2$-agonist**. The dose of **albuterol** (the most commonly used of these agents) is 0.15 mg/kg (minimum dose 2.5 mg) every 20 minutes for three doses, then 0.15–0.3 mg/kg (or 2.5–10 mg) every 1–4 hours as needed, or 0.5 mg/kg (or 5–25 mg) hourly by continuous nebulization.
   a. In patients without an immediate response, systemic steroids should be initiated. Either **methylprednisolone** (1 mg/kg every 6 hours for 48 hours, then 2 mg/kg/day in

Initial Assessment
History, physical examination (auscultation, use of accessory muscles, heart rate, respiratory rate, PEF or FEV_1, oxygen saturation, arterial blood gas of patient in extremis, and other tests as indicated)

Initial Treatment
Inhaled short-acting beta$_2$-agonist, usually by nebulization, one dose every 20 minutes for 1 hour
Oxygen to maintain SaO_2 at 95%
Systemic corticosteroids if no immediate response, if patient recently took oral steroid, or if episode is severe
Sedation is contraindicated in the treatment of exacerbations

Repeat Assessment
Physical examination, PEF, O_2 saturation, other tests as needed

Moderate Episode
PEF 50% to 70% of predicted or personal best
Physical examination: moderate symptoms, accessory muscle use
Inhaled beta$_2$-agonist every 60 minutes
Consider corticosteroids
Continue treatment 1 to 3 hours, provided there is improvement

Severe Episode
PEF < 50% of predicted or personal best
Physical examination: severe symptoms at rest, chest retraction
History: high-risk patient
No improvement after initial treatment
Inhaled beta$_2$-agonist hourly or continuously ± inhaled anticholinergic
Oxygen
Systemic corticosteroid
Consider subcutaneous, intramuscular, or intravenous beta$_2$-agonist

Good Response
Response sustained 60 minutes after last treatment
Physical examination: normal PEF > 70%
No distress
O_2 saturation > 90% (95% in children)

Incomplete Response Within 1 to 2 Hours
History: high-risk patient
Physical examination: mild to moderate symptoms
PEF > 50% but < 70%
O_2 saturation not improving

Poor Response Within 1 Hour
History: high-risk patient
Physical examination: severe symptoms, drowsiness, confusion
PEF < 30%
PCO_2 > 45 mm Hg
PO_2 < 60 mm Hg

Discharge Home
Continue treatment with inhaled beta$_2$-agonist
Consider, in most cases, oral corticosteroid
Patient education:
  Take medicine correctly
  Review action plan
  Close medical follow-up

Admit to Hospital
Inhaled beta$_2$-agonist ± inhaled anticholinergic
Systemic corticosteriod
Oxygen
Consider intravenous aminophylline
Monitor PEF, O_2 saturation, pulse, theophylline level

Admit to Intensive Care
Continuous inhaled beta$_2$-agonist ± anticholinergic
Intravenous corticosteroid
Consider subcutaneous, intramuscular, or intravenous beta$_2$-agonist
Oxygen
Consider intravenous aminophylline
Possibly intubate and provide mechanical ventilation

Improve   **Not Improve**

Discharge Home
If PEF is > 70% of predicted or personal best and sustained on oral/inhaled medication

Admit to Intensive Care
If no improvement within 6 to 12 hours

2 doses until PEF is 70%) or **prednisone** (2 mg/kg loading dose, then 2 mg/kg/day until PEF is 70%) is used.
   b. In patients who do not have a complete response to inhaled beta-agonists, **anticholinergics** should be considered. The dose of **ipratropium bromide** is 250 µg up to every 20 minutes for three doses, then 250 µg every 2–6 hours.

D. Adjuvant therapies
   1. Intravenous terbutaline (2–10 micrograms/kg loading dose over 10 minutes, then 0.1–0.4 micrograms/kg/min) is considered for patients who fail to respond to hi-dose nebulized albuterol or in those who develop respiratory insufficiency ($P_{CO_2} > 55$ mm Hg).
   2. The use of aminophylline therapy continues to be somewhat controversial. Most studies have not shown significant benefit beyond inhaled beta-agonist therapy, and there are significant risks due to the narrow therapeutic index.
   3. Intubation is a **last resort** and should be avoided unless the patient becomes obtunded or apneic. The introduction of an additional fixed obstruction (i.e., the endotracheal tube itself) often worsens blood gas values. If intubation is used, a volume-limited ventilator is preferred. Settings should allow for a shortened i-time, longer e-time, lower rates, higher positive inspiratory pressure, and higher tidal volumes. To reduce the risk of seizure, care should be taken that the P_{CO_2} does not decrease more than 10 mm Hg/h.

E. Ongoing management. As shown in the management nomogram (see Figure 47–1), frequent evaluation of response to therapy drives further management. It is vital to reassess the condition of a patient with status asthmaticus frequently.

References
Cohen NH, Eigen H, Shaughnessy TE: Status asthmaticus: common issues in pediatric and adult critical care. *Crit Care Clin* 13(3):459–476, 1997.
Murphy SJ, Kelly HW: Advances in the management of acute asthma in children. *Pediatr Rev* 17(7):227–234, 1996.
Nichols DG: Emergency management of status asthmaticus in children. *Pediatr Ann* 25(7):394–400, 1996.

Figure 47–1. Nomogram for the management of an acute exacerbation of asthma in the emergency department and hospital. PEF = peak expiratory flow. (Reprinted with permission from the *International Consensus Report on Diagnosis and Management of Asthma*, PHS #92–3091, NIH Publication No. 92–3091 National Institutes of Health, Bethesda, Md., March, 1992.)

48. Status Epilepticus

I INTRODUCTION

A. **Background.** Status epilepticus (SE) is a medical emergency that requires immediate intervention. Without prompt control of seizures, neuronal damage may occur.

B. **Definition.** Status epilepticus is characterized by a prolonged seizure (lasting more than 15 minutes) or multiple seizures without intercurrent regaining of consciousness for more than 1 hour.

C. **Pathogenesis.** For patients with epilepsy, seizures may be precipitated by poor compliance with medications, fever, sleep deprivation, or alcohol withdrawal. For patients who do not have epilepsy, cerebral pathologies (e.g., stroke, tumor, trauma, anoxia, meningitis, drug or alcohol withdrawal, metabolic disorders) are potential causes.

D. **Epidemiology.** Approximately 33% of patients who present with SE do not have a history of seizures.

II CLINICAL MANIFESTATIONS

A. Classically, **convulsive SE** is tonic/clonic and easily identifiable.

B. **Nonconvulsive SE** with complex partial or absence seizures may present with a history of confusion or stupor that sometimes lasts for days. These forms of SE are not medical emergencies, but do require an immediate electroencephalogram (EEG) for diagnosis.

III APPROACH TO THE PATIENT

A. **History and physical examination**
1. **History.** After the patient's condition is stabilized, the physician should inquire about fevers, medication history, the possibility of ingestions, and trauma. A description of the features and frequency of any previous seizures should be obtained.
2. **Physical examination.** The patient should be assessed for evidence of increased intracranial pressure (e.g., posturing, asymmetric pupils, papilledema, papillary dilation) and muscle tone. Abnormal neurologic signs (e.g., abnormal tone, pupillary changes) are common during and immediately after a seizure.

B. Laboratory tests. Electrolytes, calcium, magnesium, blood urea nitrogen (BUN), creatinine, liver function tests, glucose, serum and urine toxicology screen, and antiepileptic drug levels should be evaluated. Blood should be drawn for a complete blood count (CBC) with differential and blood culture, if indicated. Arterial blood gases may show hypercapnia and hypoxemia or an anion gap metabolic acidosis as a result of lactic acidosis.

C. Initial therapy. Treatment should follow a logical, stepwise approach.

  1. The **airway** should be secured, the oropharynx should be suctioned, and supplemental oxygen should be administered. Vital signs should be monitored closely.

  2. Intravenous access should be obtained. The need for intraosseous access or a central line should be anticipated if peripheral intravenous access cannot be obtained rapidly.

  3. A loading dose of **phenytoin** (15–20 mg/kg intravenously at 1 mg/kg/min), **lorazepam** (0.1 mg/kg intravenously), and 25% **glucose** (2–4 ml/kg intravenously) should be administered immediately. Lorazepam is preferred over diazepam because it provides longer action and less respiratory depression. Diazepam can be given rectally (0.2–0.5 mg/kg) if intravenous access is difficult to obtain. Fosphenytoin can be loaded three times faster (up to 3 mg/kg/min) than phenytoin because there are no cardiac side effects. It is also useful because it can be given intramuscularly.

  4. Additional phenytoin (up to a total of 30 mg/kg intravenously) and lorazepam (0.1 mg/kg every 5–10 minutes intravenously to a maximum of 5 mg/kg) may be administered if seizures continue. Intubation is probably needed at this point.

  5. Phenobarbital (15–20 mg/kg intravenously, to a maximum of 40 mg/kg) may be added if seizures continue.

  6. Recalcitrant seizures may require **paraldehyde** (5–10 ml rectally), lidocaine (1–2 mg/kg intravenously), or **chloral hydrate** (30 mg/kg rectally).

  7. If seizures continue for 45–60 minutes, SE is considered refractory. The patient should be intubated. General anesthesia with an isoflurane anesthetic or a pentobarbital-induced coma should be considered.

 HOT KEY Recalcitrant seizures may be caused by any of the three "hypos": hypoxemia, hyponatremia, or hypoglycemia. These causes should be considered if there is not a rapid response to medication.

D. Adjuvant therapies
  1. Intubation should be considered if the patient has received

multiple combinations of drug boluses or is unable to protect his or her airway. If intubation is required, a nondepolarizing paralytic drug should be used during the rapid-sequence intubation to minimize increases in intracerebral pressure. As seizures are controlled, resumption of normal breathing and correction of hypoventilation may be expected.

  2. Immediate ceftriaxone administration (100 mg/kg intravenously) should be given if meningitis is suspected. Ceftriaxone should still be administered even if lumbar puncture is delayed.

HOT KEY If meningitis is suspected, no more than 30 minutes should elapse between the initial suspicion and the beginning of treatment with antibiotics.

---

  3. Rectal administration of acetaminophen should be considered if the patient is febrile ($> 38°C$).
  4. Pyridoxine (100 mg intravenously) should be considered for infants who have intractable seizures. This treatment is both diagnostic and therapeutic for pyridoxine deficiency.

E. Ongoing management. A neurologist should always be consulted for assistance in the management of ongoing seizures.

  1. Admission to the intensive care unit is required for patients whose seizures are not immediately controlled.
  2. Maintenance intravenous solutions should be isotonic to keep cerebral edema to a minimum. Glucose is always added to maintenance fluids.
  3. An emergent computed tomography (CT) scan with cervical spine precautions should be obtained if head trauma is suspected. CT scans also are indicated for patients who have residual deficits or a history of partial seizures.
  4. Lumbar puncture should be performed in all patients who have suspected meningitis without clinical signs of increased intracranial pressure.
  5. Patients who require multiple doses of benzodiazepines or phenobarbital subsequently have a depressed level of consciousness and may require an EEG to assess the adequacy of therapy.

References

Kliegman RM: *Practical Strategies in Pediatric Diagnosis and Therapy*. Philadelphia, WB Saunders, 1996, pp 638–640.

McMillan JA, DeAngelis CD, Feigin RD (eds): *Oski's Pediatrics: Principles and Practice,* 3rd ed. Philadelphia, Lippincott Williams & Wilkins, 1999, pp 578–579.

49. Syncope

I INTRODUCTION

A. Syncope is the transient loss of consciousness and postural tone that results from inadequate cerebral perfusion.

B. Pathophysiology

1. Cerebral perfusion is compromised by impaired cerebral vascular tone or decreased cardiac output. In most cases, there is an imbalance in parasympathetic and sympathetic tone, with peripheral vasodilation and venodilation. Preload and stroke volume are impaired. Increased vagal tone causes bradycardia, and, as a result, cardiac output is sharply diminished.

2. A primary or secondary dysrhythmia also can cause an abrupt decrease in cardiac output and cerebral perfusion.

C. Epidemiology

1. Approximately 15% of children experience a syncopal event before the end of adolescence.

2. Before 6 years of age, vaso-vagal syncope is unusual. It usually results from seizures, breath-holding spells, or primary arrhythmias.

II APPROACH TO THE PATIENT

A. It is important to determine whether dizziness is a result of presyncope (caused by impaired cerebral perfusion), lightheadedness (due to anxiety, depression, certain medications, and hyperventilation), vertigo (due to vestibular disorders), or disequilibrium (caused by neurologic disorders).

B. Differential diagnosis. Although the most common type of syncope in children and adolescents is neurocardiogenic syncope (also known as vasodepressor syncope, vasovagal syncope, and common fainting), the differential diagnosis is broad **(Table 49–1).**

HOT KEY

Cardiac syncope is caused by either primary or secondary arrhythmia, is a predictor of sudden death, and may be an episode of aborted sudden death.

TABLE 49-1. Syncope: Differential Diagnosis

Diagnosis	History	Symptoms	Description	Postsyncope
Neurocardiogenic (vasodepressor)	At rest, upright posture	Pallor, nausea, visual changes	Brief ± convulsion	Residual pallor, sweaty, hot, recurs on standing
Other vagal				
Vasovagal	Needle stick, see blood	Pallor, nausea	Brief, convulsions rare	Residual pallor, may recur on standing
Micturition	Postvoiding	Pallor, nausea	Brief, ± convulsion	Fatigue or baseline
Cough (deglutition)	Paroxysmal cough	Cough	Abrupt onset	Fatigue or baseline
Carotid sinus	Tight collar, turned head	Vague, visual changes	Sudden onset, pallor	Relieved by eating only
Hypoglycemia	Fasting, insulin use	Gradual hunger, weakness, sweating	Pallor, sweating, LOC rare	
Neuropsychiatric				
Hyperventilation	Anxiety	SOB, fear, claustrophobia	Agitated, hyperpneic ± Pallor	Fatigue or baseline
Syncopal migraine	Headache	Aura, migraine, nausea		Headache, often occipital
Seizure disorder	Any time	± Aura	Convulsion ± incontinence	Postictal lethargy + confusion
Hysterical	Always an "audience" present	Psychological distress	Gentle, graceful swoon	Normal baseline
Breath-holding (hypoxic)	Agitation or injury	Crying	Cyanosis ± convulsion	Fatigue, residual pallor

Cardiac syncope

LVOT obstruction	Exercise	± Chest pain, SOB	Abrupt during or after exertion, pallor	Fatigue, residual pallor and sweating
Pulmonary hypertension	Any time, especially exercise	SOB	Cyanosis and pallor	Fatigue, residual cyanosis
Myocarditis	Postviral, exercise	SOB, chest pain, palpitations	Pallor	Fatigue
Tumor or mass	Recumbent, paroxysmal	SOB ± chest pain	Pallor	Baseline
Coronary artery	Exercise	SOB ± chest pain	Pallor	Fatigue, chest pain
Dysrhythmia	Any time	Palpitations ± chest pain	Pallor	Fatigue or baseline

Reprinted with permission from Lewis DA: Syncope and dizziness. In *Practical Strategies in Pediatric Diagnosis and Therapy.* Edited by Kleigman RM. Philadelphia, WB Saunders, 1996, p 680.

LOC = loss of consciousness; ± = with or without; LVOT = left ventricular outflow tract; SOB = shortness of breath.

HOT KEY

Seizures are the most likely cause of syncope in the recumbent patient.

C. Evaluation

1. **History** is paramount. Inquiries should be made about the time of the event, the last meal, activities leading up to the event, duration of the event, position before and after the event, and medication history. The patient's appearance before and after the event should be determined. The patient should also be asked about associated symptoms, such as diaphoresis, palpitations, shortness of breath, rapid heart rate, chest pain, nausea, and hearing or visual changes.

HOT KEY

Syncope without warning (no prodrome) or syncope during exercise suggests a cardiac etiology.

2. **Family history.** Inquiries should be made about syncope, sudden death, dysrhythmia, congenital heart disease, seizures, and metabolic disorders in family members.
3. **Drugs.** Accidental drug ingestion with antihypertensive medications, diuretics, antidepressants, anticonvulsants, phenothiazine, benzodiazepines/hypnotics, antipsychotics, histamine (H_2) blockers, or other drugs can induce syncope.
4. On **physical examination,** particular attention should be paid to the cardiovascular and neurologic systems.

HOT KEY

Hypotension, either supine or orthostatic, is a red flag for a cardiac etiology.

D. Diagnostic studies

1. All patients who present with syncope need an **electrocardiogram (ECG)** with careful determination of rhythm, intervals (PR, QRS, QTc), and voltages for hypertrophy or enlargement. The ECG should be examined closely for delta waves, which may be evidence of Wolf-Parkinson-White syndrome as well as long QT syndrome (**Figures 49–1** and **49–2**).
2. **Screening laboratory values,** such as electrolytes and

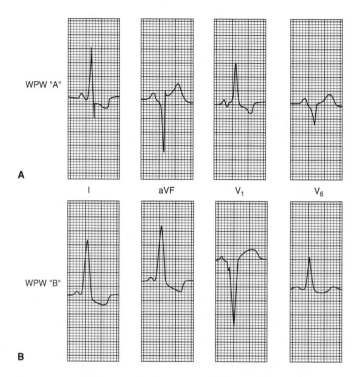

Figure 49–1. Wolff-Parkinson-White syndrome. **(A)** Rosenbaum type A and **(B)** Rosenbaum type B. An accessory path between the atria and ventricles (Kent bundle) causes a fusion complex (delta wave) and a characteristically short PR interval. (Reprinted with permission from Garson A Jr: *The Electrocardiogram in Infants and Children.* Philadelphia, Lea & Febiger, 1983, p 139.)

glucose, usually contribute little to the diagnosis. Anemia occasionally is discovered.

3. **Holter monitoring** can be useful if the syncope is recurrent or is associated with palpitations or tachycardia.

4. **Treadmill testing** may be indicated if syncope is associated with exercise.

5. **Echocardiography** should be performed if indicated by the history, examination, or ECG findings.

6. **Electroencephalography (EEG)** is appropriate if the patient has prolonged loss of consciousness, seizure activity, or a post-ictal state.

7. **Tilt-table testing** uses orthostatic stress to attempt to elicit

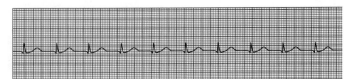

Rhythm strip - Lead III

Figure 49–2. Electrocardiogram of a patient with the Romano-Ward syndrome at age 6 years shows the longest QTc interval (0.56 second). The precordial leads are not shown. (Adapted with permission from Park MK: *Pediatric Cardiology for Practitioners,* 4th ed. Philadelphia, Mosby, 2002, p 457.)

physiologic responses associated with neurocardiogenic syncope. It is useful in cases of noncardiac recurrent syncope. It is not very specific, but its sensitivity is 85%.

E. Treatment. Therapy is determined by the cause of the event.
  1. Neurocardiogenic syncope
    a. Volume expansion, including increased fluid and salt intake with or without a low-dose mineralocorticoid (e.g., fludrocortisone acetate), usually is the initial treatment for neurocardiogenic syncope.
    b. Beta-adrenergic antagonists (e.g., atenolol) block vagal output by mimicking increased parasympathetic tone.
    c. Alpha-adrenergic agonists (e.g., pseudoephedrine) increase heart rate and peripheral vascular tone. Serotonin agonists (e.g., sertraline) are used in refractory syncope.
  2. Long QT syndrome. Immediate consultation with a cardiologist is mandatory because of the risk of sudden death. Initiation of medications should not be delayed.

References
McHarg ML, Shinnar S, Rascoff H, et al: Syncope in childhood. *Pediatr Cardiol* 18(5):367–371, 1997.
Lewis DA, Dhala A: Syncope in the pediatric patient. The cardiologist's perspective. *Pediatr Clin North Am* 46(2):205–219, 1999.

50. Refusal to Bear Weight

I. INTRODUCTION

A. Background
1. A refusal to bear weight is a common presenting complaint in emergency departments and primary care clinics.
2. Making a diagnosis is challenging because the patient often is nonverbal and uncooperative.
3. The risk of a misdiagnosis (e.g., septic arthritis, cancer) is potentially devastating.
4. Most children can "cruise" (i.e., walk while holding on to a table or another object) by 12 months and walk independently by 18 months. A mature walking pattern usually develops by 3 years.

HOT **KEY**
An important diagnosis to rule out in children who refuse to bear weight is septic arthritis, which is an orthopedic emergency.

B. Definitions
1. **Normal gait** consists of a stance phase and a swing phase. In the **stance phase,** the foot is in full contact with the ground and is supporting all body weight. The **swing phase** begins with toe push-off and ends with heel strike of the same foot.
2. **Antalgic gait** is characterized by a shortened stance phase on the affected limb.
3. **Trendelenburg gait** is characterized by the pelvis tilting away from the involved extremity in an attempt to minimize transmitted forces through the injured limb.

C. Pathogenesis and epidemiology.
Although the potential causes for a child refusing to bear weight are extensive, the most important causes of refusal to bear weight can be easily remembered using the mnemonic "the joint STARTS HOT."

"STARTS HOT"

Septic arthritis
Trauma
Acute rheumatic fever
Rheumatoid arthritis
Tumor (including leukemia)
Slipped capital femoral epiphysis (and Legg-Calvé-Perthes disease)
Henoch-Schönlein purpura
Osteomyelitis and **O**sgood-Schlatter disease
Toxic synovitis

II DIFFERENTIAL DIAGNOSIS

A. Infectious
1. The knee and hip are the joints most often affected. If the condition is misdiagnosed or if treatment is delayed, loss of joint function may result. Fifty percent of all cases develop in children younger than 3 years of age.
2. **Osteomyelitis** is an infection of the bone. The most common locations are the distal femoral metaphysis and proximal tibial metaphysis. There is a bimodal peak in infancy and preadolescence (9–11 years of age).
3. **Acute rheumatic fever or poststreptococcal reactive arthritis** is an autoimmune disorder that is caused by antibody response to the group A streptococcus antigens. It is a nonsuppurative condition that occurs after an upper respiratory infection by group A streptococci. Rheumatic fever affects large joints and is migratory. The affected joint is swollen, red, hot, and tender, but responds quickly to salicylates. Usually, rheumatic fever leaves no lasting sequelae on the affected joint.

B. Inflammatory
1. **Transient (toxic) synovitis** is a self-limited inflammatory condition of the hip joint. It is a common cause of limping and leg pain in children. The incidence peaks at 3–6 years of age. The cause is unknown, but it often occurs after upper respiratory tract infections.
2. **Henoch-Schönlein purpura** is an idiopathic vasculitis that affects multiple systems in previously well children. There is a classic palpable purpuric rash involving the lower extremities and buttocks. The arthritis is nonmigratory and periarticular and usually lacks significant warmth or erythema.
3. **Juvenile rheumatoid arthritis (JRA)** has a mean age at onset of 1–3 years. Fatigue, low-grade fever, anorexia, weight

loss, morning stiffness, night pain, and rheumatoid nodules may be present. Joints are tender, and there is pain on movement. Some forms have uveitis. Nonsteroidal anti-inflammatory drugs (NSAIDs), hydroxychloroquine, and methotrexate may be used in treatment. Each of the three types of JRA has a different set of characteristics.

C. Orthopedic

1. **Toddler's fracture** is a subtle, oblique, nondisplaced fracture through the tibial diaphysis. Minimal swelling may be present. These fractures occur in children who are just beginning to walk (9 months to 3 years of age). The fractures are believed to result from a combination of the toddler's clumsy gait and bones that have just begun to accommodate new forces. The event that causes the fracture may not be severe (e.g., changing direction suddenly, jumping and falling with a twist).

2. **Traumatic fracture.** Active toddlers are at risk for accidental trauma. Midshaft femoral fractures become more common as a child grows. However, most midshaft femur fractures in children younger than 1 year of age are caused by abuse.

3. **Developmental hip dysplasia (DHD).** The acetabulum and other hip joint structures develop during gestation and continue to develop after birth. Abnormalities in intrauterine position (e.g., breech position), or joint cartilage may result in hip dysplasia. The incidence of true dislocation at birth is 1.5 per 1000 births. This condition is six times more common in girls. Hip dysplasia usually is detected at birth or soon after, but some cases are missed and present at a later age. All newborns should be examined for the Barlow sign (subluxation during adduction and posterior pressure) and the Ortolani sign (hip relocation during abduction).

4. **Legg-Calvé-Perthes disease (LCP) or coxa plana** is a form of ischemic necrosis of the femoral head. Its cause is uncertain. The peak incidence is between 4 and 9 years of age, and it is four times more common in boys. Patients may present with a Trendelenburg gait; when standing on the affected limb, these patients cannot maintain a level pelvis. Internal rotation during flexion and abduction is especially limited.

5. **Slipped capital femoral epiphysis (SCFE)** is a disorder of puberty. It usually occurs in obese boys; 25% of cases are bilateral. The femoral head is displaced through the epiphyseal plate from the femoral neck. In more severe cases, the femoral head is displaced posteriorly and inferiorly from the proximal femur. Patients may have hip, knee, or thigh pain. Patients often have persistent external rotation with flexion.

6. **Osgood-Schlatter disease** tends to occur during the adoles-

cent growth spurt. It is believed to be due to a difference in growth rate between the osseous and soft tissue structures, combined with stress on the apophysis from vigorous physical activity. It is often bilateral. Affected patients have pain and swelling over the tibial tubercle and cannot walk on their knees.

D. Oncologic
1. **Leukemia.** Pain and loss of function may result from leukemic infiltration of the marrow cavities of the lower extremities.
2. Patients with **solid tumors** (e.g., Ewing sarcoma) also can present with pain.

III CLINICAL MANIFESTATIONS

A. History
1. **Age of child.** Common diagnoses often are age-dependent.
2. **Onset of pain.** Was the pain sudden or insidious?
3. **Duration of pain.** Is the pain constant or intermittent?
4. **Quality of pain.** Is the pain severe or mild?
5. **Location of pain.** The location of the pain often is difficult to pinpoint in nonverbal children. A change in the quality of a child's cry as a suspected area is palpated can be helpful in pinpointing a fracture.
6. **Associated symptoms** include fever, rash, vomiting, weight loss, and recent infections.
7. **Aggravating and alleviating factors.** Does tactile stimulation to the painful area make it better?

> **HOT KEY** Given the clumsiness of most toddlers, there often is a history of trauma before the onset of symptoms. Parents and physicians may mistakenly attribute the refusal to bear weight to such an event.

B. Physical examination
1. **Vital signs.** Infectious or inflammatory processes are eight times more likely to present with a temperature higher than 38°C.
2. **Observation at rest.** Does the child appear uncomfortable? Children with swollen joints rest the leg in the position that allows for the largest joint space volume. For example, a child with a septic hip will hold the leg in flexion and external rotation.
3. A **general examination** should be performed to assess the patient for rash, signs of trauma, hepatosplenomegaly, and pallor.
4. **Observation of gait** (stance and swing phases). Can the child walk on his or her knees?

HOT KEY Ask the child to walk on his or her knees. If the child cooperates and can bear weight on the knees without pain, the involved area has been isolated to the shin or below.

5. **Inspection of extremities.** Does the patient have erythema, ecchymoses, or puncture wounds? The joints and extremities should be palpated for swelling, tenderness, and warmth.
6. **Passive and active ranges of motion should be tested,** particularly for the hips. Abnormalities of internal and external hip rotation limited by pain are early indicators of hip pathology.
7. A **neurovascular evaluation** should be performed to test reflexes and capillary refill and to perform a thorough sensory examination.

IV APPROACH TO THE PATIENT

 HOT KEY "Growing pains" are common in children but should be considered a diagnosis of exclusion. Growing pains rarely present with loss of function.

A. **Diagnosis**
1. The findings on physical examination guide which, if any, laboratory tests are needed to help determine a definitive diagnosis.
2. An afebrile child without localizing findings on examination has a very low risk for an infectious process.
3. Any findings that suggest infection mandate a complete workup because of the potentially devastating consequences.
4. Differentiating transient synovitis from septic arthritis can be difficult. In one study, 97% of children with septic arthritis had a temperature higher than 37.5°C and an erythrocyte sedimentation rate of 20 mm or greater.
B. **Laboratory tests**
1. **Complete blood cell count (CBC)** should be ordered in all patients in whom an inflammatory, infectious, or leukemic disorder is suspected. Although the CBC often is elevated in infectious conditions, it may be normal.
2. The **erythrocyte sedimentation rate (ESR)** should be ordered for all patients in whom an inflammatory or infectious disorder is suspected.
3. **C-reactive protein (CRP)** is elevated in most infectious and

inflammatory disorders and may show an increase earlier in the process than ESR. It also can be used to monitor the response to therapy.

4. **Blood cultures** should be ordered if an infectious process is suspected. Cultures are positive in 30%–60% of children with osteomyelitis.

5. **Synovial fluid analysis and culture** should be performed in all patients suspected of having septic arthritis. Gram stain, culture, cell count, glucose, and protein measurements should be performed on the synovial fluid. Typically, synovial fluid culture is positive in only 30%–50% of patients with septic arthritis. Patients with septic arthritis have a white blood cell count in excess of $25,000/mm^3$, a predominance of polymorphonuclear cells, a decreased glucose level, and an increased protein level.

6. **Rheumatologic workup.** Juvenile rheumatoid arthritis usually is a diagnosis of exclusion. However, if rheumatologic disease is suspected, the following tests should be obtained: antinuclear antibodies (ANA), rheumatoid factor, ESR, and CRP. In addition, patients with JRA may have anemia of chronic inflammation, with a hemoglobin level as low as 7–10 g/dl.

C. **Imaging studies**

1. **Plain radiographs.** Bilateral films should be obtained for comparison. At least two views in perpendicular planes should be ordered. Both anteroposterior and frog-leg lateral views should be ordered if hip pathology is suspected. A complete skeletal survey should be performed if child abuse is suspected. Plain radiographs are helpful in diagnosing hip pathology and most fractures. Abnormal findings may be seen in patients with LCP (e.g., subchondral crescents, collapse of the femoral head), transient synovitis and septic arthritis (i.e., widening of the joint space), and leukemia (i.e., lytic lesions). In DHD, anteroposterior radiographs show migration of the femur; a shallow, more vertical, acetabulum; and delayed appearance of the femoral ossific nucleus.

2. **A bone scan** should be obtained if plain films are normal but nondisplaced fracture, osteomyelitis, avascular necrosis, or metastatic disease is suspected. It may be difficult to interpret findings near the epiphyses.

3. **Ultrasound scans** may be helpful to assess for fluid or pus within the hip joint.

D. **Treatment**

HOT KEY Septic arthritis, osteomyelitis, LCP, developmental hip dysplasia, malignant neoplasms, and injuries from child abuse all require immediate consultation with a specialist.

1. **Transient synovitis.** With anti-inflammatory medications and rest, symptoms should resolve within 1–2 weeks.
2. **Toddler's and traumatic fractures.** Nondisplaced fractures are splinted. Complicated fractures require orthopedic consultation. If child abuse is suspected, consultation with a specialist should be obtained and local child protective services should be contacted.
3. **Developmental hip dysplasia.** Bracing will not correct dysplasia in a toddler, although it will in a newborn. A toddler with hip dysplasia requires orthopedic consultation and surgical correction with osteotomy.
4. **LCP** requires immediate orthopedic referral for further management, which may include rest, bracing, or surgery.
5. **Slipped capital femoral epiphysis** requires referral to an orthopedic surgeon because surgery may be needed, especially in severe cases. The child's condition should be monitored longitudinally because SCFE may develop in the opposite limb.
6. **Osgood-Schlatter disease**. Treatment is not needed if the condition does not interfere with daily activities. NSAIDs, rest, and daily stretching of quadriceps and hamstrings are usually sufficient. If the pain is severe, a short course of casting or splinting may be useful.

V PROGNOSIS

A. If diagnosed and treated early, **septic arthritis and osteomyelitis** have no long-term sequelae.
B. **LCP** may result in osteoarthritis later in life, but study results are not conclusive.
C. **Transient synovitis** typically resolves without sequelae; however, some studies show a slight increase in the incidence of LCP after an episode of transient synovitis.
D. Given the healing abilities of children's bones, **fractures** rarely present any long-term complications.
E. **DHD** patients treated in a timely manner do well. Untreated patients may suffer from recurrent dislocation, gait abnormality, or avascular necrosis of the femoral head.

References
Lawrence LL: The limping child. *Emerg Med Clin North Am* 16:911–929, 1998.
Myers MT, Thompson GH: Imaging the child with a limp. *Pediatr Clin North Am* 44: 637–658, 1997.

PART VI

GENERAL CARDIOLOGY

51. Normal Murmurs

I **INTRODUCTION.** Many children have benign murmurs. Most start after S_1 and end before S_2. All of these murmurs are ejection murmurs (diamond-shaped) and have a maximum grade of III. Most can be heard in the neck; they are almost never heard in the back. All other parts of the cardiac examination are normal.

II **PRESCHOOL-AGE CHILDREN (AORTIC EJECTION MURMUR)**

A. **Physiology.** An aortic ejection murmur arises from the root of the aorta. It is heard in infants who are a few months old and in children of preschool age. It is also known as a Still's murmur.

B. **The murmur.** A normal physiologic split is heard during S_2. In contrast, in aortic stenosis, the S_2 split is narrow.
   1. **Systolic component.** The murmur has no ejection click; it is described as vibratory. The quality of this murmur is similar to the sound made by a musical instrument; some describe it as a plucked violin string or a vibrating tuning fork.
   2. The murmur has a low-to-middle frequency.
   3. The area of greatest intensity is the left lower sternal border. It also is heard well along the midclavicular line. The murmur is accentuated when listening with the bell of the stethoscope.
   4. **Differential diagnosis** includes subvalvular aortic stenosis and aortic coarctation.

III **ADOLESCENT-AGE CHILDREN (PULMONIC EJECTION MURMUR)**

A. **Physiology.** This murmur is heard in teens to young adults. It arises from the right ventricular outflow tract.

B. **The murmur.** A normal S_2 split occurs with respiration. In contrast, in valvular pulmonic stenosis, the S_2 split is prolonged.

   1. Systolic component. An ejection murmur is heard, but there
      is no ejection click.
   2. The frequency of the murmur is high.
   3. The area of greatest intensity is the upper left sternal border.
C. The **differential diagnosis** includes pulmonic stenosis and
     atrial septal defect.

IV VENOUS HUM

A. Physiology. A venous hum occurs because of the sharp angle
   between the subclavian vein and the superior vena cava. The
   sound is created by turbulent passive venous inflow.
B. The murmur. A venous hum is a medium-frequency continuous
   murmur that is best heard in the sitting position. Its intensity
   changes as the child moves his or her head from side to side; it
   disappears when the child lies down or when the jugular vein is
   gently compressed.

HOT KEY

A venous hum is best heard just below the clavicles.

C. The **differential diagnosis** includes patent ductus arteriosus.

V PERIPHERAL PULMONIC STENOSIS

A. Physiology. Peripheral pulmonic stenosis occurs because of the
   sharp angles at the branches of the pulmonary arteries. It is
   characteristically found in newborns.

HOT KEY

If peripheral pulmonic stenosis persists for longer than 6 months,
it is considered pathologic, and branch pulmonic artery stenosis
should be considered.

B. The murmur. This high-frequency murmur is heard well in the
   axilla and the back. It is maximal at the upper sternal borders,
   with good transmission into the axillae. Peripheral pulmonic
   stenosis is heard well over a wide area of the precordium.

References
Liebman J: Diagnosis and management of heart murmurs in children. *Pediatr Rev* 3:
    321–329, 1982.
Nadas AS, Fyler DC: *Nadas' Pediatric Cardiology*. Philadelphia, Hanley & Belfus,
    1992.

52. Bacterial Endocarditis

INTRODUCTION

A. Background. Bacterial endocarditis in childhood is rare, but causes substantial morbidity and mortality. Before the advent of antibiotic therapy, bacterial endocarditis was fatal. Treatment continues to be challenging and includes prolonged parenteral antibiotics and occasionally surgery. Primary prevention of endocarditis is essential.

> **HOT** **KEY**
>
> Endocarditis must be excluded in persistently febrile children, particularly those with congenital heart disease (CHD), previous cardiac surgery, and indwelling vascular catheters.

B. Definitions
1. **Bacterial endocarditis** is infection of the endocardium or cardiac endothelium.
2. **Vegetation** refers to a semiorganized fibrin thrombus that contains high concentrations of bacteria and adheres to the endocardium.

C. Pathogenesis
1. A **damaged endothelium** increases the risk of developing endocarditis during periods of bacteremia. Damage to the endothelial wall usually is secondary to high-pressure jets. This occurs most commonly with ventricular septal defects (VSDs) and aortic stenosis. Alterations in the dynamics of blood flow, also associated with CHD, lead to flow eddies, allow bacterial stasis, and increase the risk of endocarditis.
2. **Bacteremia** may occur spontaneously. It also may complicate focal infection or instrumentation of the oral cavity or the respiratory, gastrointestinal, or genitourinary tract. Indwelling vascular catheters also increase the risk of bacteremia.
3. Bacteria, platelets, and fibrin adhere to the damaged endothelium, and a **vegetation** is formed. Vegetations in the path of turbulent flow can embolize anywhere in the body. The constant presence of foreign antigen causes an immunologic response. Rheumatoid factor and circulating immune complexes are found in approximately half of patients.

D. Microbiology

1. **Alpha-hemolytic streptococci** (e.g., *Streptococcus viridans, S. sanguis*), ***Staphylococcus aureus,*** and **coagulase-negative staphylococci** cause approximately 50% of cases of childhood endocarditis. Unlike *Streptococcus viridans,* which usually causes an insidious course, *Staphylococcus aureus* is a particularly aggressive organism. Enterococci are an uncommon cause of endocarditis in children.

2. **HACEK organisms** (*Haemophilus, Actinobacillus, Cardiobacterium, Eikenella,* and *Kingella*) have become more frequently seen pathogens, particularly among immunocompromised patients and neonates. This group of fastidious organisms accounts for most cases of gram-negative endocarditis.

3. **Fungal endocarditis** usually is caused by *Candida* species. It typically occurs in neonates who have indwelling vascular catheters for prolonged periods of time. Fungal endocarditis is associated with a very poor prognosis.

4. **Culture-negative endocarditis** is clinical endocarditis in patients who have consistently negative blood culture results. It accounts for 5%–20% of cases. It is associated with organisms that are difficult to grow and cases in which there was antibiotic pretreatment.

E. Epidemiology

1. The reported incidence of bacterial endocarditis in children ranges from 1:1000 to 1:10,000. The incidence seems to be increasing.

2. The affected population is changing, with few cases associated with rheumatic fever and more cases associated with cardiac surgery and the long-term use of venous catheters in immunocompromised patients.

II CLINICAL MANIFESTATIONS include the following symptoms:

A. Very common: fever

B. Common: malaise, headaches, and myalgias

C. Uncommon: new or changing murmur, petechiae, splenomegaly, neurologic changes, hematuria, and symptoms of congestive heart failure (CHF)

D. Rare: Osler nodes (i.e., tender subcutaneous nodules on distal extremities), Janeway lesions (i.e., nontender hemorrhagic plaques on palms and soles), Roth spots (i.e., pale/hemorrhagic retinal lesions), and splinter hemorrhages

III APPROACH TO THE PATIENT

A. Diagnosis

1. **Laboratory findings**

   a. **Very common:** positive blood cultures as well as elevated sedimentation rate and C-reactive protein level
   b. **Common:** anemia, leukocytosis, hematuria, and rheumatoid factor
2. **Echocardiography.** Vegetations or an oscillating mass can be identified by echocardiography in 75%–80% of patients. Transesophageal echocardiography is more sensitive than transthoracic imaging in older children and in those with prosthetic valves or shunts. Diagnosing endocarditis can be problematic when echocardiography does not identify a vegetation.
3. **Blood cultures**
   a. Persistent bacteremia is sufficient evidence for diagnosis. Persistent bacteremia is present if multiple blood culture results from separate blood samples are positive for the same organism. Daily cultures taken over several days or three cultures taken over a 24-hour period are sufficient.
   b. Cultures should be allowed to grow for extended periods in appropriate media.
B. **Antibiotic therapy**
   1. Bacteria in the semiorganized thrombus are difficult to eradicate because they are protected from host defenses.
   2. Prolonged therapy (at least 4 weeks) with high serum concentrations of bactericidal antibiotics is required.
   3. Therapy is always guided by the sensitivities of specific organisms. General guidelines are given in **Table 52–1**.
C. **Adjuvant therapy.** Surgical intervention may be required if infection persists despite appropriate antibiotic therapy. Abscess formation, valve destruction, progressive CHF, and the potential for life-threatening embolization are also potential indications for surgery. Surgery is often required for fungal endocarditis.
D. **Prevention.** Approximately 10% of cases of endocarditis are attributable to a procedure. The American Heart Association makes recommendations according to risk stratification by procedure and cardiac condition. Prophylaxis is recommended for essentially all forms of unrepaired CHD, with the exception of isolated secundum atrial septal defects (ASDs), mitral valve prolapse without regurgitation, and repaired ASDs, ventricular septal defects (VSDs), and patent ductus arteriosus (without residua beyond 6 months) **(Tables 52–2, 52–3, 52–4, and 52–5).**

 PROGNOSIS. Reported mortality rates range from 13%–30%. Significantly higher mortality rates are reported among children without CHD or with mild anomalies, children with a rapid course of illness, and children younger than age 3 years.

Table 52-1. Guidelines for Antibiotic Therapy in Patients with Bacterial Endocarditis

Organism(s)	Antibiotic(s) Administered	Duration of Course (weeks)
Streptococci	Penicillin + gentamicin or ceftriaxone or vancomycin (if allergic)	4
Staphylococci	Nafcillin or vancomycin (if allergic or if methicillin-resistant *Staphylococcus aureus*); if prosthetic materials, vancomycin + gentamicin + rifampin	6
Enterococci	Vancomycin + gentamicin	6
HACEK organisms	Ceftriaxone	6
Culture-negative endocarditis	Nafcillin + gentamicin	6
Fungal	Amphotericin	6

Data from Brook MM: Pediatric bacterial endocarditis. Treatment and prophylaxis. *Pediatr Clin North Am* 46(2):275–287, 1999.

HACEK = *Haemophilus, Actinobacillus, Cardiobacterium, Eikenella,* and *Kingella.*

TABLE 52-2. Endocarditis Prophylaxis

	Recommended*	Not Recommended
Dental procedures	Dental extractions Periodontal procedures, including surgery, scaling and root planing, probing, and routine maintenance Dental implant placement and reimplantation of avulsed teeth Endodontic (root canal) instrumentation or surgery only beyond the apex	Restorative dentistry† (operative and prosthodontic) with or without retraction cord‡ Local anesthetic injections (nonintraligamentary) Intracanal endodontic treatment; postplacement and build-up Placement of rubber dams Postoperative suture removal Fluoride treatments *(continued)*

TABLE 52-2. Endocarditis Prophylaxis (*Continued*)		
	Recommended*	**Not Recommended**
Dental procedures (*continued*)	Subgingival placement of antibiotic fibers or strips Initial placement of orthodontic bands but not brackets Intraligamentary local anesthetic injections Prophylactic cleaning of teeth or implants during which bleeding is anticipated	Taking of oral radiographs Placement of removable prosthodontic or orthodontic appliances Taking of oral impressions Orthodontic appliance adjustment Shedding of primary teeth
Respiratory tract	Tonsillectomy, adenoidectomy, or both Surgical operations that involve respiratory mucosa Bronchoscopy with a rigid bronchoscope	Endotracheal intubation Bronchoscopy with a flexible bronchoscope, with or without biopsy§ Tympanostomy tube insertion
Gastrointestinal tract‖	Sclerotherapy for esophageal varices Esophageal stricture dilation Endoscopic retrograde cholangiography with biliary obstruction Biliary tract surgery Surgical operations that involve intestinal mucosa	Transesophageal echocardiography§ Endoscopy with or without gastrointestinal biopsy§

Genitourinary tract	Prostatic surgery
	Cystoscopy
	Urethral dilation
		Vaginal hysterectomy§
		Vaginal delivery§
		Cesarean section
		In uninfected tissue:
		    Urethral catheterization
		    Uterine dilatation and curettage
		    Therapeutic abortion
		    Sterilization procedures
		    Insertion or removal of intrauterine devices

(*continued*)

TABLE 52-2. Endocarditis Prophylaxis (*Continued*)	
Recommended*	**Not Recommended**
Other	Cardiac catheterization, including balloon angioplasty
	Implanted cardiac pacemakers, implanted defibrillators, and coronary stents
	Incision or biopsy of surgically scrubbed skin
	Circumcision

Adapted with permission from the Committee on Infectious Diseases, American Academy of Pediatrics: *2000 Red Book: Report of the Committee on Infectious Diseases*, 25th ed. Elk Grove Village, IL: American Academy of Pediatrics, 2000, pp 737–738.

*Prophylaxis is recommended for patients with high- and moderate-risk cardiac conditions.

†This includes restoration of decayed teeth (filling cavities) and replacement of missing teeth.

‡Clinical judgment may indicate antibiotic use in selected circumstances that may create significant bleeding.

§Prophylaxis is optional for high-risk patients.

‖Prophylaxis is recommended for high-risk patients; optional for medium-risk patients.

TABLE 52-3. Cardiac Conditions Associated with Endocarditis		
Recommended		**Not Recommended**
High Risk	**Moderate Risk**	**Negligible Risk***
Prosthetic cardiac valves, including bioprosthetic and homograft valves	Most other congenital cardiac malformations (other than those in the high-risk and negligible-risk categories)	Isolated secundum atrial septal defect
Previous bacterial endocarditis	Acquired valvular dysfunction (e.g., rheumatic heart disease)	Surgical repair of atrial septal defect, ventricular septal defect, or patent ductus arteriosus (without residua and beyond 6 months of age)

(continued)

TABLE 52-3. Cardiac Conditions Associated with Endocarditis (*Continued*)

Recommended		Not Recommended
High Risk	**Moderate Risk**	**Negligible Risk***
Complex cyanotic congenital heart disease (e.g., single ventricle states, transposition of the great arteries, tetralogy of Fallot) Surgically constructed systemic pulmonary shunts or conduits	Hypertrophic cardiomyopathy Mitral valve prolapse with valvular regurgitation and/or thickened leaflets[†]	Previous coronary artery bypass graft surgery Mitral valve prolapse without valvular regurgitation[†] Physiologic, functional, or innocent heart murmurs[†] Previous Kawasaki disease without valvular dysfunction Previous rheumatic fever without valvular dysfunction Cardiac pacemakers (intravascular and epicardial) and implanted defibrillators

Adapted with permission from the Committee on Infectious Diseases, American Academy of Pediatrics: *2000 Red Book: Report of the Committee on Infectious Diseases,* 25th ed. Elk Grove Village, IL: American Academy of Pediatrics, 2000, p 736.

*No greater risk than in the general population.

[†]For further details, see Dajani AS, Tabuert KA, Wilson W, et al. Prevention of bacterial endocarditis: recommendations by the American Heart Association. *JAMA* 277:1794–1801, 1977.

TABLE 52-4. Prophylactic Regimens for Dental, Oral, Respiratory Tract, or Esophageal Procedures

Situation	Agent	Regimen*
Standard general prophylaxis	Amoxicillin	Adults: 2.0 g; children: 50 mg/kg orally 1 h before procedure
Unable to take oral medications	Ampicillin	Adults: 2.0 g intramuscularly or intravenously; children: 50 mg/kg intramuscularly or intravenously within 30 min before procedure
Allergic to penicillin	Clindamycin	Adults: 600 mg; children: 20 mg/kg orally 1 h before procedure
	OR	
	Cephalexin† or cefadroxil†	Adults: 2.0 g; children: 50 mg/kg orally 1 h before procedure
	OR	
	Azithromycin or clarithromycin	Adults: 500 mg; children: 15 mg/kg orally 1 h before procedure
Allergic to penicillin and unable to take oral medications	Clindamycin	Adults: 600 mg; children: 20 mg/kg intravenously within 30 min before procedure
	OR	
	Cefazolin†	Adults: 1.0 g; children: 25 mg/kg intramuscularly or intravenously within 30 min before procedure

Adapted with permission from the Committee on Infectious Diseases, American Academy of Pediatrics: *2000 Red Book: Report of the Committee on Infectious Diseases*, 25th ed. Elk Grove Village, IL: American Academy of Pediatrics, 2000, p 739.

*Total children's dose should not exceed adult dose.

†Cephalosporins should not be used for people with immediate-type hypersensitivity reaction (urticaria, angioedema, or anaphylaxis) to penicillins.

TABLE 52-5. Prophylactic Regimens for Genitourinary and Gastrointestinal Tract (Excluding Esophageal) Procedures

Situation	Agents*	Regimen†
High-risk patients	Ampicillin PLUS Gentamicin	Adults: ampicillin 2.0 g IM or IV plus gentamicin 1.5 mg/kg (not to exceed 120 mg) within 30 min of starting the procedure; 6 h later, ampicillin 1 g IM or IV or amoxicillin 1 g orally
		Children: ampicillin 50 mg/kg IM or IV (not to exceed 2.0 g) plus gentamicin 1.5 mg/kg within 30 min of starting the procedure; 6 h later, ampicillin 25 mg/kg IM or IV or amoxicillin 25 mg/kg orally
High-risk patients allergic to ampicillin or amoxicillin	Vancomycin PLUS Gentamicin	Adults: vancomycin 1.0 g IV over 1–2 h plus gentamicin 1.5 mg/kg IV or IM (not to exceed 120 mg); complete injection/infusion within 30 min of starting the procedure
		Children: vancomycin 20 mg/kg IV over 1–2 h plus gentamicin 1.5 mg/kg IV or IM: complete injection or infusion within 30 min of starting the procedure
Moderate-risk patients	Amoxicillin OR Ampicillin	Adults: amoxicillin 2.0 g orally 1 h before procedure, or ampicillin 2.0 g IM or IV within 30 min of starting the procedure
		Children: amoxicillin 50 mg/kg orally 1 h before procedure, or ampicillin 50 mg/kg IM or IV within 30 min of starting the procedure

(continued)

TABLE 52-5. Prophylactic Regimens for Genitourinary and Gastrointestinal Tract (Excluding Esophageal) Procedures (Continued)

Situation	Agents*	Regimen†
Moderate-risk patients allergic to ampicillin or amoxicillin	Vancomycin	Adults: vancomycin 1.0 g IV over 1–2 h; complete infusion within 30 min of starting the procedure Children: vancomycin 20 mg/kg IV over 1–2 h; complete infusion within 30 min of starting the procedure

Adapted with permission from the Committee on Infectious Diseases, American Academy of Pediatrics: *2000 Red Book: Report of the Committee on Infectious Diseases*, 25ed. Elk Grove Village, IL: American Academy of Pediatrics, 2000, p 740.

IM = intramuscularly; IV = intravenously.

*Total children's dose should not exceed adult dose.

†No second dose of vancomycin or gentamicin is recommended.

References
Brook MM: Pediatric bacterial endocarditis. Treatment and prophylaxis. *Pediatr Clin North Am* 46(2):275–287, 1999.
Dajani AS, Taubert KA, Wilson W, et al: Prevention of bacterial endocarditis. Recommendations by the American Heart Association. *JAMA* 277(22):1794–1801, 1997.

53. Kawasaki Disease

I INTRODUCTION

A. **Pathogenesis.** Kawasaki disease (KD) is an acute vasculitic process. The exact pathogenesis is not known.

B. **The clinical course** of untreated KD is divided into three phases:
1. **The acute phase (0–13 days)** includes arrhythmias, pericarditis, myocarditis (a nearly universal feature—tachycardia and a gallop rhythm are hallmark findings), cardiac failure, valve damage, and extremity gangrene. The coronary arteries are inflamed, although aneurysms have yet to form.
2. **The subacute phase (14–25 days)** involves the development of aneurysms, with thrombosis or rupture of coronary, cerebral, mesenteric, or peripheral arteries.
3. **The convalescent phase (25+ days)** involves the thrombosis or healing of aneurysms, with possible stricture formation. Myocardial, cerebral, or mesenteric infarction may occur during this phase.

C. **Epidemiology**
1. KD is the leading cause of acquired heart disease in children in the United States.
2. The peak incidence occurs at 1–2 years of age; 85% of cases occur in patients younger than age 5 years. The disease is rare in patients younger than age 3 months.
3. KD is more prevalent in boys than in girls (1.5:1). The incidence in Asian American children is six times the incidence in Caucasian children.
4. The recurrence rate in Japan is estimated at 3.9%.
5. Recent exposure to cleaned carpets is associated with KD.

II CLINICAL MANIFESTATIONS. The diagnosis of KD is primarily clinical.

A. **Criteria for diagnosis. Fever** lasting 5 days or longer is a requirement for diagnosis. In addition, four of the following five criteria must be present:
1. **Bilateral nonpurulent conjunctival injection.** Perilimbic sparing is a classic finding.
2. **Oral membrane changes.** These changes may include injected or fissured lips, injected pharynx or buccal mucosa, or strawberry tongue.
3. **Polymorphic rash.** The rash usually appears as raised ery-

thematous plaques. A maculopapular eruption is the second most common rash. Marginated or erythrodermic eruptions occur, but are less common. The rash is rarely bullous or vesicular.

4. **Extremity change.** Erythema of the palms or soles and edema of the hands or feet occurs in 3–5 days. Desquamation of the skin on the fingers and toes occurs at 2–3 weeks.

5. **Acute nonsuppurative cervical lymphadenopathy.** Adenopathy usually is unilateral. At least one node should be greater than 1.5 cm in diameter.

B. **Other findings** include arthralgia or arthritis (33%), perineal rash (often desquamating), anterior uveitis (83%, can be identified by slit-lamp evaluation and is helpful in differentiating KD from other viral illnesses that present with conjunctivitis), urethritis with a sterile pyuria (70%, esterase-negative), hepatic dysfunction (40%), aseptic meningitis (25%), hydrops of the gallbladder, and diarrhea, vomiting, and abdominal pain.

HOT

KEY
Nearly all children with KD are strikingly irritable.

C. **Atypical KD in younger children.** The strict criteria for KD may be met, but the symptoms may be spread out over a longer-than-usual time frame. This distinction is important because younger children are at greater risk for the development of coronary artery aneurysms. Echocardiography should be considered in cases of prolonged, unexplained fever and signs of KD, especially in a child younger than age 6 months. Children younger than 18–24 months of age tend to present with the following symptoms:

1. Fever, which often is intermittent and can last longer than 5 days
2. Minimal lymphadenopathy
3. Vague, transient rash
4. Prominent gastrointestinal symptoms

HOT

KEY
Always think of KD in a fussy child with fever that lasts longer than 5 days!

III APPROACH TO THE PATIENT

A. Workup

1. The **electrocardiogram** may show abnormalities consistent with myocarditis (e.g., prolonged PR interval, changes in the ST segment or T waves). Evidence of arrhythmia also should be sought.

2. The **echocardiogram** is helpful in identifying coronary aneurysms and myocardial dysfunction. The results should be interpreted by a pediatric cardiologist.

3. **Laboratory tests**

   a. **Complete blood count** usually shows leukocytosis with a left shift as well as normochromic and normocytic anemia. The platelet count usually is high after the 10th day of illness and peaks in the 3rd to 4th week.

   b. **C-reactive protein (CRP)** usually is high early in the course of the disease.

   c. **Erythrocyte sedimentation rate (ESR)** usually increases after the fever resolves. This finding may help to distinguish KD from common viral illnesses.

   d. **Liver function tests** usually show a twofold to fourfold increase. A cholestatic pattern, with elevated bilirubin and alkaline phosphatase levels, also may be seen.

B. The differential diagnosis includes measles, streptococcal infection, adenoviral infection, Stevens-Johnson syndrome, toxic shock syndrome, scalded skin syndrome, juvenile rheumatoid arthritis, leptospirosis, mercury poisoning, and Reiter syndrome. An antistreptolysin O titer, liver function tests, and a throat culture should be performed. A red-top tube of blood should be saved before the patient is treated with intravenous immunoglobulin (IVIg) in case the diagnosis later comes into question.

C. Therapy

1. **IVIg therapy.** IVIg therapy is given as a single dose at 2 g/kg over 10–12 hours. Volume overload, especially in small infants, can be a complication. The value of IVIg therapy after the 10th day of illness is uncertain. IVIg therapy reduces the formation of giant aneurysms and is more effective than aspirin therapy alone. It reduces the incidence of aneurysms by threefold at 2 weeks and by fivefold at 7 weeks. IVIg also speeds the resolution of left ventricular systolic dysfunction, inflammation, and fever. Its mechanism of action is unknown, but it may block immune activation.

2. **Acetylsalicylic acid (ASA; aspirin) therapy**

   a. **High-dose ASA therapy. ASA** is given for its anti-inflammatory effect. The initial dose is 80–100 mg/kg/day divided into four daily doses, until the patient is afebrile or until the 14th day of illness.

   b. Low-dose ASA therapy. Low-dose ASA therapy is used for its antiplatelet effect. The dose is tapered to 3–5 mg/kg/day after the fever abates. This dose is continued for 6–8 weeks or until the platelet count and ESR return to normal. Low-dose ASA therapy is continued indefinitely if coronary artery aneurysms are present. Dipyridamole may be used if ASA is contraindicated.

3. **Treatment failure.** Two-thirds of patients defervesce and have improved symptoms 24 hours after receiving IVIg. Of those who remain febrile after their first dose of IVIg, two thirds improve after a second dose. If defervescence does not occur or if symptoms progress, the viability of the diagnosis is considered and a rheumatologist is consulted.

4. **Ongoing management**

   a. Follow-up. Echocardiograms are performed at the 1st, 2nd, and 4th weeks. Consultation with a pediatric cardiologist is essential.

   b. Salicylate levels are monitored during the high-dose phase of ASA therapy because absorption may be variable. Serum levels of 20–30 mg/dl are desirable.

   c. Strict bed rest is essential.

   d. IVIg may reduce the effectiveness of the measles-mumps-rubella (MMR) and varicella zoster (VZV) vaccines. Administration of the MMR vaccine is delayed for 11 months, and administration of the VZV is delayed for 5 months.

   e. A yearly influenza vaccine is administered to patients who receive long-term ASA therapy.

IV PROGNOSIS

A. **Mortality.** The mortality rate from KD is low (0.1%–0.3%). Seventy-five percent of deaths occur in the first 6 weeks, usually as a result of coronary artery occlusion. Myocardial infarction is most common in the first year; 22% of initial myocardial infarctions are fatal.

B. **Morbidity.** Approximately 20% of patients with untreated KD develop coronary artery aneurysms. Those with giant aneurysms (> 8 mm) have the worst prognosis because these do not regress. Risk factors for the formation of coronary artery aneurysms include male gender, age < 1 year, hemoglobin count < 10 g/dl, white blood cell count > 30,000 cells/mm^3, ESR > 101 mm/h, elevated CRP level, persistent elevation of CRP for more than 30 days, and prolonged fever. Factors associated with regression of aneurysms include age younger than 1 year, saccular morphology, and distal aneurysms. The long-term effect on coronary arteries is unclear.

References
Kawasaki disease. In *2000 Red Book Report of the Committee on Infectious Diseases,* 25th ed. Elk Grove Village, IL, American Academy of Pediatrics, 2000.
Melish ME: Kawasaki syndrome. *Pediatr Rev* 17(5):153–162, 1996.
Nadas AS, Fyler DC: *Nadas' Pediatric Cardiology*. Philadelphia, Hanley & Belfus, 1992, pp 319–327.

54. Hypertension

I INTRODUCTION

A. Background. Hypertension among children is more common than was previously recognized and may reflect underlying renovascular, cardiovascular, or endocrine disease. Essential hypertension, which is the most common type of adult hypertension, often presents during adolescence. The likelihood of identifying a secondary cause of hypertension is related inversely to the patient's age and directly to the severity of the hypertension. The causes of hypertension vary widely among children in different age groups **(Table 54–1).**

B. Definitions
   1. **Normal blood pressure.** Systolic and diastolic blood pressure are less than the 90th percentile for age, gender, and height.
   2. **High normal blood pressure.** The systolic or diastolic blood pressure is between the 90th and 95th percentile for age, gender, and height.
   3. **Hypertension.** The systolic or diastolic blood pressure is greater than or equal to the 95th percentile for age, gender, and height when measured on at least three occasions **(Tables 54–2 and 54–3).** For term infants, the 95th percentile of systolic blood pressure is 95 mm Hg at 4 days of age and 113 mm Hg at 6 weeks of age. In children younger than 12 months of age, systolic blood pressure is used to define hypertension.
   4. **Essential hypertension** is primary hypertension or hypertension of unknown etiology.

C. Epidemiology
   1. Approximately 2% of children younger than 13 years of age have hypertension.
   2. The prevalence of hypertension is increased among Asian and African-American children.

HOT KEY

Obesity is the major risk factor for essential hypertension.

II CLINICAL MANIFESTATIONS.
The most common symptom is frontal headache, which may be throbbing. Blurred

TABLE 54-1. Causes of Hypertension in Children

Newborn	Age Less Than 1 Year	Age 1–6 Years	Age 6–12 Years	Age 12–18 Years
Renal artery thrombosis	Aortic coarctation	Renal parenchymal disease	Renal parenchymal disease	Essential hypertension
Renal artery stenosis	Renovascular disease	Renovascular disease	Renovascular disease	Iatrogenic
Renal vein thrombosis	Renal parenchymal disease	Aortic coarctation	Essential hypertension	Renal parenchymal disease
Congenital renal defects		Endocrine causes (e.g., Cushing disease, thyroid disease, pheochromocytoma)	Aortic coarctation	Renovascular disease
Aortic coarctation		Essential hypertension	Endocrine causes	Endocrine causes

Bartosh SM, Aronson AJ: Childhood hypertension: an update on etiology, diagnosis, and treatment. *Pediatr Clin North Am* 46(2):243–44, 1999.

TABLE 54-2. Blood Pressure Levels for the 90th and 95th Percentiles for Boys Aged 1–17 Years

Age (y)	Blood Pressure Percentile*	Systolic Blood Pressure by Percentile of Height (mm Hg)†							Diastolic Blood Pressure by Percentile of Height (mm Hg)†						
		5%	10%	25%	50%	75%	90%	95%	5%	10%	25%	50%	75%	90%	95%
1	90th	94	95	97	98	100	102	102	50	51	52	53	54	54	55
	95th	98	99	101	102	104	106	106	55	55	56	57	58	59	59
2	90th	98	99	100	102	104	105	106	55	55	56	57	58	59	59
	95th	101	102	104	106	108	109	110	59	59	60	61	62	63	63
3	90th	100	101	103	105	107	108	109	59	59	60	61	62	63	63
	95th	104	105	107	109	111	112	113	63	63	64	65	66	67	67
4	90th	102	103	105	107	109	110	111	62	62	63	64	65	66	66
	95th	106	107	109	111	113	114	115	66	67	67	68	69	70	71
5	90th	104	105	106	108	110	112	112	65	65	66	67	68	69	69
	95th	108	109	110	112	114	115	116	69	70	70	71	72	73	74
6	90th	105	106	108	110	111	113	114	67	68	69	70	70	71	72
	95th	109	110	112	114	115	117	117	72	72	73	74	75	76	76
7	90th	106	107	109	111	113	114	115	69	70	71	72	72	73	74
	95th	110	111	113	115	116	118	119	74	74	75	76	77	78	78
8	90th	107	108	110	112	114	115	116	71	71	72	73	74	75	75
	95th	111	112	114	116	118	119	120	75	76	76	77	78	79	80
9	90th	109	110	112	113	115	117	117	72	73	73	74	75	76	77
	95th	113	114	116	117	119	121	121	76	77	78	79	80	80	81

(continued)

TABLE 54-2. Blood Pressure Levels for the 90th and 95th Percentiles for Boys Aged 1–17 Years (Continued)

Age (y)	Blood Pressure Percentile*	Systolic Blood Pressure by Percentile of Height (mm Hg)†							Diastolic Blood Pressure by Percentile of Height (mm Hg)†						
		5%	10%	25%	50%	75%	90%	95%	5%	10%	25%	50%	75%	90%	95%
10	90th	110	112	113	115	117	118	119	73	74	74	75	76	77	78
	95th	114	115	117	119	121	122	123	77	78	79	80	80	81	82
11	90th	112	113	115	117	119	120	121	74	74	75	76	77	78	78
	95th	116	117	119	121	123	124	125	78	79	79	80	81	82	83
12	90th	115	116	117	119	121	123	123	75	75	76	77	78	78	79
	95th	119	120	121	123	125	126	127	79	79	80	81	82	83	83
13	90th	117	118	120	122	124	125	126	75	76	76	77	78	79	80
	95th	121	122	124	126	128	129	130	79	80	81	82	83	83	84
14	90th	120	121	123	125	126	128	128	76	76	77	78	79	80	80
	95th	124	125	127	128	130	132	132	80	81	81	82	83	84	85
15	90th	123	124	125	127	129	131	131	77	77	78	79	80	81	81
	95th	127	128	129	131	133	134	135	81	82	83	83	84	85	86
16	90th	125	126	128	130	132	133	134	79	79	80	81	82	82	83
	95th	129	130	132	134	136	137	138	83	83	84	85	86	87	87
17	90th	128	129	131	133	134	136	136	81	81	82	83	84	85	85
	95th	132	133	135	136	138	140	140	85	85	86	87	88	89	89

Reprinted with permission from *Pediatrics* 98:653, 1996.

*Blood pressure percentile was determined by a single measurement.

†Height percentile was determined by standard growth curves.

TABLE 54-3. Blood Pressure Levels for the 90th and 95th Percentiles for Girls Aged 1-17 Years

Age (y)	Blood Pressure Percentile*	Systolic Blood Pressure by Percentile of Height (mm Hg)†							Diastolic Blood Pressure by Percentile of Height (mm Hg)†						
		5%	10%	25%	50%	75%	90%	95%	5%	10%	25%	50%	75%	90%	95%
1	90th	97	98	99	100	102	103	104	53	53	53	54	55	56	56
	95th	101	102	103	104	105	107	107	57	57	57	58	59	60	60
2	90th	99	99	100	102	103	104	105	57	57	58	58	59	60	61
	95th	102	103	104	105	107	108	109	61	61	62	62	63	64	65
3	90th	100	100	102	103	104	105	106	61	61	61	62	63	63	64
	95th	104	104	105	107	108	109	110	65	65	65	66	67	67	68
4	90th	101	102	103	104	106	107	108	63	63	64	65	65	66	67
	95th	105	106	107	108	109	111	111	67	67	68	69	69	70	71
5	90th	103	103	104	106	107	108	109	65	66	66	67	68	68	69
	95th	107	107	108	110	111	112	113	69	70	70	71	72	72	73
6	90th	104	105	106	107	109	110	111	67	67	68	69	69	70	71
	95th	108	109	110	111	112	114	114	71	71	72	73	73	74	75
7	90th	106	107	108	109	110	112	112	69	69	69	70	71	72	72
	95th	110	110	112	113	114	115	116	73	73	73	74	75	76	76
8	90th	108	109	110	111	112	113	114	70	70	71	71	72	73	74
	95th	112	112	113	115	116	117	118	74	74	75	75	76	77	78
9	90th	110	110	112	113	114	115	116	71	72	72	73	74	74	75
	95th	114	114	115	117	118	119	120	75	76	76	77	78	78	79

(continued)

TABLE 54-3. Blood Pressure Levels for the 90th and 95th Percentiles for Girls Aged 1–17 Years (Continued)

Age (y)	Blood Pressure Percentile*	Systolic Blood Pressure by Percentile of Height (mm Hg)†							Diastolic Blood Pressure by Percentile of Height (mm Hg)†						
		5%	10%	25%	50%	75%	90%	95%	5%	10%	25%	50%	75%	90%	95%
10	90th	112	112	114	115	116	117	118	73	73	73	74	75	76	76
	95th	116	116	117	119	120	121	122	77	77	77	78	79	80	80
11	90th	114	114	116	117	118	119	120	74	74	75	75	76	77	77
	95th	118	118	119	121	122	123	124	78	78	79	79	80	81	81
12	90th	116	116	118	119	120	121	122	75	75	76	76	77	78	78
	95th	120	120	121	123	124	125	126	79	79	80	80	81	82	82
13	90th	118	118	119	121	122	123	124	76	76	77	78	78	79	80
	95th	121	122	123	125	126	127	128	80	80	81	82	82	83	84
14	90th	119	120	121	122	124	125	126	77	77	78	79	79	80	81
	95th	123	124	125	126	128	129	130	81	81	82	83	83	84	85
15	90th	121	121	122	124	125	126	127	78	78	79	79	80	81	82
	95th	124	125	126	128	129	130	131	82	82	83	83	84	85	86
16	90th	122	122	123	125	126	127	128	79	79	79	80	81	82	82
	95th	125	126	127	128	130	131	132	83	83	83	84	85	86	86
17	90th	122	123	124	125	126	128	128	79	79	79	80	81	82	82
	95th	126	126	127	129	130	131	132	83	83	83	84	85	86	86

Reprinted with permission from *Pediatrics* 98:654, 1996.
*Blood pressure percentile was determined by a single measurement.
†Height percentile was determined by standard growth curves.

vision, seizures, and facial palsy are findings consistent with malignant hypertension. Left ventricular hypertrophy, congestive heart failure, and retinopathy may result from chronic hypertension.

III APPROACH TO THE PATIENT

A. Diagnosis

1. The **history** should include questions about any neonatal procedures (use of umbilical catheters may cause renal vessel disease), renal or urologic disorders (pyelonephritis and vesicoureteral reflux), and medications (including contraceptives). The physician should ask about symptoms that might indicate an endocrine disorder, such as flushing, weight loss, palpitations, and weakness. **A family history** of essential hypertension and its complications or genetic disorders associated with secondary hypertension should also be identified.

2. All children 3 years of age and older should have their blood pressure recorded at all emergency and health maintenance visits.

   a. The **right arm** should be used for consistency. An appropriate cuff has a bladder width that is approximately 40% of the midarm circumference. The bladder should cover 80%–100% of the circumference. The stethoscope should be placed over the brachial artery proximal to the cubital fossa and distal to the cuff.

   b. Measurements should be taken after 5 minutes of rest, with the patient sitting (or supine, in infants and toddlers) and with the cubital fossa supported at heart level.

   c. The cuff should be deflated at a rate of 2–3 mm Hg/sec. Systolic blood pressure is determined by the onset of tapping sounds (the first Korotkoff sound). As recently established by the American Heart Association, diastolic blood pressure is determined by the disappearance of sounds (i.e., the fifth Korotkoff sound). In some children, this may occur at 0 mm Hg. In such cases, diastolic hypertension is excluded.

3. **Table 54–4** provides a reasonable stepwise approach for evaluation of patients with hypertension.

B. Treatment includes pharmacologic and nonpharmacologic modalities.

1. **Essential hypertension.** The goal is to reduce blood pressure to below the 95th percentile. Prevention of obesity, decreasing sodium intake, and exercise are effective nonpharmacologic interventions.

2. **Secondary hypertension.** Antihypertensive medications, including angiotensin-converting enzyme inhibitors (capto-

---

TABLE 54-4. Evaluation of the Child with Hypertension

Phase 1
　Complete blood count
　Urinalysis
　Urine culture (if secondary hypertension is suspected)
　Blood urea nitrogen, creatinine, electrolytes, calcium, uric acid
　Lipid panel (if primary hypertension is suspected)
　Renal ultrasound
　Echocardiography

Phase 2
　Renal scan with angiotensin-converting enzyme inhibitor
　Renin profiling (with or without loop diuretic)
　Urine collection for catecholamines
　Plasma and urinary steroids

Phase 3
　Renal artery imaging or renal vein renin sampling
　Metaiodobenzlguanidine scan of adrenals
　Caval sampling for catecholamines

Bartosh SM, Aronson AJ: Childhood hypertension: an update on the etiology, diagnosis, and treatment. *Pediatr Clin North Am* 46(2):244, 1999.

---

pril), β-adrenergic antagonists (labetalol), vasodilators (hydralazine), and diuretics (furosemide, chlorothiazide) often are required.

　3. Medications for hypertensive emergencies include nifedipine, captopril, labetalol, nitroprusside, and hydralazine.

C. Ongoing management
　1. Patients with blood pressure in the 95th–98th percentile and no target organ damage should not be restricted from competitive athletics, but they should have their blood pressure checked every 2 months.
　2. Patients with severe hypertension (> 98th percentile) should be restricted from athletics.

References

Bartosh S, Aronson A: Childhood hypertension: an update on etiology, diagnosis and treatment. *Pediatr Clin North Am* 46(2):235, 1999.

National High Blood Pressure Education Program Working Group on Hypertension Control in Children and Adolescents: Update on the 1987 Task Force Report on High Blood Pressure in Children and Adolescents: A Working Group from the National High Blood Pressure Education Program. *Pediatrics* 98:649, 1996.

55. Myocarditis

I **PATHOGENESIS.** **Myocarditis** (inflammation of the myocardium) often is assumed to be caused by viral infection. There are other causes, however, such as collagen vascular disease, Takayasu arteritis, drug reactions, and Kawasaki disease. Myocarditis usually presents as a dilated cardiomyopathy.

A. Damage to the myocardium may occur by direct viral destruction of myocardial cells, by T-cell–mediated inflammation, or by damage to the coronary arteries.

B. **Viral agents** associated with viral myocarditis include coxsackievirus B (associated with more than 50% of all cases), coxsackievirus A, echoviruses, polioviruses, adenoviruses, cytomegalovirus, influenza types A and B, rubeola, rubella, mumps, hepatitis A, hepatitis B, varicella zoster virus, rabies, and lymphocytic choriomeningitis viruses.

II **CLINICAL MANIFESTATIONS**

A. **Symptoms** are secondary to congestive heart failure (CHF), and presentations vary widely. Some patients are asymptomatic, whereas others have overt cardiac failure. Myocarditis often is part of a systemic illness that may include severe hepatitis or encephalitis. The patient also may have respiratory distress, pallor, irritability, tachypnea, and sweating (especially during feeding). Arrhythmias, syncope, seizures, abdominal pain, and fever are less common symptoms.

B. **Physical examination** may show liver enlargement, wheezes, rales, a quiet precordium, or a murmur consistent with mitral regurgitation secondary to cardiomegaly. A gallop rhythm with an S3 and an S4 is often heard. Because many of the symptoms are protean, it is important to have a high index of suspicion for myocarditis, especially when there is sudden onset of unexplained tachypnea, arrhythmia, or tachycardia.

HOT

KEY
Suspicion should be raised when CHF develops after multiple fluid boluses or when a euvolemic patient is tachycardic at rest.

III APPROACH TO THE PATIENT

A. **Diagnosis.** The diagnosis of myocarditis is confirmed histologically by obtaining a sample of cardiac tissue through catheter-
directed biopsy. The histologic findings of profuse, interstitial
round cell infiltration and necrotic myocyte degeneration are
diagnostic of myocarditis. Myocardial infiltrates can be divided
into four categories. Causes by type of infiltrate are as follows.
1. **Lymphocytic.** Infectious (viral, fungal, protozoal, rickettsial,
chlamydial, mycoplasmal), postinfectious, or lymphoma
2. **Granulomatous.** Collagen vascular disease, histiocytosis,
sarcoidosis, infectious, hypersensitivity reactions, foreign
body reactions, or metabolic disorders (e.g., gout oxalosis,
granulomatous disease of childhood)
3. **Eosinophilic.** Drug hypersensitivity, Löffler syndrome, parasitic infestation, or Wegener granulomatosis
4. **Neutrophilic.** Early phase of viral infection, bacterial infection, diphtheria toxin, or infarction
B. The **differential diagnosis** of dilated cardiomyopathy includes
defects in fatty acid metabolism, primary carnitine deficiency,
carnitine transferase enzyme disorders, glycogen storage disease
type II (Pompe disease), and disorders of lysosomal enzymes.
C. **Additional tests**
1. **Creatine kinase-MB** levels may be elevated if a significant
amount of myocyte necrosis is present.
2. The **electrocardiogram** may show changes in the ST segment, T waves, or generalized low voltage. There may be left
ventricular hypertrophy and an inferior QRS axis. The T
waves may be very large in patients with carnitine deficiency.
3. **Liver enzymes and lactate dehydrogenase** levels may be elevated as a result of associated hepatitis or liver injury secondary to CHF.
4. **Viral titers (acute and convalescent)** may be used, but may
be difficult to interpret because viral infections are common
during childhood; even a fourfold increase does not necessarily indicate causation.

IV INITIAL THERAPY

A. Administration of high-dose **intravenous immunoglobulin** in
the acute phase is associated with improved recovery of ventricular function and increased survival time after the first year
following the illness.
B. Treatment with **steroids or nonsteroidal anti-inflammatory drugs**
may worsen outcome, especially in the early stages of disease.
Some physicians use steroids in patients with persistent ventricular dysfunction, with varying degrees of success.

V ONGOING MANAGEMENT

A. **Inotropes, diuretics, vasodilators, and antiarrhythmics** may be needed if the patient becomes hemodynamically unstable. In extreme cases, intra-aortic balloon pump therapy or extracorporeal membrane oxygenator support may be needed.

B. **Cardiac transplantation** is needed in some patients; however, even those who are desperately ill may eventually recover fully. For this reason, transplantation is problematic.

C. After recovery, a period of **bed rest** for weeks or even months is recommended.

D. **Follow-up** should always be managed by a cardiologist.

VI PROGNOSIS

A. **Morbidity and mortality.** Patients with a granulomatous infiltrate or diphtheritic myocarditis have a particularly poor prognosis. Newborns are particularly susceptible, and severe myocarditis may develop. Approximately 25% of patients with myocarditis are asymptomatic.

   1. Fifty percent of patients recover completely.
   2. The overall mortality rate is 10%–25%.
   3. In newborns, the overall mortality rate is nearly 75%.

References

Feigin RD, Cherry JD: *Textbook of Pediatric Infectious Diseases,* 3rd ed. Philadelphia, WB Saunders, 1992, pp 357–375.

Nadas AS, Fyler DC: *Nadas' Pediatric Cardiology.* Philadelphia, Hanley & Belfus, 1992, pp 329–363.

56. Introduction to Congenital Heart Disease

I **PHYSIOLOGY AND PATHOPHYSIOLOGY.** An understanding of prenatal and postnatal blood flow and the normal development of the pulmonary vascular bed is essential to understanding the natural history of congenital heart lesions.

A. Prenatal and postnatal circulation

    1. Prenatal. Blood is shunted around the liver and lungs through the **ductus venosus** and **ductus arteriosus,** respectively. The lungs remain deflated.

    2. Postnatal

        a. Closure of the foramen ovale occurs soon after birth, owing to increased pressure in the left atrium induced by changes in the pulmonary circulation.

        b. Closure of the ductus arteriosus usually occurs within 15 hours of birth, as a result of the postnatal increase in the arterial oxygen tension. The **ligamentum arteriosum** is the remnant of the fetal ductus arteriosus.

B. Pulmonary vascular bed. In utero, the pulmonary arteries are muscular and thick-walled, making the pulmonary vascular resistance high. After birth, the pulmonary vessels undergo a dramatic change; the walls become thinner and more compliant, thereby decreasing pulmonary vascular resistance. In the presence of a significant left-to-right shunt or other lesion characterized by increased pulmonary blood flow, the rate at which the pulmonary vascular resistance decreases may be delayed. In this case, heart failure and flooding of the lungs is delayed as well.

C. Eisenmenger syndrome. In cases of uncorrected left-to-right shunt defects [e.g., large ventricular septal defects (VSDs)], pulmonary blood flow goes unchecked and the pulmonary vasculature may develop increased resistance to blood flow (pulmonary hypertension). Histologically, the vessels undergo medial hypertrophy. An element of vasoconstriction also may contribute to the hypertension. If significant pulmonary hypertension occurs, a right-to-left shunt may develop, and the patient will become cyanotic (Eisenmenger syndrome). Once this occurs, surgery may not be possible. The only effective treatment is prevention through timely repair of lesions that put the patient at risk for pulmonary hypertension.

D. Ventricular mass. Before birth, pulmonary pressures are greater than systemic pressures; therefore, the right ventricle is as large as or larger than the left ventricle at birth. At birth, loss of the placenta (a low-resistance circuit) leads to increased aortic and left-sided pressures, and a decrease in pulmonary vascular resistance leads to decreased right-sided pressures. Eventually, the right ventricle loses and the left ventricle gains mass.

II TYPES OF CONGENITAL HEART DISEASE (CHD). CHD commonly is classified into cyanotic and noncyanotic lesions (Table 56–1).

A. Noncyanotic lesions. Noncyanotic lesions may be characterized by either an increased pressure load or an increased volume load (see Table 56–1).

B. Cyanotic lesions can result from a **right-to-left shunt** (in which the blood bypasses through the lungs) or **obstructed pulmonary blood flow.** Patients with cyanotic lesions fall into four major categories:

 1. **Cyanosis alone.** These patients usually have small, quiet hearts. Pulmonary blood flow is decreased, but there is no evidence of low cardiac output or respiratory distress.
 2. **Cyanosis and systemic venous congestion.** Systemic venous congestion results from right ventricular failure or an anatomic obstruction to inflow. Patients have slightly larger hearts, signs of right ventricular failure, and hepatosplenomegaly.
 3. **Cyanosis and moderate respiratory distress.** These patients have small (but hyperdynamic) hearts. Respiratory distress is related primarily to pulmonary venous hypertension and pulmonary congestion. There is no evidence of low cardiac output and only mild systemic venous congestion.
 4. **Cyanosis, respiratory distress, and low cardiac output.** These patients have large, hyperdynamic hearts. Pulmonary blood flow may be increased, and systemic venous congestion is present. Signs of diminished cardiac output include poor pulses, mottled skin, hypotonia, and a slight cyanosis.

HOT **KEY** The following lesions may present with cyanosis immediately after birth: obstructed total anomalous pulmonary venous return, atrioventricular malformations, Ebstein anomaly, severe coarctation of the aorta, and severe aortic stenosis.

TABLE 56-1. Types of Congenital Heart Disease

Noncyanotic
    Lesions characterized by an increased pressure load
        Simple coarctation of the aorta
        Aortic stenosis
        Pulmonic stenosis
        Mitral valve prolapse
    Lesions characterized by an increased volume load
        Aortic regurgitation
        Mitral regurgitation
        Ventricular septal defect
        Atrial septal defect
        Patent ductus arteriosus
Cyanotic
    Lesions characterized by cyanosis alone
        Hypoplastic right ventricle
        Tetralogy of Fallot
        Early truncus arteriosus
    Lesions characterized by cyanosis and systemic venous congestion
        Ebstein anomaly
        Pulmonic stenosis with intact ventricular septum
    Lesions characterized by cyanosis and moderate respiratory distress
        Transposition of the great arteries
        Truncus arteriosus
        Total anomalous pulmonary venous return
    Lesions characterized by cyanosis, respiratory distress, and low
        cardiac output
        Hypoplastic left ventricular syndrome
        Complicated coarctation of the aorta
        Severe aortic stenosis

*Note that there are many more cyanotic lesions than the "4 Ts": Tetralogy of Fallot, Truncus arteriosus, TAPVR (total anomalous pulmonary venous return), and Tricuspid atresia!

Four Cardinal Signs of Cyanotic Heart Disease ("4 Cs")

Cyanosis
Cannot breathe (respiratory distress)
Congestion of the systemic venous system (e.g., hepatosplenomegaly, right atrial or right ventricular enlargement)
Cardiac output diminished (poor peripheral pulses, cool or mottled skin)

APPROACH TO THE PATIENT

A. Patient history
  1. **Birth history**
     a. When was the murmur first heard?
     b. Was the infant cyanotic initially, or did the cyanosis develop after a few days?
     c. Did oxygen therapy improve the situation?
  2. **Growth.** Is the child meeting appropriate growth expectations?
  3. **Exercise tolerance**
     a. **Infants.** Does the baby feed well? How long can the baby nurse before tiring? Does the baby sweat excessively or develop cyanosis during feedings?
     b. **Older children**
        (1) How much exertion can the child tolerate? Can he or she keep up with peers?
        (2) Does the child become fatigued after easy exertion or at rest?
        (3) Does the child squat when tired?
        (4) Does the child experience chest pain or syncope during exercise?

B. Physical examination
  1. **General examination**
     a. **Visual inspection.** Is the patient visibly cyanotic? Is there evidence of clubbing on inspection of the nail beds?

HOT

KEY
In newborns, the degree of desaturation may be underestimated by visual inspection alone.

---

  b. **Chest examination**
     (1) Does a hand placed on the patient's chest detect a parasternal heave or a hyperdynamic left sternal border? These findings could indicate a left-to-right shunt.
     (2) The carotids and suprasternal notch also should be palpated to check for a thrill.
     (3) Listen to the lungs carefully. Are there rales or the signs of pulmonary overcirculation (tachypnea or dyspnea)?
  c. **Abdominal examination.** Is the liver enlarged?
  2. **Cardiac examination.** An organized and systematic approach to the cardiac examination is essential.
     a. **Heart sounds**
        (1) **First heart sound (S_1).** The S_1 is best auscultated at the

apex. It may be split, owing to slightly delayed closure of the tricuspid valve. There is no change with respiration.

(2) Second heart sound (S_2). The S_2 is best heard at the upper left and right sternal borders and is physiologically split into aortic (A_2) and pulmonic (P_2) components.

    (a) The time between the A_2 and the P_2 varies with respiration; normally it is longer with inspiration and shorter with expiration.

    (b) A person with an experienced ear can easily tell whether the S_2 is single, normally split, or wide.

    (c) A widely split S_2 may indicate pulmonic stenosis or an atrial septal defect (ASD); a narrowly split S_2 may indicate aortic stenosis or pulmonary hypertension. A paradoxical split occurs when A_2 advances past P_2 and the split narrows with inspiration; this most commonly occurs in severe aortic stenosis.

(3) Third heart sound (S_3). The S_3, a midsystolic, low-frequency sound, is caused by sudden filling of the ventricles. The S_3 is best heard using the bell of the stethoscope over the apex (if the left ventricle is the origin) or the lower left sternal border (if the right ventricle is the origin).

    (a) The finding of a soft S_3 at the apex is usually normal in children; it can be heard because the chest wall is thin.

    (b) A single S_3 with no other associated murmurs may indicate a left-to-right shunt, or, less commonly, cardiomyopathy.

(4) Fourth heart sound (S_4). The S_4 is heard rarely in children, although opening snaps may be heard in children with rheumatic mitral stenosis.

b. Murmurs

    (1) Determine the maximal location of the murmur (Figure 56–1). It is also important to listen in the axillary region, over the back, and on the fontanel.

    (2) The qualities of the murmur are noted.

        (a) What is the timing? Murmurs are either **systolic** (occurring between S_1 and S_2), **diastolic** (occurring after S_2), or **continuous** (beginning in systole and continuing into diastole without interruption).

        (b) At what point during the cardiac cycle (e.g., early, late, throughout the cycle, or midcycle) does the murmur occur?

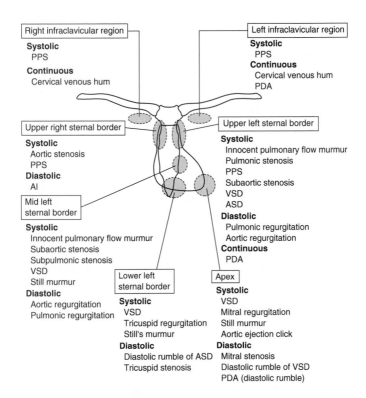

Figure 56–1. Locations of common murmurs. ASD = atrial septal defect; PDA = patent ductus arteriosus; PPS = peripheral pulmonic stenosis; VSD = ventricular septal defect. (Adapted with permission from Phoon CKL, Stanger P: *A Guide to Pediatric Cardiovascular Physical Examination. (Or, How to Survive an Outreach Clinic).* Philadelphia, Lippincott Williams & Wilkins, 1998, p 15.)

      (c) What is the shape of the murmur [e.g., plateau, decrescendo, or ejection (diamond-shaped)]?

      (d) What is the quality and pitch of the murmur (e.g., harsh, vibratory)?

C. Electrocardiography (Tables 56–2 and 56–3) . The ability to identify ventricular **hypertrophy** is critical in reading pediatric electrocardiograms (ECGs). Hypertrophy can be caused by a **ventricle pumping against increased resistance,** such as a stenotic valve or pulmonary hypertension (vascular disease). Hypertrophy can also be governed by **increased volume work** (e.g.,

TABLE 56-2. Normal Range and Mean Values for Selected Electrocardiogram (ECG) Measurements in Children*								
	0–7 Days	1 Week–1 Month	1–6 Months	6–12 Months	1–5 Years	5–10 Years	10–15 Years	>15 Years
Heart rate (beats/min)	90–160 (125)	100–175 (140)	110–180 (145)	100–180 (130)	70–160 (110)	65–140 (100)	60–130 (90)	60–100 (80)
PR interval (sec) lead II			0.08–0.15 (0.10)		0.08–0.15 (0.12)—		0.09–0.18 (0.14)	0.10–0.20 (0.16)
QRS interval (sec)			0.03–0.07 (0.05)		0.04–0.08 (0.06)—		0.04–0.09 (0.07)	0.06–0.09 (0.08)
Maximum QT$_c$ (sec)		0.45			0.44			0.43
QRS axis (degrees)	70–180 (120)	45–160 (100)	10–120 (80)				5–110 (60)	
QRS complex, lead V$_1$								
Q (mm)	0	0	0	0	0	0	0	0
R (mm)	5–25 (15)	3–22 (10)	3–20 (10)	2–20 (9)	2–18 (8)	1–15 (5)	1–12 (5)	1–6 (2)
S (mm)	0–22 (7)	0–16 (5)	0–15 (6)	1–20 (6)	1–20 (10)	3–21 (12)	3–22 (11)	3–13 (8)
QRS complex, lead V$_5$								
Q (mm)	0–1 (0.5)	0–3 (0.5)	0–3 (0.5)	0–3 (0.5)	0–5 (1)	0–5 (1)	0–3 (0.5)	0–2 (0.5)
R (mm)	2–20 (10)	3–25 (12)	5–30 (17)	10–30 (20)	10–35 (23)	13–38 (25)	10–35 (20)	7–21 (0.5)
S (mm)	2–19 (10)	2–15 (8)	1–16 (8)	1–14 (6)	1–13 (5)	1–11 (4)	1–10 (3)	0–5 (2)

(continued)

TABLE 56-2. Normal Range and Mean Values for Selected Electrocardiogram (ECG) Measurements in Children* (Continued)

	0-7 Days	1 Week-1 Month	1-6 Months	6-12 Months	1-5 Years	5-10 Years	10-15 Years	>15 Years
QRS complex, lead V$_6$								
Q (mm)	0-2 (0.5)	0-2 (0.5)	0-2 (0.5)	0-3 (0.5)	0-4 (1)	0-4 (1)	0-3 (1)	0-2 (0.5)
R (mm)	1-12 (5)	1-17 (7)	3-20 (10)	5-22 (12)	6-22 (14)	8-25 (16)	8-24 (15)	5-18 (10)
S (mm)	0-9 (3)	0-9 (3)	0-9 (3)	0-7 (3)	0-6 (2)	0-4 (2)	0-4 (1)	0-2 (1)
T wave, lead V$_1$								
T (mm)	0-4 days = -3 to +4 (0) 4-7 days = -4 to 2 (-1)	-6 - -1 (-3)				-6 - +2 (-2)	-4 - +3 (-1)	-2 - +2 (+1)

Adapted with permission from Fyler DC: Nadas' Pediatric Cardiology. Philadelphia, Hanley & Belfus, 1992, p 126.

*Values reported as 2%-98% (mean), except for QTc (given as the maximum value only).

$$QTc = \frac{\text{measured at QT (seconds)}}{\sqrt{\text{R-R interval}}}$$

TABLE 56-3. Electrocardiogram Findings and Their Commonly Associated Cardiac Malformations

Electrocardiogram Findings	Commonly Associated Lesion
Left ventricular hypertrophy	Patent ductus arteriosus, aortic stenosis, subvalvular atrial stenosis, cardiomyopathy, coarctation after infancy, anomalous origin of the left coronary artery, mitral regurgitation, severe mitral valve prolapse, aortic regurgitation, systemic arterial fistula, coronary arterial fistula, hypoplastic right ventrical (RV) with tricuspid atresia, hypoplastic RV with pulmonary atresia
Right ventricular hypertrophy	Atrial septal defect, pulmonary stenosis, total anomalous pulmonary venous return, hypoplastic left heart syndrome, coarctation, transposition, tetralogy of Fallot, mitral stenosis, Eisenmenger syndrome
Biventricular hypertrophy	Ventricular septal defect, atrioventricular canal, large patent ductus arteriosus, AP window, left ventricle–to–right atrial shunt, truncus arteriosus

in a VSD, the left ventricle does increased volume work because of the left-to-right shunting of blood).

1. **Right ventricular hypertrophy (Figure 56–2).** Because the right ventricle sits anteriorly in the chest wall, depolarizations from the right ventricle contribute an upward deflection in V_1 and a downward deflection in V_6. The following criteria are used to identify right ventricular hypertrophy:

   a. **R wave amplitude higher than the 98th percentile in V_1.** This criterion is most useful outside of the newborn period.

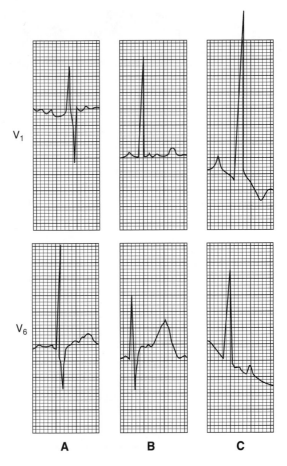

Figure 56-2. Electrocardiogram patterns with varying degrees of right ventricular pressure load hypertrophy. **(A)** Mild right ventricular hypertrophy in a 9-month-old child suggested by an upright T wave in V_1, but without excess R-wave voltage. **(B)** Moderate right ventricular hypertrophy in a 4-year-old child with an upright T wave and excess R-wave voltage in V_1. **(C)** Marked right ventricular hypertrophy in a 7-year-old child showing a very tall R wave with an inverted T wave (strain pattern) in V_1. (Adapted with permission from Fyler DC: *Nadas' Pediatric Cardiology*. Philadelphia, Hanley & Belfus, 1992, p 131.)

    b. S wave depth lower than the 98th percentile in V_6.

    c. An RSR' pattern in the right chest leads also may be a clue to right ventricular hypertrophy if it is combined with large S waves in the left chest leads **(Figure 56–3).**

2. Left ventricular hypertrophy (Figure 56–4).

    a. In general, an ECG is less sensitive for left ventricular hypertrophy and may not detect it in 50% of cases. The left ventricle sits posteriorly with its apex to the left. Therefore, depolarizations from the left ventricle contribute a downward deflection in V_1 and an upward deflection in V_6. The following criteria are used to identify left ventricular hypertrophy:

        (1) S wave depth lower than the 98th percentile waves in V_1

        (2) R waves amplitude higher than the 98th percentile in V_6

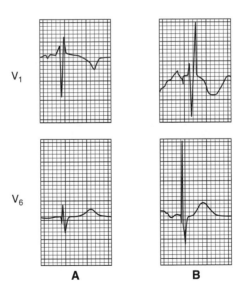

Figure 56–3. The RSR' pattern in lead V_1. **(A)** Normal patient without heart disease. **(B)** Patient with increased right ventricular volume load caused by large atrial septal defect. Note the tall R' wave in the abnormal trace. (Adapted with permission from Fyler DC: *Nadas' Pediatric Cardiology.* Philadelphia, Hanley & Belfus, 1992, p 132.)

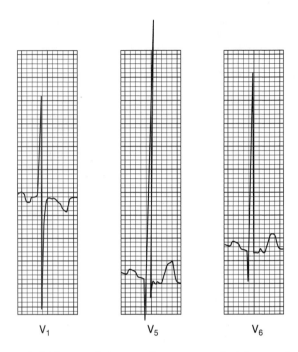

Figure 56–4. The typical electrocardiogram pattern for left ventricular hypertrophy caused by a large volume load, with deep Q waves in V_5 and V_6 in an infant with a large ventricular septal defect. (Adapted with permission from Fyler DC: *Nadas' Pediatric Cardiology.* Philadelphia, Hanley & Belfus, 1992, p 132.)

    b. Severe (Figure 56–5). It is important to identify evidence of left ventricular strain associated with more severe left ventricular hypertrophy. This is represented by **T wave abnormalities** (upright in right chest leads, inverted in left chest leads), **ST segment depression in the left chest leads,** or **Q waves.** Evidence of myocardial infarction should prompt an investigation for an anomalous left coronary artery.

3. Biventricular hypertrophy
    a. Right ventricular hypertrophy plus increased inferior vector (R-wave in Avf). These criteria are valid if the right ventricular hypertrophy is moderate and the left chest potential is adequate.
    b. Biventricular hypertrophy can also be seen as **tall R and S**

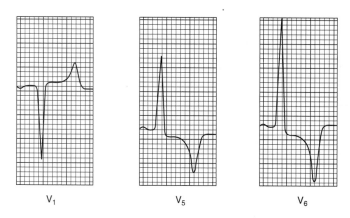

V₁   V₅   V₆

Figure 56–5. Left ventricular hypertrophy with strain pattern in a patient with aortic stenosis. The T-wave inversion is dramatic even though the R-wave voltage does not exceed normal limits. (Adapted with permission from Fyler DC: *Nadas' Pediatric Cardiology.* Philadelphia, Hanley & Belfus, 1992, p 132.)

         waves in the midchest leads (Katz-Wachtell phenomenon) [Figure 56–6].
D. Chest radiography can be an important adjunct in the evaluation of a patient with suspected CHD. Normal radiographic anatomy is shown in **Figure 56–7.** The following features should be noted when examining the chest film:

   1. Hypertrophy. Left ventricular hypertrophy is best seen on the lateral view because most of the left ventricle lies posteriorly.

   2. Atrial enlargement. Right atrial enlargement is evidenced by an enlarged right atrial shadow.

   3. Great vessels. Look for right aortic arches, evidence of post-stenotic dilatations, and enlargement of the right and left pulmonary arteries.

   4. Lung fields

      a. Increased pulmonary vascularity may suggest a left-to-right shunt with increased pulmonary blood flow.

      b. A **paucity of pulmonary vascular markings** may indicate pulmonary stenosis or tetralogy of Fallot.

      c. Pulmonary edema may suggest left ventricular failure or obstruction, as in total anomalous pulmonary venous return.

      d. The **cardiac silhouette** should be characterized. A "tear-

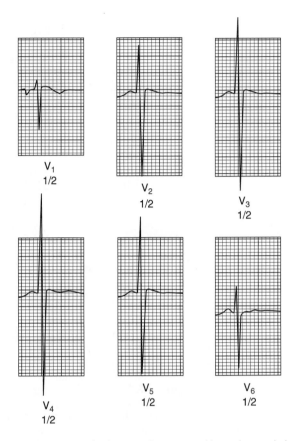

Figure 56–6. Biventricular hypertrophy suggested by midprecordial voltages above the 98th percentile. The combined R and S waves in lead V_4 are 95 mm (trace is shown at half of standard size). (Adapted with permission from Fyler DC: *Nadas' Pediatric Cardiology*. Philadelphia, Hanley & Belfus, 1992, p 133.)

drop shape" suggests transposition of the great arteries, a "boot shape" suggests tetralogy of Fallot, a "box shape" suggests Ebstein anomaly, and a "snowman shape" suggests supradiaphragmatic total anomalous pulmonary venous return.

5. **Ribs.** Rib notching may suggest longstanding coarctation of the aorta.

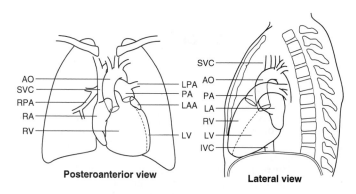

Figure 56–7. Normal radiographic anatomy. AO = aorta; IVC = inferior vena cava; LA = left atrium; LAA = left atrial appendage; LPA = left pulmonary artery; LV = left ventricle; PA = pulmonary artery; RA = right atrium; RPA = right pulmonary artery; RV = right ventricle; SVC = superior vena cava. (Adapted with permission from Park MK: *Pediatric Cardiology for Practitioners.* St. Louis, Mosby-Year Book, 1996, p 53.)

E. Echocardiography is the cornerstone of diagnosis in CHD. All patients with suspected cyanotic or noncyanotic heart lesions should receive an echocardiogram.

References

Phoon CKL, Stanger P: *A Guide to Pediatric Cardiovascular Physical Examination (Or, How to Survive an Outreach Clinic).* Philadelphia, Lippincott, Williams & Wilkins, 1998.

Walsh EP, Saul JP: Cardiac Arrhythmias. In: Fyler DC: *Nadas' Pediatric Cardiology.* Philadelphia, Hanley & Belfus, 1992, pp 377–434.

Liebman J, Diagnosis and Management of Heart Murmurs in Children. *Pediatrics in Review* 3:321–329, 1982.

57. Coarctation of the Aorta

I INTRODUCTION

A. **Definition.** Coarctation is a narrowing of the aorta, usually near the origin of the left subclavian artery and the insertion of the ligamentum arteriosum **(Figure 57–1).** Coarctation may also be subvalvular.

B. **Natural history.** Because the coarctation is located across from the ductus arteriosus, flow becomes further restricted when the ductus closes (i.e., coarctation is a **ductal-dependent** lesion). Coarctation of the aorta is progressive; the stenosis worsens and collateral formation increases over time.

II SIMPLE COARCTATION

A. **Approach to the patient**

1. **Natural history.** Most patients (50%–60%) are asymptomatic as infants, but present later (either as older children or adults) with hypertension. This condition is often discovered when the clinician finds diminished or absent femoral or dorsalis pedis pulses. In an infant with severe coarctation, low cardiac output, respiratory distress, and cyanosis may be seen. One fourth of patients present with congestive heart failure (CHF).

2. **Physical examination**

   a. **Blood pressure.** Typically, higher pressures are seen in

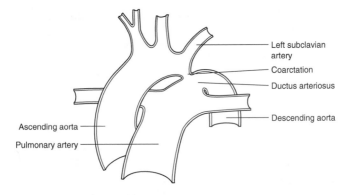

FIGURE 57–1. Coarctation of the aorta.

the arteries arising from the aorta proximal to the coarctation (i.e., those that supply the head and upper extremities) than are seen in the arteries distal to the coarctation (i.e., those that supply the lower extremities). Therefore, findings include **diminished** or **absent femoral pulses** or **dorsalis pedis pulses** and **hypertension in the upper extremities.**
  b. **Cardiac examination**
    (1) An **abnormal left ventricular impulse** and **increased intensity of the A₂** are noted.
    (2) Tracings of the **murmur** (Figure 57–2) are diamond-shaped, and the murmur is most often heard anteriorly near the left sternal border.

HOT **KEY**

The murmur of coarctation is at least as loud posteriorly as it is anteriorly.

---

3. **Electrocardiography.** In infants, right ventricular hypertrophy (caused by the increased workload imposed on the right ventricle during fetal life as it works to propel blood through the coarctation) may be seen. Biventricular hypertrophy develops as the child ages. ST and T wave changes are usually absent.
4. **Echocardiography** permits visualization of the coarctation, particularly in the high left parasternal view.
5. **Chest radiography.** Findings include:
  a. A **prominent aortic knob**
  b. The **figure 3 sign** (caused by the prestenotic and poststenotic portions of the aorta pressing against the esophagus), seen on overpenetrated films
  c. **Rib notching,** caused by erosion of the inferior aspects of

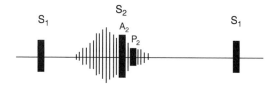

FIGURE 57–2. In coarctation of the aorta, the murmur is systolic and diamond-shaped. Often, it is late-peaking, sometimes extending into diastole.

the ribs by collateral arteries (seen only after children have
reached school age)

B. Treatment. The defect is repaired by end-to-end anastomosis.
Although surgery is usually performed when the child reaches
1 year of age, it should be considered earlier if the child's systolic blood pressure is greater than 140 mm Hg or if the difference between the right arm and leg systolic pressures is more
than 20 mm Hg.

III COMPLICATED COARCTATION is coarctation of the aorta
in association with aortic stenosis, aortic arch hypoplasia,
ventricular septal defect (VSD), or patent ductus arteriosus
(PDA). In patients with concomitant VSD or PDA, the
blood flows preferentially from left to right rather than into
the systemic circulation. The patient's condition is thereby
exacerbated because of the diminished systemic blood flow.

A. Approach to the patient
   1. Natural history. Infants are very ill and present with CHF,
   low cardiac output, respiratory distress, and moderate cyanosis.
   2. Chest radiography reveals right ventricular hypertrophy.
B. Treatment is with **end-to-end anastomosis** or **patch aortoplasty.**
   Conduits may be used for long obstructions.

References
Nadas AS, Fyler DC: *Nadas' Pediatric Cardiology.* Philadelphia, Hanley & Belfus,
   1992, pp 535–556.
Fyler DC: Nadas' Pediatric Cardiology. Philadelphia, Hanley & Belfus, 1992, pp 535–
   556.

58. Aortic Valve Disorders

AORTIC STENOSIS

A. Introduction

1. **Definition.** In valvular aortic stenosis, fusion of the cusps (resulting in a bicuspid or monocuspid valve and a small, irregular orifice) or hypoplasia of the valve components leads to aortic stenosis and left ventricular outflow obstruction. Aortic stenosis may also be subvalvular.

2. **Epidemiology.** The prevalence of aortic stenosis peaks in the 20- to 30-year age group. Boys are affected more often than girls.

B. Approach to the patient

1. **Natural history.** "Aortic stenosis begets aortic stenosis" (i.e., the lesion tends to worsen over time). The primary goal is to preserve left ventricular function. If aortic stenosis is left untreated, left ventricular dysfunction is inevitable.

   a. **Infants.** Symptoms rarely appear in the neonatal period unless the stenosis is extremely tight. Infants with severe aortic stenosis present at the age of 1 month with low cardiac output, respiratory distress, and cyanosis.

   b. **Older children and adults.** Most patients have no symptoms. When symptoms occur, they include chest pain, fainting, and exercise intolerance. These symptoms are suggestive of left ventricular dysfunction and are ominous.

2. **Physical examination**

   a. The **murmur (Figure 58–1)** is typically heard along the upper right sternal border and may radiate to the carotids.

   b. **S_2 split.** A narrow S_2 split occurs because of prolonged left ventricular systole and delayed closure of the aortic valve. In patients with severe aortic stenosis, a paradoxical split may be heard.

HOT KEY The differential diagnosis of a paradoxical split includes critical aortic stenosis, left bundle branch block, and severe pulmonary hypertension.

---

   c. **Aortic ejection click**

   (1) In aortic stenosis, the aortic ejection click is well-

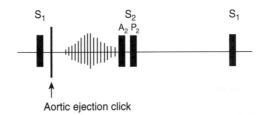

FIGURE 58-1. The murmur of aortic stenosis is a harsh systolic ejection murmur, often accompanied by an aortic ejection click. The length of the murmur increases and the S_2 split narrows as the severity of the lesion worsens.

        separated from the S_1, and it does not vary with respiration.

      (2) It is best heard at the apex and along the lower left sternal border, extending to the anterior axillary line.

  d. A **palpable thrill** at the suprasternal notch or the second right intercostal space is often present.

3. Electrocardiography (see Figures 56–4, 56–5)

  a. QRS complex. The initial cardiac activation vector is more likely to be left and posterior (as opposed to right, anterior, and superior). Hypertrophy of the left ventricle causes deep S waves in lead V_1 and tall R waves in leads V_5 and V_6.

  b. T wave. In patients with severe left ventricular hypertrophy, the T waves may be upright in the right chest leads and inverted in the left chest leads. These T wave changes may become more prominent during exercise.

HOT

KEY

  ST segment. ST segment depression may be present at rest or, like T wave changes, may develop during exercise.

---

4. Chest radiography. The ascending aorta may be prominent if there is a poststenotic dilatation. Cardiomegaly is generally not seen.

C. Treatment

  1. Interim therapy. Although immediate intervention is usually not necessary, patients should be followed up by a cardiologist regularly so that progression of the lesion can be monitored.

HOT **KEY** Symptomatic patients, patients with S-T segments or T wave abnormalities, and patients with a gradient greater than 40 mm Hg should be restricted from strenuous activity because of the risk of sudden death.

   2. **Definitive therapy. Valvuloplasty** is indicated when the patient develops symptoms, when there is a pressure gradient of more than 50 mm Hg across the valve, or when ST segment or T wave changes become apparent on the electrocardiogram. **Balloon valvuloplasty** is an effective means of relieving the gradient, although a residual pressure gradient can be expected. Some patients will require repeat balloon valvuloplasty. Valve replacement surgery is required if the valve is calcified or is grossly deformed, or if there is significant coexisting aortic regurgitation.

II AORTIC REGURGITATION

A. **Introduction**
   1. **Definition.** Aortic regurgitation results in the backflow of blood into the ventricle. Aortic regurgitation may be congenital in origin (e.g., bicuspid aortic valve, leaflet prolapse associated with ventricular septal defect), immune-mediated (rheumatic fever), or iatrogenic (e.g., a complication of balloon valvuloplasty).

 HOT **KEY** Always consider rheumatic heart disease in a patient with aortic regurgitation, especially if there is a history of arthralgia, chorea, suspicion of untreated streptococcal infection, or evidence of mitral valve disease.

   2. **Natural history.** Moderate or severe regurgitation is usually progressive. In cases caused by rheumatic heart disease, even minor regurgitation can progress if reinfection occurs. Significant aortic regurgitation increases the left ventricular volume and can lead to congestive heart failure (CHF).

 HOT **KEY** The development of CHF portends death within 2 years if left untreated.

B. **Approach to the patient**
   1. **Patient history.** Symptoms include syncope, chest pain, and left-sided CHF.

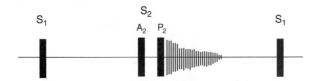

FIGURE 58–2. The murmur of aortic regurgitation is an early diastolic decrescendo murmur.

2. **Physical examination.** The diastolic decrescendo murmur **(Figure 58–2)** is of high frequency and is best heard along the left sternal border. The pulse pressure is characteristically wide. Because other lesions are often present in association with aortic regurgitation, it may be difficult to discern this murmur.
3. **Electrocardiography**
   a. **QRS complex.** Left ventricular hypertrophy is likely because of the increased work imposed on the left ventricle.
   b. **ST segment and T wave abnormalities.** T waves of increased magnitude (but oriented in the normal direction) are not cause for alarm, but other ST segment and T wave abnormalities (like those seen in severe aortic stenosis) are cause for concern.
4. **Chest radiography.** The heart size is proportional to the amount of regurgitation.
C. **Treatment.** Surgery (usually valve replacement) is required for patients with a history of syncope, CHF, or electrocardiographic changes suggestive of progressive left ventricular enlargement.
D. **Follow-up.** Patients with rheumatic heart disease require antibiotic prophylaxis to prevent recurrent infection.

References
Ankeney JL, Tzeng TS, Liebman J: Surgical therapy for congenital aortic valvular stenosis: a 23 year experience. *Cardiovasc Surg* 85:41–48, 1983. (classic article)
Fyler DC: Nadas' Pediatric Cardiology. Philadelphia, Hanley & Belfus, 1992, pp 459–471.

59. Pulmonary Valve Disorders

I PULMONIC STENOSIS

A. Introduction

1. **Definition.** In valvular pulmonic stenosis, malformation of the pulmonary valve (e.g., fused or absent commissures) leads to right ventricular outflow obstruction **(Figure 59–1).**

2. **Natural history.** Patients with pulmonic stenosis usually are well and grow normally; a murmur may be detected during a

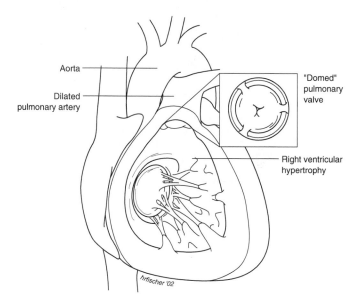

Aorta

Dilated pulmonary artery

"Domed" pulmonary valve

Right ventricular hypertrophy

hrfischer '02

FIGURE 59–1. Pathologic changes in severe pulmonic stenosis. Thickening and loss of the commissures between the cusps give the valve a "domed" appearance. Associated right ventricular hypertrophy further contributes to the obstruction. The jet of blood that spurts through the stenotic valve often leads to poststenotic dilatation of the main and left pulmonary arteries. (Adapted with permission from Fyler DC: *Nadas' Pediatric Cardiology*. Philadelphia, Hanley & Belfus, 1992, p 460.)

Chapter 59

routine examination. Patients with severe lesions present early in life with cyanosis and systemic venous congestion. Generally, only moderate or severe stenoses worsen over time.

B. Approach to the patient
  1. Physical examination
   a. The **murmur (Figure 59–2)** is best heard along the upper left sternal border.
   b. A **pulmonary ejection click** is heard almost simultaneously with S_1.
    (1) The click increases in intensity with expiration.
    (2) The pulmonary ejection click is best heard along the upper left sternal border. S_1 is not heard well at the upper left sternal border, so a loud first heart sound at that location might be a pulmonary ejection click.
  2. Electrocardiography. Pure pressure overload leads to right ventricular hypertrophy, which is proportional to the severity of the obstruction.
   a. Right atrial enlargement is seen as a result of decreased compliance of the hypertrophied right ventricle. Right atrial hypertrophy is evidenced by tall or a diphasic P wave in V_1. The P wave is narrow and peaked in lead II.
   b. **QRS complex.** The electrocardiogram (ECG) shows right-axis deviation and right ventricular hypertrophy.
    (1) An increased anterior QRS vector leads to large R waves in lead V_1 **(see Figure 56–2).**

HOT ▶ **KEY**   Multiply the R wave amplitude (in millimeters) by 5 to estimate the approximate peak systolic pressure in the right ventricle. (This formula is valid only in patients with isolated pulmonic stenosis.)

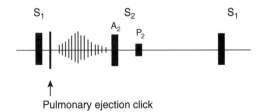

S_1 S_2 S_1
          A_2 P_2

↑
Pulmonary ejection click

FIGURE 59–2. The murmur of pulmonic stenosis is a short systolic ejection murmur, often accompanied by a pulmonic ejection click. The S_2 split often is prolonged (because the stenotic valve takes longer to close), and the intensity of the P_2 may be increased.

(2) An increased rightward terminal QRS vector, evidenced on the ECG by large S waves in lead V_6, is a very sensitive indicator of right ventricular hypertrophy.

c. **ST segment.** In patients with severe pulmonic stenosis, ST segment depression in the right chest leads may be seen. The T waves may be inverted in the left chest leads, and upright in the right chest leads.

HOT KEY

Upright T waves in the right chest leads in a neonate older than 72 hours may indicate right ventricular hypertrophy, even if the QRS complex is normal.

---

3. **Chest radiography.** Minimal cardiomegaly may be seen. The pulmonary artery and its proximal branches usually are prominent.

C. **Treatment**
   1. **Mild pulmonary stenosis.** Most patients do not need further evaluation after diagnosis. Antibiotic prophylaxis before dental procedures is recommended, but there are no limitations to physical activity.
   2. **Moderate to severe pulmonary stenosis.** These patients may require **balloon valvuloplasty.** This technique is remarkably effective; few patients require a repeat procedure.

II **PULMONIC REGURGITATION.** Isolated congenital incompetence of the pulmonary valve is rare. Pulmonic regurgitation may occur secondary to pulmonary hypertension, or as a complication of balloon valvuloplasty for the treatment of pulmonic stenosis.

References
Plansky DB, Clark EB, Doty DB: Pulmonary stenosis in infants and young children. Ann Thorac Surg 39:159–164, 1985. (classic article)
Fyler DC: Nadas' Pediatric Cardiology. Philadelphia, Hanley & Belfus, 1992, pp 493–512.

60. Mitral Valve Disorders

 MITRAL VALVE PROLAPSE

A. **Introduction**
   1. **Definition.** In mitral valve prolapse, the leaflets of the mitral valve prolapse into the left atrium during systole as a result of excessive mitral valve tissue, lengthening of the chordae tendineae, or both.
   2. **Natural history.** Mitral valve prolapse is nearly always a benign abnormality.
B. **Approach to the patient**
   1. **Patient history.** Patients are usually asymptomatic, although some patients report chest pain, faintness, and fatigue. It is not believed that mitral valve prolapse is responsible for those symptoms; often, the symptoms abate when the patient is reassured that no significant cardiac abnormality is present.
   2. **Physical examination.** The murmur is variable and is initiated by a midsystolic nonejection click, heard one third of the way into systole. The click may be loud or soft, single or multiple. The murmur is most intense at the apex, and may be loud or soft.

HOT   **KEY** The murmur of mitral valve prolapse is usually louder when the patient is standing (decreased venous return leads to increased prolapse and a louder murmur).

---

   3. **Electrocardiography.** Although the electrocardiogram (ECG) is usually normal, **T wave inversion** or **U waves** (possibly signaling papillary muscle dysfunction) may be seen.
   4. **Echocardiography** will reveal the prolapsed leaflets, but auscultation is usually sufficient for diagnosis.
C. **Treatment.** No specific treatment is necessary. Antibiotic prophylaxis should be given before dental procedures only if there is significant mitral regurgitation. Patients should be reassured that their "abnormality" is benign.

II MITRAL REGURGITATION

A. Introduction

1. **Definition.** In mitral regurgitation, part of the left ventricular stroke volume is propelled backward into the left atrium, instead of forward into the aorta. Insufficiency of the mitral valve is usually a consequence of rheumatic heart disease, but it may also result from congenital abnormalities or an anomalous left coronary artery (the left coronary artery arises from the main pulmonary artery).

2. **Natural history.** Because the lesion does tend to progress over time, all patients with mitral regurgitation need to be followed up. Mitral regurgitation, even when it is severe, can be tolerated for many years if it develops gradually. Patients with minor mitral regurgitation are usually asymptomatic. Those with more severe cases may complain of dyspnea or show signs of retarded growth. Patients with an anomalous left coronary artery may present in infancy with poor feeding, respiratory distress, or irritability.

B. Differential diagnosis.

Anomalous left coronary artery must be ruled out by echocardiogram or cardiac catheterization. Left coronary arteries arising from the pulmonary artery are subject to inadequate perfusion as pulmonary vascular resistance decreases. This leads to myocardial ischemia. Mitral regurgitation occurs as a result of ischemic damage to the papillary muscles. Ischemia can be seen on ECG as Q waves or ST segment changes.

HOT

KEY

Always consider an anomalous left coronary artery in patients who develop mitral regurgitation.

C. Approach to the patient

1. **Physical examination.** The murmur of mitral regurgitation **(Figure 60–1)** is best heard at the apex, radiating into the axilla.

2. **Electrocardiography.** Regurgitation leads to a threefold increase in volume in the left atrium, which in turn results in **left atrial enlargement.** Left atrial enlargement is seen as a broad notched P wave in lead II or as a biphasic P wave in V_1 with a deep slurred terminal portion. The increased workload imposed on the ventricle also results in **left ventricular**

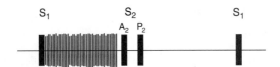

FIGURE 60–1. The murmur of mitral regurgitation is a high-frequency, holosystolic murmur that peaks in late systole. If the regurgitation is severe, a middiastolic low-frequency murmur at the apex may be heard, and the S_2 split may be decreased (owing to pulmonary venous backflow, which can flood the lungs and increase the pulmonary arterial pressure, thereby decreasing the split).

hypertrophy. Rarely, dilatation of the left atrium leads to **atrial fibrillation.** Patients with anomalous left coronary artery show evidence of anterolateral myocardial infarction (i.e., Q waves in left chest leads and aVL).

HOT KEY

Mitral regurgitation related to Marfan syndrome may cause very severe left ventricular hypertrophy in infancy.

3. **Chest radiography** may reveal cardiomegaly and increased pulmonary vascularity if the lesion is severe.
D. **Treatment.** Afterload reduction is effective for most patients. Patients with growth retardation or severe symptomatic disease require valve replacement. Those with anomalous left coronary arteries need immediate surgical repair.

References
Nishimura RA, McGoon MD, Shub C, et al: Echocardiographic documented MVP: long term follow up of 237 patients. *N Engl J Med* 313:1305–1309, 1985.
Fyler DC: Nadas' Pediatric Cardiology. Philadelphia, Hanley & Belfus, 1992, pp 609–622.

61. Ventricular Septal Defects

I INTRODUCTION

A. Definition. The interventricular septum, which has both muscular and membranous parts, separates the left ventricle from the right ventricle. Ventricular septal defects (VSDs) can be **classified according to their location** on the septum (Figure 61–1). **VSDs vary widely in size.** They may be the size of a pinhead, or they may be so large that they (in effect) obliterate the interventricular septum.

B. Eisenmenger syndrome is the development of a right-to-left shunt and cyanosis owing to significant pulmonary hypertension. In Eisenmenger syndrome, the unchecked increase in pulmonary blood flow (caused by the left-to-right shunting) leads to fibrosis of the pulmonary vessels, which in turn leads to pulmonary hypertension. The pulmonary hypertension causes the shunt to reverse to a right-to-left shunt, resulting in cyanosis.

HOT KEY

Eisenmenger syndrome can occur in any condition associated with a significant left-to-right shunt or increased pulmonary blood flow. Once the syndrome develops, it often cannot be reversed. Therefore, the only effective therapy is prevention through the timely repair of lesions that place the patient at risk for pulmonary hypertension.

C. Natural history of VSDs

1. Large VSDs. In infants with large VSDs, the right- and left-sided ventricular pressures are initially equal and the pulmonary vasculature does not rapidly mature from its muscular, noncompliant, high-resistance state to its thin-walled, compliant, low-resistance state. During this time, there may not be a murmur because there is no left-to-right shunt. As the child grows, the pulmonary beds mature, pulmonary vascular resistance decreases, and **left-to-right shunting begins**. Pulmonary vascular resistance is lowest and congestive heart failure (CHF) is maximal by 1 month of age. This left-to-right shunting causes an overload on the right-sided circulation; if uncorrected, Eisenmenger syndrome may result. Large VSDs (i.e., VSDs that are at least half as wide as the diameter of the aorta) are more often associated with Eisenmenger syndrome.

349

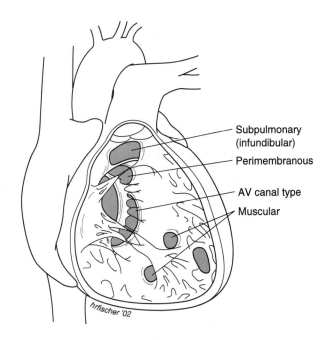

FIGURE 61–1. Ventricular septal defects (VSDs), as viewed from the right ventricle. Subpulmonary (infundibular) defects are located just below the aortic and pulmonary valves. Perimembranous defects are adjacent to the aortic valve on the left and the tricuspid valve on the right. Muscular defects are often multiple and can be found anywhere on the septum. AV = atrioventricular. (Adapted with permission from Fyler DC: *Nadas' Pediatric Cardiology.* Philadelphia, Hanley & Belfus, 1992, p 437.)

2. **Small VSDs.** In infants with small VSDs, the pulmonary vasculature matures normally, leading to **left-to-right shunting and an audible murmur in the newborn period.** If they are small enough, membranous and muscular VSDs will often close spontaneously within 6 months.

HOT KEY Children with small VSDs are protected from developing pulmonary hypertension because there is restricted flow across the smaller defect and the pulmonary vascular bed is compliant.

HOT
KEY

> Subpulmonary (infundibular), endocardial cushion, and mal-
> alignment VSDs do not close spontaneously.

D. Development of complications: aortic valve disease. Approximately 5% of patients with a subpulmonary (infundibular)
VSD develop aortic regurgitation (after prolapse of the aortic
valve leaflets through the defect). Patients with perimembranous VSDs are prone to developing subaortic stenosis.

II APPROACH TO THE PATIENT

A. Symptoms. Infants with large VSDs may develop CHF and present with poor growth, cyanosis or perspiration during feedings,
tachypnea, and a susceptibility to lower respiratory tract infections. Children with small VSDs are generally asymptomatic.

B. Physical examination

  1. Large VSDs

   a. An **enlarged liver** and **signs of pulmonary congestion**
   (rales, tachypnea) may be noted on physical examination.

   b. The characteristic **murmur** (Figure 61–2) may not be de-

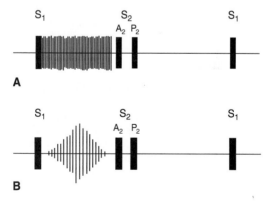

FIGURE 61–2. **(A)** In patients with large ventricular septal defects (VSDs),
a high-frequency, holosystolic, plateau-shaped murmur is heard. The S_1
is obscured because there is flow across the defect before closure of the
mitral valve. A low-frequency murmur may be heard during diastole
because of increased flow through the mitral valve. **(B)** In patients with
small VSDs, a variably pitched, diamond-shaped murmur that may continue into late systole is heard.

tectable until pulmonary vascular resistance decreases and left-to-right shunting begins. The systolic component is heard best at the third, fourth, or fifth intercostal space, depending on the location of the defect; the diastolic component is heard best at the apex.

   c. **Heart sounds**

      (1) **S_1.** The S_1 may be obscured because of flow across the defect before closure of the mitral valve.

      (2) **S_2.** A narrow S_2 split indicates an increased pulmonary artery pressure; a loud, single S_2 is worrisome for pulmonary hypertension.

      (3) **S_3.** The S_3 is present because of increased return to the left side of the heart.

2. **Small VSDs.** A murmur (see Figure 61–2) is often detectable during the newborn period.

3. **Murmur intensity.** In VSDs, the intensity of the murmur depends more on the amount of flow across the VSD rather than on the size of the defect. Minimal flow can be associated with very small defects, which do not allow much blood to traverse the defect, or with large defects occurring in the presence of high pulmonary vascular resistance. Heavy flow occurs when the gradient between the left- and right-sided circulations is high (i.e., when pulmonary vascular resistance is low).

HOT KEY

Small lesions do not necessarily mean low flow through the defect. Small lesions may still be associated with significant left-to-right shunting if the pulmonary vascular resistance is low.

C. **Electrocardiography** may reveal left, right, or biventricular hypertrophy.

   1. **Left ventricular hypertrophy.** The VSD is likely to be small, with minimal pulmonary vascular resistance. Volume overload is responsible for the left ventricular hypertrophy.

   2. **Right ventricular hypertrophy.** The VSD is likely to be large, with increased pulmonary vascular resistance and minimal left-to-right shunting. The increased pressure in the pulmonary vascular bed leads to the right ventricular hypertrophy.

   3. **Biventricular hypertrophy.** The VSD is likely to be large, with significant left-to-right shunting and high right-sided pressures. Biventricular hypertrophy is classically seen in children older than 1 month with large VSDs. This is the classic case of a child with a nonrestrictive VSD presenting at 4–6 weeks of age.

D. Chest radiography may reveal cardiomegaly, enlargement of the left atrium and pulmonary artery, and increased pulmonary vascularity.

III TREATMENT

A. Interim therapy. Patients require antibiotic prophylaxis before dental or invasive medical procedures. The risk of endocarditis is highest in patients with small VSDs.

B. Definitive therapy. Surgery is undertaken to prevent pulmonary vascular disease in patients with significantly large defects (only 15% of VSDs are large enough to necessitate surgery). The development of aortic insufficiency or subaortic stenosis is also an indication for surgery.

 HOT KEY Pulmonary vascular disease is evidenced by pruned pulmonary vasculature on the chest radiograph, right ventricular hypertrophy, and a loud single S_2.

---

1. **Before 6 months of age.** The main indication for surgery before the age of 6 months is failure to thrive. Before surgery, symptomatic infants may be treated with digoxin or furosemide. In addition, nasogastric feedings are sometimes used to maximize growth.
2. After 6 months of age, surgery is indicated if there is excessive pulmonary pressure or excessive pulmonary blood flow.

References
Corone P, Doyon F, Gaudeau S, et al: Natural history of ventricular septal defect: a study involving 790 cases. *Circulation* 55:908–915, 1977. (classic article)
Liebman J: Diagnosis and Management of Heart Murmurs in Children. *Pediatrics in Review* 3:321–329, 1982. (classic article)

62. Atrial Septal Defect

 INTRODUCTION

A. Definition. Atrial septal defect (ASD) results from the faulty formation of the interatrial septum. There are three general types. ASDs are of varying size and may be multiple (Figure 62–1).

1. **Ostium primum defects** are associated with defects of the **endocardial cushion,** a structure that contributes to the interventricular septum, the mitral and tricuspid valves, and the interatrial septum.

HOT

KEY

Ostium primum defects are often associated with mitral regurgitation.

---

2. **Ostium secundum defects** are often located in the center of the septum, near the fossa ovale.

3. In **sinus venosus defects,** one or more of the pulmonary veins drains anomalously into the superior vena cava. The hemodynamic consequences and electrocardiogram (ECG) findings are similar to those found in ostium secundum defects.

B. Natural history

1. During the newborn period, the right ventricle remains enlarged and less compliant so no left-to-right shunting occurs (i.e., the right ventricle does not accept blood as easily as the more compliant left ventricle). The pulmonary vasculature matures normally.

2. Left-to-right shunting begins only after the left ventricle increases in size (i.e., becomes less compliant) and the right ventricle decreases in size (i.e., becomes more compliant). The left-to-right shunting places a volume load on the right ventricle, but because the compliance of the right ventricle decreases slowly and the right ventricle has time to hypertrophy, the patient is protected against congestive heart failure (CHF).

3. Approximately 5%–10% of adults with uncorrected ASD develop pulmonary hypertension.

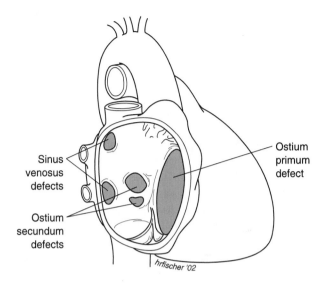

Sinus
venosus
defects

Ostium
secundum
defects

Ostium
primum
defect

hrfischer '02

FIGURE 62–1. Atrial septal defects (ASDs), as viewed from the right atrium. Ostium primum defects typically are caused by defects in the endocardial cushion, and therefore are located adjacent to the mitral and tricuspid valves. Ostium secundum defects are located near the fossa ovalis. (Adapted with permission from Fyler DC: *Nadas' Pediatric Cardiology.* Philadelphia, Hanley & Belfus, 1992, p 514.)

II APPROACH TO THE PATIENT

A. **Patient history.** Usually patients are asymptomatic. Those with large defects or significant mitral regurgitation may have exercise intolerance or recurrent pulmonary infections.

B. **Physical examination.** Blood flows through the defect from left to right, leading to volume overload of the right-sided circulation. Note that there is no murmur associated with blood flowing through the defect because blood flow through the defect is not restricted. Rather, the murmurs are functional ones, associated with increased flow across the right ventricular outflow tract and tricuspid valve **(Figure 62–2).** Because the murmur may be subtle, it is not uncommon for ASD to go undetected until adulthood. The murmurs disappear if pulmonary hypertension, right-to-left shunting, and cyanosis oc-

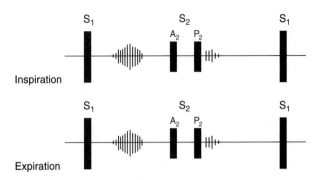

FIGURE 62–2. Diagram of the murmur of atrial septal defect (ASD). During systole, increased flow across the pulmonic valve produces a pulmonary ejection murmur, best heard at the upper left sternal border. No pulmonary ejection click is present. During early to middiastole, a short murmur of medium frequency occurs because of increased flow across the tricuspid valve. The diastolic component is best heard at the lower left sternal border. The overloaded right-sided circulation causes delayed pulmonary valve closure, leading to a wide S_2 split. The split persists throughout respiration because the communication between the atria allows pressure equilibration between the systemic and pulmonary circulations.

cur. These events usually do not occur until adolescence or adulthood.

C. Electrocardiography

    1. Ostium primum ASD. The ECG reveals an abnormally superior vector, which is a result of the endocardial cushion defect. Usually, there is left axis deviation and right ventricular hypertrophy **(Figure 62–3).**

    2. Ostium secundum ASD. The right ventricle is compliant (albeit somewhat thicker than normal) and dilated. The hypertrophy is usually mild. The ECG reveals right ventricular hypertrophy with a **typical RSR′ pattern** in the right precordial leads **(see Figure 56–3).**

D. Chest radiography reveals cardiomegaly. The pulmonary artery is enlarged, and pulmonary vascularity is increased.

III   **TREATMENT.** Surgical repair is indicated when the ratio of pulmonary blood flow to systemic blood flow is greater than 1.5:1 to prevent right ventricular failure and CHF, Eisenmenger syndrome, and paradoxical emboli. Surgery is usually delayed until the child is at least 3 years of age because

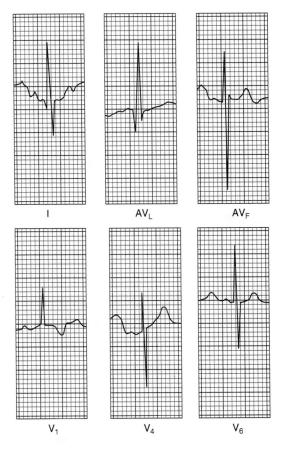

FIGURE 62-3. An electrocardiogram typical of the endocardial cushion defects. Note that the QRS axis is leftward and superior. (Adapted with permission from Fyler DC: *Nadas' Pediatric Cardiology*. Philadelphia, Hanley & Belfus, 1992, p 582.)

the ASD may spontaneously close. Catheter closure with an occlusion device is an investigational procedure with a long-term outcome that is not yet known.

References

Craig RJ, Selzer A: Natural history and prognosis of atrial septal defect. *Circulation* 1968;37:805. (classic article)

Liebman J: Diagnosis and Management of Heart Murmurs in Children. *Pediatrics in Review* 3:321–329, 1982. (classic article)

63. Patent Ductus Arteriosus

I INTRODUCTION

A. **Definition.** Patent ductus arteriosus (PDA) occurs when the ductus arteriosus, a normal fetal structure, fails to close after birth. Blood flows from the aorta through the PDA into the pulmonary artery and then into the pulmonary vascular bed, where it is returned to the left atrium **(Figure 63–1),** leading to overload of the left-sided circulation.

B. **Predisposing factors** include prematurity, congenital rubella infection, intrauterine hypoxia, and severe pulmonary disease.

C. **Pathophysiology**
   1. **Full-term infants.** "True" PDAs behave much like ventricular septal defects (VSDs) except that systemic-level pulmonary hypertension usually does not occur because the ductus is more restrictive than a large VSD. Congestive heart failure (CHF) takes slightly longer (2 months) than in VSDs.
   2. **Premature infants.** Because pulmonary vascular resistance is lower, left-to-right shunting and CHF may develop quickly. In premature infants with respiratory distress syndrome, atelectasis induces high pulmonary vascular resistance and a right-to-left shunt occurs; left-to-right shunting develops only after the pulmonary vascular resistance decreases.

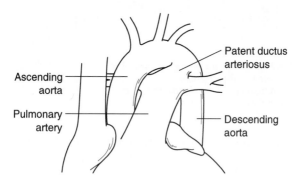

FIGURE 63–1. Patent ductus arteriosus (PDA). Blood flows from the aorta, through the PDA, and into the pulmonary artery. (Adapted with permission from Fyler DC: *Nadas' Pediatric Cardiology.* Philadelphia, Hanley & Belfus, 1992, p 526.)

D. Natural history. In full-term infants, the course depends on the size of the lesion. Larger defects induce heart failure more rapidly.

II APPROACH TO THE PATIENT

A. Physical examination
  1. A **hyperactive precordium** (e.g., abnormal left ventricular impulse, hyperdynamic left sternal edge), **increased pulse pressure,** and **bounding pulses** are typical.
  2. **Murmur.** Increased blood flow (as much as three times normal) across the mitral and aortic valves produces functional murmurs. Blood flow through the open ductus also contributes to the murmur **(Figure 63–2).**
B. Electrocardiography. In patients with smaller PDAs, the electrocardiogram (ECG) is usually normal. In those with a large PDA, left ventricular hypertrophy and left atrial enlargement may be seen. In premature infants, the ECG is not helpful because of low voltages and fluxing hemodynamics, which may cause the ductus to open and close.
C. Chest radiography reveals cardiomegaly, enlargement of the pulmonary artery and aorta, and increased pulmonary vascularity.

III TREATMENT. All PDAs should be corrected.

A. Indomethacin, a powerful prostaglandin inhibitor, is used to encourage ductal closure in infants.

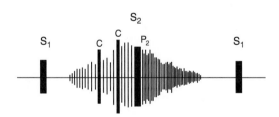

FIGURE 63–2. The continuous "machinery" murmur of patent ductus arteriosus (PDA). The systolic component is uneven, like water flowing over rapids. The initial soft systolic component is caused by increased flow through the aortic valve and is best heard at the upper right sternal border. Flow through the PDA causes the murmur to peak in late systole. The late systolic component is best heard over the upper left sternal border. Increased flow across the mitral valve results in a middiastolic rumbling murmur, best heard at the apex. Clicks **(C)** during systole contribute to the mechanical sound of this murmur.

B. Surgery. If medical therapy fails, ligation can be performed, in even the smallest babies. Catheter closure using a coil device is possible if the PDA is small enough to accommodate the device.

References

Gittenberger-De Groot AC, Van Ertbruggen I, Moulaert AJMG, et al. The ductus arteriosus in the preterm infant; histologic and clinical observations. *J Pediatr* 1980;96:88. (classic article)

Liebman J: Diagnosis and Management of Heart Murmurs in Children. *Pediatrics in Review* 3:321–329, 1982. (classic article)

64. Tricuspid Atresia and Pulmonary Atresia

I TRICUSPID ATRESIA

A. Introduction

1. **Definition.** The tricuspid (right atrioventricular) valve is atretic and the right ventricle is rudimentary. An atrial septal defect (ASD) or more commonly a patent foramen ovale (PFO) and a ventricular septal defect (VSD) are present, allowing perfusion of the lungs. The ductus arteriosus does provide blood flow to the lungs, but usually closes soon after birth. Hypoplastic right ventricle with tricuspid atresia is often associated with transposition of the great arteries. In this case, pulmonary blood flow is excessive and congestive failure results **(Figure 64–1).**

2. **Natural history.** Most infants with right ventricular hypoplasia and tricuspid atresia do not live longer than 6 months if palliative therapy is not initiated. Patients present with cyanosis as pulmonary blood flow diminishes. This may occur soon after birth when the ductus closes or some months later when the VSD begins to close. Those with excessive pulmonary flow present with congestive failure, which increases as pulmonary vascular resistance decreases.

B. Approach to the patient

1. **Physical examination** reveals a murmur characteristic of VSD (see Figure 61–2). This murmur is not always present.

2. **Electrocardiography** reveals **left ventricular hypertrophy** (owing to volume overload) and **hypoplasia of the right ventricle (Figure 64–2).** There is an associated left ventricular conduction abnormality (wide QRS), although this is not from a left bundle branch block.

C. Treatment

1. **Interim therapy**

   a. If there is inadequate pulmonary flow, prostaglandin or a Blalock-Taussig shunt (connecting the left subclavian artery to the left pulmonary artery) may be required. However, pulmonary overcirculation should be avoided. Flooding of the lungs as a result of increased flow through the ductus arteriosus or Blalock-Taussig shunt can cause pulmonary vascular disease, making future definitive surgery difficult. In addition, increased flow through the ductus

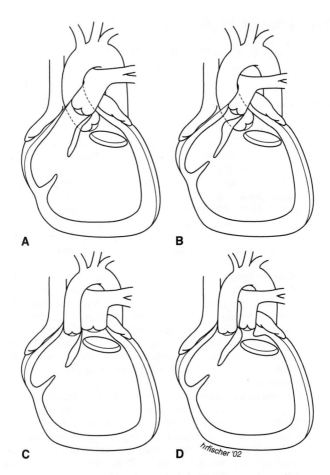

FIGURE 64-1. Tricuspid atresia is usually classified according to the absence (**A, C**) or the presence (**B, D**) of pulmonary stenosis and the presence of transposition of the great arteries (**C, D**). The ventricular septal defect varies considerably in size, and over time tends to get smaller. It may provide obstruction to pulmonary blood flow (**B**) or in the presence of transposition obstruct outflow to the aorta (functional subaortic stenosis). (Adapted with permission from Fyler DC: *Nadas' Pediatric Cardiology.* Philadelphia, Hanley & Belfus, 1992, p 659.)

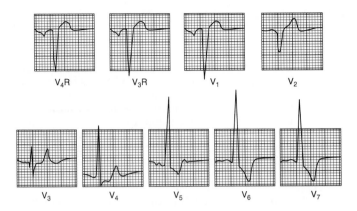

FIGURE 64–2. Absent right ventricular forces (no R wave in right chest leads) in a patient with tricuspid atresia. (Adapted with permission from Fyler DC: *Nadas' Pediatric Cardiology.* Philadelphia, Hanley & Belfus, 1992, p 134.)

    arteriosus or Blalock-Taussig shunt places extra stress on the left ventricle. If the left ventricle hypertrophies, it will not be able to accept pulmonary blood flow, again increasing the risk that definitive surgical therapy will fail.

    b. Infants with transposition of the great arteries and tricuspid atresia may have excessive pulmonary flow that requires pulmonary artery banding. However, banding may cause distortion of the pulmonary arteries or early VSD closure. Closure of the VSD causes a subaortic stenosis, which leads to left ventricular hypertrophy, thereby making future Fontan procedures difficult.

2. Definitive therapy is the **Fontan procedure.** This surgery is difficult to perform in infants; it is best to wait until the patient reaches the age of 4 or 5 years. The Fontan procedure involves anastomosing the superior vena cava and the inferior vena cava to the pulmonary artery. In essence, the right-sided circulation is bypassed and the remaining ventricle is used for the systemic circulation.

HOT KEY

Because the patient who has undergone a Fontan procedure relies solely on venous flow to feed the lungs, it is important that there is no pulmonary vascular disease or pulmonic stenosis. In addition, the left ventricle must not be hypertrophied; otherwise, it will be unable to accept pulmonary blood flow.

II PULMONARY ATRESIA WITH INTACT VENTRICULAR SEPTUM

A. Introduction

1. **Definition.** The pulmonary valve is atretic, and the right ventricle is rudimentary. An ASD, but no VSD, is present. Pulmonary flow is dependent on the ductus arteriosus.

2. **Natural history.** After physiologic closure of the ductus arteriosus, infants destabilize within 24 hours. Cyanosis and dyspnea develop as the ductus arteriosus closes. These infants may be cyanotic immediately after birth. Death occurs within a few days unless pulmonary blood flow is restored surgically.

B. Approach to the patient

1. **Physical examination.** Obstruction of the right ventricular outflow tract increases the right ventricular pressure and induces marked tricuspid regurgitation. The tricuspid regurgitation produces a systolic murmur, best heard at the lower left sternal border. In some cases, however, no murmur is heard.

HOT **KEY**

Be careful not to confuse the murmur of tricuspid regurgitation with that of VSD.

---

2. **Electrocardiography** reveals **left ventricular hypertrophy** (as a result of volume overload) and **hypoplasia of the right ventricle.** Sometimes the electrocardiogram (ECG) will be difficult to interpret because of an abnormal position of the heart.

C. Treatment.

The primary goal is to increase the pulmonary blood flow. Methods include atrial balloon septostomy (if the ASD is small), creation of a Blalock-Taussig shunt, anastomosis of the aorta to the pulmonary artery, and the administration of prostaglandin.

References

De Brux JL, ZanniniL, Binet JP, et al: Tricuspid atresia: results of treatment in 115 children. *J Thorac Cardiovasc Surg* 85:440–446, 1983. (classic article)

Liebman J: Diagnosis and Management of Heart Murmurs in Children. *Pediatrics in Review* 3:321–329, 1982. (classic article)

65. Tetralogy of Fallot

I INTRODUCTION

A. Definition. As the name suggests, tetralogy of Fallot has four hallmark features (Figure 65–1).

   1. **Hemodynamics.** Most often, **right-to-left shunting** occurs because blood shunts across the ventricular septal defect (VSD), rather than through the obstructed right ventricular outflow tract. Heart failure does not occur because the volume work of the heart is less than normal. Left-to-right shunting can occur if the pulmonic stenosis is mild and the VSD is large.

   2. **Associated anomalies.** In 40% of cases, tetralogy of Fallot occurs with atrial septal defect (ASD), patent ductus arteriosus (PDA), or tricuspid atresia. Approximately 25% of patients have a right aortic arch.

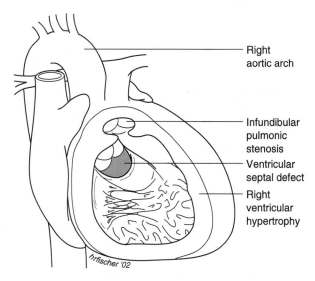

Right
aortic arch

Infundibular
pulmonic
stenosis

Ventricular
septal defect

Right
ventricular
hypertrophy

hrfischer '02

FIGURE 65–1. Tetralogy of Fallot. The pulmonic stenosis is usually infundibular, but may be valvular. Note that the aortic valve leaflets can be seen through the ventricular septal defect (VSD). (Adapted with permission from Fyler DC: *Nadas' Pediatric Cardiology.* Philadelphia, Hanley & Belfus, 1992, p 471.)

366   Chapter 65

B. Natural history. Most patients are identified at birth as having a
significant murmur. Cyanosis may or may not be present at
birth, depending on the degree of pulmonic stenosis. Because
pulmonic stenosis gradually worsens over time, total surgical
correction is required. A higher incidence of infective endocarditis, cerebrovascular accident (CVA), and brain abscess is
seen in children with untreated tetralogy of Fallot.

>
> **HOT KEY**
> Only 25% of patients with tetralogy of Fallot are cyanotic at
> birth; 75% will have become cyanotic by 1 year of age.

II APPROACH TO THE PATIENT

A. Symptoms. The severity of symptoms depends most on the degree of pulmonic stenosis.
1. **Cyanosis,** caused by right-to-left shunting, is the outstanding
   feature.
2. **"Tet spells"** are acute episodes of cyanosis, tachypnea, and
   inconsolable crying that can be induced by exercise or any
   event that is stressful to an infant. These episodes may also
   occur spontaneously. A decrease in systemic vascular resistance causes an increase in right-to-left shunting and a concomitant decrease in pulmonary blood flow. Spells are often
   followed by periods of deep sleep.
   3. **Squatting.** Older children with tetralogy of Fallot often
   squat after exercise (or even while at rest). Squatting increases the systemic vascular resistance and partially relieves
   the right-to-left shunt.
B. Physical examination
1. The second heart sound is single and loud because of the increased proximity of the anteriorly displaced aorta.
2. A **pulmonic ejection murmur** is heard in patients with mild
   to moderate pulmonic stenosis. The more severe the pulmonic stenosis, the softer the murmur. In patients with tetralogy of Fallot and pulmonary atresia, this murmur is not
   heard. In this case, a continuous murmur from collateral circulation may be heard.

>
> **HOT KEY**
> Note that there is no murmur associated with the blood shunt-
> ing right to left through the VSD.

3. In patients with chronic cyanosis, there may be digital clubbing and growth retardation.

C. **Electrocardiography** reveals right ventricular hypertrophy. However, if the VSD is large and there is minimal pulmonic stenosis (PS), there may be biventricular hypertrophy.

D. **Chest radiography.** In older children with tetralogy of Fallot, the classic boot-shaped heart (caused by right ventricular enlargement and absence of the main pulmonary artery shadow) may be seen.

III TREATMENT

A. **Interim therapy** focuses on managing tet spells and hypoxemia and on preventing infectious complications (e.g., infectious endocarditis, brain abscess). Prolonged episodes of hypoxemia are related to future cognitive deficits.

1. **Management of tet spells.** Knee–chest positioning should be attempted first, and oxygen may be administered via a face mask. If this fails, more invasive steps may need to be taken.

HOT KEY

Keep in mind that needle sticks and intravenous line starts can make the situation worse!

---

a. **Morphine sulfate,** administered intramuscularly, decreases fear, catecholamine levels, and pulmonary vascular resistance.

b. If morphine does not resolve the episode, an intravenous line may be established and a β **blocker** (e.g., propranolol) may be administered to decrease contractility and heart rate, thereby decreasing the dynamic subvalvular obstruction. **Phenylephrine** may also be administered to increase the systemic vascular resistance.

c. Intravenous administration of **bicarbonate** may be needed if there is significant acidosis.

d. **Emergent surgical intervention** is rarely required.

2. **Interim management.** Although placement of a palliative **Blalock-Taussig shunt** is a widely accepted practice, shunt placement may distort the pulmonary arteries, making future definitive correction more complicated. Some practitioners prefer early complete surgical correction.

B. **Definitive therapy.** In patients with severely impaired oxygenation, complete repair of the VSD and pulmonic stenosis is necessary in infancy. Most patients require definitive therapy by the age of 6–12 months.

IV FOLLOW-UP. Because patients who have undergone surgery have a higher incidence of ventricular arrhythmias, periodic Holter monitoring and stress tests are indicated.

> **HOT KEY**
>
> After surgical repair, electrocardiogram (ECG) findings include a right bundle branch block because the right ventricular wall is incised to correct the VSD. On physical examination, there are murmurs consistent with residual pulmonic stenosis and pulmonic insufficiency (caused by manipulation of the right ventricular outflow tract).

References

Murphy JG, Gersh BJ, Mair DD, et al. Long-term outcome in patients undergoing surgical repair of tetralogy of Fallot. *N Engl J Med* 1993; 329:593.

Fyler DC: Nadas' Pediatric Cardiology. Philadelphia, Hanley & Belfus, 1992, pp 471–492.

66. Ebstein Anomaly

I INTRODUCTION

A. Definition. The tricuspid valve is distorted and regurgitant (the posterior and septal leaflets are fused to the ventricle wall below the annulus). There is often an element of tricuspid stenosis. A stretched foramen ovale and a small right ventricle are also present.

B. Natural history. In the first weeks of life, flow to the lungs is restricted, owing to the insufficient valve and the high pulmonary vascular resistance. A right-to-left shunt occurs through the stretched foramen ovale, leading to right ventricular failure, cyanosis, and systemic venous congestion. As the infant grows and the pulmonary vascular resistance decreases, pulmonary flow increases and right-to-left shunting decreases, leading to an improvement in the clinical condition. Morbidity is highly variable and depends on the severity of the lesion, degree of cyanosis, and degree of congestive heart failure.

II APPROACH TO THE PATIENT

A. Patient history. Fifty percent of patients present as infants with right ventricular failure, cyanosis, and systemic venous congestion; the remainder present later in life with arrhythmias, heart failure, and complications of cyanosis.

HOT **KEY**

The incidence of Ebstein anomaly is higher in children who were exposed to lithium in utero.

B. Physical examination
1. During systole, a harsh (sandpaper-like), full-length **tricuspid regurgitation murmur** can be heard along the lower left sternal border. During diastole, a **tricuspid stenosis** murmur is heard.
2. Both the S_1 and the S_2 **are split,** the latter widely and persistently.

C. Electrocardiography (Figure 66–1). Electrocardiogram (ECG) findings are variable:

369

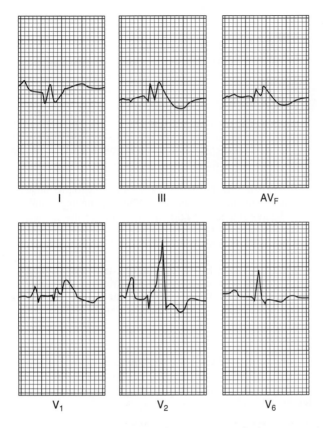

FIGURE 66–1. An electrocardiogram from a patient with Ebstein anomaly. Note the large and bizarre P waves, the wide and bizarre QRS complexes, and delta waves. (Reprinted with permission from Fyler DC: *Nadas' Pediatric Cardiology.* Philadelphia, Hanley & Belfus, 1992, p 672.)

1. Right atrial hypertrophy can cause very large, bizarre P waves.
2. Right bundle branch block may be seen, owing to abnormal development and position of the bundle.
3. The P-R interval may be shortened.
4. Wolff-Parkinson-White syndrome occurs in 10% of patients **(see Figure 66–1).** In this syndrome, the P-R interval is short. The QRS complex shows a delta wave, most often in V_2–V_4. This condition may lead to ventricular arrhythmias, which may cause seizures or syncope.

III 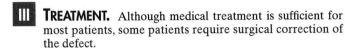 **TREATMENT.** Although medical treatment is sufficient for most patients, some patients require surgical correction of the defect.

A. **Interim therapy.** During infancy, the goal is to maintain the infant until pulmonary vascular resistance decreases. Prostaglandin may be needed if cyanosis is severe.

B. **Surgical therapy.** Surgery is used only for patients who have congestive heart failure or unremitting cyanosis.

References
Radford DJ, Graff RF and Neilson GH: Diagnosis and natural history of Ebsteins Anomaly. *Br Heart J* 54:517–522, 1985. (classic article)

67. Transposition of the Great Arteries

I INTRODUCTION

A. Definition. The great arteries are switched (Figure 67–1), so that the systemic and pulmonary circulations are parallel, rather than in series.

1. Fetal development is possible because the ductus arteriosus and the foramen ovale provide a means for oxygenated blood to reach the fetal body.

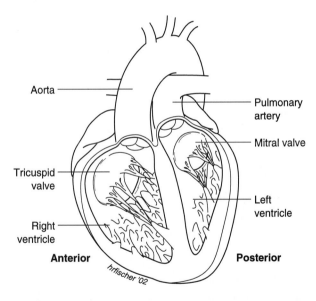

Aorta

Pulmonary artery

Mitral valve

Tricuspid valve

Left ventricle

Right ventricle

Anterior

Posterior

hrfischer '02

FIGURE 67–1. Transposition of the great arteries. The aorta arises anteriorly from the right ventricle, and the pulmonary artery arises posteriorly from the left ventricle. In this diagram, there is no connection between the pulmonary and systemic circulations, a situation that is incompatible with life. For survival, there must be a communication between the two circulations, usually in the form of a patent ductus arteriosus, a ventricular septal defect, or an atrial opening. (Adapted with permission from Fyler DC: *Nadas' Pediatric Cardiology.* Philadelphia, Hanley & Belfus, 1992, p 559.)

2. Postnatal survival depends on the degree of connection between these parallel circulations [ventricular septal defect (VSD), atrial septal defect (ASD), patent ductus arteriosus (PDA), patent foramen ovale (PFO)] as well as on the ability of the right ventricle to maintain systemic flow.

B. Natural history. The degree of cyanosis depends on the size of the VSD; the larger the opening, the greater the amount of mixing between the parallel circuits and the less cyanosis. Children with intact ventricular septums may present in the first hours of life with severe cyanosis after their ductus arteriosus closes. Those with VSDs may present later in life with congestive heart failure, tachypnea, and mild cyanosis. These children are cyanotic without being dyspneic. They are often described as "happily tachypneic," but may have a history of dyspnea and tiring with feeds. Transposition of the great arteries is more common in infants of diabetic mothers.

II CLINICAL MANIFESTATIONS

A. Physical examination. A soft pulmonary ejection murmur may be heard. Higher oxygen saturation in the lower extremities versus upper extremities (reverse differential cyanosis) on administration of oxygen is highly suggestive of transposition of the great arteries.

B. Electrocardiography reveals right ventricular hypertrophy. Although the volume work of both the right and left ventricles is increased, the left ventricle pumps against low pulmonary resistance, whereas the right ventricle pumps against higher systemic resistance.

C. Chest radiography. The heart may have the characteristic egg-on-a-string shape in as many as one third of patients.

D. Echocardiography. Look for continuity of the pulmonic and mitral valves and discontinuity of the aortic and tricuspid valves (see Figure 67–1).

E. Cardiac catheterization. Right-sided pressures are often greater than left-sided pressures.

III TREATMENT

A. Interim therapy. The goal of interim therapy is to limit severe hypoxemia by maintaining a communication between the right and left sides of the heart. **Prostaglandins** are given to maintain patency of the ductus arteriosus. Atrial septostomy may be needed if there is limited connecting between the parallel circulations.

B. Definitive therapy
 1. Jatene (switch) procedure. In this procedure, the transposed

great arteries are divided and reattached to restore the proper ventriculoarterial connections. The coronary arteries are also switched. Intramural coronary arteries and pulmonic or subpulmonic stenosis may be contraindications to the Jatene procedure.

2. **Mustard procedure.** This procedure involves inserting baffles into the atria to redirect systemic venous and pulmonary venous flow. Venous drainage is directed through the mitral valve and into the pulmonary artery, whereas pulmonary venous drainage is directed through the tricuspid valve and into the aorta. The Mustard procedure is no longer performed because of the high incidence of postoperative arrhythmias.

References

Kirklin JW, Colvin EV et al.: Complete transposition of the great arteries: treatment in the current era. *Pediatr Clinic North Am* 1990;37;171.

Fyler DC: Nadas' Pediatric Cardiology. Philadelphia, Hanley & Belfus, 1992, pp 557–576.

68. Truncus Arteriosus

▮ I INTRODUCTION

A. **Definition.** In truncus arteriosus, a single vessel gives rise to the aorta, the pulmonary artery, and the coronary arteries. There is a truncal valve with a variable number of leaflets that may be stenotic or regurgitant. There is almost always a malaligned ventricular septal defect (VSD).

B. **Classification.** Although Collett and Edwards were the first to propose a classification scheme in 1949, the classification scheme devised by van Praagh in 1964 is generally considered to be more accurate and complete **(Figure 68–1).**

C. **Natural history.** At birth, the pulmonary vascular resistance is high; there is moderate hypoxemia, but the child is well. As the

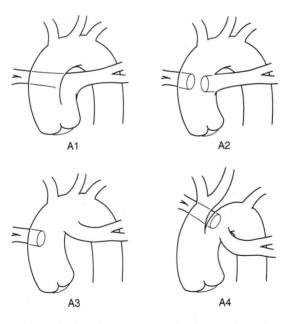

FIGURE 68–1. Van Praagh classification of truncus arteriosus. The pulmonary arteries may arise from the truncus as a single vessel or as two vessels. Type A4 is associated with an interrupted aortic arch.

pulmonary vascular resistance decreases, pulmonary blood flow increases dramatically. The hypoxia disappears, but maximal congestive heart failure (CHF) ensues. Pulmonary hypertension and a right-to-left shunt occur as the patient ages. Without treatment, most affected children die before reaching age 1 year.

II APPROACH TO THE PATIENT

A. Physical examination
 1. The **peripheral pulses** are bounding.
 2. A **systolic ejection murmur** or **regurgitant murmur** may be heard, depending on the status of the truncal valve. There may also be an aortic ejection click. The first (S_1) and second (S_2) heart sounds are loud.
B. Electrocardiography may show left, right, or biventricular hypertrophy.

HOT

KEY

Right ventricular hypertrophy is an ominous sign because it denotes pulmonary vascular disease.

C. Chest radiography reveals an enlarged heart with increased pulmonary vascularity. There may be a right aortic arch.

III TREATMENT

A. Interim management. Treatment focuses on control of CHF with diuretics, digoxin, fluid restriction, and afterload reduction. Administering 100% oxygen to these patients will decrease the pulmonary vascular resistance and worsen the CHF.
B. Surgical management. Early surgical repair involves detaching the pulmonary artery from the truncus, patching the aorta and the associated VSD, and installing a conduit from the right ventricle to the pulmonary artery. Surgery must be accomplished before the development of pulmonary vascular disease. Surgery may be necessary as early as age 6 months, especially if CHF cannot be controlled.

References
Mc Goon DC, Rastelli GC, Ongley PA. An operation for the correction of truncus arteriosus. *JAMA* 1968;205:59. (classic article)
Fyler DC: Nadas' Pediatric Cardiology. Philadelphia, Hanley & Belfus, 1992, pp 675–682.

69. Total Anomalous Pulmonary Venous Return

....

I INTRODUCTION. In total anomalous pulmonary venous return (TAPVR), the pulmonary veins drain into the systemic venous circulation, leading to mixing of deoxygenated and oxygenated blood at the level of the right atrium **(Figure 69–1).** Blood enters the systemic circulation by passing from the right atrium to the left atrium via a patent foramen ovale (PFO) or through a ductus.

A. **Nonobstructed TAPVR.** The pulmonary venous drainage is returned to the right atrium via the superior vena cava.

B. **Obstructed TAPVR.** The pulmonary venous drainage enters the systemic venous circulation at a level below the diaphragm and is returned to the right atrium via the portal vein and the inferior vena cava. Obstructed TAPVR is associated with severe pulmonary hypertension and decreased pulmonary blood flow, owing to high vascular resistance in the portal circulation.

II NONOBSTRUCTED TOTAL ANOMALOUS PULMONARY VENOUS RETURN

A. **Approach to the patient**
1. **Natural history.** Infants usually present at approximately 1 month of age with cyanosis on exertion and tachypnea. There is a history of poor growth.
2. **Physical examination**
   a. The precordium is hyperdynamic, and cyanosis is minimal.
   b. A systolic murmur may be heard at the upper left sternal border, owing to increased flow through the pulmonary artery. Increased flow through the tricuspid valve may produce a diastolic rumbling murmur, best heard at the lower left sternal border.
   c. The S_2 is loud and widely split; it varies only slightly with respiration. A gallop rhythm may be heard.
3. **Hyperoxia test.** The patient's low arterial O_2 level increases with a hyperoxia test because of the large amount of pulmonary blood flow.
4. **Electrocardiography** reveals right ventricular hypertrophy. Two factors contribute to this:
   a. The right side of the heart receives blood from the body and the lungs, leading to a tremendous volume overload.

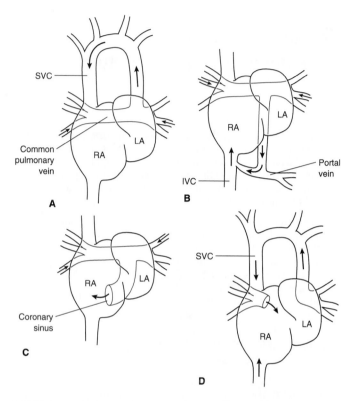

FIGURE 69–1. Variations of the anatomy in total anomalous pulmonary venous return (TAPVR). **(A)** Instead of draining into the left atrium, the pulmonary veins collect in a common channel behind the left atrium. From there, the blood is returned to the right atrium via the superior vena cava. **(B)** As in **A**, the pulmonary veins collect in a common channel behind the left atrium, but they drain below the diaphragm into the portal circulation. Blood is returned to the right atrium via the inferior vena cava. **(C)** In this variation, the pulmonary veins collect in a common channel behind the left atrium and enter the coronary sinus, which empties into the right atrium. **(D)** In this variation, drainage from the left pulmonary veins passes into the right atrium via the superior vena cava, and the right pulmonary veins drain directly into the right atrium. Note that in all cases, all of the blood entering the left atrium passes from the right atrium through an atrial septal defect. IVC = inferior vena cava; LA = left atrium; RA = right atrium; SVC = superior vena cava. (Adapted with permission from Fyler DC: *Nadas' Pediatric Cardiology*. Philadelphia, Hanley & Belfus, 1992, p 684.)

(Keep in mind that the pulmonary vasculature usually matures normally, so there is typically no increase in the right ventricular pressure.)

    b. Decreased blood flow to the left side of the heart in utero leads to underdevelopment of the left atrium and ventricle.

  5. Chest radiography reveals cardiomegaly and increased pulmonary vascularity.

B. Treatment. The mortality rate after surgery is 2%.

III OBSTRUCTED TOTAL ANOMALOUS PULMONARY VENOUS RETURN

A. Approach to the patient

  1. Natural history. Difficulty occurs in the first few days of life. Babies present with cyanosis and respiratory distress. In general, the more severe the obstruction, the earlier the presentation. If left untreated, most patients will die before reaching the age of 1 year. Babies who are symptomatic early have a poorer prognosis.

  2. Physical examination reveals a small, quiet heart. No murmur is present, but the S_2 is loud.

  3. Electrocardiography. As in nonobstructed TAPVR, obstructed TAPVR is characterized by right ventricular hypertrophy on the electrocardiogram (ECG).

    a. In utero, the pulmonary venous pressure is increased because of passage of blood through the portal circulation. The increase in the right ventricular pressure leads to right ventricular hypertrophy.

    b. As in nonobstructed TAPVR, the left ventricle and atrium are small.

  4. Cardiac catheterization. The right-sided (i.e., pulmonary) pressures may exceed the left-sided (i.e., systemic) pressures in patients with obstructed TAPVR.

  5. Chest radiography. Hallmark findings include a small heart, intense pulmonary edema, and poorly visualized pulmonary structures.

HOT **KEY**

The chest radiograph findings of obstructed TAPVR are often mistakenly attributed to primary lung disease.

HOT **KEY**

The right-sided (i.e., pulmonary) pressures may exceed the left-sided (i.e., systemic) pressures in patients with obstructed TAPVR.

B. Treatment. Patients with obstructive TAPVR require emergency surgery. The mortality rate after surgery is 10%–25% because of cardiovascular decompensation and persistently high
pulmonary artery pressures during the postoperative period.

References

Hammon JW. Total anomalous pulmonary venous connection in infancy. Ten years'
    experience including studies of post-operative ventricular function. *J Thorac
    Cardiovasc Surg* 1980;80:544. (classic article)
Fyler DC: Nadas' Pediatric Cardiology. Philadelphia, Hanley & Belfus, 1992, pp 682–
    692.

70. Hypoplastic Left Heart Syndrome

INTRODUCTION. Definition. Hypoplastic left heart syndrome encompasses a variety of malformations, all associated with significant underdevelopment of the left side of the heart **(Figure 70–1)**.

A. Specific abnormalities include:
1. An extremely small and nonfunctional left ventricle

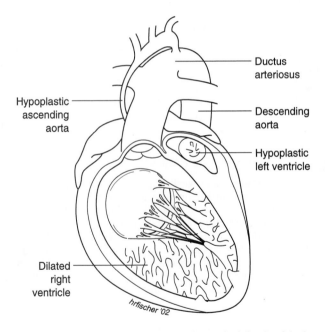

FIGURE 70–1. In hypoplastic left heart syndrome, the left side of the heart is underdeveloped and the right side is dilated and hypertrophied. Blood passes from the small left atrium to the right atrium via a patent foramen ovale, and from the right atrium to the right ventricle. The right ventricle then delivers blood to the systemic circulation through the patent ductus arteriosus. (Adapted with permission from Fyler DC: *Nadas' Pediatric Cardiology.* Philadelphia, Hanley & Belfus, 1992, p 623.)

   2. Atresia or hypoplasia of the aortic valve, the mitral valve, or both

   3. Marked hypoplasia of the ascending aorta

B. Blood flows from the pulmonary veins to the left atrium and passes from the left atrium to the right atrium via a patent foramen ovale (PFO). From the right atrium, the blood flows to the right ventricle and then to the pulmonary artery. Systemic flow is entirely dependent on the ductus arteriosus, which allows blood to pass from the pulmonary artery into the aorta.

C. **Natural history.** After birth, the ductus arteriosus closes, thereby markedly reducing systemic blood flow. In addition, pulmonary vascular resistance decreases, and the blood flow to the lungs increases dramatically. Symptoms result from the combination of excessive pulmonary flow, poor systemic output, reduced coronary artery perfusion, and pulmonary venous hypertension. The smaller the atrial connection, the more severe the left atrial and pulmonary venous hypertension. Without treatment, most infants die within 1 month of birth.

HOT **KEY** The infant appears well initially, but then presents suddenly with circulatory collapse (evidenced by cool, mottled skin and poor peripheral pulses), metabolic acidosis, cyanosis, and respiratory distress after the ductus arteriosus closes and pulmonary vascular resistance decreases.

II APPROACH TO THE PATIENT

A. **Physical examination** reveals weak or absent peripheral pulses, a hyperdynamic cardiac impulse, and murmurs associated with increased flow across the pulmonic and tricuspid valves. There may also be a tricuspid regurgitation murmur.

B. **Electrocardiography** reveals significant right ventricular hypertrophy owing to volume overload from left-to-right shunting at the atrial-level and hypoplasia of the left ventricle. However, because normal infants are right-ventricular dominant at birth, the electrocardiogram (ECG) findings are not, by themselves, diagnostic.

C. **Chest radiography** often reveals increased pulmonary vascularity and pulmonary venous congestion.

D. **Arterial blood gases** reveal significant metabolic acidosis.

III TREATMENT

A. **Initial stabilization.** The goal is to balance the systemic and pulmonary vascular resistances to maintain an acceptable amount

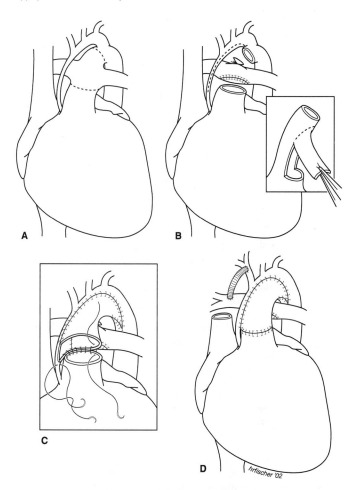

FIGURE 70–2. The Norwood procedure for hypoplastic left heart syndrome. **(A)** Typical anatomy for hypoplastic left heart syndrome. **(B)** Main pulmonary artery transected at bifurcation. Ductus arteriosus ligated and all ductal tissue removed. **Dotted line** shows incision down to base of ascending aorta. **(C)** Wedge-shaped patch cut from pulmonary homograft. **(D)** Reconstruction of new aortic root with pericardial patch with side-to-side connection of aortic root to pulmonary artery. **(E)** Completed operation showing modified Blalock-Taussig shunt of polytetrafluoroethylene tube between innominate artery and left pulmonary artery. (Adapted with permission from McMillan JA, DeAngelis CD, Feigin RD, et al.: *Oski's Pediatrics: Principles and Practice,* 3rd ed. Philadelphia, Lippincott Williams & Wilkins, 1999, p 306.)

of pulmonary and systemic blood flow. Because pulmonary blood flow is usually excessive, measures are taken to increase the systemic flow and decrease the pulmonary flow. The patient should be intubated.

1. **Increasing systemic flow.** The administration of **prostaglandins** maintains patency of the ductus arteriosus, thereby increasing systemic flow.

2. **Decreasing pulmonary flow.** Hypoxemia and hypercarbia diminish pulmonary blood flow by increasing the pulmonary vascular resistance.

   a. The fraction of inspired oxygen (FIO_2) should be decreased to 21%, with the goal being to bring the arterial oxygen tension (PaO_2) down to 30 mm Hg. In some cases, extra nitrogen can be weaned in to further decrease the FIO_2.

   b. The arterial carbon dioxide tension ($PaCO_2$) should be allowed to increase to 40 mm Hg, while maintaining an arterial blood pH of 7.35–7.40.

   c. Positive end-expiratory pressure (PEEP) may be helpful in increasing the pulmonary vascular resistance.

B. Definitive therapy entails either reconstructive surgery or cardiac transplantation.

1. **Reconstructive surgery** occurs in three stages.

   a. The **Norwood procedure (stage 1)** is associated with a 70% survival rate **(Figure 70–2).**

   b. The **hemi-Fontan procedure (stage 2)** is performed when the patient reaches 6–12 months of age. Stage 2 is associated with a 6% mortality rate.

      (1) A cavopulmonary shunt is created by removing the superior vena cava from the right atrium and anastomosing it to the pulmonary artery.

      (2) The systemic to pulmonary shunt created during the Norwood procedure is then removed.

   c. The **Fontan procedure (stage 3)** is performed 4 months later and is associated with a mortality rate of 7%. During stage 3, the inferior vena cava is removed from the right atrium and anastomosed to the pulmonary artery.

2. **Cardiac transplantation** is required if the right ventricle fails to function.

References

Lang P, Fyler DC: Hypoplastic Left heart Syndrome, Mitral Atresia and Aortic Atresia. In: Fyler DC: Nadas' Pediatric Cardiology. Philadelphia, Hanley & Belfus, 1992, pp 623–633.

Norwood WI Jr. Hypoplastic left Heart Syndrome. *Ann Thorac Surg* 199;52:688.

71. Complete Atrioventricular Canal (Endocardial Cushion Defect)

I INTRODUCTION

A. **Definition.** In complete atrioventricular canal defects, halted development of the endocardial cushion gives rise to:
  1. An ostium primum atrial septal defect (ASD)
  2. A ventricular septal defect (VSD), usually located in the posterior portion of the septum
  3. A common atrioventricular valve, a single sail-like structure with a common anterior leaflet and a common posterior leaflet
B. **Pathophysiology**
  1. A nonrestrictive VSD can lead to equal left- and right-sided pressures; therefore, the pressure in the pulmonary circulation often matches that of the systemic circulation from birth.
  2. Mitral regurgitation can occur through the valve cleft, which leads to left ventricle–to–right atrium shunting if an ASD is present. This tends to lead to an increase in pulmonary blood flow early in life. Left ventricle failure may then ensue, leading to increased pulmonary venous pressure. The combination of a left-to-right shunt and increased pulmonary venous pressure secondary to left ventricle failure leads to early severe pulmonary vascular disease.
C. **Natural history.** The mortality rate associated with untreated complete atrioventricular canal defects may be as high as 50% in the first year of life. The risk of developing permanent pulmonary vascular disease is highest after the first year of life.

II APPROACH TO THE PATIENT

A. **Symptoms.** The child may present in congestive heart failure (CHF).
B. **Physical examination.** The precordium is active.
  1. The S_2 is loud. A gallop rhythm also is often present.
  2. A systolic murmur is heard best at the lower left sternal border. An apical diastolic murmur is commonly heard as well.
C. **Electrocardiography** reveals a superior axis with right or left ventricular hypertrophy.

D. Chest radiography reveals cardiomegaly and increased pulmonary vascularity.

E. Echocardiography is vital for delineating the anatomy of the defect.

▐▐▐ TREATMENT

A. Interim therapy. The administration of **oxygen** may help to slow the progression of pulmonary vascular disease.

B. Definitive therapy entails early surgical management. Surgical success depends on the overall anatomy, the degree of ventricular hypoplasia, mitral valve anatomy, and the presence of additional muscular defects.

PART VII

PULMONOLOGY

72. Upper Airway Malformations

I INTRODUCTION

A. Background. Airway and esophageal malformations can cause expiratory or inspiratory stridor, wheezing, or feeding intolerance. These disorders may occur at birth, in infancy, or later in childhood.

B. Definitions. **Stridor** is a high-pitched musical sound that is produced by airflow turbulence from partial obstruction of the airway. **Inspiratory stridor** is usually caused by supraglottic obstruction. The presence of both **inspiratory and expiratory stridor** indicates a glottic or subglottic obstruction. **Expiratory stridor alone** indicates intrathoracic tracheal obstruction.

II SPECIFIC UPPER AIRWAY MALFORMATIONS

A. Laryngomalacia
   1. **Pathogenesis.** The presence of redundant laryngeal soft tissue with inadequate cartilaginous support causes collapse of the arytenoid cartilage and epiglottis on inspiration.
   2. **Epidemiology.** Laryngomalacia is the most common cause of noisy inspiration in neonates and infants. It is strongly associated with gastroesophageal reflux disease.
   3. **Symptoms.** Inspiratory stridor may occur at birth or between the 2nd and 4th weeks of life; typically, the patient makes noisy or crowing respiratory sounds. The stridor is worse when the infant is supine or active and is exacerbated during upper respiratory infections. Some infants merely have noisy breathing, whereas others have severe distress.
   4. **Diagnosis.** Direct laryngoscopy may be required for severe cases. Concomitant testing for gastroesophageal reflux disease should be considered.

      5. Treatment. Laser surgery is considered for patients who have associated cyanosis, feeding difficulties, failure to thrive, or periods of apnea.

      6. Prognosis. Laryngomalacia usually resolves spontaneously by 18 months of age.

B. Laryngeal webs

      1. Pathogenesis. Redundant tissue between the two sides of the larynx severely compromises the airway.

      2. Epidemiology. Laryngeal webs are uncommon. They may be associated with Arnold-Chiari malformation.

      3. Symptoms include severe stridor at birth and an absent or weak cry.

      4. Treatment. Immediate surgical treatment with tracheostomy placement is required.

C. Vocal cord paralysis

      1. Pathogenesis. Vocal cord paralysis may be caused by traction on the recurrent laryngeal nerve during birth.

      2. Epidemiology. Vocal cord paralysis is the second most common cause of neonatal laryngeal obstruction.

      3. Symptoms include inspiratory stridor and a weak, muffled cry.

      4. The **diagnosis** is made by direct laryngoscopy. A magnetic resonance imaging scan is performed to rule out central nervous system causes.

      5. Treatment is primarily supportive. Intubation may be required in severe cases.

D. Subglottic stenosis

      1. Pathogenesis. Subglottic stenosis usually is iatrogenic, and occurs as a result of prolonged intubation. It also may be congenital.

      2. Symptoms include inspiratory and expiratory stridor. Subglottic stenosis should be considered in patients who are difficult to extubate after prolonged intubation.

      3. Treatment. Tracheostomy usually is required for iatrogenic cases. For congenital subglottic stenosis, conservative treatment may be adequate.

      4. Prognosis. The mortality rate may be as high as 20%.

E. Tracheoesophageal fistula

      1. Pathogenesis. The cause is unknown.

      2. Types of fistulas are illustrated in **Figure 72–1.**

      3. Epidemiology. Tracheoesophageal fistula is the most common esophageal malformation (1:2000–1:3000 births). It is associated with maternal polyhydramnios and tracheomalacia.

      4. Symptoms. Tracheoesophageal fistula causes excessive oral secretions, respiratory distress, and feeding difficulties (e.g., choking, coughing, cyanosis).

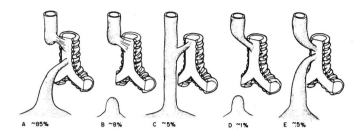

A ~85%   B ~8%   C ~5%   D ~1%   E ~5%

FIGURE 72–1. Esophageal atresia and tracheoesophageal fistula. The most common type of these esophageal anomalies is a proximal atresia with a distal fistula to the trachea. Isolated esophageal atresia is the next most common type. The remaining types are far less common. [Reprinted with permission from McMillan JA, DeAngelis CD, Feigin RD, et al (eds): *Oski's Pediatrics: Principles and Practice,* 3rd ed. Philadelphia, Lippincott Williams & Wilkins, 1999, p 310.]

5. **Diagnosis.** The diagnosis is made soon after birth, but usually not until the child aspirates. If an attempt is made to insert a nasal catheter into the stomach, the catheter stops abruptly at approximately 10 cm. A confirmatory radiograph shows the catheter coiled in the esophagus. H-type fistulas may escape detection early in life. They may cause feeding difficulties or chronic respiratory disease in later infancy or childhood. H-type fistulas require a pull-back barium esophagram for diagnosis.

6. **Treatment.** Tracheoesophageal fistula is a true surgical emergency. Aspiration can be prevented by keeping the child prone and giving nothing by mouth. Nasogastric suction keeps the esophageal pouch empty and helps to avoid aspiration.

F. **Choanal atresia**

1. **Pathogenesis.** Choanal atresia is a congenital blockage of the nasal passages. Because infants are obligate nose breathers until 4 months of age, blockage of the nares inhibits respirations.

2. **Symptoms.** The diagnosis often is made in the delivery room. Bilateral obstruction causes increased work of breathing during inspiration. The physician should suspect choanal atresia if respiratory effort is made without air entry into the lungs. Stridor is not typically present.

3. **Diagnosis.** A nasogastric catheter meets an obstruction after being inserted a few centimeters into the nares.

4. **Treatment.** An oral airway device usually is sufficient initial therapy. A pediatric otolaryngologist should be consulted

immediately. Definitive treatment involves burrowing a hole
through the nasal plate.

G. Vascular rings and slings

1. **Pathogenesis.** Vascular rings and slings occur when the trachea and esophagus become compressed as a result of malformation of the great vessels.

2. **Three major types**
   a. **Double aortic arch**. Severe symptoms are usually present
      at birth.
   b. **Right aortic arch with aberrant left subclavian and left lig-
      amentum arteriosum**. Most patients are asymptomatic.
   c. **Anomalous left pulmonary artery** (or pulmonary artery
      sling). Symptoms, which may be severe, usually occur in
      the first weeks or months of life.

3. **Symptoms**
   a. **Compression of the trachea** may cause expiratory stridor,
      chronic wheezing, cyanosis, and respiratory distress that
      are aggravated by crying, feeding, and flexion of the neck.
      Infants often arch their backs and extend their necks to re-
      lieve the compression on the trachea. Older patients some-
      times are misdiagnosed as having chronic asthma.
   b. **Compression of the esophagus** causes symptoms that are
      both less common and less severe than those of tracheal
      compression. A ring or sling should be considered if a
      child cannot tolerate solid foods. Patients also may have
      concurrent vomiting, choking, or dysphagia.

4. **Diagnosis**
   a. An **echocardiogram** is the gold-standard test. Chest CT
      scan is also a valuable diagnostic tool.
   b. A **barium esophagram** is helpful in identifying a vascular
      ring. A lateral view shows an indentation on the esophagus.
   c. A **chest radiograph** may show a right aortic arch. Pul-
      monary artery slings may cause atelectasis, hyperinflation
      of either lung, diminished left pulmonary artery branch-
      ing, or a mediastinal shift.

5. **Treatment.** Surgery is required for symptomatic patients.

References

Chung CJ, Fordham LA, Mukherji SK: The pediatric airway: a review of differential
  diagnosis by anatomy and pathology. *Neuroimaging Clin North Am* 10(1):161–180,
  2000.
Fyler DC: *Nadas' Pediatric Cardiology*. Philadelphia, Hanley & Belfus, 1992.
Sichel JY, Dangoor E, Eliashar R, et al: Management of congenital laryngeal malformations. *Am J Otolaryngol* 21(1):22–30, 2000.

73. Cystic Fibrosis

I INTRODUCTION

A. Background. Cystic fibrosis (CF) affects multiple organ systems, primarily the lung, pancreas, liver, and reproductive tract. The CF transmembrane conductance regulator (CFTR) is an apical cell membrane chloride channel that is dysfunctional in affected patients.

B. Pathogenesis

1. A defect in the CFTR causes a decrease in the efflux of apical water. As a result, luminal secretions are inadequately hydrated.
2. Inspissation, cellular hypertrophy, acute and chronic inflammation, and fibrosis occur in affected organs.
3. Salt-sensitive antimicrobial peptides, which are thought to exist in the secretions that line the airways, become ineffective. As a result, the lungs are predisposed to bacterial colonization, which leads to endobronchial infection, bronchiectasis, cyst formation, and eventual obstructive lung disease. In the pancreas, there is exocrine duct obstruction, hyperplasia, necrosis, and fibrosis.

C. Epidemiology

1. Approximately 30,000 Americans have CF. It is the most common autosomal recessive disorder in Caucasians. Four percent of the Caucasian population carries the CF gene, with a CFTR mutation in one allele.
2. Rates of disease in various ethnic groups are as follows:
   a. 1:2500 Caucasians
   b. 1:17,000 African-Americans
   c. Very rare in those of direct Asian and African descent
3. Ten percent of all cases of CF are not diagnosed until adolescence or adulthood.

D. Microbiology. Endobronchial infection by pathogenic bacteria causes serious morbidity. These infections are followed both clinically and with quantitative sputum cultures.

1. In children younger than age 10 years, typical organisms include *Staphylococcus aureus, Haemophilus influenzae* (nontypeable), and gram-negative bacteria.
2. In older children, typical organisms include *Pseudomonas aeruginosa, Burkholderia cepacia,* and *Stenotrophomonas maltophilia.*

II CLINICAL MANIFESTATIONS

A. Common presenting symptoms include failure to thrive; greasy, bulky stools; and chronic cough.

B. Other presentations

1. Meconium ileus at birth (the presenting sign for 5%–10% of children with CF)
2. Recurrent respiratory disease (e.g., sinus or pulmonary infection)
3. Cholestatic jaundice
4. Hyponatremic dehydration
5. Rectal prolapse
6. Less common presentations include portal hypertension, pancreatitis, diabetes, asthma, intussusception, and signs of specific nutrient deficiencies (e.g., fat-soluble vitamins).

HOT

KEY

A newborn with meconium ileus should always be tested for CF.

C. Manifestations of CF

1. **Respiratory**
   a. Chronic sinusitis
   b. Nasal polyposis (10% of patients)
   c. Anosmia with resultant anorexia
   d. Allergic bronchopulmonary aspergillosis
   e. Endobronchial bacterial infection
   f. Pulmonary exacerbations (see II D)

2. **Gastrointestinal**
   a. Pancreatic exocrine insufficiency (85% of patients) causes fat and protein malabsorption
   b. Meconium ileus in infancy (5%–10% of patients). The site of obstruction usually is the distal ileum. Distal intestinal obstruction syndrome (DIOS) is a similar condition in older children with CF.
   c. Rectal prolapse (up to 20% of patients)

3. **Nutrition.** Thirty-eight percent of children with CF are below the 5th percentile in weight for children their age.

4. **Hepatobiliary**
   a. Significant liver disease occurs in 3% of children with CF.
   b. Cholestasis can occur, but is rare in infancy.
   c. Gallbladder hypoplasia may occur.

5. **Reproductive**
   a. Azoospermia affects 90% of males with CF. Atresia of the vas deferens also may occur.

    b. Female infertility may occur. Women with CF have thickened cervical mucus.

 6. Endocrine

    a. Diabetes mellitus occurs in teenage patients after pancreatic involvement is advanced.

    b. Diabetic ketoacidosis is rare, but most patients depend on insulin.

 7. Metabolic

    a. Electrolyte losses

    b. Secondary hyperaldosteronism

 8. Vitamin deficiencies

    a. Vitamin K deficiency: hypoprothrombinemia and bleeding

    b. Vitamin A deficiency: bulging fontanel, night blindness

    c. Vitamin E deficiency: hemolytic anemia

D. Pulmonary exacerbations

 1. Mild exacerbations usually are caused by viral infections and are associated with increased cough and congestion.

 2. Moderate exacerbations are typified by at least 2 weeks of increased cough and sputum production, FEV_1 decrease of more than 10%, and small changes on chest radiograph.

 3. Severe exacerbations are characterized by weight loss, fever, and, occasionally, hemoptysis and pneumothorax.

III APPROACH TO THE PATIENT

A. Diagnosis

 1. Sweat chloride testing with pilocarpine iontophoresis is the most commonly used diagnostic test. A chloride concentration higher than 60 mmol/L is abnormal. In infants < 3 months of age, a concentration > 40 mmol/L is highly suggestive of CF.

 2. Genetic testing (mutational analysis). Approximately 90% of CF mutations can be detected with the polymerase chain reaction technique.

B. Additional tests may be helpful in cases in which the diagnosis is unclear.

 1. Tests of pancreatic exocrine dysfunction include fecal fat collection, stool trypsin measurement, and serum trypsinogen measurement.

 2. Nasal membrane potential difference involves measuring the electric potential difference across epithelial surfaces.

HOT KEY

The diagnosis of CF requires the presence of symptoms consistent with the disease as well as positive results on two diagnostic tests.

C. Cornerstones of therapy

1. Growth should be optimized with tube feedings if necessary for adequate caloric intake. Pancreatic enzyme replacement and vitamin supplementation (especially fat-soluble vitamins A, D, E, and K) are required.

2. The onset of lung disease should be delayed by clearing lower airway secretions and aggressively treating endobronchial infections.

D. Treatment of pulmonary exacerbations

1. High serum levels of antibiotics are required because patients with CF may have increased antibiotic metabolism. The end point of therapy is improved pulmonary function test results.

  a. Mild exacerbations. Oral antibiotics directed at *S. aureus* and *H. influenzae* are used.

  b. Moderate or severe exacerbations

    (1) Intravenous antibiotics directed at previously cultured organisms are used.

    (2) Multiple antibiotics are used to help prevent bacterial resistance.

    (3) Inhaled antibiotics (e.g., inhaled tobramycin) deliver high levels of medication to respiratory secretions.

    (4) Oral quinolones often are used as an adjunctive measure.

2. Clearance of mucus is achieved through chest physiotherapy, flutter valves, or vibrating vest devices. Recombinant human DNAase is an effective inhaled mucolytic.

3. Bronchodilation with albuterol or ipratropium is routinely used. The effectiveness of inhaled corticosteroids has not yet been well studied.

4. Nutrition. The patient's diet should provide 130% of the recommended daily caloric intake.

HOT **KEY**

Nutrition is of utmost importance in the treatment and routine care of patients with CF.

E. Health maintenance and prevention

1. Management of patients with CF includes frequent pulmonary function tests, quantitative sputum cultures, and ongoing assessment of nutritional status.

HOT KEY

Routine chest radiographs are not helpful in the management of CF.

2. The use of **prophylactic antibiotics** is controversial. They may not reduce the frequency of pulmonary exacerbations, and may contribute to the problem of bacterial resistance. However, the intermittent use of inhaled tobramycin can mitigate pulmonary disease in patients with endobronchial infection.

IV PROGNOSIS

A. Mortality
1. In 1969, the mean life expectancy for patients with CF was 14 years; in 1998, it was 29 years.
2. The most common cause of death is pulmonary disease. The second most common cause is hepatobiliary disease.

HOT KEY

Many patients with CF are now having children of their own.

B. Recent advances in therapy
1. **New medical treatments** include anti-inflammatory agents (e.g., high-dose ibuprofen), antioxidants, white blood cell enzyme antagonists, and ion transport modulators (e.g., amiloride). Long-term use of high-dose ibuprofen has been shown to decrease the rate of decline of pulmonary function.
2. **Gene therapy.** Clinical trial results have been disappointing so far.
3. **Lung transplantation**
   a. Transplantations are indicated for patients with a life expectancy of only 1–2 years.
   b. Patients with CF receive 13% of all lung transplants. The survival rate after transplantation is 75% at 1 year, 60% at 2 years, and 55% at 3 years.

References
Colin AA, Wohl ME: Cystic fibrosis. *Pediatr Rev* 15(5):192–200, 1994.
Ramsey BW: Management of pulmonary disease in patients with cystic fibrosis. *N Engl J Med* 335(3):179–188, 1996.

PART VIII

HEMATOLOGY/ONCOLOGY

74. Acute Leukemias

I INTRODUCTION

A. Background. Acute leukemias represent 97% of childhood leukemias. They are caused by clonal expansion and arrest at a specific stage of lymphoid or myeloid hematopoiesis. The two most common forms are acute lymphocytic leukemia (ALL) and acute myelogenous leukemia (AML).

B. Pathogenesis. Ionizing radiation, benzene, and alkylating agents sometimes can be implicated; however, most cases have no direct causal explanation. There is strong evidence that supports a link between genetic factors and childhood leukemias. There is an increased incidence in identical twins and siblings. The incidence also is increased in chromosomal abnormalities (e.g., trisomy 21), congenital immunodeficiencies (e.g., Wiskott-Aldrich syndrome, ataxia telangiectasia), and other genetic conditions (e.g., Klinefelter syndrome, Fanconi anemia).

C. Epidemiology

1. **ALL** affects approximately 2–4:100,000 Caucasian children. There are 2500–3000 new diagnoses in the United States each year. The peak incidence is at age 2–5 years.

2. **AML.** There are approximately 500 new diagnoses in the United States each year. There is no age predominance.

II CLINICAL MANIFESTATIONS

A. Symptoms of ALL include fever (60%), fatigue (50%), pallor (40%), bleeding (48%), bone pain (23%), lymphadenopathy (50%), splenomegaly (63%), hepatomegaly (68%), and central nervous system (CNS) involvement (< 5%). Symptoms of CNS leukemia include headache, nausea, irritability, nuchal rigidity, papilledema, and cranial nerve palsy.

B. Symptoms of AML include fever, fatigue, bleeding, and CNS involvement (5%–15%). Few have lymphadenopathy, hepatosplenomegaly, bone pain, or arthralgias.

APPROACH TO THE PATIENT

A. Diagnosis

1. **Bone marrow biopsy.** Definitive diagnosis requires a bone marrow biopsy. ALL should be suspected when bone marrow contains more than 5% blasts. Most centers require a finding of 25% blasts in the bone marrow to confirm the diagnosis; often, 80%–100% blasts are found.

2. **Blood tests**
    a. A **complete blood cell count** may reveal thrombocytopenia or normochromic, normocytic anemia with a low reticulocyte count. The white blood cell (WBC) count may be low, normal, or increased. Blasts may be abundant if the WBC count is higher than 10,000/mm^3; 20% of patients with AML have increased basophils. The diagnosis of leukemia cannot be made on the basis of the blood cell count findings alone.

 HOT Leukemia should be suspected when a patient has abnormalities in more than one hematopoietic cell line. Pancytopenia is considered leukemia until proven otherwise.
KEY

---

    b. **Hypercalcemia** is caused by leukemic infiltration of bone or by release of a parathyroid hormone–like substance from the lymphoblasts.
    c. **Hyperphosphatemia** is caused by lysis of leukemic cells and may induce hypocalcemia.
    d. **Liver function abnormalities** reflect leukemic infiltration of the liver; abnormalities usually are mild.
    e. An **elevated lactate dehydrogenase** level reflects leukemic cell lysis.

 HOT Inexperienced laboratory personnel may misread blasts on a smear as reactive or atypical lymphocytes. Be wary of smears read at nonpediatric facilities. It is always advisable to have **KEY** suspicious smears read by an experienced pathologist.

---

3. **Radiographic studies**
    a. **Chest radiograph.** A mediastinal mass may be seen, especially in T-cell leukemias.
    b. **Long bone films.** Radiographs often are obtained to evaluate bone pain. They may show transverse radiolucent metaphyseal growth arrest lines, periosteal elevation with

reactive subperiosteal cortical thickening, osteolytic lesions, or diffuse osteoporosis.

 HOT KEY Leukemic bone involvement can masquerade as osteomyelitis.

4. **Additional tests to consider**
   a. **Coagulation profile.** Coagulation study results may be abnormal in patients with AML.
   b. **Echocardiograms and electrocardiograms** are performed to assess cardiac function before chemotherapy is initiated.
   c. The **ID panel** includes cultures of cerebrospinal fluid (CSF), urine, and blood; varicella antibody titer; cytomegalovirus antibody titer; herpes simplex antibody screening; and hepatitis antibody screening.
   d. **Immunologic screening** is performed to evaluate levels of serum immunoglobulin, C3, and C4.
   e. The presence of lymphoblasts in the CSF confirms the diagnosis of CNS leukemia.
B. **Acute management.** If the WBC count is higher than 100,000/mm^3, then the patient is at risk for leukostasis. Hydration, alkalinization, and allopurinol administration should be initiated. Leukophoresis should be considered to remove the cell burden. Platelets are given when the patient is bleeding or when the platelet count is < 20,000/mm^3 (see Chapter 76 for more details). Antibiotics should be administered as indicated (see Chapter 79).
C. **Chemotherapy**
   1. **ALL.** Most standard protocols include the following phases:
      a. **Induction chemotherapy** is high-dose treatment with three to four drugs. This initial phase induces remission in 95% of patients.
      b. **Consolidation/CNS prevention** kills the majority of the remaining malignant cells. CNS prophylaxis is provided intrathecally. Cranial radiation also may be required.
      c. **Maintenance.** Extended treatment is given during remission to eliminate the final remaining leukemic cells and prevent relapse.
   2. **AML**
      a. **Aggressive chemotherapy protocols** (most include cytosine arabinoside and daunomycin) achieve a 75%–85% remission rate.
      b. **Allogenic bone marrow transplantation** usually is per-

formed after chemotherapy (for all cases except the M3 subtype).
   3. **Sequelae of treatment** include cortical atrophy, learning disabilities, growth retardation, infertility (most common in patients who receive chemotherapy after puberty and in children who receive craniospinal irradiation), and cardiac dysfunction.

IV PROGNOSIS

A. **Prognostic factors**
   1. **Standard-risk ALL** (60%–70%): age at onset 1–9 years, initial WBC count < 10,000/mm^3
   2. **High-risk ALL** (30%–40%): t(9,22) (BCR–ABL translocation), initial WBC count > 25,000/mm^3, rearranged MLL gene in a patient < 12 months old (infant ALL), induction failure
   3. **Standard-risk AML (30%):** Rapid response to induction therapy; favorable chromosomal abnormalities, t(8,21), t(15,17) and inv16; trisomy 21; FAB type M1 or M2 with Auer rods, M3, and M4eo
   4. **High-risk AML (70%):** all others who do not meet the standard risk criteria, WBC count > 100,000/mm^3
B. **Mortality**
   1. **Standard-risk ALL:** 4-year event-free survival (EFS) rate is 80%.
   2. **High-risk ALL:** 4-year EFS rate is 65%.
   3. **Standard-risk AML:** 5-year EFS rate is 45%–50%.
   4. **High-risk AML:** 5-year EFS rate is 34%.
C. **Morbidity.** Children with acute leukemias are at risk for secondary cancers (e.g., brain tumors) and complications of chemotherapy (e.g., cardiomyopathy, mucositis, infection).
D. **Relapse**
   1. **Bone marrow relapse.** The bone marrow is the most common site of relapse. Bone marrow relapse occurs in 25% to 30% of all patients with ALL. Marrow relapse usually requires bone marrow transplantation. Patients who relapse during therapy have the worst prognosis.
   2. **CNS relapse.** The CNS is the most common site of extramedullary relapse. Patients may experience symptoms of increased intracranial pressure (e.g., headache, nausea, vomiting), vision abnormalities, or nerve palsies. Intrathecal chemotherapy followed by irradiation is required.
   3. **Testicular relapse** usually presents as painless swelling. Testicular relapse sometimes heralds a bone marrow relapse.

References

Ebb DH, Weinstein HJ: Diagnosis and treatment of childhood acute myelogenous leukemia. *Pediatr Clin North Am* 44(4):847–862, 1997.

Lanzkowsky P: *Manual of Pediatric Hematology and Oncology,* 3rd ed. San Diego, Academic Press, 2000.

Pizzo PA, Poplack David G (eds): *Principles and Practice of Pediatric Oncology,* 3rd ed. Philadelphia, Lippincott-Raven, 1997.

Pui CH: Acute lymphoblastic leukemia. *Pediatr Clin North Am* 44(4):831–846, 1997.

75. Clinical Manifestations of Pediatric Tumors

I   INTRODUCTION. Familiarity with the clinical manifestations of malignant tumors leads to early diagnosis and improved prognosis. Specific treatment is always provided by a pediatric oncologist.

II   SPECIFIC TUMOR TYPES

A. Brain tumors

1. **Types** include astrocytoma, medulloblastoma, ependymoma, brain stem glioma, oligodendroglioma, craniopharyngioma, and intracranial germ cell tumor.

2. **Epidemiology.** Brain tumors account for 20% of childhood malignancies. They are the second most common childhood malignancy.

3. **Clinical manifestations.** Symptoms often are related to increased intracranial pressure (ICP). Increased ICP is suggested by headache (especially in the morning), intractable vomiting, impaired vision, cranial nerve VI palsy, papilledema, setting sun sign (downward deviation of both eyes), Parinaud syndrome (i.e., inhibited upward gaze), focal seizures, somnolence, irritability, personality changes, gait or balance disturbances, and endocrine abnormalities with evidence of hypothalamic or pituitary dysfunction [e.g., diencephalic syndrome (i.e., sudden failure to thrive at 6–36 months of age), central precocious puberty].

4. **Diagnosis.** Computed tomographic (CT) scanning detects up to 95% of tumors. Posterior fossa lesions are best evaluated with magnetic resonance imaging (MRI).

5. **Treatment** may include radiation therapy, chemotherapy, or surgery.

B. Spinal tumors

1. **Types** include astrocytoma, ependymoma, oligodendroglioma, neurofibroma, neuroblastoma, and Langerhans cell histiocytosis.

2. **Clinical manifestations.** Tumor is suggested by local back pain that is worse when recumbent or during a Valsalva maneuver and ameliorated when sitting. Other symptoms include volitional resistance to trunk flexion, spinal deformity, gait disturbance, weakness, increased lower-extremity deep

tendon reflexes (DTRs), decreased upper-extremity DTRs, sensory impairment below a given spinal root level, positive Babinski sign, sphincter impairment, midline closure defects, and nystagmus.

3. **Diagnosis.** MRI scanning is the preferred mode of imaging.
4. **Treatment.** A neurosurgeon should be consulted early. Prompt management with steroids, surgery, or emergent radiation therapy may be needed to prevent damage to the spinal cord.

C. Neuroblastoma

1. **Epidemiology.** Neuroblastoma is the most common tumor of infancy and accounts for 7% of childhood malignancies.
2. **Clinical manifestations.** Neuroblastoma usually presents as an abdominal mass; metastases often are present at diagnosis. The primary tumor may be located anywhere along the sympathetic neural pathway. Symptoms are related to the effects at the following sites:
   a. **Head:** Horner syndrome (i.e., miosis, ptosis, enophthalmos, anhydrosis)
   b. **Eyes:** exophthalmos, ecchymosis, ptosis, papilledema, strabismus, and opsoclonus
   c. **Chest:** dyspnea and recurrent infections
   d. **Abdomen and pelvis:** anorexia, vomiting, abdominal pain, constipation, urinary retention, and palpable mass on rectal examination
   e. **Paraspinal sites:** localized pain, lower-extremity weakness, paraplegia, scoliosis, and bladder and sphincter dysfunction
   f. **Olfactory bulb:** nasal obstruction, epistaxis, and rhinorrhea
   g. **Lymph nodes:** enlarged nodes
   h. **Bone:** bone pain
   i. **Excess catecholamine secretion:** episodic sweating, flushing, pallor, headaches, palpitation, and hypertension, and intractable watery diarrhea (because of secretion of vasoactive intestinal peptides)
3. **Diagnosis** usually is made by imaging studies and biopsy. Neonatal screening for neuroblastoma has no clear therapeutic benefit.
4. **Treatment.** Combinations of surgery, radiation therapy, and chemotherapy may be used.

D. Wilms tumor

1. **Epidemiology.** Wilms tumor accounts for 6% of childhood malignancies. The incidence peaks at 3–4 years of age.
2. **Clinical manifestations.** The most common presentation is a palpable abdominal mass. Hypertension and hematuria also are common. Weight loss, urinary tract infections, diarrhea, and obstipation may occur as well. Several congenital ab-

normalities are associated with Wilms tumor. One in three children with aniridia also has Wilms tumor; other conditions associated with Wilms tumor include hemihypertrophy, Beckwith-Wiedemann syndrome, genitourinary tract anomalies (e.g., horseshoe kidney, cystic disease, hypospadias, cryptorchidism, duplicated collecting system), and hamartomas (e.g., hemangiomas, multiple nevi, café au lait spots).
   3. **Treatment.** Children who have aniridia, hemihypertrophy, or Beckwith-Wiedemann syndrome should undergo serial abdominal ultrasounds (every 3 months until their 5th birthday, and then annually until adulthood) to monitor for Wilms tumor.
E. **Bone tumors**
   1. **Types** include osteosarcoma and Ewing sarcoma.
   2. **Epidemiology.** Bone tumors account for 2% of all childhood malignancies. They are the second most common tumor in adolescents and young adults. Approximately 20% of patients have metastases at diagnosis.
   3. **Clinical manifestations.** The long bones and the larger flat bones (e.g., pelvis, scapula) are most commonly affected. The ribs and vertebrae also may be involved. Local pain, swelling, and decreased range of motion are the most common symptoms. Other presentations include pathologic fracture, paraplegia, and joint effusion. Ewing sarcoma may cause fever; therefore, it is important to differentiate it from osteomyelitis. Fractures that occur in the large bones after minor injuries should raise suspicion of malignancy.
   4. **Diagnosis.** Being able to identify suspicious lesions on plain radiographic films is a crucial skill. Dense sclerosis or lytic lesions may be seen in the metaphysis of long bones. Associated findings include soft tissue extension, radiating calcifications, periosteal thickening, and lamellated periosteal reaction (onion skin).
   5. **Treatment.** Surgery, chemotherapy, and radiation therapy are used, depending on the stage of the disease. Limb-sparing procedures sometimes can be performed.
F. **Retinoblastoma**
   1. **Epidemiology.** Retinoblastoma causes 5% of childhood blindness. One third of cases are bilateral, with a median age at presentation of 18 months. The incidence of unilateral disease peaks at 2–3 years of age. The hereditary form is more likely to be bilateral.
   2. **Clinical manifestations.** Leukocoria is a white papillary reflex seen on direct ophthalmoscopic examination. All patients who have leukocoria should be evaluated for retinoblastoma. Other symptoms include strabismus and a painful, inflamed eye.

3. **Diagnosis** usually is confirmed by dilated funduscopic examination under sedation. CT or MRI scans may show calcifications.

4. **Treatment.** Surgery (enucleation), radiation therapy, and cryotherapy are the cornerstones of treatment.

III LYMPHADENOPATHY

A. **Clinical manifestations.** Enlarged lymph nodes may be benign or may signal an underlying malignancy. Signs that suggest malignancy include:

1. Nodes that are found to be fixed to the underlying fascia during palpation
2. Nodes that are enlarged for more than 4 weeks
3. Nodes that are larger than 2.5 cm
4. Nodes that continue to enlarge after 2 weeks of observation
5. Nodes that remain enlarged despite antibiotic therapy
6. Enlargement of supraclavicular or axillary nodes
7. Generalized lymphadenopathy
8. Enlarged nodes in conjunction with other evidence of malignancy (e.g., constitutional symptoms, anemia, thrombocytopenia, abdominal masses, hepatosplenomegaly)

B. **Differential diagnosis** includes lymphadenitis, cat-scratch disease, lymphoma, metastatic malignancy, collagen vascular disease, tuberculosis, Epstein-Barr virus, cytomegalovirus, HIV, malaria, and thyroglossal duct cysts.

C. **Workup.** If the cause of lymphadenopathy is not clear, workup may include a chest radiograph (to look for mediastinal adenopathy), a purified protein derivative (PPD) test, a complete blood cell count, and an erythrocyte sedimentation rate. A biopsy is required if malignancy is suspected. A bone marrow biopsy is indicated if there is evidence of marrow dysfunction. Palpable supraclavicular nodes suggest intra-abdominal malignancy, and an abdominal ultrasound is indicated.

References

Lanzkowsky P: *Manual of Pediatric Hematology and Oncology,* 3rd ed. San Diego, Academic Press, 1999.

76. Oncologic Emergencies

I **INTRODUCTION.** Several emergencies and urgent situations can be the presenting sign of malignancy in a child. After these patients are stabilized, they should be referred to a pediatric oncology center for treatment.

II **SUPERIOR VENA CAVA SYNDROME**

A. **Pathogenesis.** Obstruction or compression of the superior vena cava is caused by an anterior mediastinal mass. Potential causes include non-Hodgkin lymphoma, acute lymphoblastic leukemia (especially T-cell), Hodgkin disease, neuroblastoma, thymoma, rhabdomyosarcoma, Ewing sarcoma, and thyroid tumor.

B. **Symptoms** include shortness of breath, orthopnea, headache, facial swelling, dizziness, and pallor.

C. **Physical findings** include an edematous, plethoric face and neck; jugular venous distension; papilledema; pulsus paradoxus; adenopathy; wheezing; air hunger; and stridor.

D. **Initial workup** involves looking for an anterior mediastinal mass on chest radiograph; a computed tomographic (CT) scan is obtained to determine the location of blockage. In addition, blood samples are sent for the following tests: complete blood cell count (CBC), electrolytes, uric acid, blood urea nitrogen (BUN), creatinine, and lactate dehydrogenase (LDH). Blood typing and crossmatching for blood products are done as necessary.

E. Unless the obstruction is severe, **treatment** focuses on establishing a diagnosis and providing tumor-specific therapy. Diagnosis should be made by the least invasive route possible, because patients are at risk for circulatory collapse or respiratory failure during general anesthesia. If symptoms are life-threatening, if the patient cannot tolerate anesthesia, or if a tissue diagnosis cannot be obtained, the patient may be treated empirically for the most likely diagnosis. Biopsy is performed as soon as it is safe to do so.

III **COMPRESSION OF THE SPINAL CORD**

A. **Pathogenesis.** The spinal cord may be compressed as a result of expansion of a paravertebral tumor. As direct compression of the tumor progresses, compression of the paravertebral venous plexus may lead to cord edema, demyelination, and ischemia. The resulting damage may be permanent.

B. Symptoms. Back pain occurs in 80% of cases. In late compression, weakness, sensory loss, and incontinence may develop.

C. Physical findings. Back pain may be aggravated by straight-leg raising and neck flexion. Sensory deficits, weakness, and loss of the anal wink are late findings and are cause for concern.

D. Initial workup. Magnetic resonance imaging (MRI) is the preferred diagnostic modality. If MRI is not available, myelography is an alternative in patients who have neurologic deficits, although it is important to remember that lumbar puncture carries a risk of neurologic deterioration. Plain radiographic films show lytic lesions in 30% of cases.

E. Treatment. When spinal compression is suspected and symptoms are progressing rapidly, intravenous dexamethasone (1 mg/kg) is administered while emergent MRI scans are obtained. Surgical laminectomy can relieve the pressure and provide tissue for diagnosis. Radiation therapy or chemotherapy may be beneficial.

IV INCREASED INTRACRANIAL PRESSURE

A. Pathogenesis. Most tumors are infratentorial and block the 3rd or 4th ventricle. As the mass grows, intracranial pressure increases and displaces the brain inferiorly. A central tumor leads to progressive loss of midbrain and brain stem function. Lateral masses may lead to uncal herniation. Cerebellar masses can compress the medulla or spinal cord.

B. Symptoms. Younger children may have vomiting, lethargy, loss of developmental motor milestones, increasing occipitofrontal circumference, or seizures. Most older children have headaches that are intermittent initially and worsen as the tumor grows. Recurrent headache on arising from bed, accompanied by vomiting, suggests an intracranial mass.

   1. Uncal herniation. Mild pupillary dilation and sluggish response to light may indicate early temporal lobe herniation. Worsening herniation causes ptosis and paresis of the medial rectus muscle, which leads to a "down and out" position of the eye (cranial nerve III palsy).

   2. Midbrain or brain stem herniation may lead to decorticate (flexor) or decerebrate (extensor) posturing, irregular respirations, hypertension, or bradycardia. The last three items listed comprise "Cushing's triad."

C. Other physical findings. Posterior fossa tumors often are associated with cerebellar abnormalities on examination. Other focal neurologic findings vary depending on the location of the tumor; findings may include ataxia, weakness, dysarthria, dizziness, and lethargy.

D. Initial workup. CT scanning of the head is the most readily available diagnostic modality. MRI typically is needed to provide more detailed information, especially in posterior fossa tumors. Lumbar puncture is contraindicated unless increased intracranial pressure is ruled out.

E. Treatment. Patients who have documented masses and abnormal neurologic findings should be treated. Initial management includes fluid restriction and dexamethasone (0.5–1 mg/kg loading dose followed by 0.25–0.5 mg/kg/dose every 6 hours). Evidence of uncal, midbrain, or brain stem herniation is an ominous sign (see Chapter 104).

V HYPERLEUKOCYTOSIS

A. Pathogenesis. Leukemia may produce white blood cell (WBC) counts higher than 200,000/mm^3, which may cause hyperviscosity and subsequent aggregation of cells in the vasculature of the brain, lungs, or other organs.

B. Symptoms are related to the affected organs, but most patients are asymptomatic. Cerebral involvement may be associated with mental status changes, headache, or seizures. Pulmonary hemostasis may cause dyspnea. Involvement of other organs may lead to oliguria, priapism, or dactylitis (swelling of the digits).

C. Physical findings. Severe cerebral involvement may lead to papilledema or signs of increased intracranial pressure. Pulmonary involvement may cause hypoxemia, rales, distension of the jugular veins, or hepatomegaly.

D. Initial workup. A chest radiograph is performed to evaluate the patient for pulmonary edema or a mediastinal mass. Blood tests include electrolytes, uric acid, BUN, creatinine, prothrombin time, partial thromboplastin time, and LDH. Blood typing and crossmatching are done for appropriate blood products. An EDTA tube should be held for possible immunophenotyping of tumor cells.

E. Treatment should be considered for patients who are symptomatic or who have high, rapidly increasing WBC counts. Both exchange transfusion and leukopheresis are effective means of rapidly reducing the number of circulating WBCs. Treatment also should be initiated for tumor lysis syndrome (see VI F), and thrombocytopenia should be corrected. To limit increases in blood viscosity, the hematocrit should be maintained at less than 30% until the tumor load diminishes.

VI TUMOR LYSIS SYNDROME

A. **Pathogenesis.** Tumor lysis syndrome is associated with large tumors that are highly responsive to chemotherapy. It may occur before chemotherapy is initiated. Lysis of tumor cells leads to a release of potassium, phosphates, and nucleic acids into the circulation that may cause hyperkalemia, hypocalcemia, and the deposition of uric acid crystals in the kidneys. Urate deposition may cause renal failure.

B. **Symptoms.** Hypocalcemia causes vomiting, anorexia, and seizures. Hyperkalemia causes nausea, weakness, and paralysis.

C. **Physical findings.** When hypocalcemia is present, Chvostek sign (spasm of the facial muscle when the facial nerve is tapped) and Trousseau sign (carpopedal spasm when blood flow is impeded by a cuff that is inflated to 20 mm Hg above the systolic pressure for 3 minutes) may be elicited.

D. **Associated malignancies.** Tumor lysis syndrome most commonly occurs with Burkitt lymphoma, T-cell acute lymphoblastic leukemia, germ cell tumors, and neuroblastoma.

E. **The initial workup** includes CBC, urinalysis, and determination of electrolyte, uric acid, phosphorus, calcium, BUN, and creatinine values. The electrocardiogram (ECG) is performed if the potassium level is elevated. Hyperkalemia is associated with widening of the QRS complex and peaked T waves as the serum potassium level rises above 7.0 mEq/L. This condition can progress to ventricular arrhythmias and cardiac arrest.

F. **Treatment.** Therapy is largely preventive. Vigorous hydration is initiated as soon as possible. Intravenous fluid is given at 1.5 × maintenance rates with D5 1/4 normal saline with 50–100 mEq/L NaHCO$_3$. The added bicarbonate alkalinizes the urine. Allopurinol competitively reduces the production of uric acid and should be given at a dose of 150–300 mg/kg/day in two to three divided doses. Hyperkalemia and hypocalcemia should be treated as well **(Table 76–1).** In severe cases, dialysis may be necessary.

VII HYPERCALCEMIA

A. **Pathogenesis.** Many hematologic and solid tumors are associated with hypercalcemia (most commonly, acute lymphoblastic leukemia and alveolar rhabdomyosarcoma). These tumors may produce hormones that increase bone resorption. As hypercalcemia progresses, renal calcium excretion decreases.

B. **Symptoms** include weakness, anorexia, nausea, vomiting, constipation, abdominal pain, polyuria, and drowsiness. As levels

TABLE 76-1. Treatment of Hyperkalemia

Agent	Indication	Mechanism of Action	Dose	Side Effects/Problems
Calcium gluconate 10%	Cardiac toxicity (electrocardiogram changes)	Stabilizes membranes potential increments	1 mg/kg intravenously over 5–10 min	Hypercalcemia
Sodium bicarbonate	Emergency medication	Shifts potassium intracellularly	1 mEq/kg intravenously over 5–10 min	Sodium load
Glucose/insulin	Emergency medication	Shifts potassium intracellularly	0.25–0.5 g/kg glucose, 0.3 U insulin/kg over 30–60 min	Hyperglycemia or hypoglycemia
Kayexalate resin	Need to remove potassium from body	Binds potassium to resin in gut	1 g/kg orally/rectally in 50%–70% sorbitol	Constipation
Furosemide	Renal function intact	Removes potassium in urine	1–2 mg/kg intravenously	Often not enough renal function to be effective
Dialysis	No renal function	Removes potassium in dialysate	Hemo- or peritoneal dialysis	Risks of dialysis
Exchange transfusion	Emergency medication	Donor blood has had most potassium removed	Double volume	Risk of exchange transfusion

Reprinted with permission from Schwartz MW: *Clinical Handbook of Pediatrics*. Baltimore, Lippincott Williams & Wilkins, 1996, p 283.

increase to more than 15 mg/dl, symptoms become more severe and the patient may become comatose.

C. **Initial workup** includes determining the levels of calcium, phosphorus, and electrolytes. ECG changes may be noted, including wide T waves and a prolonged P-R interval.

D. **Treatment.** Vigorous hydration is a mainstay of therapy. Calcium levels greater than 14 mg/dl require forced diuresis with normal saline at two to three times maintenance rates and high-dose intravenous furosemide (2–3 mg/kg every 2 hours). Electrolytes must be carefully monitored during this process because hypokalemia, hyponatremia, and hypomagnesemia may result. Oral phosphate (10 mg/kg/dose two to three times daily) may reduce osteoclastic activity in patients with hypophosphatemia (< 2.5–3.0 mg/dl). Glucocorticoids, calcitonin, and mithramycin all may have a role in limiting osteoclastic activity.

References

Falk S, Fallon M: ABCs of palliative care emergencies. *BMJ* 315(7121):1525–1528, 1997.

Kelly KM, Lange B: Oncologic emergencies. *Pediatr Clin North Am* 44(4):809–830, 1997.

77. Sickle Cell Disease

I **INTRODUCTION.** Sickle cell disease is caused by a defect in the beta chain globin. A single amino acid substitution results in an absence of hemoglobin A (HbA) and the production of hemoglobin S (HbS). For sickling to occur, both beta globins must be HbS polymers; therefore, heterozygotes (sickle cell carriers) are asymptomatic.

A. Sickling. Fever, hypoxia, acidosis, and dehydration cause polymerization of HbS, which leads to sickling of red blood cells. Sickling initially is reversible, but with repeated episodes, the membrane damage becomes permanent. The abnormal shape of these cells leads to increased destruction by the spleen and resultant microvascular obstruction.

B. Manifestations are a consequence of hemolysis, a shortened red blood cell lifespan, and vaso-occlusion. Symptoms do not occur until fetal hemoglobin (HbF) production stops at 4–6 months of life.

C. Pathophysiology. Vaso-occlusion can occur anywhere in the body and without any precipitating event. A vicious cycle ensues: sickled cells create a plug, which leads to local ischemia and acidosis. This condition causes more sickling, and the block worsens, causing infarction and pain. Interestingly, during a vaso-occlusive crisis, there is no increase in the number of sickled cells seen on blood smears.

D. Epidemiology. Sickle cell disease shows an incomplete autosomal dominant inheritance pattern. In the United States, approximately 1:650 African-Americans are affected, and approximately 8% of African-Americans are heterozygous for this disease. Between 7% and 29% experience some central nervous system (CNS) sequelae, and as many as 10% experience stroke.

II **CLINICAL MANIFESTATIONS. Physical examination.** Patients often are small for their age. Many have enlarged maxillas as a result of extramedullary hematopoiesis. The conjunctiva and oral mucosa are pale, the sclera may be jaundiced, and puberty often is delayed.

III **SPECIFIC SEQUELAE OF SICKLE CELL DISEASE**

A. Pain crises. Pain crises are caused by vaso-occlusion and most commonly occur in the bone or abdomen.

1. **Workup.** Pain in the abdomen or bone must be clinically distinguished from osteomyelitis and an acute abdomen (Tables 77–1 and 77–2).

HOT **KEY** The presence of an elevated alpha-hydroxybutyric dehydrogenase level is helpful in diagnosing a true vaso-occlusive crisis and distinguishing between symptoms suggestive of both infection and vaso-occlusion.

---

2. **Treatment.** Most pain crises can be managed in the outpatient setting with increased hydration and oral analgesia. If home regimens are unsuccessful, inpatient admission is re-

TABLE 77-1. Differentiation Between Bone Infarction and Osteomyelitis

Features	Favoring Osteomyelitis	Favoring Bone Infarction
History	No previous history	Preceding painful crisis
Pain, tenderness, erythema, swelling	Single site	Multiple sites
Fever	Present	Present
Leukocytosis	Elevated band count ($> 1000/mm^3$)	Present
ESR	Elevated	Normal to low
Alpha-HBD	Normal	Elevated
Radiograph	Abnormal	Abnormal
Bone scan	Abnormal ^{99m}Tc-diphosphonate Normal ^{99m}Tc-colloid marrow uptake	Abnormal ^{99m}Tc-diphosphonate Decreased ^{99m}Tc-colloid marrow uptake
Blood culture	Positive (*Salmonella, Staphylococcus*)	Negative
Recovery	Only with appropriate antibiotic therapy	Spontaneous

Reprinted with permission from Lanzkowsky P: *Manual of Pediatric Hematology and Oncology,* 3rd ed. San Diego, Academic Press, 1999, p 162.

Alpha-HBD = alpha-hydroxybutyric dehydrogenase; ESR = erythrocyte sedimentation rate.

TABLE 77-2. Differentiation Between Painful Abdominal Crisis and Acute Abdomen

Features	Painful Crisis	Acute Abdomen
History of previous episodes	Present	Absent
Abdominal pain and distention	Present	Present
Signs of peritoneal irritation	Absent	Present
Decreased peristalsis	Present	Present
Alpha-HBD	Elevated	Normal
Leukocytosis	Present	Elevated band count ($> 1000/mm^3$)
Response to symptomatic treatment	Present	Absent

Reprinted with permission from Lanzkowsky P: *Manual of Pediatric Hematology and Oncology*, 3rd ed. San Diego, Academic Press, 1999, p 163.
Alpha-HBD = alpha-hydroxybutyric dehydrogenase.

quired. Pain management protocols should be individualized and may necessitate a patient-controlled anesthesia device. All patients should receive hydration at $1.5 \times$ the maintenance value. A partial exchange transfusion should be considered (goal Hb < 40 mg/dl) for those with refractory pain crises that last more than 5 days.

B. Hand and foot syndrome (dactylitis) is caused by vaso-occlusion.
   1. Dactylitis often is the first overt evidence of sickle cell disease, usually occurring in the first 5 years of life. Ischemic infarction of the metacarpals and metatarsals causes red, tender hands and feet. Dactylitis often is confused with a pyoderma.
   2. Dactylitis must be distinguished from osteomyelitis.
C. CNS manifestations are caused by vaso-occlusion. A high leukocyte count and acute decreases in hemoglobin are additional risk factors for stroke.
   1. CNS manifestations occur as the result of large vessel obstruction.
   2. Acute focal findings that resemble stroke may be seen. Seizures, radiculopathy, meningeal signs, blindness, vertigo, or decreased IQ, also may occur.
   3. Treatment
      a. A new focal neurologic deficit in a patient with sickle cell

disease requires immediate hydration, alkalinization, and exchange transfusion (goal HbS < 20%).

   b. After the immediate crisis is over, most recommend a follow-up head computed tomography scan or magnetic resonance imaging and angiogram.

   c. Prophylactic exchange transfusions may be required if cerebral flow is compromised.

D. Acute chest syndrome is caused by vaso-occlusion.

  1. Symptoms

    a. Acute chest syndrome is characterized by increased work of breathing, fever, and oxygen requirement.

    b. It often is associated with a painful abdominal crisis.

    c. It may be difficult to distinguish between pneumonia and pulmonary infarction (Table 77–3).

TABLE 77-3. Differentiation Between Pneumonia and Pulmonary Infarction

Feature	Favoring Pneumonia	Favoring Pulmonary Infarction
Chest pain, fever, and hypoxia	Present	Present
Age	< 5 years	> 5 years
Associated painful crisis	Absent	May be present
Chills	Present	Absent
Leukocytosis	Elevated band count (> 1000/mm^3)	Present
Blister cells on smear	Absent	Present
ESR	Elevated	Low
Alpha-HBD	Normal	Elevated
Chest radiograph	Upper lobe infiltrate	Normal
VQ scan	Normal	Positive
Cultures	Positive blood and sputum or cold agglutinins and *Mycoplasma* titers	Negative

Reprinted with permission from Lanzkowsky P: *Manual of Pediatric Hematology and Oncology,* 3rd ed. San Diego, Academic Press, 1999, p 164.

   Alpha-HBD = alpha-hydroxybutyric dehydrogenase; ESR = erythrocyte sedimentation rate; V/Q = ventilation/perfusion.

2. Workup
  a. Chest radiograph, arterial blood gases, *Mycoplasma* titers, and samples for other appropriate cultures should be drawn.
  b. Electrocardiogram and ventilation/perfusion (V/Q) scan also should be considered.
3. Treatment
  a. Aggressive hydration, O_2 support, and cefuroxime with or without a macrolide (to cover *Mycoplasma*) should be started.
  b. Exchange transfusion is indicated if the PaO_2 is below 70 or if the patient has increasing O_2 requirements or dyspnea, congestive heart failure, or right heart strain.

E. Priapism is caused by vaso-occlusion. It may be triggered by intercourse or masturbation, and prolonged erections may result in impotence. Exchange transfusion sometimes is required.

F. Splenic sequestration crisis is caused by vaso-occlusion.
  1. Splenic sequestration results from large volumes of blood pooling within the spleen. It occurs between 5 and 24 months of age.
  2. Splenic enlargement, abdominal pain, hypotension, and precipitous drops in Hb are the hallmarks of this condition.
  3. Immediate blood transfusion is required for hypotensive patients. Partial exchange transfusions and subsequent prophylactic exchange transfusion also may be required.

G. Intrahepatic vaso-occlusive crisis may occur any time after the spleen has infarcted and fibrosed.
  1. The liver is enlarged and tender to palpation.
  2. Jaundice occurs secondary to conjugated hyperbilirubinemia.
  3. Liver function test results are elevated.

H. Fever/sepsis. Before the age of 4 years, the spleen is enlarged, but is hypofunctional because of congestion. By age 4, the spleen has autoinfarcted because of massive red blood cell congestion. This increases the risk of sepsis from pneumococcus, *Haemophilus influenzae,* gram-negative enteric organisms, and *Salmonella* species.

HOT KEY

Any fever in a patient < 5 years of age with sickle cell disease must be taken seriously because it may represent sepsis.

---

  1. Workup. Blood cultures, complete blood count, chest radiograph, urinalysis, and urine culture are mandatory. Lumbar puncture, stool culture, and an evaluation for osteomyelitis should also be considered.

   2. Treatment
      a. Cefuroxime is an appropriate first-line agent.
      b. Patients should be admitted to the hospital pending culture results.
      c. Transfusion therapy may be used as an adjunctive measure.
   3. Prophylaxis. All patients should receive amoxicillin prophylaxis starting at 3–4 months of age and pneumococcal vaccine at 2 and 4 years of age. Most providers extend amoxicillin prophylaxis until at least age 16 years.
I. Hyperhemolysis may be triggered by infection or medications. G6PD may be a contributing cause. It usually is a self-limited process.
   1. Symptoms include jaundice, weakness, and increasing scleral icterus.
   2. Laboratory test results show worsened anemia and increased reticulocyte count.
   3. Transfusion therapy may be required.
J. Aplastic crises are caused by a sudden cessation of marrow function triggered by infection. The culprit often is parvovirus (B19), the virus that causes fifth disease.
   1. Profound anemia (Hb may reach 1 g/dl), which spontaneously resolves in 10–14 days, is seen.
   2. Laboratory test results show anemia with a low reticulocyte count and a low nucleated red blood cell count.
   3. Additional folate is given to prevent megaloblastic anemia.
K. Renal manifestations
   1. The medulla is an area of increased hypertonicity, so sickling in this area is common. The ability to concentrate urine is lost as a result of infarction.
   2. Symptoms include nephrotic syndrome, hematuria, loss of the ability to concentrate urine (urine has specific gravity of 1.010 or less), chronic renal failure, nocturia, and enuresis.
L. Proliferative sickle cell retinopathy (PSR)
   1. The **retina** is susceptible to hypoxia and is particularly sensitive to sickling effects.
   2. Retinal examination shows torturous retinal vessels, neovascularization, hemorrhages, exudates, and atrophy.
   3. Patients need annual ophthalmologic follow-up after age 10 years. Some patients require laser therapy to prevent blindness.
M. Skin infarction
   1. Minor traumas in the distal extremities heal very slowly. Ulcerations, particularly over the malleoli, are common secondary to thrombosis.
   2. Transfusion therapy may be necessary.
N. Cardiac dysfunction may occur from fibrosis or may be the result of hemosiderosis from chronic transfusion therapy. Both left- and right-sided cardiac failure may occur.

IV DIAGNOSIS

A. Hemoglobin electrophoresis provides the definitive diagnosis.

B. A **complete blood cell count** shows an anemia that is normo-chromic and normocytic (mean hematocrit is 22%). The reticulocyte count is elevated (5%–30%), and neutrophilia and increased platelets are common.

C. A **peripheral blood smear** shows sickle cells, polychromasia, nucleated red blood cells, and target cells. Howell-Jolly bodies indicate hyposplenism.

D. Prenatal testing includes amniocentesis or chorionic villi sampling.

E. Other laboratory findings include low folate levels, high erythropoietin levels, and hyperbilirubinemia.

V ADJUVANT THERAPIES

A. To stimulate HbF production, hydroxuria, 5-azacytidine, butyric acid analogues, and recombinant erythropoietin are used.

B. To decrease the HbS concentration in the red blood cells, monencin, gramicin, nifedipine, and verapamil are used.

C. Bone marrow transplantation can be curative, but has many inherent risks. It is considered in only the most severe cases.

D. Recombinant erythropoietin may improve anemia.

VI PROGNOSIS.
The major causes of death are **sepsis; heart, liver, and kidney failure; pulmonary thrombosis;** and **stroke.** The prognosis is improved by production of HbF that persists into adulthood.

References

Golden C, Styles L, Vichinsky E: Acute chest syndrome and sickle cell disease. *Curr Opin Hematol* 5(2):89–92, 1998.

Lanzkowsky P: *Manual of Pediatric Hematology and Oncology,* 2nd ed. New York, Churchill Livingstone, 1995, pp 117–133.

Sackey K: Hemolytic anemia: part 2. *Pediatr Rev* 20(6):204–208, 1999.

Styles LA, Vichinsky EP: New therapies and approaches to transfusion in sickle cell disease in children. *Curr Opin Pediatr* 9(1):41–45, 1997.

78. Anemia

I INTRODUCTION

A. Background. Anemia is one of the most common laboratory abnormalities seen by primary care pediatricians. The most common types of anemia in children are microcytic [mean cell volume (MCV) < 80 μm³], normocytic (MCV 81–99 μm³), and macrocytic (MCV > 100 μm³) [Table 78–1].

B. Epidemiology. Twenty percent of children in the United States have been anemic before 18 years of age.

HOT

KEY
Anemia is not a disease. It is a symptom of an underlying condition. The physician should attempt to determine the cause.

C. Definition. Anemia is present when the hemoglobin (Hb) or hematocrit level is below the 5th percentile.

II CLINICAL MANIFESTATIONS.
Symptoms include pallor, fatigue, shortness of breath, orthopnea, and syncope. Symptoms of ongoing blood loss include hematochezia and melena.

III APPROACH TO THE PATIENT.
A general approach to pallor is found in Figure 78–1.

A. History
1. **Diet.** Excessive milk intake (> 24 oz/day) after 1 year of age is a risk factor for iron deficiency anemia.
2. **Family history.** A family history of cholecystectomy or splenectomy may indicate a hereditary hemolytic process (e.g., spherocytosis).
3. **Ethnic background.** People of Mediterranean or Asian descent have a higher risk of thalassemia. People of African descent have a higher risk of sickle cell disease or sickle thalassemia, whereas those of Middle Eastern or Mediterranean descent are at higher risk for glucose-6-phosphate dehydrogenase (G6PD) deficiency.
4. **Environmental exposure.** Lead intoxication is a possible

TABLE 78-1. Normal Red Blood Cell Indices

Age (y)	Hemoglobin (g/dl)		Hematocrit (%)		Mean Cell Volume (fl)	
	Mean	Lower Limit	Mean	Lower Limit	Mean	Lower Limit
0.5–1.9	12.5	11.0	37	33	77	70
2–4	12.5	11.0	38	34	79	73
5–7	13.0	11.5	39	35	81	75
8–11	13.5	12.0	40	36	83	76
12–14						
Female	13.5	12.0	41	36	85	78
Male	14.0	12.5	43	37	84	77
15–17						
Female	14.0	12.0	41	36	87	79
Male	15.0	13.0	46	38	86	78

Reprinted with permission from Nathan DC, Oski F: Hematology of Infancy and Childhood, 4th ed. Philadelphia, WB Saunders, 1993, p 376.

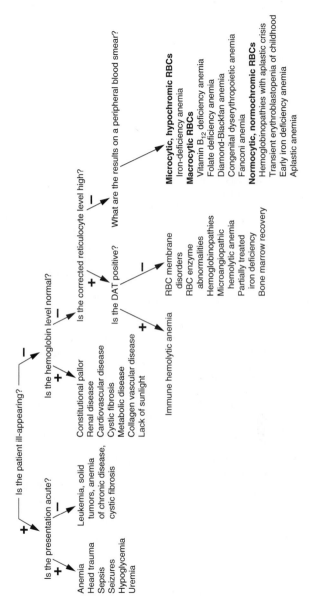

FIGURE 78-1. Evaluation of a patient with pallor. DAT = direct antibody test; RBC = red blood cell. (Reprinted with permission from Schwartz MW: *Clinical Handbook of Pediatrics,* 2nd ed. Philadelphia, Lippincott Williams & Wilkins, 1999, p 505.)

cause of anemia. Exposure to lead is most likely in children who live in older buildings.

HOT KEY

The most common cause of anemia in toddlers is poor diet, with an excessive intake of juice or milk.

B. Physical examination
   1. **Pallor** is easily evaluated by examining the deep palm creases and conjunctivae.
   2. **Bony enlargement** (e.g., frontal bossing) may indicate chronic hemolytic anemia (e.g., sickle cell disease, thalassemia major).
   3. **Splenomegaly** may be seen in congenital hemolytic anemia (e.g., hemoglobinopathies, spherocytosis). Hepatomegaly or lymphadenopathy may indicate malignancy. **Glossitis** (a red, swollen tongue) is seen in rare cases of vitamin B_{12} deficiency.
C. Laboratory evaluation. Infants reach their physiologic nadir (i.e., Hb = 10.5–11 g/dl) at 6–8 weeks of age. Children usually are screened at 9–15 months of age. A child who has pallor or an initial low hematocrit or Hb level should undergo further evaluation. Laboratory tests include the following:
   1. The **direct Coombs test** indicates immune-mediated hemolysis in hemolytic disease of the newborn, hemolytic transfusion reactions, or autoimmune hemolytic anemias.
   2. The **ferritin** level is a more sensitive indicator of iron stores than is the serum iron level. However, the ferritin level may be falsely elevated in patients who have liver or inflammatory disease.
   3. The **iron level** is decreased in patients who have iron deficiency anemia or anemia of chronic disease.
   4. The **lead level** should be determined at 9–12 months of age in children who are at risk for lead poisoning. Zinc protoporphyrin alone is an insufficiently sensitive screening tool.
   5. The **reticulocyte count** is an indicator of erythropoiesis. This count is increased in patients with acute blood loss or hemolytic anemia; it is decreased in patients with iron deficiency anemia, chronic disease, or bone marrow failure. It must be corrected for low hematocrit:

Corrected reticulocyte count =

$$\text{observed reticulocyte count} \times \frac{\text{observed hematocrit}}{\text{normal hematocrit}}$$

6. **Total iron binding capacity** helps to distinguish between anemia of chronic disease and iron deficiency anemia. Typically, it is low (fully saturated) in patients who have anemia of chronic disease and high in those with iron deficiency anemia.

IV MICROCYTIC ANEMIA

A. **Iron deficiency anemia** is the most common cause of anemia. It affects 5%–10% of all children.

   1. **Cause.** Iron deficiency anemia can be caused by insufficient dietary intake of iron or by chronic blood loss. Children older than 2 years of age are more likely than infants to have chronic intestinal blood loss. Infants are more likely to have uncomplicated nutritional anemia.

      a. **Insufficient dietary iron intake** is common between 9 and 24 months of age. Many children have a history of excessive milk intake.

      b. **Chronic blood loss** may be caused by gastrointestinal irritation from a heat-labile protein found in whole cow's milk. This irritation is relieved by reducing the quantity of whole cow's milk in the diet or by using a milk substitute such as a soy milk. Chronic blood loss also is caused by gastritis, Meckel diverticulum, polyps, or hemangioma. It is not caused by lactose intolerance.

   2. **Treatment.** Most cases of microcytic anemia are treated with 6 mg/kg/day of elemental iron in three divided doses. Treatment is continued until 2 months after the Hb level reaches the normal range. Black stools indicate compliance with treatment and appear soon after iron administration begins.

B. **Thalassemia**

   1. **β-Thalassemia** is most common in patients of Mediterranean descent. The most severe cases result from a complete lack of β-globin genes, or β^0-thalassemia. β^+-thalassemia results from partial production of β-globin genes and is less severe. These deficiencies cause anemia by 6–12 months of age. A peripheral blood smear result is markedly abnormal, and shows target cells and a high red blood cell (RBC) distribution width.

   2. **α-Thalassemia** is caused by an absence of α-globin genes; four genes code for the α-globin chain.

      a. **Deletion of one gene** results in an asymptomatic, silent carrier state.

      b. **Deletion of two genes** results in α-thalassemia trait and mild microcytic anemia. The α-thalassemia trait and silent carrier state are common in the African-American population.

    c. Deletion of three genes results in Hb H disease and more severe microcytic anemia. HbH disease affects people of Asian or Mediterranean descent almost exclusively.

    d. Deletion of all four genes causes Hb Bart disease and results in fetal death. Bart disease occurs only in people of Asian ancestry.

C. Lead poisoning

  1. Lead exposure is most common among low-income, urban populations. The most common cause is ingestion of lead-containing paint. The age and condition of housing are the best predictors for lead exposure; older houses (i.e., those built before 1975) are more likely to have surfaces with lead-containing paints.

  2. Neurotoxic effects. An estimated 890,000 American children have a blood lead level (BLL) higher than 10 μg/dl, the point at which lead has neurotoxic effects. Children with a BLL of 20 have IQs that are, on average, 2–3 points lower than those of age-matched children with a BLL of 10 μg/dl.

  3. Treatment. The most important aspect of treatment is removal of the lead source. Subsequently, treatment and follow-up depend on the initial BLL, as follows:

    a. BLL < 10 μg/dl: no action required

    b. BLL 10–14 μg/dl: The BLL is reconfirmed after 1 month. If the level still falls within this range, education is provided to reduce exposure, and testing is repeated within 3 months.

    c. BLL 15–19 μg/dl: The BLL is reconfirmed within 1 month. If the BLL remains in this range, education is provided and the BLL is repeated within 2 months.

    d. BLL 20–44 μg/dl: The BLL is reconfirmed within 1 week. If it is still within this range, education is provided and the patient is referred to the local health department. Case management also may be provided to include environmental investigation with support services. An ethylenediaminetetraacetic acid (EDTA) chelation test is performed. If the result is positive, EDTA is given (1000 mg/m^2 every 24 hours) on an outpatient basis.

    e. BLL 45–69 μg/dl: The BLL is reconfirmed within 2 days. If it remains within this range, education is provided and the patient is referred to the local health department. Chelation therapy should be initiated with EDTA (1000 mg/m^2 over 24 hours by continuous infusion for 5 consecutive days).

    f. BLL > 70 μg/dl: The patient is hospitalized for immediate medical treatment. Treatment consists of BAL 75 mg/m^2 every 4 hours, followed by EDTA 1500 mg/m^2 over 24 hours by continuous infusion for 5 consecutive days.

D. Anemia of chronic disease. Chronic inflammatory or infectious diseases may cause mild to moderate microcytic anemia because of impaired transfer of iron to the developing erythroid cells in the marrow. Iron stores are normal, ferritin levels are normal to elevated, and iron binding capacity is decreased.

V NORMOCYTIC ANEMIA (Figure 78–2)

A. Background. Normocytic anemia is caused by underproduction, increased loss, or destruction of RBCs. The cause can be distinguished by the reticulocyte count. A corrected reticulocyte count of less than 2% despite anemia is caused by underproduction. An elevated reticulocyte count indicates RBC loss or destruction.

B. Anemia of underproduction (reticulocyte count < 2%)

   1. Transient erythroblastopenia of childhood is a temporary arrest of erythropoiesis that occurs between 6 months and 5 years of age. The cause is unknown. It causes pallor and fatigue over the course of months to weeks, and recovery is spontaneous. Transfusion is indicated for those with severe, symptomatic anemia.

   2. Hematologic malignancy causes anemia when the bone marrow is infiltrated by malignant cells. It may be accompanied by thrombocytopenia and leukopenia or leukocytosis.

   3. Aplastic anemia is characterized by hypoplastic bone marrow and pancytopenia. Typically, it is idiopathic, but it may be related to previous infection or medication use.

C. Anemia as a result of hemolysis (reticulocyte count > 2%)

   1. Hereditary spherocytosis, hereditary elliptocytosis, and stomatocytosis are inherited RBC membrane defects that cause decreased RBC distensibility and increased destruction in the spleen. Newborns may have jaundice in the first day of life. Physical findings include splenomegaly and reticulocytosis. Patients are susceptible to viral-induced, transient decreases in RBC production. Cholelithiasis is a common complication; splenectomy may be required if the condition is severe.

   2. G6PD deficiency is the most common RBC enzyme defect. It is X-linked and is most common in people of African and Mediterranean descent. G6PD deficiency leads to increased susceptibility to oxidative stress. Ingestion of a variety of agents may precipitate hemolysis, including fava beans, large doses of vitamin C, antimalarial agents, nitrofurantoin, sulfonamides, and chloramphenicol. Diagnosis is made by G6PD assay.

   3. Pyruvate kinase deficiency is a rare autosomal recessive disorder that is characterized by chronic hemolysis.

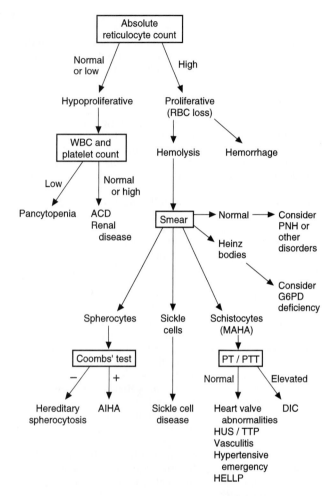

FIGURE 78–2. Determining the cause of normocytic anemia. ACD = anemia of chronic disease; AIHA = autoimmune hemolytic anemia; DIC = disseminated intravascular coagulation; G6PD = glucose-6-phosphate dehydrogenase; HELLP = hemolysis, elevated liver enzymes, and low platelet count syndrome; HTN = hypertension; HUS/TTP = hemolytic-uremic syndrome/thrombotic thrombocytopenic purpura; MAHA = microangiopathic hemolytic anemia; PNH = paroxysmal nocturnal hemoglobinuria; PT = prothrombin time; PTT = partial thromboplastin time; RBC = red blood cell; WBC = white blood cell. (Reprinted with permission from Saint S, Frances C: *Saint-Frances Guide to Inpatient Medicine.* Baltimore, Lippincott Williams & Wilkins, 1997, p 321.)

4. **Sickle hemoglobinopathy disorders** (see Chapter 77)
5. **Antibody-mediated hemolysis.** Immunoglobulin (Ig) G, or "warm," antibody-mediated hemolysis may be idiopathic or may occur secondary to collagen-vascular disease, lymphoma, Epstein-Barr virus, HIV, or drugs such as penicillin, quinine, or methyldopa. IgM, or "cold," antibody-mediated hemolysis may be idiopathic or may be caused by *Mycoplasma* infection or lymphoma. Coombs test result is diagnostic. The treatment for warm antibody-mediated hemolysis is prednisone, 2 mg/kg/day until symptoms resolve. Refractory cases may require splenectomy, intravenous Ig, immunosuppressive agents, or plasmapheresis.
6. **Mechanical hemolysis** is caused by intravascular destruction of RBCs. Misshapen schistocytes or fragmented RBCs suggest this diagnosis. This condition may occur secondary to disseminated intravascular coagulation, hemolytic-uremic syndrome, thrombotic thrombocytopenic purpura, renovascular disease, giant hemangiomata, or burns.

VI MACROCYTIC ANEMIA

A. **Folic acid deficiency.** Deficiencies of both vitamin B_{12} and folic acid are characterized by a blood smear that shows Howell-Jolly bodies, nucleated RBCs, and hypersegmented neutrophils. In addition, the serum folate level is low (< 3 ng/ml).
   1. **Characteristics.** Folic acid deficiency is characterized by anemia, granulocytopenia, and thrombocytopenia. Today, it is most prevalent in malnourished children and patients with malabsorption syndromes. It sometimes complicates trimethoprim or diphenylhydantoin therapy.
   2. **Treatment** is with folic acid, 50–100 μg/day. Concomitant vitamin B_{12} deficiency must be ruled out: although administration of folic acid will correct the hematologic findings, it will not treat the neurologic complications of vitamin B_{12} deficiency.
B. **Vitamin B_{12} deficiency** causes pancytopenia with macrocytosis. Patients also may have neurologic manifestations (e.g., ataxia, paresthesias, hyporeflexia, Babinski responses, and clonus) or gastrointestinal distress. Vitamin B_{12} deficiency may be caused by pernicious anemia, congenital absence of intrinsic factor, or ileal disease.
   1. **Diagnosis.** The diagnosis is made by checking the serum vitamin B_{12} level (normally 200–900 pg/ml). Patients with pernicious anemia have a persistently high gastric pH. The diagnosis can be confirmed by measuring antibodies to parietal cells and intrinsic factor.
   2. **Treatment** requires lifelong parenteral replacement of the

vitamin. The loading dose is 500 μg/day for 10 days, followed by 500 μg every 2 months.

C. Diamond-Blackfan anemia is a congenital red cell aplasia that may be difficult to distinguish from transient erythroblastopenia of childhood in patients younger than 1 year of age. There are elevated levels of folic acid and vitamin B_{12}. Corticosteroid treatment is beneficial if started early.

References

Graham EA: The changing face of anemia in infancy. *Pediatr Rev* 15(5):175–183, 1994.
Martin PL, Pearson HA: The anemias. In: *Oski's Pediatrics: Principles and Practice,* 3rd ed. Philadelphia, Lippincott Williams & Wilkins, 1999, p 1453–1457.
Segel GB: Anemia. *Pediatr Rev* 10(3):77, 1988.

79. Fever and Neutropenia

I INTRODUCTION

A. Background. Children with malignancies often have periods of neutropenia as a result of either their disease (e.g., leukemia) or its treatment (e.g., chemotherapy). While they are neutropenic, these children are at increased risk for life-threatening infections; often, fever is the only presenting sign. Fevers are common in children with malignancies and may result from viral syndromes, reactions to blood product transfusions, or serious bacterial or fungal infections.

> **HOT**
> ▶
> **KEY**
>
> "Harmless" and potentially life-threatening fevers are indistinguishable in the neutropenic patient.

B. Definitions. The definitions of fever and neutropenia vary among institutions. In general, the following definitions are useful:
   1. **Fever** is any single temperature higher than 38.0°C–38.5°C (100.4°F–101.3°F).
   2. **Neutropenia** is an absolute neutrophil count (ANC) < 200/μl or an ANC that is predicted to fall below 200/μl in the next 24 hours. An alternative definition is an ANC < 500/μl.
C. Pathogenesis. Children with malignancies are immunocompromised, and therefore at increased risk for serious infection for several reasons, including the following:
   1. Direct destruction of immune cells by the malignant process or chemotherapy
   2. Disruption of natural barriers to infection (e.g., skin, intestinal mucosa) as a result of chemotherapy or radiation
   3. High prevalence of indwelling central venous catheters
D. Epidemiology. Approximately 10%–20% of patients with cancer who have neutropenic fever have bacteremia. More than half of patients with bacteremia have no evidence of infection other than fever.

II APPROACH TO THE PATIENT

A. History. A thorough history is essential. Key aspects include the following:

1. **Type of malignancy,** including diagnosis, date of diagnosis, treatment protocol, and recent blood counts
2. **Medications,** including the date and type of the most recent chemotherapy, recent or current antibiotic use (including prophylaxis), and use of other medications
3. **Symptoms,** including pain (e.g., oral, abdominal, perirectal, urinary), respiratory distress, and chills or rigors
4. **Exposures,** including varicella, influenza, and other illnesses

B. Physical examination is done to identify clinically apparent sources of infection. A head-to-toe physical examination is important, with special attention paid to the following:
   1. Vital signs (e.g., temperature, evidence of septic shock such as decreased systolic or diastolic blood pressure)
   2. Oral and perirectal tissues and skin (e.g., mucositis, abscesses, skin breakdown)
   3. Lungs (e.g., areas of consolidation, evidence of respiratory distress)
   4. Abdomen (e.g., typhlitis, intra-abdominal abscess)
   5. Central venous line site (e.g., line infection)

C. Laboratory tests
   1. **Complete blood cell count** with an absolute neutrophil count should be performed.

HOT

KEY

Remember that the absolute neutrophil count includes neutrophils and bands.

---

   2. **Blood cultures.** Blood is drawn from each lumen of the central line and tested for aerobic and anaerobic organisms. Peripheral cultures that may help to distinguish sepsis from line infection also are drawn.
   3. **Both urinalysis and urine culture** should be performed, even if the results of urinalysis are negative.

D. Additional tests to consider. The findings of the history and physical examination will direct the need for additional tests. Other tests that are usually obtained include:
   1. **Chest radiograph**
   2. **Stool studies**. If diarrhea is present, a sample is evaluated for *Clostridium difficile.*
   3. **Gram stain and culture of the line site**

E. Initial therapy. Empiric, broad-spectrum antibiotics are administered as soon as possible (ideally, within 1 hour of the onset of fever).
   1. **Ceftazidime,** 150 mg/kg/day, divided and given every 8 hours

(maximum, 6000 mg/day). Alternatives include imipenem and ticarcillin/clavulanate plus an aminoglycoside.

2. If signs of sepsis (e.g., hypotension, tachycardia, changes in mental status) are present, resuscitation, including intravenous fluids, may be necessary.

F. Adjuvant therapy. Additional antibiotics may be warranted based on the history and physical findings.

1. **Nafcillin,** 100–200 mg/kg/day, divided and given every 6 hours (maximum, 8000 mg/day) if the patient has cellulitis

2. **Gentamicin,** 7.5 mg/kg/day, divided and given every 8 hours if the patient appears to be in septic shock or is hypotensive

3. **Gentamicin** plus **clindamycin,** 30 mg/kg/day, divided and given every 8 hours (maximum, 2700 mg/day) if the patient has abdominal or perirectal pain or severe oral mucositis

4. Depending on the child's clinical status and the chemotherapy protocol, **granulocyte colony-stimulating factor** may be added to stimulate neutrophil recovery.

G. Ongoing management

1. **Changes to the initial antibiotic regimen** are made for two reasons only:

    a. **Laboratory studies** (e.g., blood culture) **identify an infectious agent.** The antibiotic regimen is adjusted based on laboratory findings.

    b. **The clinical picture evolves.** For example, if abdominal pain develops, gentamicin and clindamycin are added (see II F 3).

2. **Persistent fever** alone is not an indication to change antibiotics; however, if fever persists after 7 days of empiric, broad-spectrum antibiotics, amphotericin B, 0.5 mg/kg/day every 24 hours, is added as empiric fungal coverage.

3. **Duration of antibiotic therapy**

    a. If the ANC is > 200/μl, antibiotics are discontinued when all culture results have been negative for 48 hours and the patient has been afebrile for 24–48 hours.

    b. If the ANC is < 200/μl, antibiotics may be discontinued when all culture results have been negative for 48 hours, the patient has been afebrile for 7 days (amphotericin B is not needed), and the patient has completed 14 days of empiric antibiotics.

    c. If the blood culture result is positive, 10–14 days of appropriate antibiotic therapy should be completed, starting from the time the patient is afebrile.

III PROGNOSIS. Without prompt empiric antibiotic therapy, the mortality rate for gram-negative infections in febrile patients with neutropenia approaches 80%. Appropriate therapy substantially decreases the mortality rate.

References

Alexander SW, Walsh TJ, Freifeld AG, et al: Infectious complications in pediatric cancer patients. Pizzo PA, Poplack DG (eds): *Principles and Practice of Pediatric Oncology,* 3rd ed. Philadelphia, Lippincott-Raven, 1997, pp 1084–1087.

Lanzkowsky P: *Manual of Pediatric Hematology and Oncology,* 3rd ed. San Diego, Academic Press, 1999, pp 677–686.

Rolston KV: New trends in patient management: risk-based therapy for febrile patients with neutropenia. *Clin Infect Dis* 29(3):515–521, 1999.

PART IX

UROLOGY AND NEPHROLOGY

80. Proteinuria

I INTRODUCTION

A. **Definition.** Proteinuria is a reading of 1+ or greater on dipstick or a finding of greater than 0.3 g protein in a 24-hour urine collection **(Table 80–1).**

B. **Pathogenesis.** Proteinuria may be caused by abnormalities in renal filtration, reabsorption, or secretion. It is caused by a number of syndromes or diseases that interfere with normal kidney function.

C. **Epidemiology.** Approximately 10% of school-age children have a positive proteinuria test result at any given time. If checked at four separate times, however, only 0.1% of children have consistent proteinuria.

II APPROACH TO THE PATIENT

A. **History.** The physician should ask whether the patient has a history of hypertension, oliguria, edema, or tea-colored or red

TABLE 80-1. Urine Protein Dipstick Readings	
Grade	Protein Measurement (mg/dl)
Trace	10–20
1+	30
2+	100
3+	300
4+	1000–2000

Adapted with permission from Shim HH: *Clinical Handbook of Pediatrics,* 2nd ed. Philadelphia, Lippincott Williams & Wilkins, 1999, p 545.

urine; problems with growth and nutrition; or recurrent urinary tract infections. The physician also should ask about a family history of proteinuria or renal disease. A thorough medication history should be taken to identify recent use of medications that cause kidney toxicity (e.g., gentamicin, chemotherapeutic agents, nonsteroidal anti-inflammatory drugs, heavy metals).

B. Physical examination. Blood pressure, other vital signs, and growth parameters are obtained. The patient also is examined to identify accompanying rashes, fever, arthralgias, or edema. These abnormalities necessitate immediate referral to a pediatric nephrologist.

C. Workup

   1. Dipstick. A positive dipstick finding should be rechecked because most proteinuria is transient and disappears without treatment. If the second test result is positive, the next test obtained should be a morning first void urinanalysis to rule out orthostatic proteinuria. Another positive result warrants timed collections, preferably two 12-hour collections to differentiate between nighttime and daytime excretion rates (to identify orthostatic differences). A 24-hour collection level of 0.2 g or greater warrants further workup.

   2. Other laboratory tests include measurement of electrolytes, blood urea nitrogen and creatinine levels, antistreptolysin O (ASO) and C3 titers, and albumin, lipid, and cholesterol levels. A renal ultrasound also should be obtained. An abnormal finding warrants referral to a pediatric nephrologist for probable renal biopsy **(Figure 80–1).**

D. Differential diagnosis. Proteinuria also may be caused by a variety of iatrogenic and systemic diseases.

   1. Tumors, both solid types and lymphomas, can cause proteinuria.

   2. Several **drugs** are linked to proteinuria, including penicillamine, captopril, lithium, procainamide, chlorpropamide, and phenytoin.

   3. Certain **syndromes** are linked to proteinuria, including Alport syndrome and Drash syndrome.

E. Specific causes

   1. Nonpathogenic (self-resolving) proteinuria

   a. Diagnosis. Approximately 10% of randomly tested children show detectable proteinuria. Most of these cases resolve on their own. Although the exact cause is unknown, fever, exercise, and changes in glomerular blood flow may cause transient proteinuria.

   b. Additional tests. Repeated urine dipstick readings show no proteinuria.

   c. Initial therapy. No treatment is required.

   d. Prognosis is excellent. No long-term effects are seen.

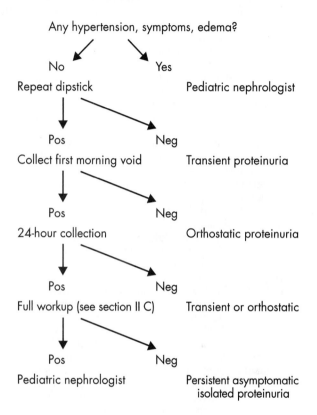

Positive dipstick

Any hypertension, symptoms, edema?

No → Yes

Repeat dipstick → Pediatric nephrologist

Pos → Neg

Collect first morning void → Transient proteinuria

Pos → Neg

24-hour collection → Orthostatic proteinuria

Pos → Neg

Full workup (see section II C) → Transient or orthostatic

Pos → Neg

Pediatric nephrologist → Persistent asymptomatic isolated proteinuria

FIGURE 80–1. Suggested workup for proteinuria.

2. **Persistent asymptomatic isolated proteinuria**
   a. **Diagnosis.** Repeated urine dipstick readings show proteinuria, but the patient is asymptomatic. The protein level should be less than 2 g/day. This condition is unrelated to activity or orthostatic positioning. For the diagnosis to be made, symptoms must be present for at least 3 months.
   b. **Additional tests.** Full laboratory workup and renal ultrasound are required to rule out other causes.
   c. **Initial therapy.** Animal studies show possible benefits of treatment with angiotensin-converting enzyme inhibitors. This approach is controversial, however.

    d. Morbidity and mortality. The prognosis is guarded. Some studies show no histologic changes. Others show glomerular changes in 50% of affected children; some of these changes lead to renal failure. Close follow-up is warranted.

3. Orthostatic proteinuria

    a. Diagnosis. Orthostatic proteinuria occurs when the patient is in an upright position. The cause is not well understood, but may be related to increased glomerular filtration in this position. Orthostatic proteinuria is the most common type of proteinuria, accounting for 60% of reproducible cases. It is more common in adolescents and in girls.

    b. Additional tests. Results of urine checks for protein on first waking should be negative. Also indicative are 12-hour collections that show much more proteinuria in the daytime than at night. Total proteinuria must be less than 1 g/day.

    c. Initial therapy. No treatment is necessary.

    d. Prognosis is excellent. No long-term effects are seen in newly diagnosed adolescents. Long-term follow-up of younger children has not been done, however, so children should be evaluated annually.

4. Nephrotic syndrome

    a. Diagnosis. Nephrotic syndrome is significant proteinuria (> 40 mg/m^2/hour) that occurs with hypoproteinemia, edema, and high levels of cholesterol. Most cases are primary; only about 10% of cases are caused by other diseases. The most common type is minimal change disease (75%–85%). The next most common types are focal segmental glomerulosclerosis and membranoproliferative glomerulonephritis. The most important symptom is edema, which may occur at any site and may progress to involve the abdomen, lungs, and scrotum.

    b. Additional tests include urinalysis, albumin level, cholesterol level, and 24-hour urine protein level.

    c. Initial therapy. Most patients with nephrotic syndrome and nearly all patients with minimal change disease respond to steroid therapy. Initially, prednisone, 2 mg/kg/day (maximum, 80 mg), is administered in divided doses. After the urine clears, steroids are tapered slowly over 4–8 weeks. Recurrence may necessitate immunosuppressive therapy. Patients who do not respond to steroids should undergo renal biopsy.

    d. Prognosis depends on the cause. Minimal change disease has an excellent prognosis, with a mortality rate of only 1%. Other causes have a more guarded prognosis. Complications include spontaneous peritonitis, other bacterial infections, and vascular thrombosis.

5. **Glomerulonephritis.** Although hematuria is the hallmark of glomerulonephritis, some proteinuria may occur. The workup, additional tests, therapy, and prognosis depend on the cause and type of the glomerulonephritis.

References

Cruz CC, Spitzer A: When you find protein or blood in the urine. *Contemp Pediatr* 15: 89–109, 1998.

Ettenger RB: The evaluation of the child with proteinuria. *Pediatr Ann* 23(9):486–494, 1994.

81. Hematuria

I INTRODUCTION

A. **Background.** Hematuria (blood in the urine) can come from any segment of the urinary tract, from the glomerulus to the urethra.

B. **Definitions**
1. **Gross hematuria** is blood in the urine detectable by the naked eye.
2. **Microscopic hematuria** is defined as five or more red blood cells per high-power field.

C. **Pathogenesis.** Most childhood hematuria originates from the glomeruli and occurs when red blood cells cross the glomerular endothelial-epithelial barrier to enter the capillary.

D. **Epidemiology.** Hematuria may be found in 5% of school-aged children. Fewer than one half of these cases still have positive results on repeat testing 1 week later.

II APPROACH TO THE PATIENT

A. **History**
1. Hematuria may be asymptomatic or may be accompanied by a number of symptoms, including pain, rash, fever, and edema.
2. A history of trauma, exercise, menstruation, or other iatrogenic manipulations of the urinary tract can lead to a quick diagnosis.
3. Recent infection, either viral or bacterial, can lead to post-infectious glomerulopathy.
4. Dysuria and abdominal pain may indicate urinary tract infection or renal calculi.
5. A complete family history also is important.

B. **Physical examination**
1. The patient's **blood pressure** must be obtained; hypertension mandates an immediate workup.
2. It is important to look for accompanying rashes, fever, or arthritis.
3. The **abdomen** should be closely examined for possible masses.

HOT KEY

All children with hematuria must have their blood pressure checked!

C. Initial workup. The initial evaluation is simple. The only tests required are a microscopic urinalysis and a dipstick test for proteinuria. If the patient also has hypertension, edema, oliguria, or significant proteinuria, other tests to consider include a complete blood cell count, throat culture, streptozyme panel, antinuclear antibody and serum C3. Renal ultrasound also should be considered.

D. Further workup. Because hematuria is a symptom, not a disease, the workup and treatment depend on the cause. Both microscopic and gross hematuria have a large differential diagnosis. A simple mnemonic for remembering this list is **"ABCDEFGHI"**.

ABCDEFGHI

Anatomic or vascular disorders
Bitty boulders (stones)
Cancer
Drugs
Exercise
Familial causes (e.g., benign familial hematuria, Alport syndrome)
Glomerulonephritis
Hematologic disorders (e.g., sickle cell disease), Hypercalciuria
Infection, Immunoglobulin A (IgA) nephropathy

---

1. **Anatomic and vascular disorders.** Although rare in children, arteriovenous malformations and hemangiomas cause gross blood in the urine, possibly with clots.
   a. **Additional tests to consider.** Angiography is the most useful study.
   b. **Urologic consultation** is required; surgery may be needed.
   c. **Prognosis** depends on the type and location of the abnormality.
2. **Stones (renal calculi).** Renal stones usually cause excruciating pain and may be found anywhere in the urinary tract. They can be formed by calcium, oxalate, urate, struvite, or cysteine.
   a. **Additional tests to consider.** Radiographs detect opaque stones, but they are not the gold standard for diagnosis. Ultrasound and intravenous pyelogram are more effective diagnostic tests, but the best test is a spiral computed tomography (CT) scan.
   b. **Initial therapy.** Fluids are the mainstay of treatment. Calculi that do not pass must be fractured with lithotripsy or removed surgically.

      c. Prognosis. After the stones are removed or passed, the prognosis is excellent if dietary changes (reduced calcium and sodium intake) are made.

3. Wilms tumor is the most common renal tumor of childhood. However, the tumor that most commonly causes hematuria in children is renal cell carcinoma, which accounts for fewer than 10% of all renal tumors in children.

      a. Additional tests to consider. Renal ultrasound and CT scan are needed to rule out tumor, and biopsy may be needed for definitive diagnosis.

      b. Initial therapy. Surgery and chemotherapy are warranted, depending on the stage and type of the tumor.

4. Drugs. A thorough medication history is essential. Several common drugs may cause hematuria, including antibiotics, which can damage tubules (e.g., penicillin, sulfonamides), and drugs that can cause cystitis (e.g., cyclophosphamide).

      a. Additional tests to consider. Depending on the drug suspected, tests to measure its levels or effects may help to confirm the diagnosis.

      b. Initial therapy. The drug must be discontinued. If applicable, steps to counteract its effects are instituted.

      c. Prognosis. In most cases, damage to the urinary tract caused by drugs is reversible.

5. Exercise. Hematuria may be caused by exercise, more commonly in boys than in girls. Usually, it is related to the intensity or duration of the exercise.

      a. Additional tests to consider. The exercise is stopped, and urinalysis is repeated in 48 hours. If the hematuria resolves, then the diagnosis can be made.

      b. Initial therapy. No therapy is required.

      c. Prognosis. Most patients have no long-term effects. If a patient has only one kidney, however, consultation with a nephrologist is recommended before exercise is resumed.

6. Familial causes (benign familial hematuria). Benign familial hematuria is an autosomal dominant condition that is not accompanied by proteinuria or other renal symptoms.

      a. Additional tests to consider. Renal biopsy may show minimal glomerular abnormalities.

      b. Initial therapy. No treatment is required.

      c. Prognosis. The prognosis is excellent, and renal failure is rare.

7. Familial causes [Alport syndrome (hereditary nephritis)]. Alport syndrome is an X-linked dominant disease that is accompanied by hearing loss, proteinuria, and renal insufficiency.

      a. **Additional tests to consider.** Diagnosis is made by biopsy or chromosomal testing.

      b. **Initial therapy.** No current treatment prevents eventual renal failure. Treatment should be directed at alleviating symptoms.

      c. **Prognosis.** The prognosis is poor, and many patients progress to end-stage renal disease.

  8. **Glomerulonephritis** (acute poststreptococcal glomerulonephritis) [see Chapter 9]

  9. **Hematologic disorders (sickle cell disease).** A family history is helpful in making this diagnosis, as are accompanying symptoms of a sickle cell crisis.

      a. **Additional tests to consider.** The workup is the same as for a sickle cell crisis: complete blood cell count, reticulocyte count, and renal function tests. The left kidney is affected five times more often than the right kidney.

      b. **Initial therapy.** Antibiotics are required.

      c. **Prognosis.** Approximately 5%–10% of affected patients progress to end-stage renal disease.

  10. **Hypercalciuria** is an idiopathic disorder that is a common cause of renal stones in children.

      a. **Additional tests to consider.** A random urine calcium:creatinine ratio greater than 0.2 requires further testing. A 24-hour urine calcium level greater than 4.0 mg/kg confirms the diagnosis.

      b. **Initial therapy.** Increased fluid intake and a low-sodium diet decreases the amount of calcium in the kidney. The use of thiazide diuretics is not widely accepted.

      c. **Prognosis.** If the hypercalciuria can be corrected, the chance that long-term renal disease will result from it is slight.

  11. **Infection (e.g., urinary tract infection, pyelonephritis)** [see Chapter 83]

  12. **Immunoglobulin A (IgA) nephropathy.** IgA nephropathy is immunologically mediated. It usually occurs after infection and can be accompanied by proteinuria, hypertension, pain, and acute renal failure.

      a. **Additional tests to consider** include complete urinalysis. The definitive diagnosis is made by the detection of immunoglobulin deposits on biopsy specimens.

      b. **Initial therapy** includes anti-inflammatory agents, including steroids and cyclosporine. Antioxidants also may be of therapeutic value.

      c. **Morbidity and mortality.** Approximately 5%–10% of affected patients progress to end-stage renal disease.

References
Cliento BG, Stock JA, Kaplan GW: Hematuria in children: a practical approach. *Urol Clin North Am* 22:(1)43–55, 1995.
Feld LG, Waz WR, Perez LM, et al: Hematuria: an integrated medical and surgical approach. *Pediatr Clin North Am* 44:(5)1191–1210, 1997.
Lieu TA, Grasmeder HM, Kaplan BS: An approach to the evaluation and treatment of microscopic hematuria. *Pediatr Clin North Am* 38(3):579–592, 1991.

82. Acute Renal Failure

I INTRODUCTION

A. **Background.** Acute renal failure (ARF) is common in critically ill or injured patients. Rapid recognition and prompt treatment can be life-saving and can prevent progression to end-stage renal disease. The most common causes of ARF by age group include perinatal asphyxia in newborns and hypovolemia from gastroenteritis in older children.

B. **Definitions**
   1. **ARF** is a rapid decline in renal function (i.e., an increase in creatinine of 0.5 mg/dl/day or more) that causes the retention of nitrogenous (azotemia) and other metabolic waste products and leads to fluid and electrolyte imbalance.
   2. **Oliguria** is urine output less than 0.5 ml/kg/h in infants or less than 300 ml/m^2/day in older children.
   3. **Anuria** is total cessation of urinary output.

C. **Pathogenesis.** The causes of ARF are classified as prerenal, renal, or postrenal. This classification helps to determine possible causes and is used to guide treatment (Table 82-1).
   1. **Prerenal** ARF is the most common type. It occurs when blood flow to the glomerulus is decreased as a result of either hypovolemia or diminished cardiac output. Initially, the glomerular filtration rate and renal blood flow are preserved by autoregulation. However, if kidney hypoperfusion is severe or prolonged, renal failure occurs.
      a. **Hypovolemia** is the most common cause of prerenal ARF. It may be attributable to dehydration as a result of

TABLE Table 82-1. Causes of Acute Renal Failure

Type	Specific Causes
Prerenal	Hypovolemia
	Maldistribution of blood volume
	Decreased cardiac output
Renal	Acute tubular necrosis
	Glomerulonephritis
	Vasculitis
	Interstitial nephritis
Postrenal	Obstruction

gastrointestinal losses, hemorrhage, burns, or renal losses from polyuria (e.g., diabetes insipidus, insulin-dependent diabetes mellitus, diuretics). Causes specific to neonates include blood loss from twin–twin transfusion, birth trauma, abruptio placentae, or severe intraventricular hemorrhage.

b. Maldistribution of blood volume leads to ineffective circulatory volume, even when total body fluid level is normal. Third spacing (e.g., from abdominal surgery, peritonitis, trauma, pancreatitis, or hypoalbuminemia) or shock (e.g., from sepsis, perinatal asphyxia, anaphylaxis, or necrotizing enterocolitis) may decrease circulatory volume and cause ARF.

c. Diminished cardiac output results from congenital or acquired heart disease that progresses to congestive heart failure, arrhythmia, tamponade, or cardiogenic shock.

d. Renal-specific causes include bilateral renal thrombosis (e.g., from indwelling umbilical arterial catheters in premature infants) and renal artery stenosis from fibromuscular dysplasia. Medications such as nonsteroidal antiinflammatory drugs and angiotensin-converting enzyme inhibitors also may contribute.

2. Renal (intrinsic) causes of ARF result from damage to a component of the kidney (e.g., glomeruli, tubules, interstitium, vessels).

a. Acute tubular necrosis (ATN) is the most common cause of intrinsic ARF. It can be caused by the following:

(1) Ischemic injury can be caused by any prolonged prerenal event, especially shock.

(2) Nephrotoxic injury can be caused by antimicrobial agents (e.g., aminoglycosides, amphotericin, cyclosporine, sulfonamides) and chemotherapeutic agents (e.g., methotrexate, cisplatin). Other toxins include ethylene glycol, heavy metals, organic solvents, and radiologic contrast dyes.

(3) Endogenous pigments include hemoglobin (e.g., from disseminated intravascular coagulation, transfusion reactions, or glucose-6-phosphate dehydrogenase deficiency) and myoglobin (e.g., from rhabdomyolysis, trauma, myositis, seizure, or carnitine palmityl transferase deficiency).

b. Glomerulonephritis. Examples include postinfectious glomerulonephritis, membranoproliferative glomerulonephritis, Henoch-Schönlein purpura nephritis, immunoglobulin A nephritis, and systemic lupus erythematosus nephritis.

c. Vasculitis of childhood can be caused by hemolyticuremic syndrome (especially from *Escherichia coli* O157:H7 infection), Kawasaki disease, and polyarteritis nodosa.

    d. Acute interstitial nephritis can be caused by drugs (e.g., beta-lactam antibiotics, rifampin, acyclovir, diuretics) and infection (e.g., infectious mononucleosis, streptococcal infection).
3. **Postrenal** ARF occurs in patients with a lower tract obstruction or bilateral upper tract obstructions. Unilateral upper tract obstruction does not lead to ARF because the unaffected kidney compensates.

    (1) Structural congenital anomalies. Examples include posterior urethral valves or an ectopic ureter.

    (2) Functional abnormalities. Examples include neurogenic bladder or anticholinergic drugs.

    (3) Obstruction can be caused by calculi or precipitated uric acid (e.g., from cell lysis before or after chemotherapy).

HOT KEY Prerenal and postrenal causes are extrarenal causes of ARF. If these conditions are not recognized and treated promptly, however, they may progress to intrinsic renal failure (ATN).

II CLINICAL MANIFESTATIONS. ARF usually occurs in the setting of decreased urine output. However, nonoliguric renal failure also occurs, especially from nephrotoxic drug injuries.

A. Nonspecific generalized symptoms, including lethargy, anorexia, vomiting, and abdominal pain, occur if ARF is prolonged or severe.
B. Electrolyte abnormalities are common [see III A 3 a (3)].
C. Hypertension occurs as a result of extracellular volume expansion and often is accompanied by peripheral and pulmonary edema.
D. Metabolic acidosis often occurs when acid–base homeostasis is lost.

III APPROACH TO THE PATIENT

A. Diagnosis. Decreasing urine output and abnormal laboratory values help to establish the diagnosis. An increase in the blood urea nitrogen level of 10–20 mg/dl/day or a creatinine level of 0.5–1.5 mg/dl/day, often accompanied by electrolyte abnormalities, suggests ARF.
1. **History.** Vomiting or diarrhea suggests a prerenal cause. A sudden decrease in urine output suggests a postrenal etiology. The patient's medication list should be reviewed for drug-related causes.

2. **Physical examination.** Tachycardia or hypotension suggests a prerenal cause. An unstable temperature may indicate sepsis. A palpable bladder suggests obstruction; urine output should be measured to determine whether renal failure is oliguric or nonoliguric.
3. **Laboratory tests**
   a. **Basic laboratory tests,** such as a complete blood cell count, electrolyte measurements, and urinalysis, differentiate between prerenal and renal causes; however, recent use of diuretics may invalidate test results (Table 82–2).
      (1) **Urinalysis**
         (a) **A specific gravity** greater than 1.016 suggests urine concentration and a prerenal etiology.
         (b) **Casts.** Red blood cell or granular casts suggest glomerulonephritis or vasculitis. White blood cell casts suggest infection or inflammation (interstitial nephritis). Tubular casts suggest acute tubular necrosis.
         (c) **Eosinophils** suggest interstitial nephritis.
         (d) **A heme-positive dipstick reading,** with few red blood cells seen microscopically, suggests myoglobinuria or hemoglobinuria.
      (2) **Complete blood cell count.** Microangiopathic hemolytic anemia with thrombocytopenia occurs with hemolytic uremic syndrome. An elevated white blood cell count is seen with infection or interstitial nephritis.
      (3) **Electrolyte levels** commonly indicate hyponatremia, hyperkalemia, hypocalcemia, hyperphosphatemia, and hypermagnesemia.

TABLE 82-2. Differentiation of Renal and Prerenal Causes of Acute Renal Failure Based on Laboratory Data

Laboratory Value	Prerenal	Renal
FENa%	< 1% (< 2.5% in newborn)	> 2.5%
Blood urea nitrogen: creatinine ratio	> 20	< 10
Urine Na$^+$	< 20	> 40
Urine osmolarity	> 400 mOsm/L (> 350 mOsm/L in newborn)	< 350

FENa, fractional excretion of sodium.

$$FENa = \frac{Urine\ Na^+/Plasma\ Na^+}{Urine\ Cr/Plasma\ Cr} \times 100\%$$

   b. **Additional laboratory testing** should be based on the suspected etiology. The creatine phosphokinase level should be determined if rhabdomyolysis is suspected. Complement levels (C3, C4), anti-streptolysin-O titer, streptozymes, and anti-DNAaseB should be considered if acute poststreptococcal glomerulonephritis is suspected. An antinuclear antibody test should be performed if nephritis caused by systemic lupus erythematosus is suspected. Antineutrophil cytoplasmic antibodies (ANCA) should be measured if vasculitis is suspected.

4. **Imaging studies.** Renal ultrasound is useful in evaluating anatomic abnormalities, kidney size, hydronephrosis, and renal blood flow. A renal nuclear scan can estimate renal perfusion and function.

5. **Renal biopsy** can help provide a definitive diagnosis if the etiology remains unknown.

B. **Treatment** usually is supportive and consists of fluid management, adjusting any medication dosages according to renal function, and avoiding nephrotoxic drugs if possible.

1. **Prerenal ARF.** Intravascular volume is restored with a 10–20 ml/kg bolus of normal saline or 5% albumin. This treatment may be repeated as needed; however, fluid status should be monitored to avoid fluid overload. If the etiology is impaired cardiac output, inotropic support with dopamine or dobutamine should be considered.

2. **Renal ARF**

   a. **Fluid restriction** often is necessary to prevent fluid overload and to allow time for the kidneys to recover. Insensible water loss of approximately 400 ml/m^2/day (approximately 700 ml/m^2/day in infants) should be replaced with D_5W–$D_{10}W$. All other losses (e.g., urine output, vomiting) are replaced with 1/2 normal saline at a 1:1 ratio. Fluid input and output as well as daily weight should be monitored closely.

   b. **Electrolyte abnormalities** must be monitored and corrected. Metabolic acidosis should be monitored; sodium bicarbonate or tris (hydroxymethyl) THAM often is used to correct acidosis.

   c. A low-salt, low-potassium, and low-protein diet should be followed.

   d. **Hypertension** is controlled with nifedipine, 0.25–1.0 mg/kg/dose. The dose may be repeated within 30 minutes and then every 3–4 hours. Diazoxide, hydralazine, labetalol, and sodium nitroprusside also are used.

   e. Loop and osmotic diuretics often are used to convert oliguric ARF to nonoliguric ARF; however, the effect of this treatment on morbidity is unclear.

   3. **Postrenal ARF.** Treatment requires removal of obstructions
      (e.g., placement of a Foley catheter, vesicostomy, ureteral
      stents, or nephrostomy tubes) and management of postob-
      structive diuresis, which can lead to hypokalemia, hypona-
      tremia, and hypotension.
C. Indications for acute dialysis can be remembered with the
   mnemonic "AEIOU."

"AEIOU"

Acidosis: Complications of metabolic acidosis (e.g.,
   arrhythmias, left ventricular dysfunction) or pH
   less than 7.2. Sodium bicarbonate can be used as
   a temporizing measure until dialysis is initiated.

Electrolytes: Severe hyperkalemia (> 6.5–7 mEq/L)
   or hyperkalemia with changes on electrocardiogram (peaked T wave, prolongation of P-R interval, and widening of QRS). The treatment can be
   remembered with the mnemonic **"C-A-BIG-K":**
   intravenous **c**alcium, **a**lbuterol, sodium **b**icarbon-
   ate, **i**nsulin, and **g**lucose and sodium polystyrene
   sulfonate (**K**ayexalate)

Intoxication: ARF from a dialyzable, toxic ingestion
   (e.g., salicylates, ethylene glycol)

Overload: Volume overload that is refractory to diuretics. Temporizing measures include nitrates
   and furosemide.

Uremia: Dialysis often is needed when blood urea
   nitrogen is greater than 100 mg/dl or when certain
   symptoms occur (altered mental status, seizures,
   pericarditis, intractable nausea and vomiting, uncontrolled bleeding as a result of platelet dysfunction).

 PROGNOSIS. If the underlying cause is recognized and
treated early, the prognosis is good. However, ARF often occurs in association with conditions that have high mortality
rates (e.g., septic shock).

References
Sehic A, Chesney RW: Acute renal failure: diagnosis. *Pediatr Rev* 16(3):101–106, 1995.
Sehic A, Chesney RW: Acute renal failure: therapy. *Pediatr Rev* 16(4):137–141, 1995.
Stewart CL, Barnett R: Acute renal failure in infants, children and adults. *Crit Care
    Clin* 13(3):575–590, 1997.
Thadhani R, Pascual M, Bonventre J: Acute renal failure. *N Engl J Med* 334(22):
    1448–1457, 1996.

83. Urinary Tract Infections

I   INTRODUCTION

A. Background. Urinary tract infection (UTI) is the most common serious bacterial infection in febrile infants and children. Recurrent UTIs can lead to renal failure in children and are a significant contributor to adult hypertension.

B. Definitions
   1. **Pyelonephritis** is a bacterial infection of the upper urinary tract with involvement of the renal parenchyma.
   2. **Cystitis** is a UTI of the bladder. It is not associated with fever or renal injury.
   3. **Asymptomatic bacteriuria** is a positive bacterial urine culture without clinical manifestations or renal sequelae (present in approximately 0.5% of children).

C. Pathogenesis. UTIs are usually caused when bacteria ascend from the perineal region to the urinary tract through the urethra. Other contributing factors include poor hygiene, pinworms, perineal irritation, dysfunctional voiding, constipation, neurogenic bladder, and sexual activity.

D. Epidemiology
   1. Half of all febrile UTIs, which are presumed to be pyelonephritis, occur in children younger than 12 months of age.
   2. In the first year of life, boys have UTIs about half as often as girls. Most UTIs in boys occur in infancy. After the first year of life, the incidence is much higher in girls than in boys.
   3. The overall incidence of UTI in infants is approximately 1%.
   4. Circumcision decreases the risk of UTI in male infants from approximately 1:100 to 1:1000.

HOT

KEY

In children younger than 12 months of age who have a fever and no obvious clinical source, approximately 5% have a UTI.

E. Microbiology. UTIs usually are caused by gram-negative bacteria, such as *Escherichia coli* (approximately 75% of all cases), *Klebsiella, Proteus* (can be associated with stone formation), and *Pseudomonas.* Occasionally, these infections are caused by gram-positive bacteria, such as *Enterococcus, Staphylococcus aureus,* or *S. saprophyticus* (especially in teenage girls).

II CLINICAL MANIFESTATIONS

A. **Symptoms** may vary, depending on which part of the urinary tract is involved.
   1. Urethritis may cause dysuria and increased frequency.
   2. Cystitis may cause dysuria and increased frequency as well as urgency and suprapubic pain.
   3. Pyelonephritis may cause all of the symptoms described for urethritis and cystitis as well as flank pain, vomiting, and systemic symptoms, such as fever. Symptoms do not reliably differentiate between cystitis and pyelonephritis in infants and young children, so pyelonephritis always must be considered in these age groups.
   4. Other symptoms may include enuresis, foul-smelling urine, and hematuria.
B. **Differential diagnosis** includes chemical urethritis, diabetes, a mass adjacent to the bladder, dehydration, appendicitis, gastroenteritis, and pelvic inflammatory disease.
C. **Complications**
   1. The greatest risk of renal damage occurs in infants and children younger than 2 years of age. Bacteremia and urosepsis occurs in as many as 30% of neonates with UTI.
   2. Repeat episodes of pyelonephritis (febrile UTIs) can lead to scarring of the renal parenchyma. As many as 50% of children with renal scarring have hypertension by 30 years of age.
   3. Some patients progress to end-stage renal disease. Approximately 10% of all pediatric renal transplantation and dialysis patients have a history of recurrent UTIs.

III APPROACH TO THE PATIENT

A. **Diagnosis**
   1. Table 83–1 shows the advantages and disadvantages of **various urine collection methods**.
   2. **Urinalysis** consists of biochemical tests and microscopy. The findings can suggest the presence of a UTI, but a specimen must be sent for urine culture (by catheterization in an infant or young child) before presumptive antibiotic treatment is begun. Urine dipsticks are useful for home screening in patients who have a history of recurrent UTIs.
      a. **Leukocyte esterase** has a sensitivity and specificity of approximately 80%. A positive leukocyte esterase test result may suggest UTI, but it is not by itself reliable for diagnosis.
      b. **Nitrite** test results are not sensitive (approximately 50%), but are very specific (approximately 98%). This test is less

TABLE 83-1. Urine Collection Methods

Method	Diagnostic of UTI If:	Advantages	Disadvantages
Bag specimen	Usually not considered diagnostic because of high likelihood of contamination	Noninvasive UTI extremely unlikely if urine culture is negative (sensitivity almost 100%)	Must wait until patient voids Contamination causes unacceptable false-positive rate (specificity < 15%)
Clean-voided specimen	> 100,000 cfu/ml of a single organism	Noninvasive	Requires toilet-trained, cooperative patient (mid-stream specimen is best)
Transurethral catheterization	> 1,000 cfu/ml	Contamination very unlikely with good sterile technique	Invasive (but safe) May not be possible in children with labial adhesion or phimosis
Suprapubic aspiration	Any gram-negative organism > 1,000 cfu/ml of a gram-positive organism	Contamination very unlikely	Invasive (but safe) Urine may be difficult to obtain if the patient has recently voided

cfu = colony-forming units; UTI = urinary tract infection.

sensitive in young children because urine must remain in the bladder for several hours for nitrite production to occur.

c. **Pyuria** is diagnosed if more than 10 white blood cells/mm^3 are noted in an unspun specimen or if more than 5 white blood cells/high-power field are noted in a spun specimen.

d. **Bacteriuria** is identified by Gram stain and microscopy. It may occur as asymptomatic bacteriuria.

HOT KEY

About 10% of infants with a UTI have a completely negative urinalysis; a urine culture should always be performed.

B. Therapy

1. **Cystitis.** In **school-age children,** a short course (3 days) of an oral antibiotic usually is sufficient.

2. **Presumed pyelonephritis**

   a. **Infants (< 6 weeks of age).** A full 14-day course of a parenteral antibiotic is recommended.

   b. **Infants and young children (6 weeks–2 years of age)**

      (1) **Parenteral antibiotics** are used if the child appears ill, is dehydrated, is vomiting, or if compliance cannot be ensured. Parenteral antibiotics are continued until the patient is afebrile for a period of 24 to 48 hours. Oral antibiotics are then given to complete a total of 14 days of therapy.

      (2) Treatment may be initiated with **oral antibiotics** if the patient appears well. Many experts prefer a 14-day course of therapy.

3. **Appropriate antibiotic agents**

   a. **Parenteral antibiotics**

      (1) **Ampicillin** often is used in combination with gentamicin to treat infection with gram-positive organisms.

      (2) **Aminoglycosides (e.g., gentamicin)** achieve adequate therapeutic levels in the bloodstream and in renal tissue, but may be nephrotoxic.

      (3) **Cephalosporins** also achieve therapeutic levels in tissue. Ceftriaxone is administered once daily and is convenient for outpatient parenteral therapy.

   b. **Oral antibiotic treatment** is based on the susceptibility of bacteria identified by urine culture.

      (1) **Amoxicillin** is well concentrated in the urine. *E. coli* resistance to amoxicillin is increasing.

      (2) **Trimethoprim-sulfamethoxazole.** Although bacterial

resistance to *E. coli* is increasing, trimethoprim-sulfamethoxazole is still an appropriate first-line agent for *E. coli.*

(3) **Cephalosporins.** Cefixime may be adequate treatment for pyelonephritis, even in children younger than age 2 years.

HOT **KEY**   Repeat urine culture is unnecessary unless the clinical response to treatment is inadequate or the cultured organism is resistant to the administered antibiotic.

C. Evaluation
  1. A careful **radiologic evaluation** is necessary for several reasons:
      a. Pyelonephritis may be difficult to diagnose in infants and young children on the basis of symptoms alone.
      b. Infants and young children with UTIs are at significant risk for renal scarring.
      c. Vesicoureteral reflux (VUR) is common in children with UTIs (30%–50%). Even without VUR, pyelonephritis may occur.
  2. **Renal ultrasound** should be performed in all children with first-time febrile UTI to rule out anatomic abnormalities. This test is noninvasive and can identify renal obstruction. However, it does not reliably detect pyelonephritis, VUR, or renal function.
  3. **Voiding cystourethrogram (VCUG)** [Table 83–2] is recommended in all boys who have a UTI and in all girls younger than age 6 years who have pyelonephritis. It shows both the presence and the severity of VUR as well as bladder and urethral abnormalities. The voiding phase of a VCUG is important in the identification of VUR and should be performed as soon as a UTI clinically resolves.

HOT **KEY**   All first-time febrile UTIs require a renal ultrasound. A girl younger than age 6 years with pyelonephritis or any boy with a UTI should undergo VCUG.

---

  4. **Radionuclide cystogram** is useful in the follow-up of children with known VUR and should be considered in asymptomatic siblings of children with VUR. It does not reliably detect grade I VUR and shows less anatomic detail than VCUG.
  5. **Dimethylsuccinic acid (DMSA) scan.** The role of DMSA

TABLE 83-2. Grading of Vesicoureteral Reflux	
Grade I	Reflux into a ureter without dilatation
Grade II	Reflux into the upper collecting system without dilatation
Grade III	Reflux into a dilated ureter and/or blunting of calyces
Grade IV	Reflux into a grossly dilated ureter
Grade V	Massive reflux with significant dilatation and tortuosity of the ureter and loss of calyceal appearance

scan in the evaluation of children with UTI is unclear. A DMSA scan is used to detect renal scarring in children with VUR as well as in the follow-up of children with known renal scarring. This test is also sensitive in the detection of acute pyelonephritis. However, it does not detect renal obstruction.

D. Prevention
1. Regulation of voiding habits and treatment of constipation may help decrease the risk of UTI.
2. Avoidance of back-to-front wiping and bubble baths does not decrease the risk of UTI.
3. Prophylactic antibiotics are indicated in children with VUR and may be indicated in children with recurrent UTIs who do not have VUR. Antibiotics that do not select for resistant fecal flora (e.g., nitrofurantoin, trimethoprim-sulfamethoxazole) can be used.

 HOT KEY After antibiotic treatment of a UTI is completed, empiric antibiotic prophylaxis should be given until the radiologic evaluation is complete. This is especially important for patients who are less than 2 years old.

IV PROGNOSIS

A. Resolution of VUR
1. **Grades I and II.** Approximately one third of cases resolve each year; approximately 80%–90% resolve completely.
2. **Grades IV and V.** Approximately 40%–45% of cases resolve completely.

HOT KEY

High-grade VUR (grades IV–V) warrants referral to a urologist.

B. The likelihood of renal scarring increases with each subsequent UTI. The likelihood of recurrent UTI is as follows:
   1. 30% if the patient has had one previous UTI
   2. 60% if the patient has had two previous UTIs
   3. 70% if the patient has had three previous UTIs

References

Committee on Quality Improvement, AAP: Practice parameter: the diagnosis, treatment, and evaluation of the initial urinary tract infection in febrile infants and young children. *Pediatrics* 103(4 Pt 1):843–852, 1999.

Rushton HG: Urinary tract infections in children: epidemiology, evaluation, and management. *Pediatr Clin North Am* 4(5):1133–1169, 1997.

Todd JK: Management of urinary tract infections: children are different. *Pediatr Rev* 16(5):190–196,1995.

84. Swollen Scrotum

I **INTRODUCTION.** Acute scrotal pain is a rare but potentially serious presenting symptom. Acute scrotal pain is a potential surgical emergency that may lead to loss of the testicle. The typical causes of acute scrotal pain are epididymitis, testicular torsion, and torsion of the appendix testis.

A. Pathogenesis

1. **Epididymitis** is inflammation of the epididymis. It usually occurs secondary to bacterial infection, but also may result from trauma.
2. **Testicular torsion** occurs when the testis rotates within the tunica vaginalis, kinking off venous and arterial blood flow. It often results from a congenital deformity in which the testis is not attached to the enveloping fascia.
3. **Torsion of the appendix testis.** The appendix testis is an embryologic remnant of the Müllerian duct system. It is located at the superior pole of the testis. Through unknown mechanisms, these remnants are susceptible to torsion that results in inflammation and edema.

B. Epidemiology

1. **Epididymitis** previously was thought to occur most commonly in association with gonorrhea and chlamydia in sexually active adolescents and adults. However, recent research casts doubt on this belief. An episode of infectious epididymitis in a prepubescent boy usually signifies an anatomic malformation (ureteral and vasal abnormalities).
2. **Testicular torsion** most commonly occurs in prepubertal and pubertal boys. It is rare in infancy. The incidence is 1:160 boys. It is the cause of 14%–38% of cases of acute scrotal pain in children.
3. **Torsion of the appendix testis** is most common in prepubertal boys (7–12 years of age). Appendiceal torsion is the final diagnosis in 14%–46% of patients with acute scrotal pain.

II **CLINICAL MANIFESTATIONS**

A. History

1. **Epididymitis.** Pain typically is insidious in onset, and the patient may have associated fever, urinary frequency, and dysuria.

HOT KEY

Although a thorough history is always important, none of these conditions can be diagnosed based on history alone.

2. **Testicular torsion.** The classic presentation is that of a pubertal boy with sudden onset of severe, unilateral scrotal pain, often accompanied by nausea and vomiting. The pain may occur during activity, at rest, or after trauma. Boys with testicular torsion tend to seek medical care earlier than do boys with other scrotal conditions.

3. **Torsion of the appendix testis.** Typically, the pain is not debilitating and appears gradually over a few days. Often, the boy has experienced similar pain for brief, intermittent episodes over the preceding few weeks. Nausea, vomiting, and fever are rare.

B. **Physical examination.** A thorough examination begins with an overall assessment of the patient's level of discomfort. The patient should stand while the scrotum is examined for erythema, swelling, and lie of the testis (the testis normally lies in the scrotum with its long axis perpendicular to the frontal plane). The cremasteric reflex should be assessed bilaterally; however, it is not consistently present after the onset of puberty.

HOT KEY

Some boys are embarrassed by the source of the pain and complain only of vague abdominal or "groin" pain. All boys with such complaints require a thorough genital examination.

1. **Epididymitis.** The patient may be febrile, with scrotal erythema and edema as well as an exquisitely tender epididymis. Scrotal erythema and swelling progress without treatment.

2. **Testicular torsion.** A few hours after the onset of pain, examination typically shows a tender, swollen, transverse-lying testis with overlying scrotal erythema. Swelling and erythema increase with time. The cremasteric reflex is usually absent.

3. **Torsion of the appendix testis.** Examination early in the course of illness shows little or no edema and erythema of the involved hemiscrotum. Tenderness usually is limited to the superior pole of the testis. The appearance of a small blue dot under the scrotal skin overlying the superior pole of the testis is pathognomonic for torsion of the appendix testis.

C. Differential diagnosis. Other diagnoses to consider include idiopathic scrotal edema, hydrocele, Henoch-Schönlein purpura,
varicocele (collection of enlarged veins of the pampiniform
plexus, with a characteristic "bag of worms" feel), and inguinal
hernia. Testicular cancer is rare in adolescence, but any scrotal
mass (except an obvious varicocele) should be imaged.

III APPROACH TO THE PATIENT

HOT KEY Acute scrotal pain that occurs after trauma and persists for
longer than 1 hour mandates further evaluation and diagnostic imaging.

A. Diagnosis. Making a definitive diagnosis in patients with acute
scrotal pain can be challenging. Urinalysis and culture should be
obtained if epididymitis is suspected. The viability of the testis
depends on the length of time that it is torsed; 12 hours is the
upper limit of survivability. Therefore, patients whose history
and examination suggest testicular torsion should go directly to
the operating room. However, these patients are few because
there are few pathognomonic findings in the history or physical
examination. Patients with equivocal findings on physical examination should undergo diagnostic imaging.

B. Diagnostic imaging. Color Doppler ultrasound is helpful in determining the need for surgery in patients who have acute scrotal pain. In patients with testicular torsion, color Doppler ultrasound shows decreased or absent blood flow. In patients with
torsion of the appendix testis and epididymitis, there is normal
or increased blood flow. Color Doppler ultrasound is not available in all hospitals, and its sensitivity is dependent on the skill
of the operator. In addition, results are unreliable for children
younger than age 6 years because of the small size of the testis.

HOT KEY A definitive diagnosis is difficult to make without imaging or
surgery. Therefore, a urologic consultation must be obtained.

C. Treatment
  1. Epididymitis. Febrile patients with severe epididymitis are
    admitted to the hospital and treated initially with broad-
    spectrum antibiotics to prevent the formation of abscesses

that could result in loss of the testis. Outpatient treatment consists of oral antibiotics, anti-inflammatory medications and analgesics, scrotal elevation, and bed rest. Antibiotic coverage is tailored based on the results of urine culture, and treatment is continued for 2 weeks. Symptoms usually resolve within 1 week.

2. **Testicular torsion.** If the findings of the history and physical examination indicate testicular torsion, the patient should proceed directly to the operating room. During surgery, the testis is detorsed and its viability assessed. If the involved testis is viable, both testes are secured within the tunica vaginalis to prevent recurrence. If the testis is not viable, it is removed.

3. **Torsion of the appendix testis.** With anti-inflammatory and analgesic medications, bed rest, and scrotal elevation, symptoms usually resolve within 1 week.

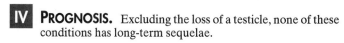 **PROGNOSIS.** Excluding the loss of a testicle, none of these conditions has long-term sequelae.

References

Kadish HA, Bolte RG: A retrospective review of pediatric patients with epididymitis, testicular torsion, and torsion of testicular appendages. *Pediatrics* 102(1 Pt 1): 73–76, 1998.

Kass EJ, Lundak B: The acute scrotum. *Pediatr Clin North Am* 44(5):1251–1266, 1997.

PART X

GASTROENTEROLOGY

85. Vomiting During Infancy

I **INTRODUCTION.** Vomiting during infancy is caused by a wide range of conditions **(Table 85–1).** Although the cause of vomiting usually is not serious, a high index of suspicion is necessary to ensure prompt referral and management of potentially life-threatening conditions.

II **VOMITING IN THE NEWBORN PERIOD.** This may be caused by intestinal atresia or obstruction. Immediate surgical consultation is required whenever intestinal obstruction is suspected. The infant should be given nothing by mouth, and a nasogastric catheter should be placed on low intermittent suction.

A. **Esophageal atresia** causes regurgitation of saliva and difficulty feeding immediately after birth. The diagnosis can be made by

TABLE 85-1. Conditions That Cause Vomiting in Infants	
Conditions	**Age at Onset**
Intestinal atresia or obstruction	Newborn period
Esophageal atresia	
Duodenal atresia	
Hirschsprung disease	
Meconium ileus	
Malrotation (midgut volvulus)	
Pyloric stenosis	First month of life (usually 3 weeks)
Gastroesophageal reflux	First month of life
Intussusception	5–9 months of age
Incarcerated inguinal hernia	2–12 months of age

gently attempting to introduce a catheter into the stomach. If the esophagus ends in a blind pouch, the catheter will not pass into the stomach. A radiograph confirms that the catheter has remained coiled in the esophagus.

B. Duodenal atresia causes bilious vomiting shortly after birth. As with all intestinal atresias, there often is a history of polyhydramnios in utero. The classic radiographic finding is a "double bubble," with air noted in the stomach and proximal duodenum, separated by the pylorus. This sign may disappear after a nasogastric tube is inserted to evacuate gastric air.

C. Hirschsprung disease varies in severity. The most severely affected infants have profuse vomiting and enterocolitis.

D. Meconium ileus. Approximately 10% of newborns with cystic fibrosis have inspissated meconium. Constipation may progress to vomiting if it is not relieved by enemas. Surgical intervention occasionally is required.

E. Malrotation (midgut volvulus)

 1. **Pathogenesis.** Malrotation with volvulus is a dangerous obstructing lesion that requires a high index of suspicion to diagnose. Usually, the axis points of the midgut are on the duodenum, which is held in place by the ligament of Treitz (in the upper left quadrant), and the cecum, which is held in place by Ladd bands (in the lower right quadrant). These two bands provide a long axis on which the bowel cannot rotate. In malrotation, incomplete rotation of the developing bowel can leave the cecum higher than normal. Both of the axis points are located in the upper right quadrant, providing a short axis on which the small bowel can twist. Persistent volvulus leads to ischemia of the intestine and eventual sepsis.

 2. **Epidemiology.** Malrotation occurs in 1:500 live births. Approximately 40% of cases occur during the first week of life, 50% in the first month, and 80% in the first year.

 3. **Symptoms.** Bilious vomiting is the hallmark of malrotation. Typically, there is a sudden onset of bilious vomiting and pain in a previously normal infant.

 4. **Physical findings.** In the earliest stages, few patients have tenderness to palpation. Findings on abdominal examination are normal in approximately 50% of patients. As ischemia progresses, however, fever, sepsis, and peritonitis may occur.

 5. **Workup.** Upper gastrointestinal radiographs or ultrasound can be used to determine the location of the ligament of Treitz.

 6. **Treatment.** Fluid resuscitation is required, a nasogastric tube is placed, and the patient is given broad-spectrum antibiotics. Immediate laparotomy is indicated. The bowel is untwisted and assessed for viability. Necrotic bowel is resected, and a Ladd procedure is performed to correct the malrotation.

>
> **HOT**
> **KEY**
>
> Bilious (green) vomiting in a neonate is malrotation with volvu-
> lus until proven otherwise. Quick intervention is essential to
> prevent bowel necrosis and death.

III VOMITING IN THE FIRST MONTH OF LIFE

A. **Pyloric stenosis**
  1. **Pathogenesis.** The etiology of pyloric stenosis is unknown.
     There is marked hypertrophy of the muscular layers of the
     pyloric sphincter. The stomach becomes dilated and hyper-
     trophied from the constant effort to propel its contents
     through the stenotic sphincter.
  2. **Epidemiology.** Pyloric stenosis is common, occurring in
     1:400 births. There is a strong male predominance (5:1) and
     a strong genetic association, especially in the maternal line.
     Pyloric stenosis occurs in infants between 1 and 10 weeks of
     age. The average age at presentation is 3 weeks.
  3. **Symptoms.** Pyloric stenosis is characterized by progressively
     worsening, nonbilious vomiting. The emesis occasionally is
     bloody. Vomiting usually occurs 30–60 minutes after a
     feeding, and the infant typically remains hungry.
  4. **Physical findings.** The finding of an "olive" (a 1- to 2-cm, ob-
     long, smooth, firm mass in the epigastrium) is diagnostic for
     pyloric stenosis and warrants surgical correction. The exam-
     ination is best performed on a quiet, relaxed infant with the
     legs elevated and flexed. After feeding, gastric peristaltic
     waves sometimes are seen.
  5. **Workup.** Two thirds of infants with pyloric stenosis have
     hypochloremic, hypokalemic, metabolic alkalosis. Sonogra-
     phy is a useful adjunct when the findings on clinical exami-
     nation are unclear. Ultrasound may reveal a thickened, elon-
     gated pylorus. An upper gastrointestinal study may show the
     classic "string sign," but this test should be reserved for cases
     in which ultrasound findings are inconclusive.
  6. **Treatment.** Surgery is nonemergent. Initial medical man-
     agement consists of correction of dehydration and elec-
     trolyte abnormalities. Patients with dehydration are given an
     isotonic saline bolus, and D_5 1/2 normal saline at 1.5 × main-
     tenance is continued until the child is euvolemic. The oper-
     ative treatment is **Ramstedt pyloromyotomy,** which involves
     splitting the hypertrophied pyloric muscle.
B. **Gastroesophageal reflux** (see Chapter 91) is the most common
   treatable cause of vomiting in infants. Reflux often is associated
   with irritability, nonbilious vomiting, poor weight gain, stridor,
   wheezing, or arching of the back and turning of the neck (Sandifer

syndrome). The differential diagnosis includes pyloric stenosis, malrotation, and metabolic disorders.

IV VOMITING AFTER THE FIRST MONTH OF LIFE

A. **Intussusception,** or telescoping of a proximal portion of bowel into a distal portion, is a common surgical emergency in infants. Classically, there is a history of severe, colicky abdominal pain every 5–30 minutes. The episodes may be separated by periods of normal behavior or lethargy. Vomiting may progress to become bilious. In some cases, stools become dark red and mucoid (like currant jelly). Most cases occur in children who are 5–9 months old.

B. **Incarcerated inguinal hernia**

1. **Pathogenesis.** Incomplete obliteration of the processus vaginalis leaves a passage through which abdominal contents can enter the groin. Incarceration is the most serious complication; unrelieved incarceration can progress to strangulation and ischemia.

2. **Epidemiology.** The hernia may occur at any age, but 70% of incarcerated hernias occur before 1 year of age.

3. **Symptoms.** The patient may have a history of a bulge in the groin. In addition to swelling and discoloration of the groin area, infants typically have irritability and vomiting. Prolonged incarceration may cause fever and abdominal distension.

4. **Treatment.** Intermittent inguinal herniation requires prompt referral to a surgeon. An incarcerated hernia requires immediate surgical evaluation; attempts at manual reduction should not be postponed. Manual reduction is most successful if the patient is sedated and in the Trendelenburg position. If the hernia cannot be reduced manually, immediate surgery is required.

References

Garcia VF, Randolph JG: Pyloric stenosis: diagnosis and management. *Pediatr Rev* 11(10):292–296,1990.

Irish MS, Pearl RH, Caty MG, et al: The approach to common abdominal diagnoses in infants and children. *Pediatr Clin North Am* 45(4):729–772, 1998.

Ross AJ: Intestinal obstruction in the newborn. *Pediatr Rev* 15(9):338–347, 1994.

86. Intussusception

I INTRODUCTION

A. Background. Intussusception is a common cause of bowel obstruction in children younger than age 2 years. It typically occurs between ages 3 months and 1 year.

B. Definition. Intussusception is telescoping of a proximal segment of bowel (intussusceptum) into a distal segment (intussuscipiens).

C. Pathogenesis

   1. Associated illness. Intussusception is believed to be associated with viral processes (e.g., upper respiratory infections or acute gastroenteritis). Hypertrophied Peyer patches may act as lead points of intussusception.

   a. As the proximal segment telescopes into the distal segment, pressure on the associated mesentery leads to edema, venous and lymphatic congestion, and possible vascular compromise.

   b. The telescoped bowel becomes obstructed, leading to abdominal pain and vomiting. The vascular congestion leads to bloody, mucoid stools ("currant jelly stool").

   c. If the obstruction is not corrected, vascular compromise and necrosis of the intussuscepted bowel may occur.

   2. Anatomic anomalies. In neonates or in children older than age 5 years, intussusception may be caused by anatomic anomalies [e.g., Meckel diverticulum, polyps, vascular malformations, Hirschsprung disease (see Chapter 87), meconium ileus secondary to cystic fibrosis, Henoch-Schönlein purpura, lymphoma].

D. Epidemiology

   1. More than 75% of cases of ileocolic intussusception are idiopathic.

   2. There is a predominance in males (2:1).

   3. Approximately 60% of patients are younger than 1 year of age; 80% of patients are younger than 2 years of age.

   4. As many as 5% of cases may recur in the first 24 hours. No reliable clinical indicators are predictive of recurrence.

II CLINICAL MANIFESTATIONS

A. Symptoms

   1. Emesis initially is clear, but may become bilious or even fecaloid. Pain often precedes vomiting.

2. Sudden onset of **intermittent, crampy abdominal pain** (screaming, inconsolable crying, pulling the legs to the chest) is characteristic.

3. Between episodes, the child appears normal and has no pain. Eventually, however, the patient may become lethargic. Symptoms may resemble those of sepsis or meningitis.

4. Normal stools are passed within the first few hours. After this, stool output is scant, and there is little or no flatus.

5. **Bloody, mucous stool** usually occurs within the first 12 hours but may be delayed as much as 48 hours. Sixty percent of patients with intussusception have bloody, mucous stools.

HOT

Always consider intussusception in lethargic patients who have a history of severe crampy abdominal pain.
KEY

B. **Physical examination.** Patients may have a palpable, sausage-shaped abdominal mass in the midepigastric region or hepatic flexure. (It is important to remember that the mass may not be palpable if it is positioned under the liver.) Classically, there is an absence of bowel in the right lower quadrant (Dance sign).

III APPROACH TO THE PATIENT

A. **Diagnosis.** The diagnosis is suggested based on the history and physical examination. It often is confirmed by abdominal radiography.

1. Upright and supine abdominal films may show a range of findings, from nonspecific bowel gas patterns, to ileus with air-fluid levels, to a clearly obstructive small bowel pattern.

2. **Free air** may be seen if perforation occurs. Plain films may show an empty sigmoid or rectum or a soft tissue mass outlined by air.

3. An "**adipose rose,**" which represents the intussusception in cross-section in the upper right quadrant, is a classic finding.

B. **Differential diagnosis**

1. In **neonates,** the differential diagnosis includes malrotation with volvulus, necrotizing enterocolitis, hernia, and meconium ileus.

2. In **older children,** the differential diagnosis includes acute gastroenteritis, appendicitis, Meckel diverticulum, and hernia.

C. **Medical management**

1. A nasogastric tube is placed, and intravenous access is obtained for hydration, sedation, and antibiotic administration.

   2. Barium, air, or water-soluble **contrast enema** is both diag-
      nostic and therapeutic.
      a. All methods use less than 120 mm Hg pressure for brief
         periods (2–5 minutes). Reduction is confirmed by passage
         of contrast material into the terminal ileum (30%–80%
         success rate).
      b. Most physicians administer a dose of cefoxitin and obtain
         a surgical consultation before the procedure in case per-
         foration occurs.
D. Surgical management
   1. In patients who have evidence of free peritoneal air or signs
      of peritonitis or who have had symptoms for more than 5
      days, surgical reduction is appropriate after fluid resuscita-
      tion and administration of broad-spectrum antibiotics.
   2. If the intussusception is not reducible (approximately 20%
      of cases), the patient should undergo resection and reanas-
      tomosis.

References
Champoux AN, Del Beccaro MA, Nazar-Stewart V: Recurrent intussusception: risks
   and features. *Arch Pediatr Adolesc Med* 148:474–478, 1999.
Orenstein J: Update on intussusception. *Contemp Pediatr* (17)3:180–191, 2000.
West DW, Grosfeld JL: Intussusception in infants and children. In *Pediatric Gastrointestinal Disease*. Edited by Wyllie R, Hyams JS. Philadelphia, WB Saunders, 1999,
   pp 472–477.

87. Hirschsprung Disease

I | INTRODUCTION

A. Background. Hirschsprung disease is a disorder of enteric neuronal migration. It leads to congenital bowel dysfunctions that range from constipation to enterocolitis and death.

B. Pathogenesis. Hirschsprung disease occurs when the craniocaudal migration of ganglion cell precursors along the gastrointestinal tract does not reach the anus. If normal migration occurred, these ganglion cells would become parasympathetic (inhibitory) nerves. These nerves regulate relaxation of the bowel wall and sphincters. An imbalance in sympathetic and parasympathetic muscle tone occurs and functionally blocks the movement of stool. The result is proximal dilation and hypertrophy of the colon.

C. Epidemiology
1. Hirschsprung disease occurs in approximately 1:5000 live births.
2. The male:female predominance is 4:1.
3. Diagnosis usually is made within the first year of life.
4. Hirschsprung disease is found in approximately 10% of children with Down syndrome.

D. Extent of disease
1. Approximately 75% of cases are limited to the rectum and sigmoid colon.
2. Only 8% of cases involve the entire colon.

II | CLINICAL MANIFESTATIONS

A. Clinical presentation. The most common symptoms are constipation, vomiting, and abdominal distension. Older children with short-segment Hirschsprung disease do not have significant encopresis, as do those with functional constipation. However, those with Hirschsprung disease have abdominal distension and evidence of malnutrition. In patients who have short-segment disease, diagnosis may be delayed for years.

HOT KEY More than 90% of children with Hirschsprung disease did not pass meconium in the first 24 hours of life. More than 90% of unaffected infants pass meconium on the first day of life.

B. Physical examination shows abdominal distension (83%) and an empty rectum on digital examination (61%). The anal reflex is absent. In patients with short-segment disease, a rapid expulsion of liquid stool often occurs after digital examination.

III APPROACH TO THE PATIENT

A. Diagnosis. The diagnosis is suggested by characteristic symptoms and by the findings on physical examination. Useful studies include:

    1. Rectal biopsy. Biopsy with histochemical staining for acetylcholinesterase is the standard diagnostic method. Full-thickness rectal biopsy is the gold standard for diagnosis, but many studies show that suction rectal biopsy also is reliable.

    2. Radiograph. The absence of gas in the pelvis on plain radiograph suggests Hirschsprung disease and indicates the need for further studies.

    3. Barium enema can assess for the transition zone between aganglionic and dilated ganglionic bowel; this is diagnostic in 80% of patients. Delayed passage of barium on 24- to 48-hour film suggests Hirschsprung disease, even without a transition zone.

    4. Anal manometry detects Hirschsprung disease in 75%–95% of patients. This test shows a tonic contraction of the internal sphincter.

B. Differential diagnosis includes meconium plug syndrome, microcolon, hypothyroidism, sepsis, cystic fibrosis, incarcerated inguinal hernia, colonic atresia, and functional constipation.

C. Management. The role of medical intervention is to stabilize the child by restoring the fluid and electrolyte balance. Broad-spectrum antibiotics are used in patients with suspected enterocolitis.

D. Surgical treatment

    1. Procedures. The general principle of surgical treatment of Hirschsprung disease is to place bowel with normal peristalsis at the anus and to eliminate the tonic contraction of the internal sphincter. Three basic surgical approaches are used for reanastomosis. All three have similar success and complication rates.

        a. The **Swenson procedure** directly reanastomoses normal bowel to the distal anal canal.

        b. The **Duhamel procedure** connects the normal bowel to a segment of distal aganglionic bowel in a side-to-side fashion. For children who have longer-segment (less functional colon) disease, the **Martin modification** provides a longer segment of side-to-side anastomosis for fluid absorption.

    c. The **Soave procedure** pulls the normal proximal ganglionic bowel through a muscular sleeve of retained rectum from which the aganglionic mucosa has been removed.

2. Long-term results. After surgery, one third to one half of all patients have normal stooling patterns. The remainder of patients reported either loose stools or constipation. Enterocolitis is a potential complication of surgery because of the possible formation of postoperative rectal stricture.

References

Adzick NS, Nance ML: Pediatric surgery (part I). *N Engl J Med* 342(22):1651–1657, 2000.

Kirschner BS: Hirschsprung's disease. In *Pediatric Gastrointestinal Disease: Pathophysiology, Diagnosis, Management.* Edited by Allan W, Walker MD, Durie PR, Hamilton JR, Walker SM, Watkins JB. St Louis, Mosby, 1996, pp 980–983.

88. Inflammatory Bowel Disease

I INTRODUCTION

A. Definitions

1. **Crohn disease** is a chronic, transmural, inflammatory process that involves the entire gastrointestinal tract (mouth to anus). It usually involves the distal small bowel (terminal ileum), colon, and perianal region. Crohn disease is best known for its patchy involvement of the bowel (skip lesions) as well as a high frequency of intestinal fistula formation and obstruction.

2. **Ulcerative colitis** is an inflammatory disease that involves the mucosal layer of the colon. It almost always affects the rectum and extends proximally, without skip lesions. Patients are at increased risk for colon cancer.

B. Epidemiology

1. **Crohn disease** has an incidence of 8–26 per 100,000 population. The peak age of onset is in the midteens to twenties. Both sexes are affected equally. There is a familial predisposition, and 20% of patients with Crohn disease have an affected first-degree relative. The incidence is higher in people of middle European origin as well as in Ashkenazi Jews. Smoking is associated with an increased risk of Crohn disease by a factor of between 2 and 5.

2. **Ulcerative colitis** has an incidence of 3–15 per 100,000 population. The peak incidence is in young adults (20–40 years of age), but it can present as early as in the first year of life. Both sexes are affected equally. Approximately 10% of patients with ulcerative colitis have an affected first-degree relative. The highest incidence is in the United States, United Kingdom, northern Europe, and Australia. The incidence is higher among Jewish people. Interestingly, smoking may provide some protection against the development of ulcerative colitis. Seventy percent of patients with ulcerative colitis are positive for a perinuclear staining antineutrophil cytoplasmic auto-antibody (pANCA).

II CLINICAL MANIFESTATIONS

A. Crohn disease. The most common initial symptom is abdominal pain (often postprandial and periumbilical), with or without vomiting and diarrhea. Aphthous oral ulcers may be present as well as perirectal findings (skin tags, fissures, and fistulas). Fever, malaise, anorexia, and weight loss also are common. The diagnosis is delayed an average of 14 months because of the protean presentation.

HOT **KEY**	Crohn disease should always be considered in patients who have a history of chronic abdominal pain and weight loss. Extraintestinal manifestations, which can be a clue to the diagnosis, should be sought.

B. Ulcerative colitis. The most common initial symptoms are abdominal pain and diarrhea (often bloody). Bloody diarrhea also may accompany Crohn disease if the colon is involved. Anorexia and weight loss may occur, but are much less common in patients with ulcerative colitis than in those with Crohn disease. Fever often is a sign of fulminant ulcerative colitis. Approximately 10%–15% of patients have fulminant disease, which is characterized by the following symptoms:
   1. Six or more bloody stools daily
   2. Abdominal distension and tenderness
   3. Fever and tachycardia
   4. Anemia (hematocrit < 30%)
   5. Hypoalbuminemia
C. Toxic megacolon is the primary cause of death in patients who have ulcerative colitis; among patients who develop toxic megacolon, the mortality rate is 40%. Toxic megacolon occurs when inflammation extends through the bowel wall. It most commonly affects the anterior transverse colon. The patient presents with systemic toxicity, fever, diarrhea, dehydration, abdominal distension, and electrolyte abnormalities (e.g., hypokalemia, hypomagnesemia). Perforation and peritonitis most commonly occur with the first episode. If perforation occurs, radiographic examination shows free air or dilated segments of large bowel. This is an emergency; broad-spectrum antibiotics and colonic resection are needed. However, surgery often is difficult because the mucosa is friable.
D. Extraintestinal manifestations in both Crohn disease and ulcerative colitis are shown in **Table 88–1**.

III APPROACH TO THE PATIENT
A. Physical examination
   1. **Head, ears, eyes, nose, and throat (HEENT).** Aphthous oral ulcers (stomatitis)
   2. **Abdomen.** Abdominal distension or tenderness, abdominal mass, or hepatosplenomegaly

TABLE 88-1. Extraintestinal Manifestations of Inflammatory Bowel Disease

Skin
  Erythema nodosum
  Pyoderma gangrenosum
  Perianal disease
Joints
  Arthralgia
  Arthritis
  Ankylosing spondylitis
  Sacroiliitis
  Hypertrophic osteoarthropathy
    (clubbing)
Eyes
  Uveitis
  Episcleritis
  Keratitis
  Retinal vasculitis
  Cataract
Hematologic
  Iron deficiency
  Anemia of chronic disease
  Folate deficiency
  Vitamin B_{12} deficiency
  Thrombocytosis
  Neutropenia

Liver/biliary tract
  Sclerosing cholangitis
  Chronic hepatitis
  Gallstones
  Cirrhosis
Bone
  Osteopenia
  Osteonecrosis
Renal/urologic
  Stones
  Hydronephrosis
  Enterovesical fistula
Vascular
  Thrombophlebitis
  Vasculitis
Extraintestinal cancer
  Lymphoma
  Acute myelocytic leukemia

Reprinted with permission from Altschuler SM, Liacouras CA: *Clinical Pediatric Gastroenterology.* Philadelphia, WB Saunders, 1998, p 215.

3. **Rectum.** Fistulas, fissures, or skin tags
4. **Skin.** Pyoderma gangrenosum or erythema nodosum
5. **Extremities.** Clubbing
B. **Growth.** The patient's height and weight should be plotted, and previous growth parameters should be obtained for comparison. Sexual maturity may be delayed as a result of chronic disease.
C. **Laboratory data**
  1. **Complete blood cell count with differential** shows anemia, thrombocytosis, and an elevated white blood cell count, with or without a left shift.
  2. **Erythrocyte sedimentation rate and C-reactive protein level** usually are elevated; however, these test results may be inaccurate when the hematocrit is lower than 30%.

3. **Total protein albumin level** may be low, especially in patients who have fulminant disease.

4. **Stool guaiac test result** is positive; stools may be grossly bloody. Stool should be sent for Gram stain and culture. A *Clostridium difficile* toxin assay should be performed on all patients, regardless of previous treatment with antibiotics.

D. Radiologic data

1. **Barium enema** is not commonly used in the diagnosis of inflammatory bowel disease because of the risk of perforation and exacerbation of colitis.

2. An **upper gastrointestinal series** with small bowel follow-through is a sensitive study for the initial diagnosis of small bowel disease in patients with Crohn disease.

   a. **Small bowel involvement** rules out the diagnosis of ulcerative colitis and suggests Crohn disease. An exception is the occasional "backwash" ileitis of ulcerative colitis.

   b. Skip lesions, fistulas (e.g., enteric, enterovaginal), and the string sign suggest Crohn disease.

3. **Plain abdominal films** occasionally show evidence of ulcerative colitis (i.e., thickening of the bowel wall, colonic distension with loss of haustra).

E. Endoscopy

1. **History of bloody diarrhea.** Patients who have bloody diarrhea should undergo flexible sigmoidoscopy or colonoscopy before contrast studies are performed. Flexible sigmoidoscopy can be performed with minimal bowel preparation and may show colonic involvement.

   a. **Ulcerative colitis.** The colonic mucosa appears ulcerated, friable, and granular, with loss of the normal vascular pattern.

   b. **Crohn disease.** Rectal sparing is common. The colonic mucosa has an irregular pattern, with a patchy distribution of linear ulcers. Biopsy specimens of normal and abnormal tissue should be obtained to look for microscopic inflammation and granulomas that may be present in Crohn disease.

2. **No history of bloody diarrhea**

   a. **Esophagogastroduodenoscopy (EGD)** may precede colonoscopy to search for esophageal, gastric, or small bowel involvement.

   b. **Flexible sigmoidoscopy or colonoscopy** can be performed to define the extent of disease (if EGD findings are positive) or to rule out colonic pathology (if EGD results are inconclusive).

F. Management

1. **Medications**

   a. **5-Aminosalicylates (5-ASA)**

HOT KEY No current therapy can cure inflammatory bowel disease. The goal of treatment is to relieve symptoms and improve the quality of life.

    (1) Indications. 5-ASAs are used to treat mild to moderate Crohn colitis and ulcerative colitis. 5-ASAs are used to induce remission of active colonic disease and also as maintenance therapy after remission is achieved. They may be given orally or as an enema. Mesalamine (a delayed-release form of 5-ASA) is used to treat both ulcerative colitis and Crohn disease.

    (2) Mechanism. Sulfasalazine is composed of sulfapyrazine azo-bonded to 5-ASA; it is particularly useful in patients with distal colitis. This bond causes poor absorption of the compound in the small bowel. The bond is cleaved by colonic bacteria, where the 5-ASA moiety interferes with the synthesis of prostaglandins by the colonic mucosa. Sulfasalazine (50 mg/kg/day) may cause nausea and vomiting, abdominal pain, and bone marrow toxicity.

  b. Corticosteroids. Steroids are the mainstay of treatment for patients who have moderate symptoms that do not respond to 5-ASA compounds. Steroids also are used to treat severe symptoms of Crohn disease and ulcerative colitis. Once remission is achieved, treatment is tapered slowly (alternate-day therapy or decreasing dosages). The dosage of prednisone is 1–2 mg/kg/day (maximum, 40–60 mg/day).

  c. Antibiotics. Metronidazole and ciprofloxacin are commonly used in the treatment of inflammatory bowel disease. Both may be effective in the treatment of pouchitis, which may occur after colectomy in patients with ulcerative colitis.

    (1) Metronidazole (10–20 mg/kg/day) is useful in treating perirectal fistulas and severe colitis in patients with Crohn disease.

    (2) Ciprofloxacin (250–500 mg twice daily) may be used to treat perirectal disease in adolescents.

  d. Immunosuppressive therapy is used in patients who are dependent on steroids or whose disease does not respond to steroid treatment. Relief of symptoms may not be evident for 3–9 months after the initiation of therapy. 6-Mercaptopurine and azathioprine are the most commonly used agents (1–2 mg/kg/day, to a maximum of 100 mg/day). Cyclosporine occasionally is used in patients who have fulminant ulcerative colitis.

   e. **Antidiarrheal agents.** Loperamide sometimes is used to control the frequency of diarrhea.

HOT
▶
KEY

The use of any antimotility agent is contraindicated in patients who have fulminant inflammatory bowel disease or toxic megacolon.

---

2. **Surgery.** Indications for surgical management include severe fistula formation, obstruction, perforation, uncontrolled hemorrhage, and significant failure to thrive. Common procedures include colectomy, mucosal proctectomy, the formation of an ileal–anal pouch reservoir (30% incidence of pouchitis), and stricturoplasty.
   a. Approximately 10%–25% of children who have **ulcerative colitis** require colectomy within 5 years of diagnosis. Colectomy is curative.
   b. Approximately 50%–75% of all patients who have **Crohn disease** require surgical intervention within 15 years of diagnosis.
3. **New therapies** include an antitumor necrosis factor antibody **(infliximab).** Tumor necrosis factor is a proinflammatory cytokine that plays a major role in the pathogenesis of Crohn disease. Recent multicenter trials in adults showed improvement in both clinical symptoms and endoscopic findings in patients with refractory Crohn disease. The use of this treatment in children is under investigation.
4. **Nutrition.** Evidence supports the use of elemental diets to induce remission of Crohn disease. However, controlled trials do not show the efficacy of parenteral nutrition or elemental diets in ulcerative colitis.

IV PROGNOSIS

A. **Colon cancer and ulcerative colitis.** The risk of colon cancer in patients with ulcerative colitis is 1% at 10 years after diagnosis, with an increase of 1%–2% for every subsequent year. Some studies show up to a 50% risk of colon cancer 20 years after diagnosis. Greater colonic involvement leads to earlier development of cancer. In patients whose involvement is limited to the descending colon, the onset of cancer is delayed by approximately 10 years.
   1. Total colectomy virtually eliminates the risk of colon cancer, but is not indicated solely to prevent cancer.
   2. Ten years after diagnosis, the patient should undergo colonoscopy and rectal biopsy. These tests should be repeated every 6 months.

B. Malignancy and Crohn disease. The risk of all malignancies is increased 20 times in patients with Crohn disease who are diagnosed before 21 years of age. The risk of small bowel and colon cancer is lower overall compared with that for patients who have ulcerative colitis. However, when colonic involvement with Crohn disease is extensive, the risk is similar to that for ulcerative colitis. Therefore, patients who have extensive Crohn colitis should undergo surveillance colonoscopy.

References

Hyams JS: Inflammatory bowel disease. In *Clinical Pediatric Gastroenterology*. Edited by Altschuler SM, Liacouras CA. Philadelphia, Churchill Livingstone, 1998, pp 213–221.

Jewell DP: Ulcerative colitis. In *Sleisenger and Fordtran's Gastrointestinal and Liver Disease: Pathophysiology/Diagnosis/Management,* 6th ed. Edited by Feldman M, Scharschmidt BF, Sleisenger MH. Philadelphia, WB Saunders, 1998, pp 1735–1761.

Kornbluth A, Sachar DB, Salomon P: Crohn's disease. In *Sleisenger and Fordtran's Gastrointestinal and Liver Disease: Pathophysiology/Diagnosis/Management,* 6th ed. Edited by Feldman M, Scharschmidt BF, Sleisenger MH. Philadelphia, WB Saunders, 1998, pp 1735–1761.

89. Appendicitis

I INTRODUCTION

A. **Pathogenesis.** Appendicitis is caused by obstruction of the appendiceal lumen by lymphoid hyperplasia secondary to viral infection (55%), a fecalith (40%), a foreign body (4%), or a stricture or tumor (1%). Obstruction leads to stasis, bacterial overgrowth, and inflammation. Unrecognized appendicitis may progress to perforation and peritonitis. A periappendiceal abscess may occur when perforations are walled off by loops of small bowel or omentum. Periappendiceal abscesses usually are caused by fecaliths.

B. **Epidemiology.** Approximately 1% of all children have appendicitis before 15 years of age. Appendicitis is rare in infancy. The incidence peaks in early childhood and the teen years.

II CLINICAL MANIFESTATIONS

A. **Symptoms**
   1. **First hour.** Periumbilical pain occurs because the nerve plexus from the appendix enters at the same level of somatic afferents from the periumbilical level.
   2. **After 4 hours.** Nausea, vomiting, and anorexia occur when peristaltic waves hit the obstruction and are reflected retrograde.
   3. **After 8 hours.** Pain becomes localized to the lower quadrants. If perforation occurs, peritoneal signs and fever ensue. Occasionally, an inflamed appendix irritates the colon and causes diarrhea.

HOT **KEY** Unlike adults, children who have appendicitis may not have prominent anorexia!

B. **Physical examination.** Because the appendix is a mobile structure, pain does not always occur in the classic anterior location.
   1. **McBurney point.** If the appendix is located anteriorly, pain occurs at the point located one third of the distance along the line from the anterior superior iliac spine to the pubic symphysis.

HOT KEY An attempt to elicit rebound tenderness offers little benefit and may simply cause the patient unnecessary pain. Asking a child to jump can be a good test for peritoneal inflammation. If the child grabs her lower quadrant and refuses to jump again, the test result is positive.

2. **Psoas sign.** The patient is rolled on the left side, and the right leg is hyperextended at the hip. Pain on hip extension indicates a retrocecal appendix.
3. **Obturator sign.** Pain on flexion and internal rotation of the hip also indicates an inflamed retrocecal appendix.
4. **Rovsing sign.** Pain that occurs in the right lower quadrant when the left lower quadrant is palpated indicates peritonitis.

 APPROACH TO THE PATIENT

A. Diagnosis

HOT KEY Repeating the basics (i.e., history and physical examination) leads to the correct diagnosis more often than sophisticated diagnostic testing.

1. **Laboratory tests** that help to refine the diagnosis of appendicitis include the following:
   a. **White blood cell count.** Leukocytosis with a left shift (i.e., > 10% bands) is a classic finding. One third of patients with appendicitis have a normal white blood cell count, but most children have a left shift.
   b. A **human chorionic gonadotropin** test is performed in teenage girls to rule out pregnancy.
   c. **Urinalysis.** An inflamed appendix lying over a ureter can produce pyuria or hematuria. As a result, the findings of the urinalysis may lead to an incorrect diagnosis of pyelonephritis.
2. **Imaging tests**
   a. **Abdominal ultrasound** is useful in children, with a sensitivity of 86% and a specificity of 98%. Classically, abdominal ultrasound shows a distended or noncompressible appendix. It also may show obstetric pathology that might preclude laparotomy. However, the success of this test depends on the skill of the operator.
   b. **Abdominal radiograph** may show a fecalith (small, round, radiopaque object) or a distended gas-filled appendix with an air-fluid level. Supporting signs include localized gas in

the cecum or terminal ileum, scoliosis as a result of right psoas muscle spasm, and loss of the right properitoneal fat line. Free air under the diaphragm is visible if perforation has occurred.

    c. Appendiceal computed tomography scan with rectal contrast recently has been shown to be an excellent test for appendicitis (94% sensitivity and specificity).

B. Differential diagnosis
1. Pharyngitis with mesenteric adenitis
2. Constipation
3. Mittelschmerz
4. Pelvic inflammatory disease
5. Pyelonephritis
6. Diabetic ketoacidosis
7. Lower lobe pneumonia (can refer pain to the right lower quadrant)

HOT

KEY
Always obtain a chest radiograph in patients suspected of having appendicitis to rule out pneumonia.

C. Therapy. Surgery is the mainstay of therapy. Broad-spectrum antibiotics are required if perforation occurs. A combination of ampicillin and gentamicin with clindamycin or metronidazole is appropriate.

D. Ongoing management. In cases in which the diagnosis is in question, vital signs are checked hourly, serial examinations are performed at least every 2 hours, and a white blood cell count is performed every 6 hours. It is important to remember that potent analgesics may mask signs of peritonitis.

IV PROGNOSIS

A. Mortality rate. Appendicitis has a very low mortality rate (< 1%). The mortality rate increases at the extremes of age and with perforation.

B. Morbidity rate. Approximately 5% of cases of infertility in women result from a perforated appendix.

References
Garcia Pena BM, Mandl KD, Kraus SJ, et al: Ultrasonography and limited computed tomography in the diagnosis and management of appendicitis in children. *JAMA* 282(11):1041–1046, 1999.
Kliegman RM, Nieder ML, Super DM: *Practical Strategies in Pediatric Diagnosis and Therapy.* Philadelphia, WB Saunders, 1996, pp 269–270.

Lawrence PF, Bell RM: *Essentials of General Surgery,* 2nd ed. Philadelphia, Lippincott Williams & Wilkins, 1992, pp 205–206.

McMillan JA, Deangelis CD, Feigin RD (eds): *Oski's Pediatrics: Principles and Practice,* 3rd ed. Philadelphia, Lippincott Williams & Wilkins, 1999, pp 1702–1703.

Wong ML, Casey SO, Leonidas JC, et al: Sonographic diagnosis of acute appendicitis in children. *J Pediatr Surg* 29(10):1356–1360, 1994.

90. Gastrointestinal Bleeding

I DEFINITIONS

A. **Hematemesis** is blood in the vomitus. This symptom signifies an upper gastrointestinal source of bleeding (i.e., proximal to the ligament of Treitz). A "coffee-ground" appearance indicates that blood has been denatured by gastric fluids.

B. **Melena** is black, tarry stool. This symptom suggests an upper gastrointestinal source of bleeding proximal to the ileocecal valve. Occasionally, it represents bleeding from the right colon with a slow transit time.

C. **Hematochezia** is bright red or maroon blood in the stool. It implies either a lower gastrointestinal source (bleeding distal to the ileocecal valve) or brisk upper gastrointestinal tract bleeding.

D. **Factitious hematochezia** is red, maroon, or black discoloration of the stool that is caused by ingestion of food (e.g., licorice, spinach, beets) or medications (e.g., bismuth, ampicillin). It may also be caused by nongastrointestinal sources of bleeding (e.g., menstruation, hematuria).

E. **Occult gastrointestinal bleeding** is blood that cannot be seen in the stool, but is detected by a stool guaiac test. False-negative test results most often are caused by ingestion of vitamin C or prolonged specimen storage (> 4 days). False-positive test results may be caused by ingestion of certain foods, including red meat, horseradish, turnips, cauliflower, and tomatoes, or by iron supplementation.

II CLINICAL MANIFESTATIONS

A. **Symptoms.** Patient presentations may range from fatigue and pallor (occult gastrointestinal blood loss), to occasional maroon stools, to massive and hemodynamically significant rectal bleeding or hematemesis. The immediate goal is to identify a hemodynamically unstable patient.

B. **Physical examination**
   1. **Vital signs.** Particular attention should be paid to the blood pressure and heart rate. Tachycardia is the initial sign; a decrease in blood pressure is a late finding. Orthostatic hypotension (a decrease in diastolic blood pressure of > 15 mm Hg, along with a 10% increase in heart rate when the patient stands from a recumbent position) also is a sign of decreased intravascular volume.

> **HOT** ▶ **KEY** In patients who have obvious gastrointestinal bleeding, tachycardia is considered hypovolemic in origin until proven otherwise.

2. **General appearance.** Altered mental status is an ominous sign of hypovolemia.
3. **Head, ears, eyes, nose, and throat (HEENT).** The nares and oropharynx are examined for new or old blood, and the mucous membranes are checked for pallor. Evidence of dental trauma or gingival bleeding should be sought. Facial petechiae may indicate violent coughing or retching.
4. **Abdomen.** Rebound tenderness, guarding, or the presence of ascites should be assessed. The abdomen should be palpated for masses and hepatosplenomegaly.
5. **Skin.** The skin and mucous membranes are checked for pallor and prolonged (> 2 seconds) capillary refill. Skin hemangiomas are associated with intestinal or hepatic hemangiomas, and axillary, buccal, or lip freckles may indicate Peutz-Jeghers syndrome.
6. **Anus and rectum.** A digital examination and stool guaiac test should be performed. The physician should assess the patient for condylomata or perianal bruising (indicating sexual abuse), fissures, and perianal fistulas (indicating Crohn disease).

III APPROACH TO THE HEMODYNAMICALLY UNSTABLE PATIENT

A. **Initial management.** Patients who are hemodynamically unstable require immediate attention. Stabilization, not identification of the source of the bleeding, is paramount. Admission to the intensive care unit is mandatory.
  1. **Supplemental oxygen** is administered to maximize both the oxygen-carrying capacity of available red blood cells and oxygen delivery to tissues.
  2. **Airway protection.** Endotracheal intubation is indicated in patients with altered mental status and persistent emesis or hematemesis.
  3. At least **two peripheral intravenous lines** are placed (the larger bore, the better), and a bolus of 20 ml/kg isotonic fluids (normal saline or lactated Ringer solution) is administered rapidly to maintain perfusion until blood products arrive. Placement of a central venous catheter should be considered as well.
  4. **Blood products.** At least one unit of O-negative packed red

blood cells or whole blood should be available for immediate transfusion. Transfusion should be done quickly if brisk ongoing gastrointestinal bleeding occurs; the hematocrit should be maintained near 30%. Multiple units of blood should be crossmatched in case uncontrolled bleeding occurs.

B. Laboratory studies. A complete blood cell count and platelet count should be obtained as well as coagulation studies, liver function tests, and renal function tests. The hematocrit does not decrease immediately in the setting of acute gastrointestinal bleeding; it can take several hours to reflect the true amount of bleeding.

HOT

In a patient who has clinical evidence of hypovolemia, a "normal" hematocrit is not a reassuring finding.

KEY

IV APPROACH TO THE HEMODYNAMICALLY STABLE PATIENT

A. Initial steps
  1. Once the patient is stable, efforts are made to identify the source of bleeding.
  2. A nasogastric tube is placed, and a gastric aspirate is obtained. If blood is found, an upper gastrointestinal source is suspected. A negative result suggests lower gastrointestinal bleeding, but does not rule out upper gastrointestinal bleeding.
B. Management of suspected upper gastrointestinal bleed (i.e., gastric aspirate is positive)
  1. Diagnostic studies
    a. Esophagogastroduodenoscopy is indicated in cases of uncontrolled upper gastrointestinal hemorrhage and recurrent upper gastrointestinal bleeding. This test is potentially therapeutic (sclerotherapy, endoscopic variceal ligation) for variceal bleeding. In 90% of cases, the source of bleeding can be determined if endoscopy is performed within the first 24 hours. Biopsy specimens should be obtained as well.
    b. The Apt-Downey test is helpful in cases of hematemesis in a newborn. It distinguishes red cells of fetal origin from those of maternal origin.
    c. *Helicobacter pylori* infection can be identified by histopathologic tissue studies. Noninvasive testing methods include antibody testing and breath testing with ^{13}C-labeled urea. Antibody testing cannot distinguish between past and current infection. The sensitivity and specificity of breath testing are unknown in children.

2. **Differential diagnosis of upper intestinal bleeding.** The site of the bleeding often can be inferred from the patient's history:
   a. **Esophagus.** Paroxysmal retching may indicate superficial mucosal injuries or Mallory-Weiss tears. Gastroesophageal reflux may indicate esophagitis. A history of jaundice, pruritus, or chronic liver disease may indicate varices.
   b. **Peptic ulcer disease.** A patient with ulcers has a history of intermittent nausea and midepigastric pain. The patient should be asked about recent use of nonsteroidal antiinflammatory drugs (NSAIDs) or steroids. A very ill child (e.g., with extensive burn injury) may have gastric or duodenal ulcers or gastritis.

3. **Therapeutic interventions**
   a. Ongoing volume resuscitation is administered as needed.
   b. A nasogastric tube is placed and maintained at low intermittent suction in an effort to remove blood from the stomach. Blood in the stomach nearly always causes emesis.
   c. Antacids or histamine-2 blockers can be administered empirically to maintain pH at greater than 4.5.
   d. NSAIDs, alcohol, and tobacco should be avoided.
   e. If brisk upper gastrointestinal hemorrhage occurs, nasogastric lavage can be performed with room-temperature normal saline. Iced fluids, which were previously thought to promote local vasoconstriction, now are believed to increase the risk of hypothermia.
   f. If varices are present, octreotide can be used to decrease portal pressure. A Sengstaken-Blakemore tube (an esophageal and gastric balloon) may be placed, or injection sclerotherapy through an endoscope may be performed.

C. **Management of lower gastrointestinal bleeding** (gastric aspirate is negative)
   1. **Diagnostic studies.** A directed approach, based on history and symptoms, is best.
      a. **Flexible sigmoidoscopy** is performed in patients who have hematochezia. This test identifies mucosal lesions from the distal descending colon to the rectum. Positive findings (e.g., polyps, distal colitis) are an indication for full colonoscopy.
      b. **Meckel scan** is performed in patients who have a history of painless rectal bleeding (homogenously maroon or bright red stool). It uses ^{99m}Tc pertechnetate to localize the ectopic gastric mucosa found in Meckel diverticula. Sensitivity may be enhanced with the use of histamine-2 blockers or pentagastrin. A negative finding does not preclude surgical exploration if the index of suspicion is high.
      c. **Stool cultures and testing for fecal leukocytes** are performed when an infectious cause is suspected. Symptoms

include abdominal pain, vomiting, and fever. *Salmonella, Shigella, Campylobacter, Yersinia, Escherichia coli, Clostridium difficile,* and *Entamoeba* are potential pathogens.
   d. Scans and angiography are used in patients who have persistent blood loss from an unidentified source.
   (1) During a bleeding scan, the patient's blood is labeled with ^{99m}Tc and injected into the patient under a gamma counter. Images detect extravasation of the labeled cells into the intestinal lumen. This test is reliable if the bleeding rate is 0.1–0.3 ml/min (500 ml/day).
   (2) Angiography is performed in patients who have brisk bleeding (= 0.5 ml/min). A vascular "blush" identifies the source. Angiography also is potentially therapeutic.
2. Differential diagnosis
   a. Premature infants and neonates
   (1) Well-appearing patient. Anal fissure, swallowed maternal blood, and milk protein allergy
   (2) Ill-appearing patient. Necrotizing enterocolitis, infectious enterocolitis, Hirschsprung enterocolitis, and intussusception
   (3) Rare causes. Intestinal duplication, coagulopathy, and vascular lesions (e.g., Dieulafoy erosion)
   b. Older infants and children
   (1) Well-appearing patient. Anal fissures, intestinal polyps, Meckel diverticulum, and inflammatory bowel disease
   (2) Ill-appearing patient. Infectious enterocolitis, intussusception, coagulopathy (i.e., in the setting of sepsis), and *Clostridium difficile* enterocolitis
   (3) Rare causes. Vascular lesions (e.g., Dieulafoy erosion), intestinal duplication, hemorrhoids (rare in an otherwise healthy child), sexual abuse, and rectal trauma

References
Laine L: Acute and chronic gastrointestinal bleeding. In *Sleisenger & Fordtran's Gastrointestinal and Liver Disease: Pathophysiology, Diagnosis, Management.* Edited by Feldman M, Scharschmidt BF, Sleisenger M. Philadelphia, WB Saunders, 1998, pp 198–219.
Squires RH Jr: Gastrointestinal bleeding. In *Clinical Pediatric Gastroenterology.* Edited by Altschuler SM, Liacouras CA. New York, Churchill Livingstone, 1998, pp 31–42.

91. Gastroesophageal Reflux Disease

I. INTRODUCTION

A. Definition. Gastroesophageal reflux disease (GERD) is the pathogenic effortless retrograde movement of gastric contents into the esophagus.

B. Types

1. **Physiologic GERD** is associated with delayed maturation of the gastrointestinal structure and function in infants younger than 3 months of age. Weight gain is normal, and no blood or bile is present in regurgitated material. Some patients have positive results on pH probe tests.

2. **Uncomplicated pathologic GERD.** Regurgitation is greater in quantity and frequency than in patients with physiologic GERD. Frank vomiting also may occur.

3. **Complicated GERD.** Patients are irritable, and a wide range of complications may occur (see IV).

4. **Secondary GERD** is caused by another condition, such as neurologic disease, pulmonary disease, or congenital malformation (e.g., tracheoesophageal fistula). Secondary GERD often is intractable and responds poorly to standard therapy.

HOT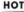

KEY

The term reflux often is used to describe normal infant regurgitation. This normal regurgitation is not the same as GERD.

C. Pathogenesis. One or more of the following abnormalities can lead to GERD. These factors are developmental immaturities commonly found in infants younger than 4 months of age.

1. Low esophageal motility
2. Decreased lower esophageal sphincter (LES) pressure
3. Episodic LES relaxations
4. Delayed gastric emptying

D. Epidemiology. Approximately 10% of children have GERD. It is the third most common reason for surgery in pediatric centers.

II   CLINICAL MANIFESTATIONS

A. Unusually high frequency or volume of regurgitation
B. Painful or uncomfortable regurgitation
C. Refusal of feedings even when hungry
D. Crying during and after feedings
E. Dyspnea, cyanosis, wheezing, hoarseness
F. Excessive crying or fussiness
G. Excessive hiccupping
H. Back arching
I. Poor weight gain

III   APPROACH TO THE PATIENT

A. **Differential diagnosis.** After physiologic GERD is ruled out,
   the list of diagnoses in **Table 91–1** should be considered.
B. **Diagnosis**
   1. A **careful history** should be obtained. Often, the history
      alone provides adequate information to guide therapy. An

---

TABLE 91-1. Diagnoses That May Be Confused With Gastroesophageal Reflux Disease

Parenting or psychosocial factors
Overfeeding
Infantile colic
Munchausen syndrome by proxy
Anatomic abnormalities
Hypertrophic pyloric stenosis
Malrotation with intermittent volvulus
Antral or duodenal web
Annular pancreas
Intestinal duplication
Tracheoesophageal fistula
Other gastrointestinal diseases
Milk protein allergy
Hirschsprung disease
Achalasia
Peptic ulcer disease
Respiratory diseases
Asthma
Obstructive apnea
Central apnea
Pneumonia

intercurrent respiratory infection may temporarily worsen symptoms.

2. pH Probe testing is the definitive and most sensitive test for GERD. This test is invasive and usually requires an overnight hospital admission.

    a. Indications for pH probe testing

        (1) Moderate or severe symptoms

        (2) Suspected complications

        (3) Failure of empiric medical therapy

    b. If apnea is present, a pH probe test can be accompanied by a **pneumogram** that measures the duration and number of episodes during which esophageal pH is less than 4.

    c. Upper and lower esophageal pH can be monitored if secondary aspiration is suspected.

3. Additional tests to consider

    a. Upper gastrointestinal contrast study is used to rule out anatomic abnormality (e.g., malrotation, web, or vascular abnormality); this test is best for examining structure, not function. However, this test can identify severe GERD in some patients.

    b. Endoscopy is useful in assessing esophagitis or ulcer formation. This test should be considered if the patient is excessively irritable or anorexic.

    c. Scintigraphy (nuclear scan) can provide proof that aspiration is present and can demonstrate delayed gastric emptying.

    d. LES manometry can be performed if a motility disorder is suspected.

C. Initial therapy

    1. Reassurance is helpful, especially if GERD seems to be physiologic.

    2. Small, frequent feedings should be given. Formula should be thickened with 1 tablespoon of dry cereal per ounce.

    3. Positioning

        a. The patient's head should be elevated at a 30° angle during sleeping and for 1 hour after each feeding. A wedge can be placed under the upper part of the mattress to elevate the head.

        b. The use of an infant seat should be avoided because it increases intra-abdominal pressure, as does changing diapers with the infant's feet held up in the air. The prone position is best; the supine position is worst.

    4. Empiric medical therapy includes a histamine (H_2) blocker (e.g., ranitidine, 1.25–2 mg/kg every 12 hours).

D. Adjuvant therapies

    1. Proton pump inhibitors (e.g., omeprazole) can reduce acid formation. Dosing for patients younger than age 2 years has not been established. For patients older than age 2 years, the dosage for omeprazole is 0.3–2.0 mg/kg/day given in a single dose.

2. Promotility agents (e.g., erythromycin) may be useful for patients who have delayed gastric emptying.

HOT KEY Cisapride is no longer used in children due to the risk of cardiac conduction abnormalities.

3. Surgical therapy. Gastric (Nissen) fundoplication is indicated if the child has had multiple episodes of aspiration pneumonia, severe esophagitis, or recalcitrant weight loss. In fundoplication, a portion of the stomach is wrapped around the lower esophageal sphincter to prevent reflux mechanically. This procedure has a 10%–20% rate of complication or failure.

IV PROGNOSIS

A. Complications
1. **Esophagitis.** In severe cases, esophageal stricture may occur.
2. **Failure to thrive**
3. **Respiratory complications,** including the following:
   a. Coughing, choking
   b. Central apnea secondary to vagal stimulation
   c. Obstructive apnea, including frank choking or reflex laryngospasm
   d. Reflex bronchospasm
   e. Aspiration or microaspiration, which can lead to chemical pneumonitis or bacterial pneumonia
   f. Sudden infant death syndrome (this link is controversial)
4. **Sandifer syndrome.** Torticollis and back-arching motions may be associated with GERD.

HOT KEY GERD and respiratory disease may interact. GERD may cause respiratory disease, which in turn may exacerbate GERD.

B. Morbidity. Approximately 1 per 200 children with GERD require gastric fundoplication. If reflux persists after 1 year of age, the rate of complication increases dramatically.

C. Outcome

1. In two thirds of infants with GERD, symptoms resolve within 6 weeks without intervention.
2. In approximately 90% of cases, symptoms resolve by age 18 months.

References

Faubion WA Jr, Zein NN: Gastroesophageal reflux in infants and children. *Mayo Clin Proc* 73(2):166–173, 1998.

Hebra A, Hoffman MA: Gastroesophageal reflux in children. *Pediatr Clin North Am* 40(6):1233–1251, 1993.

PART XI

ENDOCRINOLOGY AND METABOLIC DISORBERS

92. Diabetes Mellitus

I INTRODUCTION

A. Background. Diabetes mellitus is the most common endocrine disorder of childhood. It is a lifelong illness with many potential complications, and it demands a carefully monitored lifestyle. Diabetes is characterized by elevated levels of blood glucose and is caused by an absolute or relative deficiency of insulin secretion or action.

B. Pathogenesis

1. **Type I diabetes** is also known as insulin-dependent diabetes mellitus (IDDM), or juvenile diabetes. Patients have extremely low circulating insulin levels as a result of pancreatic islet β-cell destruction. β-cells are likely destroyed by autoimmune mechanisms. Possible triggers for destruction are viral infections (e.g., mumps, rubella, coxsackievirus) and early exposure to cow's milk proteins. Insulin-producing capacity progressively decreases, resulting in eventual glucose intolerance and fasting hyperglycemia. Regulatory hormones become imbalanced, leading to a catabolic state and ketosis.

2. **Type II diabetes** is also known as non–insulin-dependent diabetes mellitus (NIDDM), or adult-onset diabetes. Insulin resistance occurs and is not compensated for by adequate insulin secretion. Autoantibodies are rarely present. Ketosis and the need for exogenous insulin are less common in patients with type II diabetes. Ketosis usually occurs in conjunction with a supervening illness. Most patients with type II diabetes are obese.

3. **Maturity-onset diabetes of the young (MODY)** is a dominantly inherited form of type II diabetes that involves less insulin resistance and may require insulin treatment.

4. **Other causes** of diabetes include cystic fibrosis, pancreatectomy, Cushing syndrome, and exposure to toxins.

C. Epidemiology
   1. The risk of type I diabetes is greater in children who have a first-degree relative with type I diabetes (2%–5%). The concordance rate in identical twins is 25%–35%.
   2. The risk of type II diabetes is increased in children of patients who have type II diabetes. The concordance rate in identical twins is nearly 100%.
   3. The overall incidence of diabetes among school-age children is 1.9:1000. It is 1:1500 by 5 years of age and 1:360 by 16 years of age.
   4. The incidence of new cases peaks at 5–7 years of age and also in adolescence. It also increases in the fall and winter months, suggesting possible viral triggers.

II CLINICAL MANIFESTATIONS

A. Symptoms include polyuria, secondary enuresis, polydipsia, weakness, polyphagia, blurred vision, and weight loss despite adequate caloric intake.

B. Presentations
   1. **Insidious onset of lethargy, weakness, and weight loss, with polyuria and polydipsia.** In patients with type I diabetes, these symptoms usually occur less than 1 month before diagnosis. In contrast, type II diabetes produces lower levels of hyperglycemia, and these symptoms may be milder and may persist for months or years before diagnosis.
   2. **Incidental hyperglycemia** can be a normal finding in the setting of another illness. However, 30% of well children with hyperglycemia discovered incidentally will develop diabetes.
   3. **Incidental glucosuria** may indicate a renal tubular abnormality. However, it may also reveal impaired glucose tolerance or provide the first clue that a child has diabetes.
   4. **Diabetic ketoacidosis** (see Chapter 93)

III APPROACH TO THE PATIENT

A. Diagnosis
   1. **Diabetes mellitus** is diagnosed by any of the following criteria:
      a. Symptoms of diabetes (see II A) and a random plasma glucose level of 200 mg/dl or greater
      b. Fasting plasma glucose level greater than 125 mg/dl
      c. Oral glucose tolerance test with a 2-hour plasma glucose level of 200 mg/dl or greater
   2. **Impaired glucose tolerance** is a risk factor for future diabetes. It is diagnosed by the presence of both of the following criteria:

     a. Fasting plasma glucose level of 125 mg/dl or less
     b. Oral glucose tolerance test with a 2-hour plasma glucose level of 140–199 mg/dl
  3. Glucosuria occurs when the plasma glucose level is greater than approximately 180 mg/dl, which exceeds the renal threshold for glucose reabsorption.
B. Additional tests to consider
  1. Anti-islet cell antibodies and anti-insulin antibodies
  2. Thyroid-stimulating hormone should be measured if autoimmune hypothyroidism is suspected. This condition is associated with type I diabetes.
  3. Glycosylated hemoglobin (HbA$_{1c}$) level indicates the chronicity and severity of hyperglycemia.
C. Goals of therapy are to prevent symptoms and long-term complications of diabetes, promote normal growth and development, and avoid hypoglycemic episodes.

HOT **KEY**   Tight glucose control (maintenance of plasma glucose at < 150 mg/dl) is associated with improved long-term outcome. However, it increases the risk of hypoglycemia and requires a demanding daily regimen.

D. Initial treatment of type I diabetes
  1. If present, diabetic ketoacidosis should be treated (see Chapter 93).
  2. The transition phase involves establishing an insulin regimen with subcutaneous injections.
    a. Insulin requirements. Most children require approximately 0.5 U/kg/day insulin. The requirement may be as high as 0.7 U/kg/day for a child or as high as 1.5 U/kg/day for an adolescent who is hospitalized and inactive or ketonuric.
    b. Insulin preparations (Table 92–1). Human insulin comes in many preparations with various activity profiles.
      (1) The estimated daily requirement can be divided into four doses of **regular insulin** given before meals.
      (2) Additional **rapid-acting insulin** can be added to a premeal dose in an amount proportional to the premeal blood glucose level ("sliding scale").
      (3) Neutral protamine Hagedorn (NPH) insulin and lente insulin are forms of **intermediate-acting insulin,** which can be given instead of regular insulin at the bedtime dose.
      (4) Once the total daily requirement is refined, two injections of a **mixture of rapid-acting (usually regular)**

TABLE 92-1. Types of Insulin and Their Effects

Duration	Type	Time to Onset	Peak Effect	End of Effect
Rapid-acting	Lispro	15–30 min	1–2 h	2–3 h
Rapid-acting	Regular	30–60 min	2–3 h	3–6 h
Intermediate-acting	Neutral protamine Hagedorn (NPH)	2–4 h	4–10 h	10–16 h
Intermediate-acting	Lente	3–4 h	4–12 h	12–18 h
Long-acting	Ultralente	6–10 h	Evenly released	18–20 h

and intermediate-acting insulin can be given, one before breakfast and one before dinner.
   (a) Two thirds of the total insulin requirement is given before breakfast, and one third is given before dinner.
   (b) The ratio of NPH insulin:regular insulin or lente insulin:regular insulin is approximately 2:1.
   (c) Young children may need less rapid-acting and more intermediate-acting insulin.
   (5) Total daily insulin requirements can be increased or decreased by 10%–20%, depending on the level of control desired, activity level, or amount of food intake.
   (6) The blood glucose level is monitored at least four times daily at first: before meals and at bedtime. An early morning (approximately 3:00 AM) blood glucose check also may be needed.

HOT   Most children receive at least two daily injections of insulin.
▶   The doses may be adjusted to compensate for typical childhood variations in diet and activity. The regimen is adjusted to
KEY   maximize both glycemic control and compliance.

---

   3. **Remission: the "honeymoon" period.** Approximately 75% of patients with diabetes require less insulin in the weeks to months after diagnosis. The reason for this residual islet cell function is unclear, but this phase must be anticipated to avoid hypoglycemia. A single daily dose of intermediate-acting insulin may be appropriate during this period. Approximately 5% of patients require no exogenous insulin during this period, and approximately 2% remain in complete remission for years.
E. **Initial treatment of type II diabetes** includes weight loss through diet and exercise, combined with oral agents.
   1. **Biguanides** (e.g., metformin) are oral agents that enhance peripheral insulin sensitivity. These agents usually are the first choice of therapy.
   2. **Sulfonylureas** are oral hypoglycemic medications that stimulate insulin production, but can cause weight gain.
F. **Maintenance treatment and monitoring.** Continued refinement of insulin regimen and blood glucose monitoring occurs throughout childhood and adolescence.
   1. **Hypoglycemic episodes.** Signs and symptoms include trembling, diaphoresis, tachycardia, and confusion. Fruit juice can be given. If the patient is unstable, however, glucagon 0.02–0.03 mg/kg (up to 1 mg total) can be administered subcutaneously or intramuscularly.
   2. **Hyperglycemic episodes.** Signs and symptoms include

polyuria, polydipsia, and blurred vision. Rapid-acting insulin can be given to treat these episodes.

   a. Somogyi phenomenon is hyperglycemia that occurs after hypoglycemia and subsequent release of catecholamines.

   b. Dawn phenomenon is early-morning hyperglycemia caused by diurnal release of growth hormone.

3. Effects of illness. Insulin requirements usually increase as a result of inactivity and the stress of illness. Urine should be checked for ketones. Some patients require hospital admission.

4. Exercise. Vigorous exercise can precipitate hypoglycemia or exacerbate uncontrolled hyperglycemia. However, regular exercise can reduce insulin requirements. In patients with type II diabetes, exercise promotes both weight loss and peripheral insulin sensitivity.

5. Diet. Consistency is important. Stable caloric intake, with planned snacks between meals, helps to prevent hypoglycemia. A basic nutrient guideline is to obtain 55% of calories from carbohydrates (mostly complex carbohydrates), 30% from fat, and 15% from protein. The American Diabetic Association (ADA) "exchange" system is a helpful tool for nutritional management.

HOT

KEY

For children up to 12 years of age, the daily caloric requirement is approximated as follows: $1000 + (100 \times \text{age in years})$.

---

6. Monitoring

   a. The **HbA_{1c} level** should be measured every 3 months. A level of approximately 6%–9% indicates reasonable glycemic control.

   b. The patient should be evaluated for **ketonuria** during illness or when the blood glucose level is high.

   c. Periodic urine tests for **microalbuminuria** should be performed to screen for nephropathy.

   d. The patient should undergo an annual **ophthalmologic evaluation**.

   e. A **multidisciplinary approach** is essential and should include a primary care provider, an endocrinologist, a diabetic nurse specialist, a dietician, and a psychologist.

IV PROGNOSIS

A. Complications

1. Microvascular complications include retinopathy, nephropathy, and neuropathy. Atherosclerosis of larger vessels and cataracts can also occur.

2. **Lipohypertrophy** may occur as a result of repeated subcutaneous injections. Rotating injection sites can help avoid this complication.

3. **Mauriac syndrome** includes short stature, delayed puberty, and hepatomegaly.

4. **Psychosocial issues** include overprotection by parents, stigmatization during adolescence, and noncompliance.

B. **Morbidity.** The Diabetes Control and Complication Trial (1993) showed that improved glucose control, achieved with intensive diabetes therapy, decreases the risk of long-term complications. This study found that for every 1% reduction in the HbA_{1c} level, a 40% reduction in long-term complications occurs. However, a 20% increase in hypoglycemic episodes also occurs with every 1% reduction in the HbA_{1c} level. Even with improvements in glucose control, children with diabetes are still at risk for delayed puberty and short stature.

HOT

KEY
Young children may be more sensitive to severe hypoglycemia and may be at risk for related long-term neurocognitive effects.

V RECENT ADVANCES

A. Many new **glucose meters** have a memory system that can store glucose measurements and insulin doses.

B. **Continuous insulin infusion** with a subcutaneous pump is now available. This technology permits careful control of plasma glucose levels. Current pump systems require patients to calculate insulin dosages based on serial blood glucose measurements. A motivated patient with good support is the best candidate for an insulin pump.

C. The ongoing United States Diabetes Prevention Trial I is examining the use of **exogenous insulin** to delay or prevent diabetes in healthy children who are at risk for diabetes (e.g., siblings of patients with diabetes).

D. **Screening** children who are at increased risk for diabetes (e.g., postprandial plasma glucose testing or oral glucose tolerance testing) seems to offer little benefit.

References
Glaser NS: Non–insulin-dependent diabetes mellitus in childhood and adolescence. *Pediatr Clin North Am* 1997;44(2):307–337.
Kaufman FR: Diabetes mellitus. *Pediatr Rev* 1997;18(11):383–393.
Sperling M: Diabetes mellitus. In *Clinical Pediatric Endocrinology.* Edited by Kaplan S. Philadelphia, WB Saunders, 1990, pp 127–164.

93. Diabetic Ketoacidosis

I. INTRODUCTION

A. Definitions
1. **Diabetic ketoacidosis (DKA)** is defined as hyperglycemia (> 250 mg/dl) with hyperketonemia/ketonuria and acidosis (serum pH < 7.3).
2. **Hyperosmolar nonketotic coma** is defined as a coma with a very high serum glucose level and mild ketosis.

B. Pathogenesis. DKA is caused by insulin deficiency, which may result from any of the following situations:
1. Failure to take insulin
2. Acute stress leading to an increase in hormones that have an anti-insulin effect (e.g., glucagon, epinephrine, cortisol, growth hormone)
3. Acute illness (e.g., bacterial or viral infection)

 HOT KEY

In acute illness, some patients make the mistake of using too little insulin because they are not eating as usual; this decrease in insulin dosage may precipitate DKA.

C. Epidemiology. DKA is the most common reason for hospitalization in children with diabetes. Approximately 20%–40% of children with type I diabetes have DKA at some point.

II. APPROACH TO THE PATIENT

A. History. The physician should ask about infections, recent acute illnesses, previous insulin therapy, time and amount of last dose of insulin, change in weight as a result of illness before DKA, polyuria, and polydipsia.

B. Physical examination. The physician should note the patient's cardiovascular status, state of hydration, respiratory rate, and mental status.

C. Symptoms
1. **Dehydration.** Patients often are dehydrated as a result of increased urine output secondary to an osmotic diuresis. They also may have increased insensible losses as a result of hyperventilation secondary to ketosis.
2. **Ketosis.** Tachypnea occurs to compensate for metabolic acidosis. The patient's breath may have a "fruity" ketone odor.

3. **Abdominal pain.** Abdominal tenderness is common and should improve as the patient's condition stabilizes. The patient also may have significant nausea and vomiting.

HOT
▶
KEY

Patients with DKA may be misdiagnosed as having appendicitis.

4. **Acute cerebral edema** may occur from excessive fluid resuscitation, a too-rapid decrease in serum glucose level, or failure of serum sodium level to increase during therapy. Symptoms include decreasing level of consciousness, incontinence, severe headache, agitation, combativeness, vomiting, apnea, ophthalmoplegia, unequal or sluggish pupils, papilledema, and seizures.

5. **Changes in vital signs** also may occur. These include hypothermia, hypotension or hypertension, and tachycardia or bradycardia.

HOT
▶
KEY

A high index of suspicion is needed to diagnose DKA in infants and young children.

D. Laboratory tests
   1. **Initial blood tests** include levels of glucose, sodium, potassium, phosphate, calcium, magnesium, bicarbonate, blood urea nitrogen, creatinine, and arterial or venous blood gases.
   2. **Urinalysis** is performed, and urine is tested for ketones at each void.
   3. **Follow-up tests.** Blood glucose levels should be measured hourly. Electrolytes and pH should be measured every 2 hours for 8 hours, and then every 4 hours as the patient's condition stabilizes.
   4. **Interpreting electrolyte values**
      a. The **sodium (Na) level** may be spuriously low because of dilution from the high serum glucose level. Most patients have a total-body sodium deficit, however. The true serum sodium level can be determined with the following formula:

$$\text{Corrected Serum Sodium} = \text{Measured Na} + \left[1.6 \times \frac{\text{Glucose (mg/dL)} - 100}{100} \right]$$

      b. **Potassium.** Total body potassium (K) almost always is de-pleted. Initially, the serum potassium level may be misleadingly elevated because of the patient's acidosis.

c. Calculating osmolality. The patient is at risk for cerebral edema if the initial serum osmolality is greater than 320 mOsm/L:

$$\text{Serum osmolality} \atop (\text{mOsm/kg})} = \left(2 \times (\text{Na}(\text{mmol/L}) + \text{K}(\text{mmol/L})\right) + \left(\frac{\text{BVN}}{2.8}\right) + \left(\frac{\text{Glucose mg/dl}}{18}\right)$$

HOT
KEY

Meningitis should be considered in patients who are confused or comatose and are suspected of having DKA, but whose serum osmolality is < 320 mOsm/L.

 III **TREATMENT.** The mnemonic "ADMIT" is a useful way to remember the findings that suggest the need to admit a patient with DKA to the pediatric intensive care unit.

"ADMIT"

Age < 2 years
Decreased pH to < 7.1
Mental status changes or obtundation
Instability of cardiovascular status or severe dehydration
T waves or other significant electrocardiogram findings related to hypokalemia or hyperkalemia

---

A. Fluids and electrolytes

1. **Initial resuscitation.** The patient will be dehydrated by 5% to 10%. The best estimate of dehydration can be made by noting the patient's premorbid and current weights. An initial bolus of normal saline or lactated Ringer solution (10–20 ml/kg) is given over a period of 1 hour. The smallest possible volume should be given to prevent cerebral edema. Albumin (5%) at 20–25 ml/kg may be used if the patient is severely dehydrated or in shock. The patient should receive nothing by mouth initially. Boluses of large volumes of hypotonic fluids must be avoided because they increase the risk of cerebral edema.

2. The **fluid deficit** should be estimated by clinical criteria **(Table 93–1).** To minimize the risk of cerebral edema, rapid changes in serum osmolality should be avoided by ensuring that the serum sodium level increases as the serum glucose level decreases. The deficit can be replaced with 1/2 normal

TABLE 93-1. Evaluation of Severity of Dehydration			
Examination	Older Child 3%, Infant 5%	Older Child 6%, Infant 10%	Older Child 9%, Infant 15%
Skin turgor	Normal	Tenting	None
Skin, touch	Normal	Dry	Clammy
Buccal mucosa/ lips	Moist	Dry	Parched/ cracked
Eyes	Normal	Deep set	Sunken
Crying, tears	Present	Reduced	None
Fontanel	Flat	Soft	Sunken
Central nervous system	Consolable	Irritable	Lethargic
Pulse	Regular	Slightly increased	Tachycardia
Urine output	Normal	Decreased	Anuria

Reprinted with permission from McMillan JA, DeAngelis CD, Feigin RD (eds): *Oski's Pediatrics: Principles and Practice*, 3rd ed. Philadelphia, Lippincott Williams & Wilkins, 1999, p 69.

saline over 36 hours if the serum osmolality is greater than 320 mOsm/L. If the serum osmolality is greater than 340 mOsm/L, the deficit should be replaced over a period of 48 hours. In such a case, it probably is safest to correct the fluid deficit with normal saline over a 48-hour period.

3. **Potassium.** When the serum potassium level is in the normal range and the patient has urinated, 40 mEq/L potassium [half as potassium chloride (KCl) and half as potassium phosphate (KPO_4)] may be administered.

B. Insulin therapy

HOT KEY

Subcutaneous insulin has no place in the initial treatment of DKA. Initiation of an intravenous insulin infusion should not be delayed.

1. **Intravenous insulin infusion.** The standard solution is composed of 50 units of regular insulin in 250 ml normal saline, which provides 0.1 U/kg/h at 0.5 ml/kg/h. The tubing must be flushed initially with 50 ml insulin solution to compensate for insulin that adheres to the tubing.

2. **Intravenous infusion rates**
   a. Unlike adults, children do not need a bolus of insulin. A

continuous infusion of insulin achieves a steady state within 15–20 minutes. The infusion rate should begin at 0.1 U/kg/h. Blood glucose level should not decrease more than 75–100 mg/dl/h; too rapid a decline promotes cerebral edema.

b. The rate of insulin infusion should be reduced only if the patient's pH responds satisfactorily. Intravenous administration of insulin should continue until urine ketone values are negative for two measurements, or until the patient is consuming a normal diet orally.

3. Addition of dextrose

a. When the blood glucose level is less than 250 mg/dl, 5% dextrose should be added to the maintenance fluids.

b. Intravenous dextrose should be increased as needed to maintain a blood sugar level greater than 100 mg/dl.

HOT KEY

A common pitfall is reducing the insulin infusion rate when the blood glucose decreases and the patient is still acidemic (pH < 7.25). The patient requires intravenous insulin to prevent ketosis. The appropriate maneuver is to increase the dextrose concentration of the maintenance fluids.

C. Bicarbonate is not used except in the following circumstances:

1. Shock that does not respond to fluid resuscitation (pH < 7.1 and serum bicarbonate level < 5 mEq/L)

2. Hyperkalemia with electrocardiographic changes. If needed, bicarbonate is given at 1–2 mEq/kg. Bicarbonate should not be administered by intravenous push, it should be given over a period of 2 hours.

IV ONGOING MANAGEMENT

A. Acute cerebral edema. The patient's neurologic status must be re-evaluated repeatedly to detect possible cerebral edema. Patients younger than 5 years of age and those with previously undiagnosed diabetes are at higher risk. Rapid rehydration, hypoxia, and precipitous drops in the blood glucose level may exacerbate the situation.

1. If acute cerebral edema occurs, it should be treated with 0.5–1 g/kg intravenous mannitol; repeat doses may be required.

2. In severe cases, intubation and hyperventilation may be needed to decrease cerebral edema.

3. Computed tomography scans are not helpful in diagnosing acute cerebral edema; the decision to treat is based on clinical grounds.

4. **Urinary losses.** Urine output should be monitored closely, and fluids should be adjusted accordingly. There are hidden sources of H_2O in patients with DKA from the oxidation of glucose and ketones and from an elevated antidiuretic hormone level. Therefore, if urine losses are replaced, 0.5 ml of normal saline per milliliter of urine should be administered after the blood glucose level decreases to less than 250 mg/dl.

B. Continuous **electrocardiographic monitoring** should be performed if the serum potassium level is less than 3 or greater than 6 mEq/L.

C. **Oral intake.** Oral feeding should be reinstated gradually, and not until the patient's ileus resolves. If fed too early, the patient may vomit.

D. **Conversion from intravenous to subcutaneous insulin** should be considered when the glucose level is less than 250 mg/dl, urine ketones are not detected, and the venous pH is greater than 7.25.

   1. Intravenous insulin should be continued for 3 hours after the initiation of subcutaneous insulin therapy to allow for absorption of the subcutaneous insulin.

   2. The usual 24-hour insulin requirement is approximately 1 U/kg for a patient who is newly diagnosed with diabetes.

     a. Two thirds of the total dose should be given in the morning, with the remaining one third given in the evening.

     b. Two thirds of each dose should be lente insulin, and one third should be regular insulin.

   3. For a patient with previously diagnosed diabetes, a sliding scale for hyperglycemia and urine ketones should be added to the normal regimen. The insulin requirements may be higher during the first day after DKA.

   4. Because of the risk of hypoglycemia, aggressive insulin doses should not be given during periods of fasting (e.g., at night).

 PROGNOSIS. DKA has a mortality rate of 1%–2%. Most deaths are caused by increased intracranial pressure. The prognosis is worse for patients who have respiratory arrest as a result of acute cerebral edema.

References

McMillan JA, DeAngelis CD, Feigin RD (eds): *Oski's Pediatrics: Principles and Practice,* 3rd ed. Philadelphia, Lippincott Williams & Wilkins, 1999, pp 1799–1802.

Rosenbloom AL, Hanas R: Diabetic ketoacidosis (DKA): treatment guidelines. *Clin Pediatr* 35(5):261–266, 1996.

94. Precocious Puberty

I **INTRODUCTION.** **Precocious puberty** is defined as the appearance of secondary sexual characteristics before 9 years of age in a boy and 8 years of age in a girl.

II **REVIEW OF NORMAL PUBESCENCE**

A. In girls
1. Girls normally enter puberty between 8 and 13 years of age. Puberty is complete in 1.5–6 years.
2. The appearance of breast buds and a growth spurt are followed by development of pubic hair and the maturation of external genitalia. Axillary hair appears 2 years after pubic hair, and menstruation begins about 2 years after the appearance of breasts.

B. In boys
1. Boys normally begin puberty between 9 and 14 years of age. Puberty is complete in 2–4.5 years.
2. Pubic hair appears 6 months after the testes enlarge. Phallic enlargement and a growth spurt occur 12 to 18 months after testicular enlargement. Axillary and facial hair develop variably, but usually about 2 years after pubic hair.

C. The **hypothalamic-pituitary-gonadal axis.** The hypothalamus releases gonadotropin-releasing hormone (GnRH) in a pulsatile fashion, stimulating the release of follicle-stimulating hormone (FSH) and luteinizing hormone (LH) from the pituitary. FSH and LH initiate estrogen production in the ovaries and testosterone production in the testes.

D. Estrogen stimulates breast development, enlargement of the ovaries and uterus, growth acceleration, and bone age advancement.

E. Androgen spurs development of pubic hair, acne, clitoral enlargement, phallic enlargement, growth acceleration, and bone age advancement.

F. Adrenal maturation. The adrenal gland produces dehydroepiandrosterone (DHA) and its sulfate (DHAS), which are responsible for androgen effects in girls. The virilizing changes seen in boys result from the androgen secreted from the testes.

III **GONADOTROPIN-DEPENDENT PRECOCIOUS PUBERTY** is also known as true, or central, precocious puberty.

A. Pathophysiology. Central precocious puberty is caused by activation of the hypothalamic-pituitary-gonadal axis.

B. General features. Secondary sex characteristics are always isosexual. The ovaries and testes are enlarged.

C. Causes

    1. Idiopathic (constitutional or functional) precocious puberty.

    2. Hypothalamic hamartoma is caused by an ectopic GnRH-secreting pulse-generating tumor often attached to the floor of the third ventricle. Rapidly progressive precocious puberty in very young children suggests hypothalamic hamartoma.

    3. Organic brain lesions [e.g., brain tumors (optic gliomas, astrocytomas, ependymomas, neurofibromas, germinomas), hydrocephalus, severe head trauma, postencephalitic scars, tuberculosis, meningitis, and tuberous sclerosis] may cause precocious puberty by an unknown mechanism. Hypothalamic signs [e.g., diabetes insipidus, adipsia, hyperthermia, unnatural crying or laughing (gelastic seizures), obesity, and cachexia] suggest an intracranial lesion.

D. Epidemiology. Central precocious puberty is more common in girls than in boys (10:1). One in three affected boys is found to have an intracranial tumor, whereas only 1 in 10 affected girls has an intracranial tumor.

E. Growth effects

    1. Height, weight, and osseous maturation are accelerated.

    2. Osseous maturation often is 2–3 standard deviations above the norm.

F. The **clinical course** follows three established patterns:

    1. Rapidly progressive. Most patients are younger than 6 years of age and show rapid osseous and physical maturation. These patients are at greatest risk for loss of height potential.

    2. Slowly progressive. Most patients are older than 6 years of age and have preserved height potential.

    3. Spontaneously regressive. The variability of the clinical course underscores the importance of longitudinal observation before the decision is made to initiate treatment.

G. Diagnosis. The diagnosis of central precocious puberty is confirmed by the presence of pubertal levels of gonadotropins and testosterone or estradiol, as well as pubertal enlargement of the testes or ovaries.

    1. GnRH stimulation test. GnRH is given, and the LH response is measured. The LH level is higher than the FSH level in boys with early precocity. A small LH response in girls is seen early in precocity, with the LH:FSH ratio increasing as puberty progresses. Prepubertal children do not secrete increased levels of LH in response to a GnRH challenge.

    2. Girls should undergo **pelvic ultrasound** to look for enlargement of the ovaries or uterus. For boys, the size of the testes is carefully noted.

3. **Bone age.** Radiographs of the patient's hands and wrists are compared with standard measurements. Any advancement > 2 standard deviations is considered abnormal.

4. **Computed tomography (CT) and magnetic resonance imaging (MRI).** A CT or MRI scan of the head is obtained if there is suspicion of central precocious puberty.

5. Because as many as one half of patients with untreated hypothyroidism show some evidence of isosexual development, thyroid screening should be considered.

H. Treatment

1. **GnRH agonists.** Continuous pituitary stimulation with a GnRH agonist is provided to down-regulate the axis. All patients with rapidly progressive courses are candidates for this treatment. Depot preparations (e.g., Lupron Depot Ped) may be given once every 4 weeks. GnRH agonists are as effective for organic brain lesions as they are for idiopathic sexual precocity, but they are not effective in treating peripheral precocious puberty.

2. **Hypothalamic hamartomas** do not require surgery unless intractable seizures develop.

IV GONADOTROPIN-INDEPENDENT, OR PERIPHERAL PRECOCIOUS PUBERTY

A. General features

1. Secondary sex characteristics may be isosexual or heterosexual. Virilization in girls is characterized by ambiguous genitalia, clitoromegaly, and hirsutism.

2. Hypothalamic-pituitary-gonadal activation does not occur. In these cases, the sex steroids are secreted autonomously.

3. As with central precocious puberty, affected children are characterized by rapid growth and advancement of skeletal age.

B. Causes

1. **In girls,** causes may be isosexual or heterosexual.

a. **Isosexual causes** include: McCune-Albright syndrome, autonomous ovarian cysts, ovarian tumors, granulosa cell tumors, gonadoblastomas, lipoid tumors, ovarian carcinomas, adrenocortical tumors, and exogenous estrogen exposure (e.g., oral contraceptives, skin creams, medications, and animal proteins—especially poultry—may be high in estrogens).

b. **Heterosexual (virilization) causes** include: congenital adrenal hyperplasia (e.g., 21-hydroxylase, 11-hydroxylase, and 3-beta-hydroxysteroid dehydrogenase deficiency), adrenal tumors, ovarian tumors, glucocorticoid receptor defect, and exogenous androgens (anabolic steroids).

2. **In boys,** causes may be isosexual or heterosexual.

   a. **Isosexual causes** include congenital adrenal hyperplasia, adrenocortical tumor, Leydig cell tumor, familial male precocious puberty, pseudohypoparathyroidism, human chorionic gonadotropin (hCG)–secreting tumors (e.g., hepatomas, hepatoblastomas, teratomas, chorioepitheliomas, germinomas), glucocorticoid receptor defect, exogenous androgens (e.g., anabolic steroids), McCune-Albright syndrome.

   b. **Heterosexual (feminization) causes** include feminizing adrenocortical tumor (rare and highly malignant), sex cord tumor, familial increased aromatase activity, and exogenous estrogens.

C. Workup

1. The possibility of unintended ingestion of **exogenous estrogens or androgens** must be investigated. If these are the culprit, the ovaries and testes will be prepubertal in size.

2. **Gonadotropins** are not elevated in peripheral precocious puberty.

3. There is no gonadotropin increase in response to GnRH stimulation testing.

4. If peripheral precocious puberty is suspected, **imaging studies** (CT, MRI, or ultrasound) should be performed to search for an ovarian or adrenal tumor. The testes must be examined carefully for any masses or irregular consistency.

5. **Virilization in girls** is a clue to an adrenal or ovarian lesion. There may be increased adrenal androgens and increased levels of 17-ketosteroids. **Feminization in boys** should prompt a search for an adrenal tumor, a testicular tumor, hepatoma, or an increase in aromatase activity.

6. **McCune-Albright syndrome** must always be considered in a patient with precocious puberty, café-au-lait spots, and fibrous dysplasia of the skull and long bones. These patients also may have elevated thyroid hormone (T3) levels.

7. **Very high testosterone levels** suggest a Leydig cell tumor.

8. **Very high estradiol levels** are found in granulosa cell tumors, gonadoblastomas, lipoid tumors, or ovarian carcinomas.

9. Patients with **increased levels of hCG** require imaging studies to search for an hCG-secreting tumor in the liver, mediastinum, or central nervous system.

V INCOMPLETE (PARTIAL) PRECOCIOUS PUBERTY

A. **Premature thelarche** is defined as unilateral or bilateral breast development in girls without any other evidence of precocious maturity. Onset is most common in the first 2 years of life.

1. **Pathophysiology.** Premature thelarche is caused by normal episodes of ovarian follicular maturation and estrogen secretion.
2. **Prognosis.** The breast enlargement may persist for 3–5 years; regression begins earlier in girls with onset before age 2 years. True precocious puberty must be ruled out in any patient with evidence of systemic estrogen effects.
3. **Symptoms**
   a. **Breast development** may fluctuate, and may be symmetric or asymmetric.
   b. **Estrogen levels** may be high enough to induce growth acceleration or bone age advancement. This condition regresses spontaneously.
4. **Diagnosis**
   a. **LH and FSH levels** usually are low.
   b. A **GnRH release test** shows an increased FSH:LH ratio (prepubertal pattern).
   c. **Estradiol levels** may be in the early adolescent or normal range, depending on the stage of ovarian follicular maturation. Persistently low levels herald the regression of breast tissue.
   d. Ultrasound may show a **functional ovarian cyst,** but ovaries are of normal size.
5. **Differential diagnosis** includes ovarian or adrenal neoplasm, the beginning of progressive true sexual precocity, and exogenous estrogen ingestion.

B. **Premature adrenarche** is defined as the appearance of pubic hair before 7 or 8 years of age without other signs of precocious sexual maturity. Like premature thelarche, this condition usually is benign and self-limited.
   1. **Pathophysiology.** Premature adrenarche results from early maturation of adrenal androgen production. The GnRH release test shows a prepubertal pattern.
   2. **Prognosis.** Girls are at increased risk for hyperandrogenism and polycystic ovarian syndrome as adults.
   3. **Symptoms.** Pubic hair begins to develop on the labia majora and progresses to the pubic region and axilla. Adult axillary odor is common.
   4. **Diagnosis**
      a. Plasma and urine 17-ketosteroid levels are in the early pubertal range.
      b. A GnRH release test shows a prepubertal pattern.
      c. **Congenital adrenal hyperplasia** must be ruled out if there is evidence of systemic androgen stimulation (e.g., clitoral or phallic enlargement, growth acceleration, or osseous maturation).

C. **Premature menarche** is defined as isolated menses without other evidence of sexual development. It probably is caused by bursts in ovarian activity. In most cases, only one to three episodes of bleeding occur.

1. **Diagnosis**
   a. Gonadotropins are at normal levels, although estradiol levels may be elevated.
   b. Ultrasound may show ovarian cysts.
2. **Differential diagnosis** includes vulvovaginitis, foreign body, urethral prolapse, and sarcoma botryoides.

D. **Gynecomastia in adolescent boys** is caused by a high estradiol:testosterone secretion ratio, which is normal in the early pubertal testes.

1. **Diagnosis.** Gonadotropin, sex steroid, and prolactin levels are normal.
2. **Differential diagnosis** includes Klinefelter syndrome; chronic marijuana use; use of ketoconazole, spironolactone, and cimetidine; untreated hyperthyroidism; renal failure; cirrhosis; choriocarcinoma; and estrogen-secreting tumors of the testes or adrenal gland.

References

Behrman RE, Kliegman RM, Arvin AM: *Nelson Textbook of Pediatrics,* 16th ed. Philadelphia, WB Saunders, 1999.

Wheeler MD, Styne DM: Diagnosis and management of precocious puberty. *Pediatr Clin North Am* 37(6):1255–1271, 1990.

95. Inborn Errors of Metabolism

I **INTRODUCTION.** Inborn errors of metabolism often present in the neonatal period. Prompt diagnosis requires a high index of suspicion based on protean symptoms.

HOT KEY Metabolic disease should be suspected in infants who suddenly become ill after appearing well for the first few days of life.

A. General features of inborn errors of metabolism
   1. Metabolic acidosis
   2. Coma that is unresponsive to intravenous (IV) glucose administration
   3. Poor feeding
   4. Hepatomegaly or liver failure
   5. Seizures
   6. Unexplained mental retardation or neurologic regression
   7. Lethargy
   8. Failure to thrive
   9. Vomiting
   10. Developmental delay

HOT KEY Neonatal sepsis, ductal-dependent cardiac malformations, and acute presentations of inborn errors of metabolism have a similar clinical picture.

HOT KEY Unexplained liver dysfunction suggests a metabolic disorder. Liver dysfunction may indicate a defect of amino acid metabolism, a urea cycle defect, or a disorder of carbohydrate metabolism.

B. General workup
   1. If a metabolic disorder is suspected, the initial laboratory workup includes:

513

    a. Serum glucose, pH, bicarbonate, ammonia (NH_3), blood urea nitrogen (BUN), and lactate as well as a complete blood count (CBC) and electrolytes

    b. Urinalysis for reducing substances and ketones

  2. Complete physical examination, with special attention paid to dysmorphic features and liver size

  3. Quantitative serum and urine amino acids and organic acid analysis are tested based on the results of the initial screening laboratory tests (see I C).

C. Preliminary diagnosis (Figure 95–1)

  1. The combination of a high or normal NH_3 level, acidosis, a low bicarbonate level, ketosis, and neutropenia indicates organic acidemia.

  2. The combination of a high NH_3 level, normal pH, and a low BUN level indicates a urea cycle defect.

  3. The initial laboratory workup may not show any abnormalities in cases of amino acid disorders or hyperglycinemia. An exception to this is the classic form of maple syrup urine disease, which presents with severe acidosis.

  4. The combination of a low glucose level, lactic acidosis, and ketosis indicates a disorder of carbohydrate metabolism.

  5. The combination of low serum glucose and low urinary ketones indicates a disorder of fatty acid oxidation.

  6. Dysmorphic features indicate peroxisomal and lysosomal disorders.

D. Empiric treatment for suspected acute metabolic disease

  1. All intake of protein, lactate, or fructose is discontinued.

  2. Acidosis and hypoglycemia are corrected.

  3. IV glucose is given as the only carbohydrate source.

  4. Patients are monitored for increased intracranial pressure and NH_3 encephalopathy.

  5. Megadose vitamin therapy may be indicated for suspected cofactor-dependent diseases.

FIGURE 95–1. Algorithm diagnosis of inborn errors of metabolism. CBC = complete blood cell count; CNS = central nervous system; GSD = glycogen storage disease; LCHAD = long-chain hydroxyacyl CoA dehydrogenase; MCAD = medium-chain acyl-CoA dehydrogenase; MELAS = mitochondrial encephalomyopathy–lactic acidosis–and stroke-like syndrome; MERRF = myoclonus epilepsy with ragged red fibers syndrome; MSUD = maple syrup urine disease; OTC = ornithine transcarbamylase; PDH = Pyruvate dehydrogenase; RBC = red blood cell; VLCFA = very-long-chain fatty acid. (Courtesy of Dr. Ronald Scott, University of Washington School of Medicine, Seattle, Washington, 2001.)

Flowchart: Diagnostic approach to acute metabolic presentation in infancy

(Lethargy, coma, acidosis, hepatomegaly)

Rule out:
- Hypoglycemia
- Hypoxic event
- Sepsis
- CNS bleed
- Congenital heart disease
- Toxins

Physical examination
- Normal phenotype
- Enlarged liver
- Dysmorphic features

Laboratory Tests
CBC
Electrolytes
Glucose

Lactate
NH3

Urine:
pH
Specific gravity
Ketones
Reducing substance

Major Disorder	Abnormal Clinical Test	Disease Example	Confirming Genetic Test
Amino acid disorder		MSUD, NKH glycinemia, Tyrosinemia-I	Plasma amino acids, Organic acids, Tissue enzymes
Urea cycle disorder	NH3 ↑	OTC, Argininosuccinate, Citrullinemia	Plasma/urine amino acids, Orotic acid, Tissue enzymes
Organic acid disorder	Acidosis, NH3 ↑ (?), Urine ketones	Methylmalonic, Propionate/isovaleric, Glutaric-II	Organic acids, Tissue enzymes
HCO3 loss	Electrolytes	Renal loss, GI loss	Plasma/urine amino acids, pH & HCO3
Lactic acidosis/mitochondria	Lactate ↑	PDH deficiency, Mitochondrial disorders, MERRF, MELAS	Pyruvate/lactate, Tissue enzymes, Muscle biopsy, DNA
Glycogen storage	Acidosis, Glucose ↓, Lactate ↑	GSD-I and III	Glucose/lactate, Cholesterol/triglycerides/uric acid, Liver biopsy, DNA
Fatty acid oxidation	Glucose ↓, Urine ketones ↓	MCAD, LCHAD	Organic acids, DNA for MCAD, LCHAD, Tissue enzymes
Galactosemia	Positive urine-reducing substance	Galactosemia	RBC gal-1-PUT, DNA genotype
Peroxisomal disease		Zellweger syndrome, Psuedo-Zellweger syndrome	Radiographs, VLCFA/plasmalogens, Liver biopsy, Tissue enzymes
Lysosomal disease		GM-1 gangliosidosis, Mucopolysaccharide disorders	Radiographs, Tissue enzymes, Mucopolysaccharide, Oligosaccharides, Electron microscopy of skin

6. A metabolic disease expert is consulted.
7. If death is imminent, samples of blood and urine are collected and held. Skin and liver biopsy specimens are obtained promptly after death.

II ORGANIC ACIDEMIAS (Table 95–1)

A. **Natural history.** Organic acidemias usually present acutely early in life, causing decreased feeding, vomiting, and lethargy. The vomiting may be severe enough that pyloric stenosis is suspected. If untreated, encephalopathy, coma, and death may ensue.
B. **General laboratory features**
   1. Findings include a normal or high NH_3 level, acidosis, a low bicarbonate level, ketonuria, and neutropenia.
   2. The specific disorder is diagnosed by detection of the appropriate organic acid or its metabolite in body fluids.
C. **Prognosis.** Patients with acute neonatal onset often have significant neurologic sequelae.
D. **Treatment of organic acidemias**
   1. Sodium bicarbonate infusions are given to normalize pH.
   2. Adequate hydration is ensured.
   3. Protein intake is restricted.
   4. A catabolic state is minimized by providing adequate calories, with 50%–60% of calories coming from glucose.
   5. The NH_3 level is monitored.
   6. Dialysis may be needed to control acidosis and hyperammonemia.

III AMINO ACID DISORDERS (Table 95–2)

A. **Natural history.** Aminoacidopathies have a spectrum of presentation and involve multiple organ systems.
B. **General laboratory features.** Presentation is varied. Most forms do not cause acidosis, ketosis, or hyperammonemia. The exact disorder is diagnosed by detecting the appropriate amino acid or its metabolite in body fluids.

IV DISORDERS OF AMMONIA METABOLISM (Table 95–3)

A. **Pathogenesis.** The breakdown of amino acids results in the production of NH_3, which normally is detoxified into urea by the urea cycle. Defects are caused by a deficiency of urea cycle enzymes and accumulation of NH_3.
B. **Natural history.** Patients usually present in the neonatal period with acute neurologic deterioration. Classically, neonates appear normal for the first 24–48 hours of life. Milder forms may present later in infancy or in childhood, with intermittent symptoms.

TABLE 95-1. Organic Acidemias

Disease	Pathogenesis	Natural History and Symptoms	Diagnosis	Adjunctive Treatments
Isovaleric acidemia	Deficiency of isovaleryl CoA dehydrogenase Accumulation of isovaleryl-CoA	Half of patients present acutely. There is a chronic intermittent form that presents in the first months to years of life.	Elevated levels of urine iso-valeric acid and its metabolites (isovalerylglycine, 3-hydroxyisovaleric acid) Elevated level of serum glycine Sweaty feet odor	Protein restriction, low dietary leucine Glycine and carnitine supplements aid in the removal of toxic metabolites.
Proprionic acidemia	Accumulation of propionyl-CoA	Most patients present acutely with neonatal coma.	Elevated levels of propionic acid and methylcitric acid in plasma and urine Elevated level of serum glycine	Protein restriction; valine, isoleucine, threonine, and methionine intake restriction Glycine and carnitine supplements may be helpful. Some patients respond to biotin.
Methylmalonic acidemia	Accumulation of methylmalonyl-CoA	Patients may present with failure to thrive with episodic acidosis.	Elevated levels of methylmalonic acid and its metabolites (3-hydroxypropionate and methylcitrate) in the urine Elevated level of serum glycine	Protein restriction; restrict valine, isoleucine, threonine, and methionine from diet Carnitine supplements may be helpful. Some patients respond to high-dose hydroxocobalamin.

CoA = coenzyme A.

TABLE 95-2. Amino Acid Disorders

Disease	Pathogenesis	Natural History and Symptoms	Diagnosis	Adjunctive Treatments
Phenylketonuria	Deficiency of phenylalanine hydroxylase leads to phenylalanine accumulation. Caucasians and Asian populations Autosomal recessive	**Natural history:** Patients are normal at birth. Severe mental retardation develops gradually; IQ drops to 60 by age 1 and to 40 by age 4. **Physical findings:** Microcephaly, widely spaced teeth, enamel hypoplasia, eczematoid rashes, pigment dilution **Symptoms:** Psychomotor retardation, hyperactive and purposeless movements, athetosis, vomiting, seizures Hyperreflexia and autistic-like behaviors ensue if untreated. Mousy or musty odor All symptoms are reversible except loss of intellectual potential. Patients whose phenylalanine is controlled by 1 month of age have the best prognosis.	Newborn screening Elevated serum and urine phenylalanine	Reduce phenylalanine intake and supplement tyrosine.

Tyrosinemia	Deficiency of fumaryl-acetoacetate hydrolase causes succinylacetone accumulation. Autosomal recessive	**Natural history:** Progressive hepatic dysfunction begins in infancy. Acute hepatic crises with neurologic crises (painful paresthesias and paralysis) are a common presentation. **Symptoms:** Failure to thrive, hepatomegaly, acute hepatic failure, developmental delay, irritability, vomiting Rancid, fishy, or cabbage-like odor	Newborn screening Serum and urine succinylacetone levels are elevated. Serum tyrosine and methionine also are increased. Elevated bilirubin (direct and indirect) and transaminase levels. Alpha-fetoprotein level usually is very high.	Reduce tyrosine, phenylalanine, and methionine intake. 2-(2-nitro-4-trifluoro-methylbenzoyl)-1,3-cyclohexanedione reduces succinylacetone formation. Most patients require liver transplantation.
Homocystinuria	Caused by a deficiency of cystathionine synthase. Level of homocystine, a degradation product of methionine metabolism, is elevated. Autosomal recessive	**Natural history:** Patients are normal at birth. The diagnosis often is made later in life. **Symptoms:** Subluxation of the lens causes severe myopia, cataracts, retinal detachment, glaucoma, astigmatism, and optic atrophy. Mental retardation occurs in ⅔ of patients; psychiatric disorders are common. Thromboembolic episodes can lead to stroke or cor pulmonale. **Physical findings:** Marfanoid appearance (tall, thin, high arched palate, pectus excavatum, pes cavus, genu valgum), fair complexion, blue eyes, and malar flush	Elevated serum and urine methionine and homocystine Low levels of cystine	Reduce methionine intake and supplement cystine. Some respond to high-dose vitamin B$_{12}$. Betaine: remethylates homocystine to methionine

(continued)

TABLE 95-2. Amino Acid Disorders (Continued)

Disease	Pathogenesis	Natural History and Symptoms	Diagnosis	Adjunctive Treatments
Maple syrup urine disease	No decarboxylation of BCAA: leucine, isoleucine, and valine More common among Mennonites from eastern Pennsylvania	There is a spectrum of presentation. The classic form is the most severe; it presents in the first days of life with acidosis, vomiting, lethargy, coma, and episodic hypertonicity, followed by flaccidity and severe opisthotonos. Less severe forms may present later in life with psychomotor handicaps, seizures, lethargy, vomiting, or metabolic decompensation with intercurrent illness.	Elevated serum and urine levels of leucine, isoleucine, valine, and alloisoleucine Decreased levels of alanine Hyperammonemia, hypoglycemia Maple syrup odor	Peritoneal dialysis is the most effective means of removing BCAA in acute cases. Remove BCAA from the diet. Supplement glutamine and alanine.

BCAA = branched chain amino acids.

TABLE 95-3. Disorders of Ammonia Metabolism/Urea Cycle Disorders

Disease	Pathogenesis	Natural History and Symptoms	Diagnosis	Adjunctive Treatments
CPS deficiency	CPS, which catalyzes the formation of carbamyl phosphate from ammonia, is absent. Autosomal recessive	Hyperammonemic coma in the neonatal period	Absent plasma citrulline and low arginine levels Elevated plasma glutamine, alanine, and glycine levels Normal urine orotic acid level	Restrict dietary protein intake. Foods should contain only essential amino acids and L-citrulline. Combined sodium benzoate and sodium phenylacetate. Liver transplantation may be required.
OTC deficiency	The most common urea cycle disorder X-linked	Hyperammonemic coma in the neonatal period Female patients have varying symptoms, depending on the degree of lyonization.	Low plasma citrulline level Elevated plasma glutamine, alanine, and glycine levels Markedly elevated urine orotic acid level	Same as for CPS Female relatives of affected patients should receive genetic counseling to determine their carrier status.
Citrullinemia	Caused by deficient activity of argininosuccinate synthetase. Autosomal recessive	Hyperammonemic coma in the neonatal period	Elevated plasma and urine citrulline levels Elevated plasma glutamine and alanine levels Absent plasma argininosuccinic acid Moderately elevated urine orotic acid level	Because citrulline is excreted well renally, management of hyperammonemia is less problematic. Otherwise, treatment is similar to that for CPS and OTC. Combined sodium benzoate and sodium phenylacetate. Supplemental L-arginine
Arginosuccinic aciduria	Caused by argininosuccinase deficiency. Autosomal recessive	May present as late as 1–2 weeks after birth.	Elevated plasma and urine argininosuccinic acid levels Elevated plasma glutamine and alanine levels Normal urine orotic acid level	Argininosuccinic acid is rapidly excreted in the urine. Patients do well with protein restriction and supplemental L-arginine. Sodium benzoate and sodium phenylacetate may be required for hyperammonemic episodes.

CPS = carbamyl phosphate synthetase; OTC = ornithine transcarbamylase.

C. General laboratory features
 1. The NH_3 level is high, the pH is normal, and the BUN level is low.
 2. The exact enzyme deficiency is determined by assays on erythrocytes, cultured fibroblasts, or liver biopsy specimens.
 3. Evidence of hepatic insufficiency is common.
D. Clinical features of hyperammonemia
 1. Initial features include lethargy, poor feeding, seizures, vomiting, anorexia, ataxia, confusion, agitation, and combativeness. Tachypnea may be striking.
 2. These symptoms may progress to circulatory collapse, seizures, cerebral edema, and coma.
E. Prognosis. Only 30% to 50% of neonates who have hyperammonemic coma survive; most survivors have significant neurologic defects.

HOT KEY

Prompt control of hyperammonemia greatly improves morbidity and mortality rates.

F. Treatment of acute hyperammonemia
 1. Comatose patients require mechanical ventilation.
 2. All protein intake is stopped.
 3. IV sodium benzoate (250 mg/kg/day) or IV sodium phenylacetate (250–500 mg/kg/day) can increase the renal excretion of nitrogenous waste.
 4. Hemodialysis is required for recalcitrant hyperammonemia (> 350 μmol). Exchange transfusion or peritoneal dialysis is far less effective than hemodialysis.
 5. Arginine is supplemented.

V DISORDERS OF CARBOHYDRATE METABOLISM (Table 95–4) The major disorders of carbohydrate metabolism involve glycogen, galactose, and fructose.

A. Natural history. Onset may be acute or chronic. The patient's presentation may be protean (e.g., growth retardation, muscle weakness, exercise intolerance). The most important physical finding often is hepatomegaly.
B. General laboratory features include a low glucose level, lactic acidosis, and hepatomegaly or hepatic dysfunction.
C. Differential diagnosis. In addition to the disorders listed in Table 95–4, adrenal insufficiency and hypopituitarism should be considered.

TABLE 95-4. Disorders of Carbohydrate Metabolism

Disease	Pathogenesis	Natural History and Symptoms	Diagnosis	Treatment
Hepatic glycogen storage disorders (e.g., Von Gierke, Pompe, Cori, Hers disease)	Enzymatic defects prevent the formation or degradation of liver glycogen. There are multiple single enzyme defects. All are autosomal recessive, except for type IX, which is X-linked. Type II (Pompe disease) has generalized muscle and liver involvement.	Patients present with lethargy, encephalopathy, and hypoglycemia at times of fasting or diminished carbohydrate intake. Hepatomegaly can be striking. Pompe disease is particularly severe, characterized by cardiac hypertrophy, hypotonia, and hepatomegaly. Patients die within the first year of life.	Fasting hypoglycemia, lactic acidosis, and ketosis. Liver biopsy needed for definitive diagnosis. Any glucose fasting or tolerance testing should be done by a specialist, with caution.	Patients require constant exogenous sources of glucose (corn starch). Enteral feeds may be required at night to prevent hypoglycemia. Hospitalization for intravenous 10% dextrose may be needed during intercurrent illnesses. Restrict intake of galactose and fructose. Liver transplantation may be required in some cases.
Muscle glycogen storage disorders	Types V (McArdle) and VII (Tarui) affect skeletal muscle glycogen metabolism.	Presentation is similar to that of hepatic glycogen storage disorders, with the addition of severe muscle cramps and myoglobinuria. Muscle wasting may be prominent. Hepatomegaly may or may not be present.	Definitive diagnosis requires a muscle biopsy. Elevated CK, LDH, and aldolase; blood lactate is normal. Ischemic exercise test: Inflate a blood pressure cuff to greater than systolic pressure and have the patient squeeze a rubber ball repeatedly. Severe muscle cramping and tetany results.	Avoidance of strenuous exercise helps avoid risk of muscle breakdown and subsequent acute renal failure. High-protein diet

(continued)

TABLE 95-4. Disorders of Carbohydrate Metabolism (Continued)

Disease	Pathogenesis	Natural History and Symptoms	Diagnosis	Treatment
Galactosemia	Deficiency of galactose-1-phosphate uridyl transferase prevents the breakdown of galactose into glucose. Galactose-1-phosphate accumulates. Most common defect of galactose metabolism Autosomal recessive	Normal at birth; problems begin when the child starts to feed. There is vomiting, diarrhea, and lethargy. *Escherichia coli* sepsis is common. Hepatomegaly and liver failure may occur. Galactosemia should be suspected in infants with conjugated hyperbilirubinemia. Central nervous system sequelae are common and can include psychomotor problems, learning disabilities, and attention deficit hyperactivity disorder. Female survivors may suffer from ovarian atrophy and amenorrhea.	Assay for galactose-1-phosphate uridyl transferase in erythrocytes is confirmatory. Non–glucose reducing substances in urine; elevated galactose and galactose-1-phosphate, abnormal liver function test results Nuclear cataracts are seen on slit-lamp evaluation; these lesions can regress with treatment.	Any infant suspected of having galactosemia should be placed on a galactose- and lactose-free diet. Soy-based formulas are the diet of choice. Adherence to this diet must be lifelong.

| Fructose intolerance | Absence of fructose-1-phosphate aldolase B causes acute hypoglycemia on ingestion of fructose. | Symptoms occur immediately after ingestion of fructose (found in citrus fruits, vegetables, and sweetened foods). Infants present when such foods are first introduced into their diets. **Symptoms:** Acute: Symptoms are more severe in infants. Sweating, trembling, emesis, lethargy, coma, seizures and shock. Chronic: Poor feeding; failure to thrive; nausea, vomiting, and diarrhea; irritability; hepatomegaly. Hepatic and renal dysfunction. | Laboratory study results are abnormal only immediately after ingestion of sucrose or fructose: hypoglycemia, lactic acidosis, fructosuria, fructosemia hypophosphatemia, hypermagnesemia, hyperuricemia, hyperkalemia. Non-glucose reducing substances in urine | Elimination of all sources of sucrose, fructose, and sorbitol Intravenous glucose infusions for acute episodes Liver transplantation may be required. |

TABLE 95-5. Disorders of Fatty Acid Oxidation

Disease	Pathogenesis	Natural History and Symptoms	Diagnosis	Treatment
MCAD deficiency, LDHAD deficiency, VLCAD deficiency	Absence of MCAD, LCHAD, or VLCAD	MCAD deficiency is the most common disorder of fatty acid metabolism; patients present between 5–24 months of age. Patients with VLCAD deficiency may present at less than 6 months of age with a dilated cardiomyopathy. Patients with LDHAD deficiency may develop a hypertrophic cardiomyopathy Infants born to mothers with acute fatty liver of pregnancy or HELLP syndrome should be screened for LCHAD deficiency.	Accumulation of acetyl-CoA compounds and dicarboxylic acids in blood and urine organic acid analysis during acute episodes Abnormal urine acylglycine or plasma acylcarnitine profiles between episodes Glucose fasting or tolerance testing should not be done because of the risk of precipitating a fatal episode.	Avoid fasting; meals should be high in carbohydrates and low in fat. The appropriate chain length triglyceride is excluded from the diet. Supplement L-carnitine. Hospitalization for intravenous D10 may be needed during intercurrent illnesses.

CoA = coenzyme A; HELLP = Hemolysis, elevated liver enzymes, low platelets; LDHAD = long-chain hydroxyacyl-CoA dehydrogenase; MCAD = medium-chain acyl-CoA dehydrogenase; VLCAD = very-long-chain acyl-CoA dehydrogenase.

TABLE 95-6. Lysosomal and Peroxisomal Disorders

Disorder	Pathogenesis	General Features
Lysosomal storage disorders Hunter, Hurler, Scheie, Sanfillippo, Morquio, Tay-Sachs, Sandhoff, Fabry, Gaucher, Farber, Neiman-Pick, Krabbe Metachromatic leukodystrophy	Lysosomes are organelles that degrade a variety of substances. In these disorders, hydrolases needed to degrade substances are absent, and the partially degraded matter accumulates, thereby disrupting cell function.	Characterized by progressive hepatomegaly, splenomegaly, neurologic regression, skeletal anomalies (e.g., dolichocephaly, thickened calvarium, boot-shaped sella, kyphosis, thickened ribs, proximally narrowed and distally widened metacarpals, coxa valga, shortened and thickened long bones), short stature, and coarse facies. Tay-Sachs and Neiman-Picks disease have characteristic cherry-red spots on the macula.
Peroxisomal disorders Zellweger syndrome, adrenal leukodystrophy, rhizomelic chondrodysplasia punctata	Peroxisomes are subcellular organelles with a variety of synthetic and degradative functions, often involving components of lipid membranes.	The hallmark of these diseases is inexorable neurodegeneration. Most have dysmorphic features. Some have adrenal, hepatic, or renal dysfunction.

VI DISORDERS OF FATTY ACID OXIDATION (Table 95-5)

A. **Pathogenesis.** During normal fasting, mitochondria produce energy from the beta-oxidation of fatty acids. The inability to do so leads to an accumulation of fatty acid metabolites. The serum glucose decreases secondarily from the failure of gluconeogenesis.

B. **Natural history.** Patients usually present at less than 2 years of age with vomiting, lethargy, encephalopathy, cardiovascular collapse, and hypoglycemia at times of fasting or diminished carbohydrate intake.

C. **General laboratory features.** The hallmark laboratory findings are hypoglycemia and absent urine ketones. There may be mild elevations of ammonia and liver enzymes; mild acidosis may also be present.

VII LYSOSOMAL AND PEROXISOMAL DISORDERS (Table 95-6)

A. Diagnosis is based on the clinical constellation of symptoms and confirmatory biochemical assays of red blood cells and fibroblasts. The presence of dysmorphic features is often the key to diagnosis.

B. Treatment for these disorders is mainly supportive. Bone marrow transplantation may be successful in some cases.

References

Barness LA: Analyzing signs and symptoms of metabolic diseases. *South Med J* 89(2): 163–166, 1996.

Bove KE: The metabolic crisis: a diagnostic challenge. *J Pediatr* 131(2):181–182, 1997.

Eichenwald HF, Stroder JS, Ginsburg CM: *Pediatric Therapy,* 3rd ed. St. Louis, CV Mosby, 1993.

McMillan JA, DeAngelis CD, Feigin RD, et al: *Oski's Pediatrics: Principles and Practice,* 3rd ed. Philadelphia, Lippincott Williams & Wilkins, 1999, pp 1823–1900.

PART XII

RHEUMATOLOGY

96. Henoch-Schönlein Purpura

I **BACKGROUND.** Henoch-Schönlein purpura (HSP), or anaphylactoid purpura, is the most common vasculitic disease of childhood. It is a vasculitis of arterioles, capillaries, and venules. It can affect any organ system, although the skin, joints, kidneys, and gastrointestinal tract are most commonly affected.

II **PATHOGENESIS**

A. The pathogenesis of HSP is unknown, but onset often occurs after an upper respiratory tract infection. Between 40% and 50% of patients have elevated antistreptolysin O (ASO) titers, suggesting a recent streptococcal infection.
B. The disease is characterized by **abnormalities in immunoglobulin A (IgA),** including increased serum IgA, IgA immune complexes (which can be found deposited in the walls of capillaries on kidney or skin biopsy), and unusual IgA autoantibodies—IgA rheumatoid factor and IgA antineutrophil cytoplasmic antibody.
C. Biopsy specimens show **granulocytic infiltration** into the walls of arterioles and venules.

III **EPIDEMIOLOGY**

A. The **incidence** of HSP in the United States is 9–18:100,000 children annually, with peaks in the winter and spring months.
B. The disease affects patients from age 6 months through adulthood. It is most common in children: 50% of cases occur in patients younger than 5 years of age, and 75% of cases occur in those younger than 10 years of age.
C. HSP is more common in boys than in girls (1.5:1), in children of lower socioeconomic groups, and in Hispanic children.

IV CLINICAL MANIFESTATIONS

A. Constitutional. Low-grade fever and malaise occur in more than 50% of patients.

B. Skin. The skin is affected in more than 90% of patients.

   1. The classic rash of HSP is a **palpable purpura** that occurs in the absence of thrombocytopenia. The lesions are red and macular when they first appear and dark, blue-purple, and palpable as they progress.

   2. Small petechial lesions may be seen at sites of skin compression (e.g., under elastic waistbands or socks), where pressure injures fragile vessels.

   3. Distribution of the rash classically is on dependent areas (e.g., legs, buttocks, arms), although other areas may be affected as well.

C. Joints

   1. Arthralgia (joint pain) occurs in 65%–84% of patients, usually involving the knees, ankles, or both.

   2. Arthritis (joint pain with swelling, warmth, and erythema) develops in approximately 30% of patients.

D. Gastrointestinal

   1. Abdominal pain, vomiting, and gastrointestinal bleeding occur in 63%–76% of patients.

   2. **Vasculitic lesions** that are similar to the classic rash (see IV B 1) develop throughout the bowel in many patients. As a result, friable areas develop and are easily sloughed and ulcerated. Bowel pain usually begins within 1 week of the onset of rash, but may occur up to 1 month later. Rarely, it precedes other symptoms.

   3. **Intussusception and hydrops of the gallbladder** also have been associated with HSP.

E. Renal

   1. Between 20% and 50% of affected patients have **nephritis,** which is characterized by **hematuria** with or without proteinuria.

   2. Nephritis often is associated with the development of significant **hypertension.**

   3. Most cases of nephritis (80%) occur within the first month of the syndrome. The rest occur in the following 2 months.

   4. Patients who have bloody stools are at increased risk for nephritis.

   5. Rapidly progressive, crescentic glomerulonephritis is rare, but can occur. Early recognition of declining renal function is critical.

F. Neurologic

   1. One third of patients have **headache,** and as many as 8% have mild encephalopathy.

  2. Rare complications, such as seizures, paresis, and coma, also
  may occur.
G. Genitourinary. Scrotal swelling and pain occur in approximately 4% of male patients. The symptoms may simulate testicular torsion.

V APPROACH TO THE PATIENT

A. Diagnosis. Diagnostic criteria established in 1990 by the American College of Rheumatology include the following:
  1. Age younger than 20 years
  2. Palpable purpura
  3. "Bowel angina" (abdominal pain typically is associated with
    bloody stools)
  4. Evidence of granulocytic infiltrates in the walls of arterioles
    or venules from skin or kidney biopsy specimens
B. The following tests also may be helpful in making the diagnosis:
  1. Complete blood cell count (CBC) to rule out thrombocyto-
    penia and evaluate hematocrit in the setting of gastrointest-
    inal bleeding
  2. Blood pressure measurement to detect renal disease
  3. Hemoccult test of stool to detect occult intestinal bleeding
  4. Urinalysis to assess hematuria and proteinuria
C. Additional tests to consider include:
  1. Skin biopsy, especially if the rash is atypical
  **2. Electrolytes, blood urea nitrogen (BUN), and creatinine
    measurement** to evaluate renal function
  3. Urine protein:creatinine ratio and **serum albumin measure-
    ment** to evaluate for nephrosis if the patient appears edema-
    tous or has a significant amount of protein in the urine
  4. Kidney biopsy if the patient has evidence of rapidly progres-
    sive glomerulonephritis
  5. ASO titer or **Streptozyme.** Although the link is unclear,
    40%–50% of patients have a history of recent streptococcal
    infection.
  6. Surgical consultation and **air-contrast enema** may be needed
    to evaluate for intussusception if the patient has symptoms
    or signs of acute abdomen.

VI ADJUVANT THERAPY

A. The efficacy of **steroids** in the treatment of HSP is a matter of
  ongoing controversy. Currently, the only clinically proven indication is for abdominal pain within the first 72 hours of onset in
  patients who cannot tolerate oral hydration.
B. Steroids do not seem to prevent nephritis, although the studies
  are too small to be conclusive. In the setting of rapidly progressive

glomerulonephritis, aggressive therapy with steroids and immunosuppressants may be indicated.

VII MANAGEMENT

A. **Urinalysis** is performed weekly for 3–6 months, then monthly for up to 3 years to screen for nephritis.
B. HSP has a 50% recurrence rate and is associated with streptococcal infection. Therefore, some practitioners advocate the use of **prophylactic antibiotics** (penicillin or amoxicillin) for 1 year at a low dosage.

VIII PROGNOSIS

A. **Mortality.** Death as a result of HSP is rare.
B. **Morbidity**
   1. The course of HSP typically is self-limited, lasting 4–6 weeks.
   2. The most significant long-term morbidity associated with HSP is nephritis. Between 1% and 5% of all patients who have nephritis go on to have significant renal morbidity, and 5%–15% of pediatric cases of end-stage renal disease are caused by HSP nephritis.

References

Szer IS: Gastrointestinal and renal involvement in vasculitis: management strategies in Henoch-Schönlein purpura. *Cleve Clin J Med* 66(5):312–317, 1999.

Szer IS: Henoch-Schönlein purpura: when and how to treat. *J Rheumatol* 23(9): 1661–1665, 1996.

Tizard EJ: Henoch-Schönlein purpura. *Arch Dis Child* 80:380–383, 1999.

97. Juvenile Rheumatoid Arthritis

I INTRODUCTION

A. Background

1. **Juvenile rheumatoid arthritis (JRA)** is the most common form of chronic childhood rheumatic disease. It originally was described as a single disorder with a spectrum of symptoms, but it is now defined as including three distinct but related childhood arthritis syndromes: pauciarticular, polyarticular, and systemic JRA.

2. The classic clinical description of lymphadenopathy, splenomegaly, a rash, and pericarditis was made in 1897 by Dr. George Frederick Still, and the systemic onset form sometimes is referred to as Still disease.

B. Definitions

1. Arthritis is joint pain combined with swelling, warmth, erythema, or limitation of motion. Joint pain alone is known as arthralgia, and should not raise concern for JRA.

2. **Onset type** is determined by the number of joints involved within the first 6 months:

   a. **Pauciarticular.** One to four joints

   b. **Polyarticular.** Five or more joints. Patients with polyarticular disease are divided into two major subgroups:

      (1) **RF-negative (Rheumatoid Factor),** with onset of symptoms in early childhood

      (2) **RF-positive,** with onset of symptoms during adolescence. This subgroup is similar to those with adult rheumatoid arthritis.

   c. **Systemic.** Any number of joints, plus the characteristic daily fever

C. Pathogenesis

1. **Chronic synovitis** (inflammation of the tissue that lines the joint) is the primary feature of JRA. Inflammation results in hyperemia, increased production of joint fluid, edema of the synovium with villous hypertrophy, and sometimes development of a synovial tissue pannus within the joint. The surrounding bone may be eroded and ultimately destroyed by the inflammation.

2. The etiology is unknown, but JRA is believed to be caused by an inciting event (e.g., infection) in a genetically susceptible

individual. Genetic associations have been made between HLA DR5 and DR8 and pauciarticular disease and between HLA DR4 and the rheumatoid factor (RF) positive subgroup of polyarticular disease.

II **CLINICAL MANIFESTATIONS** of JRA are shown in **Table 97–2.**

III **APPROACH TO THE PATIENT**

A. Diagnosis
  1. **Diagnostic criteria** from the American College of Rheumatology include:
     a. Age younger than 16 years at onset
     b. Arthritis in one or more joints
     c. Duration of disease for 6 weeks or longer
     d. Exclusion of other forms of juvenile arthritis
  2. Onset type (see I B 2; **Table 97–3**) is determined by the number of joints involved in the first 6 months.
  3. **Additional tests** that should be considered after JRA has been diagnosed include the following:
     a. **Ophthalmologic examination** to check for uveitis
     b. **Echocardiogram** or **electrocardiogram (ECG)** to evaluate pericardial effusion if JRA is the systemic onset type.
     c. **Joint aspiration** and **synovial fluid analysis.** Polymorphonuclear and mononuclear cells are present, but over a broad range (150–100,000 cells/mm^3) of concentrations.

TABLE 97-1. Epidemiology of Juvenile Rheumatoid Arthritis			
	Type of Juvenile Rheumatoid Arthritis		
	Pauciarticular	**Polyarticular**	**Systemic onset**
Proportion of all juvenile rheumatoid arthritis	40%–60%	30%–40%	10%–20%
Sex difference	4:1 female predominance	3:1 female predominance	Equal
Usual age of onset	1–3 y	1–3 y and adolescence	Any age

The estimated prevalence of juvenile rheumatoid arthritis in the United States is 113 cases per 100,000 children.

TABLE 97-2. Clinical Manifestations of Juvenile Rheumatoid Arthritis

System Affected	Type of Juvenile Rheumatoid Arthritis		
	Pauciarticular	Polyarticular	Systemic Onset
Constitutional	None	May have low-grade fever	Malaise, fatigue, and weight loss are common. Daily spiking fevers > 39°C often peak in the evening. Between episodes, temperature is normal or subnormal.
Cardiovascular	None	None	Pericarditis and, rarely, myocarditis
Pulmonary	None	None	Pleural effusions
Gastrointestinal	None	May have mild hepatosplenomegaly	Hepatosplenomegaly
Hematologic	None	Felty syndrome (splenomegaly and neutropenia) may develop in RF-positive patients	Anemia and leukocytosis
Lymphatic	None	May have mild lymphadenopathy	Generalized lymphadenopathy *(continued)*

TABLE 97-2. Clinical Manifestations of Juvenile Rheumatoid Arthritis (Continued)

System Affected	Type of Juvenile Rheumatoid Arthritis		
	Pauciarticular	Polyarticular	Systemic Onset
Bones and joints	Asymmetric arthritis of large joints. Knees and ankles are the most common sites, but fingers, elbows, and wrists also may be affected. History of morning stiffness that improves with use is classic. Cervical spine involvement is rare. Hip involvement is unusual. Leg-length discrepancy is possible because of inflammatory hyperemia in asymmetrically affected joints.	Symmetric involvement of large and small joints. Knees, wrists, and ankles are the most common sites, but joints of the hands and feet often are affected as well. Involvement of cervical spine and temporomandibular joint is common. Hip girdle may be involved. Rheumatoid nodules may develop over pressure points (e.g., elbows, fingers), particularly in RF-positive patients.	Any number of joints and any joints may be involved. Hip involvement is a major cause of disability in prolonged disease. Pain often is more severe than in other forms of juvenile rheumatoid arthritis. Systemic symptoms and arthritis may not occur simultaneously and occasionally are separated by years.

Eyes	Chronic uveitis in about 20%; can lead to blindness if untreated	Chronic uveitis in about 10%	Chronic uveitis in about 5%
Skin	None	None	Classic rash described as discrete, salmon-pink erythematous macules 2–5 cm in diameter. Migratory, evanescent, and often worst during fever. Most common on trunk and in axillae.

RF = rheumatoid factor.

TABLE 97-3. Types of Juvenile Rheumatoid Arthritis

	Pauciarticular	Polyarticular	Systemic Onset
Clinical findings			
Number of joints affected	1–4	> 5	Any
Joints involved	Large	Large and small	Any—painful arthritis
Systemic symptoms	None	Possible low-grade fever	Daily fever spikes > 39°C (key to diagnosis)
		Rheumatoid nodules	Rash, hepatosplenomegaly, anemia, pericarditis, lymphadenopathy
		Felty syndrome, splenomegaly	
Eyes	The chronic uveitis of juvenile rheumatoid arthritis usually is silent (not painful and not red). It often can be diagnosed only by a slit-lamp examination. Chronic, untreated inflammation can cause formation of synechiae between the iris and lens, which make the pupil appear jagged and poorly reactive on physical examination. The highest risk is in pauciarticular disease.		

Laboratory findings

ESR	Normal to mildly elevated	Normal to moderately elevated	Moderately to highly elevated
CRP	Normal	Normal to mildly elevated	Highly elevated
ANA-positive	30%–50%	30%	15%
RF-positive	< 5%	15%–50%, particularly with onset in adolescence	< 5%
CBC	Normal	Neutropenia (with Felty syndrome)	Anemia and leukocytosis

ANA = antinuclear antibody; CBC = complete blood cell count; CRP = C-reactive protein; ESR = erythrocyte sedimentation rate; RF = rheumatoid factor.

The concentration does not correlate with the severity of clinical disease. Glucose levels typically are low.

    d. Radiographs of affected joints may show bony destruction, particularly in the polyarticular and systemic onset forms of the disease. In patients with temporomandibular joint involvement, a Panorex study of the jaw may be useful to assess abnormalities of the mandible.

    e. A magnetic resonance imaging scan of the affected joints may be useful to evaluate the soft tissues and surrounding bony architecture.

B. Initial therapy

    1. Nonsteroidal anti-inflammatory drugs (NSAIDs) are the first-line therapy for pauciarticular and polyarticular disease.

    2. Steroids (e.g., prednisone) often are used in systemic onset disease, the polyarticular form, and Felty syndrome (characterized by splenomegaly and neutropenia).

C. Adjuvant therapies

    1. Second-line agents, such as hydroxychloroquine and sulfasalazine, may be helpful when NSAIDs are not effective.

    2. Methotrexate or cyclophosphamide may be helpful in cases that do not respond to NSAIDs or to second-line agents.

    3. Intra-articular injection of steroids can be very effective, and systemic effects may be less severe than those associated with oral or intravenous therapy.

    4. Early trials of new therapies that specifically target tumor necrosis factor (TNF) [e.g., soluble TNF-receptor preparations] are promising. These drugs may be helpful when NSAIDs and methotrexate are ineffective.

    5. Steroid eye drops are used for patients who have evidence of uveitis. Some patients also require a mydriatic agent (pupil dilator) once daily to prevent the formation of synechiae.

D. Ongoing ophthalmologic surveillance is necessary, even in patients who do not yet have uveitis. Recommended intervals for slit-lamp examinations are as follows:

    1. Pauciarticular or polyarticular disease

        a. If the patient is younger than age 7 years at onset and is antinuclear antibody (ANA)-positive: every 3 to 4 months for 4 years, then every 6 months for 3 years, then annually

        b. If the patient is younger than age 7 years at onset and is ANA-negative: every 6 months for 7 years, then annually

        c. If the patient is older than age 7 years at onset: every 6 months for 4 years, then annually, whether positive or negative for ANA

    2. Systemic disease. For patients of all ages, either positive or negative for ANA: annually

TABLE 97-4. Morbidity of Juvenile Rheumatoid Arthritis			
	Type of Juvenile Rheumatoid Arthritis		
	Pauciarticular	**Polyarticular**	**Systemic Onset**
Overall prognosis	Excellent	Good	Variable
Joint degeneration	Uncommon	RF-negative: 10%–15% RF-positive: 25%–50%	25%–50%

IV PROGNOSIS

A. Mortality

1. The risk of death from all forms of JRA is estimated at less than 1%. Most of these deaths occur in patients with systemic-onset disease.

2. The most common cause of death is overwhelming infection associated with the use of immunosuppressive medications (e.g., steroids).

B. Morbidity (Table 97–4)

1. Overall growth retardation, joint contractures, leg-length discrepancy (pauciarticular disease), and micrognathia (from temporomandibular joint involvement) are possible.

2. The risk of blindness is significant (10%–30%) in patients who have chronic uveitis that is poorly controlled or untreated.

References

Cassidy JT, Petty RE: Juvenile rheumatoid arthritis. In *Textbook of Pediatric Rheumatology*, 3rd ed. Edited by Cassidy JT, Petty RE. Philadelphia, WB Saunders, 1995, pp 384–388.

Schaller JG: Juvenile rheumatoid arthritis. *Pediatr Rev* 18(10);337–349, 1997.

Sherry DD, Mosca VS: Juvenile rheumatoid arthritis and seronegative spondyloarthropathies. In *Lovell and Winter's Pediatric Orthopaedics*, 4th ed. Edited by Raymoud T. Morrissy MD, Stuart L. Weinstein MD. Philadelphia, Lippincott-Raven, 1996, pp 393–409.

98. Systemic Lupus Erythematosus

I INTRODUCTION

A. Background

1. Systemic lupus erythematosus (SLE) is a systemic inflammatory disorder that is marked by the production of autoantibodies and immune complexes.

2. The name lupus comes from the Latin word for wolf; the malar rash resembles the facial hair pattern of a wolf.

B. Pathogenesis

1. The cause of SLE is unknown. Key features include polyclonal B cell activation, production of autoantibodies directed toward numerous self-antigens, formation of immune complexes, and complement consumption.

2. Many of the clinical manifestations of SLE are related to systemic vasculitis caused by deposition of immune complexes in blood vessel walls, complement fixation, and recruitment of inflammatory cells.

3. **Genetic predisposition** seems important. Certain human leukocyte antigen (HLA) genes are associated with a higher risk of SLE and also with producing specific autoantibodies. In addition, SLE is associated with some hereditary complement and immunoglobulin deficiencies [e.g., C2 and C4 deficiencies, C1 esterase deficiency, and selective immunoglobulin A (IgA) deficiency].

4. **Drug-induced SLE** occurs in children, most commonly in response to anticonvulsants. The specific mechanism is unknown, but this type of SLE is believed to be caused by vasculitis that occurs when immune complexes are deposited in the walls of blood vessels. Symptoms typically resolve when the drug is discontinued.

C. Epidemiology

1. The estimated incidence of SLE is approximately 0.6:100,000 children in the United States.

2. Most patients are diagnosed in adolescence; onset before age 5 years is rare.

3. **Prevalence**
   a. SLE is most common in Asians, followed by African-Americans and then by Caucasians.
   b. The female:male predominance is 3:1 before puberty and 5:1 after puberty.

▐▌ CLINICAL MANIFESTATIONS

A. Constitutional manifestations include malaise, fatigue, fever, and weight loss.

B. Skin

1. A distinctive **malar (butterfly) rash** on cheeks, usually sparing the nasolabial folds

2. A **discoid rash** characterized by raised, erythematous areas covered by thick, keratotic scale. If untreated, this rash may lead to atrophic scarring.

3. **Photosensitivity,** indicated by a rash (see II B 2) and by feeling ill after exposure to sunlight or use of a tanning bed

4. A **vasculitic rash,** which may appear purpuric, bullous, or gangrenous

5. **Painless mucocutaneous ulcers,** often oral, usually appearing on the anterior hard palate

6. **Hair loss and alopecia,** with growth of short "lupus hairs" along the forehead

C. Cardiovascular

1. **Pericarditis** occurs in approximately 25% of patients, but usually is not severe enough to cause cardiac tamponade.

2. **Myocarditis** and **vascular inflammation** may be present and increase the risk of accelerated atherosclerosis and myocardial infarction.

3. **Libman-Sacks endocarditis** is characterized by aseptic vegetations, typically on the mitral valve.

4. **Raynaud phenomenon** is peripheral vasospasm that causes blanching, cyanosis, and erythema (white, blue, red) of the fingers or toes. The diagnosis of true Raynaud phenomenon requires the presence of all three phases.

D. Pulmonary

1. **Pleuritis** with effusion is common at presentation.

2. Interstitial lung disease sometimes is discovered only with pulmonary function testing.

3. Pulmonary hemorrhage is rare in SLE, but when it occurs, the prognosis is grim.

E. Gastrointestinal

1. **Pancreatitis** may be present secondary to intrinsic involvement or to therapy.

2. **Abdominal pain** may be a sign of mesenteric arteritis, which can lead to hemorrhage, necrosis, and perforation of the bowel.

F. Renal

1. **Hypertension** is common.

2. **Hematuria** and **proteinuria** may be seen. Urinary protein excretion often is persistently greater than 0.5 g/day.

3. **Rapidly progressive glomerulonephritis** (RPGN) requires aggressive therapy and carries a poor prognosis.

G. Endocrine
   1. **Autoimmune thyroiditis** occasionally is seen.
   2. **Amenorrhea** may be present as a result of chronic disease or high doses of exogenous steroids.
   3. **Gonadal failure** may occur as a result of therapy with cyclophosphamide (Cytoxan), a commonly used chemotherapeutic agent. The risk increases in proportion to the cumulative dose.

H. Hematologic
   1. **Anemia,** either autoimmune hemolytic anemia or the anemia of chronic disease, may be the presenting sign of SLE.
   2. **Thrombocytopenia,** usually autoimmune-mediated, also may occur. Leukopenia (white blood cell count < 4000) is seen at presentation in approximately 50% of patients with SLE. It may be caused by antilymphocyte antibodies.
   3. **Hypercoagulability** as a result of circulating SLE anticoagulant may be seen. These patients are at risk for thrombophlebitis.

I. Musculoskeletal
   1. Painful **arthritis** or **arthralgia** may occur in both large and small joints and may be migratory. Typically, no joint destruction occurs.
   2. **Myositis** is common.

J. Neurologic
   1. **Impaired cognitive function** (organic brain syndrome), **seizures,** and **psychosis** are common at presentation.
   2. Chorea, aseptic meningitis, and cranial nerve palsies also are seen, but are rare.
   3. **Cerebrovascular accidents** may occur as a result of vasculitis and hypercoagulability.

K. Infectious diseases. Patients with SLE are at significantly increased risk for infection because of leukopenia, decreased complement levels, and immunosuppressive therapy.

III APPROACH TO THE PATIENT

A. Diagnosis
   1. The American College of Rheumatology lists 11 **diagnostic criteria** for SLE. The presence of any four of these criteria establishes the diagnosis.
      a. Skin findings
         (1) Malar rash (see II B 1)
         (2) Photosensitivity (see II B 3)
         (3) Discoid lesions (see II B 2)
         (4) Painless oral ulcers, often on the anterior hard palate (see II B 5)
      b. Laboratory findings
         (1) Positive result on antinuclear antibody (ANA) test, usually with a high titer (> 1:640)

   (2) Evidence of immune dysregulation: anti-DNA antibodies, Anti-Sm (Smith) antibodies, or chronically
   false-positive Venereal Disease Research Laboratories (VDRL) findings
  c. Major systems findings
   (1) Musculoskeletal. Nondeforming arthritis, with red,
   painful joints
   (2) Central nervous system. Symptoms ranging from mood
   or personality changes to seizures and frank psychosis
   (3) Renal. Renal involvement may be either nephritic or
   nephrotic
   (4) Polyserositis. Pericarditis or pleuritis, often with
   effusion
   (5) Hematologic. Hemolytic anemia (usually with a positive result on Coombs test), thrombocytopenia, leukopenia, or lymphopenia
 2. Other **physical examination findings** that suggest SLE
  a. Coarse hair that comes out easily, **alopecia,** and rows of
   short hairs near the forehead **("lupus hairs")**
  b. Inflamed gingiva
  c. Retinal "cotton wool" spots
  d. Splinter hemorrhages under nails
  e. Microinfarctions on hands and feet
  f. Urticarial or other vasculitic rash
  g. Unexplained evidence of renal disease (e.g., hypertension,
   edema, tea-colored urine)
B. Initial evaluation
 1. General. Electrolytes, including calcium, magnesium, and
  phosphate if renal disease is suspected
 2. Inflammatory studies
  a. Erythrocyte sedimentation rate (ESR) and **C-reactive
   protein (CRP)** level. Characteristically, the ESR is elevated, but the CRP level is normal. The ESR is not reliable in the setting of anemia.
  b. ANA studies
  c. Complement studies. CH5O, C3, and C4
 3. Cardiovascular studies. Electrocardiogram to evaluate cardiac rhythm and identify pericarditis or infarction
 4. Pulmonary studies. Chest radiograph to identify pleural effusion and determine heart size
 5. Gastrointestinal studies
  a. Liver function tests
  b. Lipase and amylase levels to evaluate liver and pancreatic
   involvement
 6. Renal
  a. Blood urea nitrogen and creatinine
  b. Urinalysis

7. **Hematologic**
    a. Complete blood cell count and differential
    b. Prothrombin time (PT) and partial thromboplastin time (PTT). The PT is normal, but the PTT often is prolonged and does not return to normal when mixed 1:1 with fresh plasma because of the presence of antiphospholipid antibodies.
8. **Neurologic**
    a. **Lumbar puncture,** if the patient has significant neurologic findings. Cultures and cell counts are performed, and glucose and protein levels are measured. The protein level often is elevated significantly.
    b. **Ophthalmologic evaluation** is performed to assess the degree of eye involvement
9. **Blood cultures** are performed to check for infection
C. **Additional tests to consider**
    1. **Immunologic studies**
        a. If the result of the ANA test is positive, then **anti–double-stranded DNA** and **anti-Sm (Smith) antibody titers** are checked. The anti-Sm titer is positive in only 30% of cases, but it is very specific for SLE.
        b. If the patient does not meet the classic criteria for SLE and is suspected of having an overlap syndrome [e.g., mixed connective tissue disease (MCTD)], then extractable nuclear antigen (ENA) antibody titers should be checked. ENA titers are extremely elevated in MCTD, but normal or mildly elevated in SLE.
        c. Immunoglobulin levels typically are elevated.
    2. **Cardiac**
        a. **Echocardiogram** is performed to evaluate cardiac function and identify pericardial effusion and valvular vegetations.
        b. **CK-MB** and **troponin** levels are evaluated if myocarditis or infarction is suspected.
    3. **Pulmonary function testing** is performed to evaluate interstitial lung disease in patients who have significant respiratory symptoms without a clear source.
    4. **Renal biopsy** is performed if RPGN is suspected.
    5. **Coombs test** is performed if **anemia** is suspected. Results of this test may be positive before the patient becomes anemic.
    6. **Central nervous system**
        a. **Computed tomography** or **magnetic resonance imaging scan of the head** is performed if the patient has neurologic involvement.
        b. An **electroencephalogram** is performed if the patient is having seizures.

    c. Cerebrospinal fluid complement and antineuronal antibody tests may be helpful.

7. A **biopsy of skin lesions** may be helpful if the diagnosis is unclear. Immune complexes containing IgG and C3 often are shown along the epidermal basement membrane by direct immunofluorescence, which reveals the "lupus band" (i.e., the specific immunoglobulins that immunofluoresce in SLE).

8. Infectious

    a. A tuberculin skin test and controls must be performed before treatment with high-dose steroids is initiated.

    b. The VDRL result is persistently falsely positive because antiphospholipid antibodies are present.

D. Treatment

  1. Sunscreen is needed because of the associated photosensitivity.

  2. High-dose pulse intravenous (IV) **methylprednisolone** 30 mg/kg/day for 3 days is followed by maintenance **prednisone** 1.5–2 mg/kg/day in divided doses.

  3. Cytotoxic agents (e.g., azathioprine, cyclophosphamide) are given either orally or as IV pulses in patients with significant renal or central nervous system involvement.

  4. Nonsteroidal anti-inflammatory agents are used for patients who have joint involvement.

  5. Hydroxychloroquine is given to patients who have significant skin involvement.

  6. Antihypertensive agents are given for hypertension.

E. Management

  1. Complement levels can be used to monitor the effectiveness of therapy. These levels should return to normal if treatment is successful.

  2. Patients with SLE are considered functionally asplenic and should receive pneumococcal vaccination in addition to all other immunizations.

  3. Patients who are receiving immunosuppressive and cytotoxic therapy are at increased risk for severe bacterial and fungal infection. Because the CRP level usually is normal in patients with SLE, elevated levels during an acute febrile episode suggest infection rather than a lupus flare.

  4. Patients who are receiving Cytoxan are at increased risk for gonadal failure. Boys should bank sperm before starting therapy, if time permits.

IV Prognosis

A. Mortality. The main cause of death in SLE is overwhelming infection secondary to the chronic use of steroids and cytotoxic agents. Other causes of death are myocarditis, cerebritis, and pulmonary hemorrhage.

B. Morbidity. Significant physical and psychological morbidity is associated with SLE. There is a significant risk of progression to renal failure and consequent need for kidney transplantation.

References
Cassidy JT, Petty RE: Systemic lupus erythematosus. In *Textbook of Pediatric Rheumatology,* 3rd ed. Edited by Cassidy JT, Petty RE. Philadelphia, WB Saunders, 1995, pp 384–388.
Emery H: Clinical aspects of systemic lupus erythematosus in childhood. *Pediatr Clin North Am* 33(5);1177–1190, 1986.

PART XIII

NEUROLOGY

99. Seizures

I CLINICAL MANIFESTATIONS

A. Partial seizures. Seizures are limited to one part of the cerebral hemisphere. The symptoms reflect the area of the brain affected by the seizure.

1. **Simple partial seizures**
   a. Consciousness is not impaired.
   b. Motor signs (e.g., tonic-clonic activity of a given limb, tonic deviation of the head to one side) are seen.
   c. Partial seizures may evolve to generalized tonic, clonic, or tonic-clonic seizures.

2. **Complex partial seizures**
   a. Consciousness often is impaired.
   b. Automatisms (i.e., semipurposeful movements, e.g., fidgeting with clothing, walking, running, mastication, or lingual movements). These may manifest as a continuing repetition of the activity the patient was engaged in at the onset of the seizure.
   c. Somatosensory symptoms (e.g., numbness; paresthesias; visual, auditory or gustatory phenomena).
   d. Psychic symptoms (e.g., distorted memory or time sense, déjà vu, hallucinations, distorted perceptions of the size of objects or self, depression, fearfulness) are seen if the temporal, frontal, or limbic system is involved.

B. Generalized seizures

1. **Tonic-clonic seizures**
   a. Consciousness is impaired.
   b. The **tonic phase** involves contraction of muscle groups. The **clonic phase** occurs when the contraction is interrupted repeatedly by a momentary relaxation of the muscle group.
   c. Tonic-clonic seizures often are followed by a postictal period.

   2. **Atonic seizures** involve a sudden decrease in muscle tone
      followed by a loss of consciousness. Symptoms depend on
      the muscles involved. For example, falls occur with atonic
      seizures of truncal or leg muscles, and a sudden head drop
      may occur if the neck muscles are involved.
   3. **Myoclonic seizures** are brief, random contractions of a mus-
      cle or group of muscles. There usually is no loss of con-
      sciousness. This type of seizure is often associated with a pro-
      gressive encephalopathy.
   4. **Absence seizures** are characterized by staring spells. They
      usually last for only 5 to 10 seconds. They are distinguished
      from simple "daydreaming" in that the child cannot be
      aroused from the seizure by touch or voice. After the seizure,
      the child simply continues the activity he or she was engaged
      in when the seizure began.
C. Physical examination
   1. A complete **neurologic examination** is performed to rule out
      a space-occupying lesion.
   2. Evidence of **neurocutaneous syndromes** is sought.
      a. Facial hemangiomas in the fifth cranial nerve distribution
         suggest Sturge-Weber syndrome.
      b. Adenoma sebaceum, retinal hamartomas, and "ash leaf"
         spots suggest tuberous sclerosis.
      c. Café-au-lait spots and axillary freckling suggest neurofibro-
         matosis.
      d. Verrucous yellow hyperpigmented plaques on the face
         and scalp suggest epidermal nevus syndrome.

II APPROACH TO THE PATIENT

A. Diagnosis
   1. Because of the ephemeral nature of seizures, a thorough his-
      tory, including interviews with witnesses, is vital.
   2. Although **electroencephalography (EEG)** is a standard di-
      agnostic tool, the initial EEG result is abnormal in only ap-
      proximately 50% of patients who have a seizure disorder. If
      the diagnosis is uncertain, a 24-hour video EEG study is per-
      formed.
   3. In patients with **partial seizures,** a magnetic resonance imag-
      ing scan of the head is required to rule out a space-occupying
      lesion. Furthermore, complex partial seizures are a common
      manifestation of herpes encephalitis.
   4. **Infants** require a broader initial workup. Seizures may be
      caused by any of the following:
      a. Inborn errors of metabolism
      b. Electrolyte abnormalities (e.g., hypocalcemia, hypogly-
         cemia, hypomagnesemia)

    c. Pyridoxine deficiency
    d. Hypoxic-ischemic encephalopathy
    e. Sepsis/meningitis

B. Differential diagnosis

    1. Breath-holding spells are preceded by a period of crying, prolonged expiration, and cyanosis that eventually leads to collapse.

    2. Jitteriness in infants can be distinguished from seizures by a lack of eye deviation. Jitteriness can be extinguished by gentle restraint and is stimulus-sensitive.

C. Initial therapy

    1. Most patients do not require an antiepileptic drug after the first seizure. Fifty percent of patients with a first seizure never have another seizure. Epilepsy may be diagnosed after two unprovoked seizures.

    2. The probability of epilepsy is higher if the patient has an abnormal neurologic examination, a second seizure, focal spikes on EEG, or complex partial seizures.

    3. Treatment varies according to the seizure type (Table 99-1).

        a. Simple partial seizures respond to carbamazepine, phenytoin, and phenobarbital.

        b. For **complex partial seizures,** carbamazepine is the drug of choice.

        c. For **generalized tonic-clonic, clonic, or tonic seizures,** phenobarbital, phenytoin, carbamazepine, and valproic acid are all effective.

        d. Myoclonic and atonic seizures may be controlled by valproic acid, ethosuximide, and clonazepam.

        e. The preferred therapies for **other seizure types** are listed in Table 99-1.

D. Ongoing management

    1. The patient must be monitored for **common side effects** of medications.

        a. Most agents may cause dysequilibrium and sedation.

        b. Prednisone or adrenocorticotropic hormone may cause hyperglycemia and hypertension.

        c. Carbamazepine may lead to leukopenia and liver toxicity.

        d. Phenytoin may cause gingival hyperplasia, Stevens-Johnson syndrome, a lupus-like illness, rickets, megaloblastic anemia, and hirsutism.

        e. Phenobarbital may lead to a decrease in IQ after 2 years of use. It also may cause hyperkinesis and severe behavioral changes.

        f. Ethosuximide and carbamazepine may cause psychosis.

        g. Valproic acid can lead to fatal liver toxicity, high NH_3 levels, and a Reye-like syndrome.

    2. Medication dosages typically are adjusted based on the trough

TABLE 99-1. Specific Epileptic Syndromes

Syndrome	Pathogenesis	Epidemiology	Symptoms	Prognosis	EEG	Treatment
Infantile spasms (West syndrome)	Dysgenetic, perinatal brain injury Encephalopathies Intrauterine infections Hemorrhage Toxic anabolic processes	Can occur in previously normal infants Begins in the first 3–7 months of infancy, family history–associated	Flexor, extensor, or mixed spasms (entire body appears to flex or extend suddenly)	Poor prognosis (5%–15% mortality rate) Epilepsy in 60% of affected persons Mental retardation in 70%–85% of patients Medications may preserve some IQ points	Hypsarrhythmia	Adrenocorticotropic hormone Prednisone
Lennox-Gastaut syndrome	Perinatal brain injury Dysgenetic Often preceded by infantile spasms	Infants (3%–10% of epilepsy cases) More common in boys Can occur in previously normal children	Multiple seizure types may occur: tonic, atonic, myoclonic, atypical absence May be induced by startling the patient	Poor (mortality rate, 4.2%) Mental retardation in 20%–60% of cases	Interictal, diffuse slow spike–wave pattern	Treatments usually are ineffective. They include valproic acid, ketogenic diet, and corpus callostomy.

| Typical absence seizures | Probably genetic. Differential diagnosis includes attention deficit hyperactivity disorder. Absence seizures are suspected when there is attention deficit without hyperactivity. | Peak age of onset is 3–10 y | Sudden, brief (5–15 sec), lapse in mental function, staring with turning of head and eyes. Consciousness is impaired (patient will not respond to own name or to touch). May be precipitated by hyperventilation or flashing lights. Multiple seizures may occur during the course of the day. The patient has no awareness that anything has happened. | Favorable prognosis; 80% remission rate, mean age of cessation of seizures is 10.5 y | Characteristic 3-Hz spike–wave pattern with abrupt onset and termination | Ethosuximide Valproic acid Benzodiazepines |

(continued)

TABLE 99-1. Specific Epileptic Syndromes *(Continued)*

Syndrome	Pathogenesis	Epidemiology	Symptoms	Prognosis	EEG	Treatment
Benign epilepsy of childhood with Rolandic centrotemporal spikes	Unknown May be autosomal dominant trait	Female and male prevalence is the same Onset at age 2–14 y There may be a positive family history with variable expressivity. Linked with febrile seizures and migraines.	Simple partial seizures (face, tongue, mouth, and arm) often occur when awake. Sleep-related generalized tonic-clonic ("nocturnal") seizure also can occur upon awakening.	Good; 100% remission by 17 years of age with or without medication	Paroxysmal di- or triphasic sharp waves in centro temporal area, with normal background	Carbamazepine may be used if seizures are frequent.

Juvenile myoclonic epilepsy (Janz)	Unknown Probably a genetic connection	Most common in teenage years	Sudden myoclonic jerks with no loss of consciousness. Tonic-clonic seizures begin a few years later. Seizures often occur soon after awakening. Patients may report trouble brushing their teeth or combing their hair in the morning. Adolescents sometimes deny that seizures occur.	Medication is required for remission. Requires lifelong therapy	Interictal, bilateral 4- to 6-Hz irregular spike-wave pattern. There may be photosensitivity: 20% of patients with this type experience seizures when exposed to a strobe light.	Exquisitely sensitive to valproic acid.

levels. Dosages must be changed to reflect weight gain in a rapidly growing child.

3. **Withdrawal of medications** should take place over a period of 4–6 weeks to avoid precipitating status epilepticus. Withdrawal may be considered in the following situations:
   a. The patient has been seizure-free for 2–3 years.
   b. The neurologic examination results are normal.
   c. The EEG is normal with the patient on treatment.
   d. The patient has a single type of partial or generalized seizure.

HOT
KEY

Noncompliance is the most common reason for seizures in a child with known epilepsy.

 SPECIFIC EPILEPTIC SYNDROMES are described in Table 99–1.

References
Holmes G: Benign focal epilepsies of childhood. *Epilepsia* 34:S49–61, 1993.
Kliegman RM: *Practical Strategies in Pediatric Diagnosis and Therapy*. Philadelphia, WB Saunders, 1966, pp 610–640.
McMillan JA, DeAngelis CD, Felgin RD: *Oski's Pediatrics: Principles and Practice,* 3rd ed. Philadelphia, Lippincott Williams & Wilkins, 1999, pp 1936–1952.
Wyllie E: *The Treatment of Epilepsy: Principles and Practice*. Philadelphia, Lea & Febiger, 1993.

100. Febrile Seizures

I INTRODUCTION

A. **Definitions**
   1. **A "typical" febrile seizure** is a single, generalized tonic-clonic seizure occurring in the setting of fever. Such seizures occur in neurologically normal children and last for less than 15 minutes.
   2. **Atypical, or complex, febrile seizures** last longer than 15 minutes, are focal, or recur within a 24-hour period.
B. **Pathogenesis.** The exact mechanism is unknown. Febrile seizures are associated with a rapidly rising temperature.
C. **Epidemiology**
   1. Febrile seizures are the most common type of seizures in children (3% incidence).
   2. Onset is usually between 9 months and 3 years of age. Febrile seizures are rare before 6 months and after 6 years of age.
   3. There may be a genetic predisposition.
   4. Primary human herpesvirus-6 (HHV-6) infection is associated with one third of febrile seizures.

II CLINICAL MANIFESTATIONS.
Seizures are usually generalized and tonic-clonic, although atonic seizures are also reported. The seizures usually last for less than 10 minutes, and a postictal state is often present. Most febrile seizures occur on the first day of illness.

III APPROACH TO THE PATIENT

A. **History.** Is the child otherwise normal? Is there a history of nonfebrile seizures in the child or family? What was the child's neurologic status before the seizure occurred? Was the child febrile when the seizure began? What did the seizure look like, and how long did it last?

HOT

KEY
Parents often overestimate the duration of a child's seizure.

B. Differential diagnosis includes:
1. Central nervous system (CNS) infection (e.g., meningitis, encephalitis)
2. Anoxia
3. Trauma
4. Toxic ingestion
5. Brain tumor
6. Neurocutaneous syndromes (e.g., tuberous sclerosis, Sturge-Weber syndrome, neurofibromatosis)

C. Initial therapy
1. Acutely, airway, breathing, and circulation (the ABCs) should be ensured. Usually, seizures can be observed without intervention. If the episode is prolonged (i.e., > 5 minutes), benzodiazepines (lorazepam 0.05–0.1 mg/kg) are first-line medications (see Chapter 48).
2. Antipyretics, including acetaminophen, in conjunction with ibuprofen, can be given if needed. Sponge baths also may be helpful in lowering the patient's temperature.

D. Tests
1. Lumbar puncture is performed and antibiotics are started if the possibility of meningitis is a concern, especially if the patient is younger than 12 months of age or if the seizure occurs after the second day of illness. A postictal child's mental status can be difficult to evaluate; however, if the physician is reassured that it is normal, lumbar puncture can be deferred.
2. An electroencephalogram (EEG) should be performed on a child who has atypical febrile seizures. This may be done on an outpatient basis.
3. Measurement of the blood glucose level and electrolytes should be considered for an actively seizing patient.
4. A head computed tomography (CT) scan should be done if a focal seizure is present. Some practitioners recommend a CT scan for all patients with complex febrile seizures.

HOT

KEY
Herpes encephalitis should be considered in the case of any child who has a focal febrile seizure.

E. Seizure prophylaxis. Anticonvulsant prophylaxis usually is not recommended because of the associated side effects. Drug therapy affects the recurrence rate, but not the natural history (i.e., development of epilepsy). Diazepam can be given orally at the onset of fever (0.3 mg/kg every 8 hours). Although it is effective, diazepam can mask signs of a developing CNS infection, so it should be given cautiously. Primidone, phenobarbital, and valproic acid are also effective drugs, but are generally reserved for cases of recurrent complex febrile seizures or for patients at high risk for epilepsy (e.g., children with cerebral palsy, structural brain lesions, or abnormal EEG results).

IV PROGNOSIS

A. **Morbidity.** For simple febrile seizures, the prognosis is excellent; there usually are no sequelae.

B. **Recurrence risk.** Overall, one third of children with a simple first febrile seizure have a recurrence. Four independent risk factors increase the likelihood of a recurrence:

  1. Young age at onset ($<$ 18 months). If the first seizure occurs at $<$ 1 year of age, the recurrence risk is 50%–60%; this decreases to 28% if the first seizure occurs at $>$ 1 year of age.
  2. History of febrile seizures in a first-degree relative
  3. Low degree of fever on first examination
  4. Brief duration ($<$ 1 hour) between the onset of fever and the initial seizure

C. **Risk factors for epilepsy.** The incidence of epilepsy after a febrile seizure in a normal child is slightly higher than in the general population (1% versus 0.5%) when no risk factors are present. The risk of epilepsy increases with additional risk factors. A recurrence is not an established risk factor for epilepsy. Risk factors include:

  1. Family history of epilepsy
  2. Initial febrile seizure before 9 months of age
  3. Atypical seizure
  4. Delayed developmental milestones
  5. Abnormal findings on neurologic examination
  6. Pre-existing structural brain abnormality

References

American Academy of Pediatrics Practice Parameters: Long-term treatment of the child with simple febrile illness. *Pediatrics* 103(6):1307–1309, 1999.

Berg AT, Shinnar S, Darefsky AS, et al: Predictors of recurrent febrile seizures: a prospective cohort study. *Arch Pediatr Adolesc Med* 151:371–378, 1997.

101. Headaches

I INTRODUCTION

A. Causes
1. The brain has no pain receptors. Headaches result from referred pain from structures in the head or neck.
2. Although usually benign, headache may be a symptom of another disorder, or it may be related to an underlying pathologic process.

B. Types
1. **Tension headaches** are thought to be related to pericranial muscle tension, which can be caused by stress.
2. **Migraine headaches** are vascular in origin. They usually are bilateral in children and unilateral in adults. In addition to pain, symptoms may include nausea, vomiting, anorexia, abdominal pain, irritability, photophobia, malaise, and fatigue. Migraines are classified as follows:
   a. **Common migraine** (see I B 2)
   b. **Classic migraine** has the features of common migraine (see I B 2) plus a visual aura consisting of scintillations, scatomata, or blurred vision that typically precedes the onset of pain. Pain can intensify and may last hours to days.
   c. **Complicated migraine** includes all of the features of common migraine (see I B 2) plus neurologic deficits, such as aphasia or hemiplegia.
   d. **Variant migraines** include cyclic vomiting, "Alice in Wonderland" syndrome, in which objects appear to shrink and grow, and paroxysmal vertigo.

II EPIDEMIOLOGY

A. Sixty percent of children experience a headache of some kind during the school-age years.
B. Three percent of prepubertal children experience at least one migraine.
C. Fifteen percent of adolescents experience at least one migraine.

III APPROACH TO THE PATIENT

A. **Differential diagnosis.** It is critical to determine whether the headache is benign (e.g., tension headache) or is the result of a specific physical cause.

560

1. **Infections** that may cause headache include:
   a. **Sinusitis.** Other symptoms are cough, facial pain, congestion, or nasal drainage.
   b. **Dental abscess,** characterized by tooth pain or poor dental care
   c. **Meningitis and encephalitis,** which are marked by fever, stiff neck, and photophobia
2. **Increased intracranial pressure** may be caused by:
   a. **Hydrocephalus**. The occipitofrontal circumference should be checked.
   b. **Pseudotumor cerebri.** The optic discs should be checked for an enlarging blind spot.
   c. **Subarachnoid hemorrhage,** which may be linked to a history of trauma or arteriovenous malformation
3. **Trauma**
   a. **Closed head injury** may be diagnosed by obtaining a history of the trauma.
   b. **Hematoma**
4. **Mass lesions** that may induce headache include the following:
   a. **Brain tumors.** Symptoms include focal neurologic findings, papilledema, and morning vomiting. Cerebellar signs, such as ataxia, positive Romberg sign, impaired finger-to-nose follow, and disrupted speech, are important to assess because many pediatric brain tumors involve the posterior fossa.
   b. **Brain abscess** is characterized by fever, headaches, and focal neurologic findings. Congenital heart disease is associated with 5%–10% of all cases.

B. **History**
   1. The location, duration, and character of the pain (e.g., constant, sharp, throbbing) must be established.
   2. Conditions that **trigger or exacerbate** the headaches are investigated, including foods or medications and hormonal fluctuations related to the patient's menstrual cycle.
   3. Associated **symptoms,** such as blurred vision, aura, nausea, or vomiting, are investigated.
   4. **Nonorganic causes,** such as stress at home or at school, are researched.
   5. The **family history** is investigated to establish whether anyone else in the family has migraines or has had an aneurysm.

C. **Physical examination.** Physical findings usually are normal. Blood pressure and head circumference should be measured. Special attention should be paid to the optic discs and the neurologic findings.

D. **Laboratory studies.** None are routinely indicated.

E. Imaging studies
  1. Routine imaging studies are necessary if at least one of the following indications is present:
     a. Abnormal neurologic findings
     b. Sudden drop-off in growth rate
     c. Significant change in behavior
     d. Seizures
     e. Morning vomiting
     f. Positional increases in pain

HOT

KEY
Any child who has a history of headache and focal neurologic signs should undergo an imaging study of the brain.

---

  2. Simple computed tomographic (CT) scanning or magnetic resonance imaging (MRI) is adequate to rule out structural problems. These scans also can be reassuring to the parents.
  3. MRI is more effective than CT scanning for imaging the posterior fossa (the most common location of brain tumors).
F. Therapy. Treatment for migraine headaches is divided into three categories:
  1. Symptomatic treatment is used when headaches occur and includes the analgesics acetaminophen, ibuprofen, and aspirin (for children older than 12 years of age).
  2. Abortive treatments interrupt headaches after they begin.
     a. Sumatriptan, a highly effective 5-HT agonist, is available in injection, tablet, or spray form.
     b. Ergots (e.g., ergotamine) are effective, but must be taken very early in the course of the headache. This treatment may be difficult in children because they often do not recognize or report headaches early enough.
  3. Prophylactic therapy is reserved for children who have frequent, recurrent, debilitating headaches.
     a. β-blockers usually are given as the first-line therapy, although their effectiveness is controversial.
     b. Amitriptyline is effective, but tricyclics must be used with caution in children and adolescents because of the potential for accidental overdose.
     c. Anticonvulsants are used, but their effectiveness is not established.
     d. Biofeedback and behavioral interventions are as effective as medication if children are motivated to participate.
  4. Long-term control of headaches requires regular, close **follow-up** to characterize the problem, follow its course, and establish an effective treatment regimen.

PROGNOSIS. Approximately 50% of children with migraines continue to have them as adults. The migraines may become more or less frequent or severe over time.

References
O'Hara J, Koch TK: Heading off headaches. *Contemp Pediatr* 15(3);97–112, 1998.
Rothner AD: Headaches in children and adolescents: update 2001. *Semin Pediatr Neurol* 8(1):2–6, 2001.
Smith MS: Comprehensive evaluation and treatment of recurrent pediatric headaches. *Pediatr Ann* 24:452–457, 1995.

PART XIV

TRAUMA

102. Initial Assessment and Management of the Trauma Patient

 PRIMARY SURVEY. The purpose of the primary survey is to identify and manage immediately life-threatening injuries. Patients who can talk are not likely to be in immediate jeopardy.

A. Airway and cervical spine precautions

1. **Assessment.** The patency of the airway is checked, and the patient's ability to handle secretions is assessed. The chest is auscultated for symmetric breath sounds. Chest wall rise is evaluated, and stridor is identified.

> **HOT KEY**
>
> Children who refuse to lie down may be indicating an inability to handle secretions.

2. **Actions**
   a. **The cervical spine is protected** by using a cervical collar and backboard and immobilizing the head. Cervical spine injury should be assumed in any patient with multisystem trauma, an altered level of consciousness, facial injury, or a blunt injury above the clavicle.

> **HOT KEY**
>
> The absence of neurologic defects does not preclude cervical spine injury.

   b. **Patency of the airway is ensured.**
       (1) **Oral airway.** In conscious patients, a **jaw thrust ma-
           neuver, chin lift maneuver,** or **nasopharyngeal airway**
           may be used. In unconscious patients, an **oropharyn-
           geal airway** can be used before a definitive airway is
           obtained.
       (2) **Intubation** is necessary if there is any doubt about the
           patient's ability to maintain the airway (Table 102–1).
           The procedure for **rapid sequence induction (RSI)** is
           given in Table 102–2.
   c. **Aspiration must be prevented.** If the child vomits, cricoid
       pressure is applied, the child is rolled to a left lateral de-
       cubitus position while cervical spine precautions are
       maintained, and the oral cavity is suctioned.

HOT **KEY**   Using opiates (e.g., fentanyl) and barbiturates (e.g., thiopental) in hypovolemic, hypotensive trauma patients can exacer-
bate shock.

B. Breathing. Airway patency, by itself, does not ensure adequate
   oxygenation and ventilation, and a profoundly dyspneic patient
   does not necessarily have an airway problem. In addition, infants are obligate nose breathers; therefore, occlusion of the
   nose owing to injury or a foreign body (e.g., a nasogastric tube)
   may impair ventilation.
   1. **Assessment.** Evidence of immediately life-threatening dis-
      orders (e.g., tension pneumothorax, massive hemothorax)
      should be sought (see Chapter 106 II A 1–2, 4).

TABLE 102-1. Indications for Intubation

Loss of consciousness
Severe maxillofacial fractures
Risk for aspiration from bleeding or vomiting
Risk for obstruction from neck hematoma, laryngeal injury, or
   tracheal injury
Stridor, apnea, hypoxemia, or hypercarbia
Severe closed head injury and a Glasgow Coma Scale score of
   less than 8

TABLE 102-2. Rapid Sequence Induction in Pediatric Patients

1. Preoxygenate: **100% oxygen** for 3–5 minutes
2. Prevent bradycardia: **atropine** (0.02 mg/kg)
3. Induce unawareness and sedation: **midazolam** (0.05 mg/kg)
4. **Morphine** (0.05–0.1 mg/kg)
5. Prevent aspiration: apply **cricoid pressure**
6. Induce paralysis: administer **pancuronium** (0.1 mg/kg IV) or **succinylcholine*** (2 mg/kg IV for children < 10 kg; 1 mg/kg for children ≥ 10 kg)
7. Intubate
8. Confirm tube placement and begin ventilation

Variations

For a patient with increased ICP and cardiovascular compromise

1. **Fentanyl** (1–2 μg/kg IV) or **diazepam** (0.2 mg/kg) instead of midazolam, a barbiturate or morphine, because these agents are less likely to produce hypotension
2. **Lidocaine** (1 mg/kg IV) to help prevent increases in ICP
3. **Vecuronium** (0.1 mg/kg) or other nondepolarizing agent instead of succinylcholine, to avoid increases in ICP

For a patient with increased ICP but no cardiovascular compromise

1. **Thiopental** (4–6 mg/kg) (in addition to inducing sedation, thiopental lowers the ICP by reducing cerebral blood flow)
2. **Lidocaine**
3. **Vecuronium** or other nondepolarizing agent

All drugs specified in this table are administered intravenously.
ICP = intracranial pressure; IV = intravenously; RSI = rapid sequence induction.
*This agent is contraindicated in patients with chronic renal failure, hyperkalemia, neuromuscular disease, penetrating eye injuries, major burn injury, or a closed head injury.

HOT KEY Deterioration of the patient's condition during positive-pressure ventilation may indicate an undiagnosed tension pneumothorax.

2. Actions. All patients are given 100% supplemental oxygen.

C. Circulation.

    1. Assessment. The pulse, skin color, neck veins, capillary refill time, and heart sounds are evaluated.

HOT KEY Tachycardia and/or hypotension is hypovolemic in origin until proven otherwise.

   a. Pay very close attention to the vital signs.
   b. A decreased level of consciousness or rapid, thready pulses may indicate hypovolemia.
   c. An ashen or very pale complexion is an ominous sign of hypovolemia.
   d. Patients with absent central pulses require immediate fluid resuscitation.
 2. Actions
   a. External hemorrhage is identified and controlled using direct pressure or a pneumatic splinting device.
   b. At least two large-caliber intravenous lines are placed. Although placement in the upper extremity is preferred, an intraosseous line may be considered if the child is younger than age 6 years or if peripheral intravenous access is difficult to obtain. Fluid resuscitation should be initiated as described in Chapter 107 III A 5.
D. Disability. Serial examinations are necessary because unexpected deterioration of the patient's clinical condition is not unusual in patients with closed head injuries.
E. Exposure. The patient should be completely undressed to facilitate evaluation. External heat loss should be prevented using warmed blankets and warmed intravenous fluids.

HOT KEY Hypothermia exacerbates shock! Take the patient's core temperature.

F. Adjuncts to the primary survey
 1. Electrocardiogram (ECG) monitoring is mandatory for trauma patients.
 2. Placement of a **nasogastric tube** can help reduce the risk of aspiration. If a cribriform plate fracture is suspected, an orogastric tube should be placed instead.
 3. Foley catheter placement. Patients who are unconscious or who have multiple injuries require bladder catheterization.

> **HOT**
> ▶
> **KEY**
> Do not place a Foley catheter if there is blood at the meatus, perineal ecchymosis, blood in the scrotum, a high-riding or nonpalpable prostate, or a pelvic fracture. If urethral integrity is suspect, a retrograde urethrogram must be performed before urinary catheter placement.

4. **Pulse oximetry** enables the clinician to recognize oxygen desaturation before bradycardia develops, thereby allowing time to correct the developing pulmonary or cardiovascular problem before it becomes difficult to reverse. Placement of an oxygen saturation monitor distal to the blood pressure cuff may result in spurious readings.

5. **Radiographic studies.** Patients with a history of significant trauma should undergo anterior and posterior lateral cervical spine radiographs, chest radiograph, and pelvic radiographs; and abdominal CT if abdominal injury is suspected. Views of the extremities are added if clinically indicated.

6. **Laboratory studies.** Serial hematocrit levels, a complete blood cell count, electrolyte levels, blood type and crossmatch, human chorionic gonadotropin (pregnancy) test, and urinalysis should be obtained. Arterial blood gas levels (ABGs) should be obtained if ventilation or oxygenation is in question.

II **SECONDARY SURVEY.** The secondary survey systematically identifies additional injuries and completes the patient history.

A. **Patient history**
   1. Does the patient have any allergies?
   2. What medications is she taking?
   3. What is the patient's medical history?
   4. When did the patient last eat?
   5. Is the patient pregnant?
   6. What were the circumstances surrounding the injury (e.g., mechanism of injury, caliber of the bullet, length of the knife)?

B. **Physical examination.** The patient should be evaluated methodically, from head to toe.
   1. **Head.** Visual acuity and pupillary size are assessed, and the patient is checked for hemorrhages of the conjunctiva and fundi (see Chapter 104 III C for more detail). Contact lenses are removed if the patient is wearing them.
   2. **Neck.** The neck is checked for tenderness, subcutaneous emphysema, tracheal deviation, and laryngeal fracture. Carotid bruits are noted.

TABLE 102-3. Pediatric Trauma Score			
	+2	+1	−1
Patient's weight	> 20 kg	10–20 kg	< 10 kg
Airway status	Normal	Maintainable	Nonmaintainable
Systolic blood pressure	> 90 mm Hg	50–90 mm Hg	< 50 mm Hg
Level of consciousness	Awake	Obtunded or unconscious	Comatose or decerebrate
Skeletal injuries	None	Closed fractures	Open or multiple fractures
Cutaneous injuries	None	Minor	Major or penetrating

3. **Chest.** Pulmonary contusion, rib fractures, and other disorders that may not be immediately evident are assessed (see Chapter 106 II B).

4. **Abdomen.** The patient is checked for blunt abdominal trauma (see Chapter 105 II B).

5. **Extremities.** The patient is assessed for fractures (see Chapter 103 II B).

6. **Back.** Evaluation for spinal cord injury should be carried out as described in Chapter 108 III.

III **PEDIATRIC TRAUMA SCORE.** Values range from −6 to 12 (Table 102–3). All patients with trauma scores of less than 8 must be transferred to a level I pediatric trauma center.

References

Advanced Trauma Life Support (ATLS), 6th ed. Chicago, American College of Surgeons, 1997.

Eichelberger MR: *Pediatric Trauma: Prevention, Acute Care, Rehabilitation.* St. Louis, Mosby-Year Book, 1993.

Tepas JJ III, Ramenofsky ML, Mollitt DL, et al: The pediatric trauma score as a predictor of injury severity. *J Trauma* 28:425–429, 1988.

Thompson AE: Pediatric airway management. In *Pediatric Critical Care,* 2nd ed. Edited by Fuhrman B, Zimmerman JJ. St. Louis, Mosby-Yearbook, 1997.

103. Fractures

I TYPES OF FRACTURES

A. Incomplete fractures. The bones of children are more porous than those of adults; therefore, children are more prone to incomplete fractures.

1. Torus fractures result from compression in the metaphyseal region of the long bones.

2. Traumatic bowing, commonly seen in the radius, ulna, and fibula, results from bending forces.

3. Greenstick fractures occur when a bone is bent beyond its limits. The fracture is located on the convex side of the deformity.

B. Complete fractures (Figure 103–1)

1. Transverse fractures. The fracture line is perpendicular to the longitudinal axis of the bone.

2. Comminuted fractures. The bone is fractured into three or more pieces. Comminuted fractures are associated with a great deal of energy (e.g., high-speed impact, gunshot wounds).

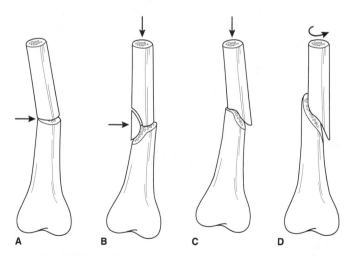

FIGURE 103–1. Complete fractures. The direction of the force causing the fracture is indicated by the **arrows.** **(A)** Transverse fracture. **(B)** Comminuted fracture. **(C)** Oblique fracture. **(D)** Spiral fracture.

   3. **Oblique fractures.** The fracture line is oriented at an angle to
      the longitudinal axis of the bone. These fractures are the re-
      sult of axial loading.
   4. **Spiral fractures.** In addition to being oblique, the fracture line
      encircles the shaft of the bone. These fractures are caused by
      rotary forces.
C. **Growth plate (physeal) fractures,** classified using the **Salter-
   Harris classification scheme** (Table 103–1), are unique to children. Because these fractures can impact future growth, all patients require follow-up with an orthopedic surgeon.

II APPROACH TO THE PATIENT

HOT KEY Focusing too much attention on the obvious fracture can lead to missed diagnoses of other, less obvious injuries. A thorough physical examination should be performed and radiographs obtained accordingly.

A. The **patient history** elicits information such as the mechanism of
   injury and sites of pain and numbness.
B. **Physical examination.** The presence of **swelling** with **point tenderness** usually indicates that a fracture is present.
   1. The patient is assessed for **surface wounds** and **deformity.**
   2. The color and perfusion of the affected limb are assessed.
      Coolness, pallor, and **paresthesia** suggest arterial compro-
      mise.
   3. The patient should always be "log-rolled" (after appropriate
      cervical and thoracic spine precautions are taken), and the
      back should be examined.
C. **Imaging.** Radiographs are obtained that include the joints both
   proximal and distal to the bone in question.

III TREATMENT

A. **Simple fractures. Splinting** or **casting** prevents further injury
   and controls pain.

HOT KEY Reduction and immobilization of a fracture should provide quick pain relief. Persistence of pain after reduction and casting is ischemia until proven otherwise; the possibility of compartment syndrome must also be considered.

B. **Complicated fractures**
   1. **Open reduction** and **internal fixation** may be necessary for

TABLE 103-1. Salter-Harris Classification of Growth Plate Fracture

Fracture		Description
I	Metaphysis Physis Epiphysis Joint surface	Separation of the metaphysis from the epiphysis through the zone of cartilage
II		Involves the physis and a triangular portion of the metaphysis
III		Involves the physis and the epiphysis
IV		Involves the physis, metaphysis, and epiphysis
V		Crush injury to the physis

patients with complicated fractures (e.g., open fractures, Salter-Harris types III or IV).

2. **Antibiotic therapy** is indicated for **open fractures,** which are surgical emergencies.
   a. The wound should not be probed. It should be covered with a sterile dressing.
   b. Tetanus prophylaxis should be ensured, and prophylactic antibiotics (e.g., cefazolin) should be administered.
   c. A culture of the wound should be obtained before surgery.

IV SPECIFIC FRACTURES

A. **Upper extremity fractures**
   1. **Clavicular fractures** usually heal well. Placing the shoulder in a figure-8 strap for 3 weeks is adequate therapy.
   2. **Proximal humeral fractures** usually result from a backward fall on an outstretched hand. Remodeling of the proximal humerus is usually good; therefore, precise reduction usually is not needed.
   3. **Distal humeral fractures.** Displaced supracondylar fractures carry a high risk of complications (e.g., ischemic contractures, brachial artery injury, radial nerve or median nerve paralysis). These injuries require careful management by an orthopedic surgeon.
   4. **Radial and ulnar fractures** usually result from falls on an outstretched hand. Complications are rare, and surgical correction usually is not necessary.
B. **Pelvic fractures** require significant forces and may be associated with injury to intraperitoneal, retroperitoneal, or vascular structures. Disruption of the pelvic ring may tear the pelvic venous plexus or disrupt the internal iliac arterial system.
   1. **Signs** include progressive flank, scrotal, or perianal swelling and bruising; a high-riding prostate; and blood at the urethral meatus.

HOT KEY A pelvic stability examination should be performed only once, because repeated testing may dislodge clots from coagulated vessels.

---

   2. **Treatment**
      a. If the patient is hemodynamically unstable and there is an open fracture, emergent surgery is needed to find the source of and to control hemorrhage.
      b. If the patient is hemodynamically unstable and has a closed

fracture, diagnostic peritoneal lavage or an ultrasound is indicated.

c. If the patient is hemodynamically stable and the fracture is closed, the fracture can be immobilized by splinting. This can be accomplished by wrapping a sheet around the pelvis (thereby placing the hips in internal rotation). A pneumatic antishock garment is used if the patient must be transferred; it is inflated only if the patient experiences hypotension during transport.

C. Lower extremity fractures

1. **Femoral shaft fractures** often are seen in "auto versus pedestrian" injuries. The femoral shaft fracture often is accompanied by injuries to the head and chest (Waddle triad). Treatment usually involves traction splinting and the application of a spica cast.

2. **Patellar fractures** should be immobilized in 10° of flexion.

3. **Tibial fractures** should be immobilized using a well-padded cardboard or metal gutter. Because nerve injuries and compartment syndrome (see V C) may complicate tibial fractures, patients with displaced tibial fractures generally require hospital admission for 24 hours to monitor for complications.

V ASSOCIATED INJURIES

A. Major arterial hemorrhage should be controlled with a pneumatic tourniquet. Clamps are applied into an open wound only if a superficial vessel is clearly identified.

B. Vascular injuries are evidenced by cold, pale, pulseless limbs. Perfusion should always be assessed before and after the fracture is immobilized. If there is evidence of vascular injury, a surgical consult should be promptly obtained.

C. Compartment syndromes occur when pressure within an osteofascial compartment compromises arterial blood flow, leading to muscle and nerve ischemia and necrosis.

1. **Classic signs** include pain greater than expected with passive stretching of the involved muscle, hypesthesia or paresthesia, and tense swelling. Weakness or paralysis and loss of pulses are late signs. After 8–12 hours, loss of muscle and nerve function occurs.

2. **Treatment.** Release all constricting devices and obtain a surgical consult promptly. Fasciotomy may be required.

D. Crush injuries. The release of byproducts from injured muscle (rhabdomyolysis) can cause acute renal failure, metabolic acidosis, hyperkalemia, hypocalcemia, and disseminated intravascular coagulation (DIC).

1. **Diagnosis.** Myoglobin gives the urine a dark amber color. A urine myoglobin assay should be obtained.
2. **Treatment.** Intravenous fluids should be administered, and the urine should be alkalinized if myoglobinuria is present.

E. **Traumatic amputation.** To prepare the amputated part for reimplantation, it is washed in an isotonic solution and then wrapped in sterile gauze soaked in aqueous penicillin (100,000 U penicillin/50 ml lactated Ringer solution). A towel is soaked in the same solution and used to wrap the gauze-wrapped body part. The entire package is then placed in a plastic bag for transport in a cooling chest with crushed ice. Patients with multiple injuries who require resuscitation and emergency surgery are not candidates for reimplantation.

References

Advanced Trauma Life Support (ATLS), 6th ed. Chicago, American College of Surgeons, 1997.

Eichelberger MR: *Pediatric Trauma: Prevention, Acute Care, Rehabilitation.* St. Louis, Mosby-Year Book, 1993.

104. Head Trauma

....

I **INTRODUCTION.** Head injuries account for 70% of all traumatic deaths in children. The **morbidity and mortality** associated with head trauma is **related to** both **the initial injury** and **the subsequent adverse effects of increased intracranial pressure (ICP).** When the ICP is increased, oxygen and substrate delivery to the neural tissue is impaired. Controlling the ICP in the hours and days after the initial injury is vital for reducing patient morbidity as a result of head trauma.

A. **Increased ICP**
1. **Monro-Kellie doctrine.** The adult skull is a nonexpansile space. The volume is equal to the sum of its compartments [i.e., cerebrospinal fluid (CSF), blood, and brain tissue]. When the volume of one of these compartments increases, another compartment must decrease if the volume is to remain constant. If this does not occur, the ICP will increase.
2. **Measurement of the ICP**
   a. The ICP is measured using an ICP monitoring device. This device is placed by a neurosurgeon in cases of severe head trauma.
   b. The **normal value** is **10 mm Hg.** A measurement of 20 mm Hg would be classified as abnormal, and one as high as 40 mm Hg would be considered severely abnormal.
B. **Cerebral perfusion pressure.** The cerebral perfusion pressure decreases as the ICP increases or the mean arterial pressure (MAP) decreases:

$$CPP = MAP - ICP,$$
where CPP = cerebral perfusion pressure, MAP = mean arterial pressure, and ICP = intracranial pressure.

1. To ensure adequate brain perfusion, a cerebral perfusion pressure of **at least 70 mm Hg** in an adult or **40 mm Hg** in a child must be maintained.
2. Adult patients are at risk if the cerebral perfusion pressure is less than 50 mm Hg for more than 3 minutes.

II DIFFERENTIAL DIAGNOSIS

> **HOT**
> ▶
> **KEY**
> Consider the possibility of child abuse, especially if the child is younger than 2 years of age or presents with an altered level of consciousness with no history of trauma or a history of minor trauma.

A. **Mild concussion.** Consciousness is preserved, but temporary neurologic dysfunction (e.g., confusion, disorientation, retrograde or anterograde amnesia) is present to some degree. Amnesia is a more serious finding.

B. **Cerebral contusion.** Consciousness is lost but usually is regained fully within 6 hours. The duration of amnesia immediately after the injury is a good measure of the severity of the injury. Most patients have no sequelae, but some develop postconcussion syndrome (characterized by memory difficulties, dizziness, nausea, anosmia, and depression).

C. **Skull fractures**
   1. The risk of intracranial hemorrhage increases with skull fractures. Fragments that are depressed more than the thickness of the skull or fractures with CSF leaks require surgery.
   2. **Basilar skull fractures** often are missed on plain films. Clinical signs of a basilar skull fracture include periorbital ecchymosis ("raccoon eyes"), retroauricular ecchymosis (Battle sign), facial nerve (cranial nerve VII) palsy, hemotympanum, and CSF otorrhea or rhinorrhea.

D. **Hematomas**
   1. **Epidural hematoma.** A lenticular-shaped bleed is seen on a computed tomography (CT) scan of the head (Figure 104–1).
      a. If managed properly, epidural hematomas are associated with a good long-term outcome because damage to the underlying brain tissue is limited. Most bleeds are arterial (middle meningeal).
      b. Approximately 60% of patients do not lose consciousness initially. Some patients may have a lucid interval, followed by a rapid decline ("talk and die"). The lucid interval can be prolonged in children.
   2. **Subdural hematoma.** A bleed that follows the contour of the brain is seen on the head CT scan (Figure 104–2). This injury often is seen in abused children.
      a. Nearly all patients have an underlying brain contusion.
      b. Subdural hematomas require aggressive surgical and medical management.
   3. **Intracerebral hematoma.** The frontal and temporal lobes are

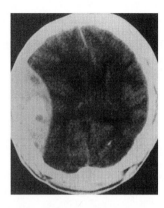

FIGURE 104–1. Epidural hematoma. This biconvex or lenticular shape typifies an epidural hematoma. Note the massive shift of the midline. (Reprinted with permission from Grossman RG, Loftus CM: *Principles of Neurosurgery,* 2nd ed. Philadelphia, Lippincott Williams & Wilkins, 1999, p 137.)

most commonly involved. This injury is highly associated with subdural hematoma.

E. Diffuse axonal injury is the result of a rapid acceleration–deceleration shear injury. Many patients do not survive this injury.

   1. Loss of consciousness is immediate. Patients often remain comatose and show decortication or decerebration. Autonomic

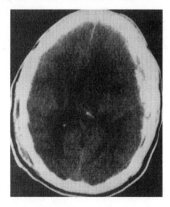

FIGURE 104–2. Subdural hematoma. Note that the hyperdense collection covers almost the entire surface of the hemisphere and has a concave inner margin. There is a 1-cm left-to-right shift of the midline. (Reprinted with permission from Grossman RG, Loftus CM: *Principles of Neurosurgery,* 2nd ed. Philadelphia, Lippincott Williams & Wilkins, 1999, p 137.)

dysfunction (manifested as hypertension, hyperhidrosis, and hyperpyrexia) may be seen.

2. A head CT scan may show punctuate hemorrhages and diffuse edema; no intracranial mass is noted.

3. The major differential diagnosis for diffuse axonal injury is hypoxic brain injury.

III APPROACH TO THE PATIENT

A. **Primary survey.** A quick preliminary assessment [airway, breathing, and circulation (ABCs)] should be performed to gain an overview of the patient's clinical status.

1. The **Glasgow coma scale (GCS)**(Table 104–1) is a helpful tool for assessing the severity of a head injury.

TABLE 104-1. Glasgow Coma Scale*		
Category	**Response**	**Score**
Eye opening	Open spontaneously	4
	Open in response to verbal command	3
	Open in response to pain	2
	No response	1
Verbal response		
In children	Smiles, oriented to sound, interacts with examiner	5
	Crying but consolable	4
	Persistently irritable	3
	Restless and agitated	2
	No response	1
In adults	Oriented	5
	Confused conversation	4
	Inappropriate words	3
	Incomprehensible sounds	2
	No response	1
Motor response	Obeys commands	6
	Responds to painful stimulus	5
	Withdraws from painful stimulus	5
	Decorticate posturing (flexion)	3
	Decerebrate posturing (extension)	2
	No response	1
Total score		3–15

*Adapted for use in pediatric patients.

2. **Head CT scan.** The CT scan should be obtained within 30 minutes if the patient is hemodynamically stable. The scan should be checked for:

    a. Shift of midline structures (> 5 mm indicates need for surgery)

    b. Hematomas

    c. Intraventricular hemorrhage (associated with parenchymal hemorrhage)

    d. Hydrocephalus (acute obstructive hydrocephalus may occur secondary to a posterior fossa hematoma; communicating hydrocephalus may be caused by blood in the subarachnoid space)

B. Initial management is based on the GCS score.

    1. Mild head injury (GCS score of 14–15). These patients are awake and alert but may be amnesic.

        a. Workup. A **head CT scan** is indicated for all patients who have experienced amnesia or a loss or decreased level of consciousness, or who have abnormal findings on neurologic examination. If the patient is awake, alert, and asymptomatic, he or she can be admitted to the hospital for 12–24 hours of observation without obtaining a CT scan.

        b. Disposition

            (1) Admission to the hospital is warranted if the CT scan is abnormal, there is a loss of consciousness, a CSF leak is detected, the patient's level of consciousness is deteriorating, there is evidence of a skull fracture, there is no reliable companion at home, the toxicology screen result is positive, or the patient has sustained penetrating head trauma. There is a small chance (3%) that the patient's clinical condition will deteriorate unexpectedly; therefore, admission for 12–24 hours of observation may be appropriate.

            (2) Discharge. If the patient is discharged, the caretaker should be advised to wake the child every 2 hours during the night. If it is difficult to rouse the child or there are other signs that the child's condition may be deteriorating (e.g., persistent nausea and vomiting, convulsions, discharge from the nose or ear, severe headache, weakness, pupil inequality, slow or rapid pulse, or unusual breathing patterns), the parent should be advised to call a physician immediately.

    2. Moderate head injury (GCS score of 9–13). These patients can follow simple commands but are confused or somnolent and may have focal neurologic deficits.

        a. Workup. A **CT scan** is always obtained.

        b. Disposition. Because 10%–20% of these patients will experience a deterioration in clinical status, all should be admitted, even if the CT scan results are normal. If the patient's clinical condition does deteriorate, he will require immediate treatment per the severe head injury protocol (see III B 3).

3. Severe head injury (GCS score of 3–8). A GCS score of less than 8 is the generally accepted definition of coma. Because hypoxemia and hypotension lead to secondary brain injury if untreated, it is imperative to diagnose and treat the patient promptly. Approximately 50%–75% of these patients develop increased ICP. Infants with open fontanels are more tolerant of an expanding intracranial mass lesion. Symptoms may be hidden until rapid decompensation occurs. Therefore, the appearance of a bulging fontanel or widened sutures is a serious finding that necessitates immediate neurosurgical consultation.

a. Airway. The patient should be intubated immediately to prevent hypoxemia. Medications are used to blunt any increase in ICP that may occur during intubation:

(1) For patients with an **increased ICP** and **cardiovascular compromise,** fentanyl (1–2 mcg/kg/dose) or diazepam (0.2 mg/kg); lidocaine (1 mg/kg); and vecuronium (0.1 mg/kg) are used for rapid sequence intubation.

(2) For patients with an **increased ICP** but **no cardiovascular compromise,** thiopental (4–6 mg/kg) can be used instead of fentanyl or diazepam.

b. Breathing

(1) Hyperventilation. If the patient has a worsening GCS score or pupillary dilatation, he or she may be cautiously hyperventilated until an arterial carbon dioxide tension ($PaCO_2$) of 25–30 mm Hg is reached.

HOT KEY "Blowing off" too much carbon dioxide ($PCO_2 < 25$) will cause vasoconstriction and worsen ischemia. Hypoventilation should always be used in moderation and for as brief a period as possible.

---

(2) Positive end-expiratory pressure (PEEP). Excessive PEEP, which can decrease cerebral venous return and increase the ICP, should be avoided.

c. Circulation. Hypotension usually is not the result of the brain injury itself; it usually is a marker of blood loss. Volume replacement is begun with isotonic fluids (e.g., lactated Ringer solution, normal saline). Often the GCS score will improve as brain perfusion from fluid resuscitation takes effect.

d. Imaging studies. Diagnostic peritoneal lavage or abdominal ultrasound is routine in comatose patients because an abdominal examination for tenderness is not possible.

   (1) Generally, if fluid resuscitation cannot maintain the blood pressure adequately, abdominal ultrasound or exploratory laparotomy takes precedence over a head CT scan.

   (2) If the patient is hemodynamically stable after fluid resuscitation, head and abdominal CT scans can be safely obtained.

  e. Neurosurgical consult. Because these patients require ICP monitoring, consult a neurosurgeon immediately.

C. Secondary survey. Serial neurologic examinations, including repeat GCS scores and eye examinations, are necessary to follow the progress of the patient with a head injury.

  1. Repeat GCS scoring. Any decline in the GCS score over time should be attributed to increased ICP until proven otherwise.

  2. Eye examination

    a. Pupillary light response. The best and worst responses and left and right sides should be reported separately.

     (1) Mild dilation and a sluggish pupillary response to light may indicate early temporal lobe herniation.

     (2) Bilaterally dilated and nonreactive pupils can be a sign of inadequate brain perfusion.

     (3) Bilaterally constricted pupils may be a sign of drug intoxication.

     (4) Concentric pupils without direct reactivity (Marcus-Gunn pupils) suggest optic nerve injury.

    b. Ocular motility. Patients with worsening temporal lobe herniation show ptosis and paresis of the medial rectus muscle (i.e., the eye will be in a "down and out" position) as a result of cranial nerve III palsy.

    c. Fundoscopic examination. Papilledema may not be present until several days after the injury.

IV ONGOING MANAGEMENT

A. Control of the ICP

  1. Intravenous fluids. If the patient is not hypovolemic, two thirds of the maintenance requirement should be administered. An isotonic solution should be used during the first 24 hours.

HOT

KEY
  Do not use hypotonic fluids, which will increase cerebral edema!

---

   2. Hyperventilation [see III B 3 b (1)]
   3. Mannitol can worsen hypovolemia and must be used with
      caution.
      a. Mannitol (1 g/kg of a 20% solution given as an intra-
         venous bolus) may be used for patients who develop
         pupillary dilatation or who have bilaterally dilated non-
         reactive pupils.
      b. If the increased ICP persists, mannitol (0.25 g/kg every
         4 hours) can be used to achieve a serum osmolality of
         310–320 mOsm/L. An osmolality greater than 320 mOsm/L
         is associated with renal injury.
   4. Furosemide (0.3–0.5 mg/kg intravenously) may be given as
      an adjunct to mannitol after consulting a neurosurgeon. An
      added benefit of furosemide is that it may decrease CSF pro-
      duction.
   5. Muscle paralysis combined with sedation can help reduce
      the ICP.
   6. Control of hyperpyrexia and **seizures** is indicated to reduce
      the cerebral metabolic demand.
   7. Reverse Trendelenburg positioning. Place the patient in a
      reverse Trendelenburg position with his head in a neutral
      position to maximize venous drainage and decrease the ICP.
      Keep in mind that elevation of the head may increase the
      ICP in some patients, and the cerebral perfusion pressure
      may decrease, especially in hypotensive patients.
B. Adjunctive therapies
   1. Anticonvulsants. Patients who have sustained head trauma
      require seizure prophylaxis for 1 week with phenytoin or
      phenobarbital. Benzodiazepines are used to acutely manage
      seizures.
   2. Insulin is used to treat persistent hyperglycemia (i.e., a serum
      glucose level greater than 250 mg/dl). Aim to achieve a nor-
      mal serum glucose level (i.e., 60–100 mg/dl).
   3. Antibiotics should be given prophylactically if pneumo-
      cephalus is present.

V PROGNOSIS. The patient's outcome can be predicted to
      some degree by:

A. The degree of dysfunction seen soon after the injury
B. The best GCS motor score
C. The presence of reactive pupils
D. The systolic blood pressure
E. The age of the patient (patients younger than age 3 years tend
      to have worse outcomes)

References

Advanced Trauma Life Support (ATLS), 6th ed. Chicago, American College of Surgeons, 1997.

Eichelberger MR: *Pediatric Trauma: Prevention, Acute Care, Rehabilitation.* St. Louis, Mosby-Year Book, 1993.

105. Abdominal Trauma

I INTRODUCTION

A. **Blunt abdominal trauma,** which can lead to rupture of a hollow viscus or bleeding from a solid organ, is not necessarily associated with clinical signs.

> **HOT** **KEY**
>
> Assume abdominal viscera injury in any patient who has sustained significant blunt force trauma to the torso.

B. **Indicators for serious abdominal injury** are listed in Table 105–1.

II APPROACH TO THE PATIENT

A. **Physical examination**
   1. **Abdomen**
      a. Evidence of **lap-belt trauma,** indicated by a characteristic abrasion pattern across the chest and abdomen, is sought.
      b. The patient is examined for evidence of **splenic injury. Kehr sign** (i.e., left shoulder pain in response to palpation of the left upper quadrant), **Grey-Turner sign** (i.e., bruis-

---

TABLE 105-1. Indicators for Serious Abdominal Injury*

Gross hematuria (seen in 52% of patients with serious abdominal injury)
Abdominal tenderness (seen in 22% of patients)
Hematocrit < 25%
Lap-belt injury
Injury from assault or abuse
Trauma score < 12 (see Table 102–3)

---

*The presence of three or more of these criteria should alert the physician to the possibility of serious abdominal injury. (Reprinted with permission from Eichelberger MR: *Pediatric Trauma: Prevention, Acute Care, Rehabilitation.* St. Louis, Mosby-Year Book, 1993, p 453.)

ing in the left flank), and **Cullen sign** (i.e., bruising in the umbilical region) are suggestive.

c. Any **tangential or superficial wounds** are examined. Approximately one third (25%–33%) of stab wounds do not penetrate the peritoneal cavity; therefore, local wound exploration may be indicated.

HOT

KEY
Diagnosis of a small bowel perforation often is delayed in children because peritoneal signs develop more slowly in children than in adults.

---

   2. Pelvic stability is assessed. The anterior superior iliac spine and the iliac crests are compressed manually.

   3. Perineal and rectal areas

     a. Guaiac test is performed on stool samples.

     b. Sphincter tone is assessed.

     c. The position of the prostate is checked (a high-riding prostate indicates urethral disruption).

   4. Gluteal region (i.e., the area extending from the iliac crests to the gluteal folds). Penetrating injuries in the gluteal region are associated with a 50% incidence of significant intra-abdominal injury.

B. Laboratory studies include a blood type and cross-match, a complete blood count (CBC), a serum electrolyte panel, urinalysis, serum amylase levels, serum liver enzyme levels, serum ethyl alcohol levels, human chorionic gonadotropin (hCG), and a hematocrit.

   1. Repeat hematocrits are essential for monitoring for ongoing hemorrhage.

   2. Increasing amylase levels are an indicator of pancreatic injury.

   3. Elevated liver enzyme levels [i.e., an aspartate aminotransferase (AST) level greater than 200 U/L and an alanine aminotransferase (ALT) level greater than 100 U/L] are likely to indicate hepatic injury. However, the degree of liver enzyme elevation does not predict the severity of the hepatic injury.

C. Imaging studies

   1. Radiographs

     a. For blunt trauma

       (1) Chest (anterior–posterior view) and pelvic x-rays, and abdominal CT should be obtained.

       (2) Lower left rib fractures, elevation of the left hemidiaphragm, pleural effusion, medial displacement of the stomach, opacification of the left hypochondrium, and downward displacement of the transverse colon can indicate splenic injury.

b. For penetrating trauma

(1) An upright chest radiograph should be obtained for **stable patients** with wounds above the umbilicus to evaluate for hemothorax, pneumothorax, or intraperitoneal air.

(2) Unstable patients should be sent to the operating room.

2. Abdominal ultrasound has the advantage of being quick, noninvasive, and immediately repeatable if changing physical findings warrant a repeat examination. Abdominal ultrasound is as sensitive as diagnostic peritoneal lavage when performed by an experienced technician.

3. Abdominal computed tomography (CT) scan is indicated only for hemodynamically stable patients. It has become the diagnostic modality of choice in the pediatric population. It has the advantage over diagnostic peritoneal lavage of diagnosing retroperitoneal injuries and specific organ injuries, but it is time-consuming.

HOT KEY The finding of free fluid on an abdominal CT scan in the absence of hepatic or splenic injuries suggests a gastrointestinal tract or mesenteric injury and mandates early surgical intervention.

D. Diagnostic peritoneal lavage is used to assess for intraperitoneal bleeding but usually is reserved for adult-sized patients. This test is 98% sensitive, although assessment of the retroperitoneal space and diaphragm is difficult.

HOT KEY Gastric tube placement is indicated before performing diagnostic peritoneal lavage in order to relieve dilatation. A gastric tube should not be placed if the patient has severe facial fractures or a basilar skull fracture, owing to the risk of passing the tube through the cribriform plate and into the brain.

---

1. Indications. Diagnostic peritoneal lavage is indicated for hemodynamically unstable patients with multiple blunt injuries. Specific indications include:

a. Changes in the patient's sensorium

b. Injury to the lower ribs, pelvis, or lumbar spine

c. An inability to assess changes in abdominal examinations reliably (when the patient is obtunded or unconscious)

   2. **Findings.** Surgery is indicated if:
      a. The aspirate contains blood, gastrointestinal contents, vegetable fibers, bile, or more than 100,000 red blood cells (RBCs)/mm^3
      b. Gram staining of the aspirate is positive for bacteria
E. **Urinary catheter placement**
   1. Patients who meet any of the following criteria should have a retrograde urethrogram to confirm that the urethra is intact before a urinary catheter is placed.
      a. Inability to void
      b. Unstable pelvic fracture
      c. Presence of blood at the meatus
      d. Scrotal hematoma or perineal ecchymoses
      e. High-riding prostate
   2. Patients with disrupted urethras require surgical suprapubic tube placement.
F. **Celiotomy** is indicated for the following patients:
   1. **Blunt trauma.** Patients who have positive findings on diagnostic peritoneal lavage or abdominal ultrasound, or who have recurrent hypotension (despite adequate resuscitation)
   2. **Penetrating trauma.** Patients who have hypotension; are bleeding from the stomach, rectum, or genitourinary tract; or who have a transversing gunshot wound
   3. **Peritonitis.** Patients with peritonitis (either early or subsequent to the initial examination)

References

Abdominal injury (Chapters 41 to 46). In *Pediatric Trauma: Prevention, Acute Care, Rehabilitation.* Edited by Eichelberger MR, St. Louis, Mosby-Year Book, 1993.

Advanced Trauma Life Support (ATLS), 6th ed. Chicago, American College of Surgeons, 1997.

106. Thoracic Trauma

I **INTRODUCTION.** The thorax contains several critical structures: the lungs and lower airways, the heart and great vessels, the esophagus, and the thoracic spine. Because respiratory compromise often is a major component of chest trauma (Table 106–1), securing the airway and maintaining breathing is of the utmost importance.

A. The **chest wall** is more pliable in children than in adults. Consequently, blunt force to the thoracic region can result in serious internal organ damage in a child even if it does not cause rib

---

TABLE 106-1. Respiratory Compromise Associated With Chest Trauma

Airway compromise
  Coma and apnea
  Intraluminal airway obstruction
  Direct injury to tracheobronchial tree
Extrapulmonary compromise
  Pneumothorax
  Hemothorax
  Tension pneumothorax
  Impaired diaphragmatic function
    Massive gastric distension
    Massive hemoperitoneum or pneumoperitoneum
Pulmonary compromise
  Aspiration
  Pulmonary contusion
  Pulmonary hematoma
Ventilatory compromise
  Fractured ribs with splinting
  Phrenic nerve injury
  Diaphragmatic rupture
  Flail chest
  Large open pneumothorax

Reprinted with permission from Flesisher GR, Ludwig S, Silverman BK: *Synopsis of Pediatric Emergency Medicine.* Baltimore, Williams & Wilkins, 1996, p 621.

fractures. The presence of rib fractures in a child implies that a great deal of force was applied to the chest wall; therefore, internal organ injury should be assumed in any child with multiple rib fractures.

B. In multiple trauma, the mortality rate among those with chest injury is dramatically higher than that among those without chest injury (26% versus 1.5%).

C. Most life-threatening thoracic injuries can be treated with a chest tube or needle.

II DIFFERENTIAL DIAGNOSIS

A. Immediately life-threatening disorders are sought during the **primary survey.**

 1. **Laryngeal fractures** lead to disruption of the airway. Signs and symptoms include hoarseness, subcutaneous emphysema, and a palpable fracture.

 2. **Tension pneumothorax** results when a tear in the lung parenchyma forms a one-way valve that allows air to leak into the thoracic cavity but not to escape. The result is shifting of the mediastinal structures, compression of the heart and lungs, and diminished venous return.

HOT **KEY**
Increased mobility of the mediastinal structures makes tension pneumothorax more common in children.

---

 a. **Causes** include mechanical ventilation, blunt or penetrating trauma, displaced thoracic spine fractures, and iatrogenic causes (e.g., complications resulting from subclavian or internal jugular line placement).

 b. **Signs and symptoms** include chest pain, air hunger, respiratory distress, tachycardia, hypotension, tracheal deviation, and a unilateral absence of breath sounds.

HOT **KEY**
Suspect a tension pneumothorax when the clinical status of a patient undergoing positive-pressure ventilation suddenly deteriorates.

---

 3. **Open pneumothorax.** In open chest wounds, if the defect is large enough, air will preferentially enter through the defect, leading to hypoxia and hypercapnia.

 4. **Flail chest** results when two or more adjacent ribs are fractured

in two or more locations, leading to disruption of normal chest wall movement. Associated pain can contribute to hypoxia. Flail chest often is associated with significant injury to the underlying viscera, such as severe pulmonary contusion and hemopneumothorax. Crepitus and paradoxical or asymmetric chest wall movements may be noted.

5. **Massive hemothorax**
   a. The source of the intrathoracic bleeding usually is the lung or the intercostal vessels, although bleeding can occur directly from the heart or great vessels.
   b. This diagnosis should be considered in a patient with shock who has absent breath sounds, dullness to percussion on one side of the chest, or both. The neck veins may be distended (if there is an associated tension pneumothorax) or flat (secondary to hypovolemia).

6. **Cardiac tamponade**
   a. **Cardiac tamponade** is the accumulation of blood in the pericardial cavity, leading to compression of the heart and inadequate ventricular filling. Only a small amount of blood is needed in the pericardium to impair cardiac filling.
   b. **Signs** include Beck triad (i.e., an elevated venous pressure, a decreased arterial pressure, and muffled heart tones), pulsus paradoxus (i.e., a decrease in blood pressure during spontaneous inspiration), and Kussmaul sign (i.e., an increase in the venous pressure with spontaneous inspiration).
   c. In the absence of hypovolemia and tension pneumothorax, **pulseless electrical activity** suggests tamponade.

HOT KEY Clinical detection of cardiac tamponade is difficult. Consider this diagnosis when the patient has a plausible mechanism of injury and does not respond to resuscitative efforts.

B. **Other disorders.** The following disorders are sought during the secondary survey.
   1. **Simple pneumothorax** results when air enters the potential space between the visceral and parietal pleurae. It usually is caused by a lung laceration. Signs include decreased breath sounds, hyperresonance to percussion, and tracheal shift.
   2. **Pulmonary contusion** is the most common potentially lethal chest injury. Common complications include lung edema, atelectasis, and hypoxemia. Respiratory failure can be subtle and may develop over time.

3. **Tracheobronchial tree injury.** Many patients with tracheo-bronchial tree injuries die at the scene of injury. Signs and symptoms include hemoptysis, subcutaneous emphysema, tension pneumothorax, and pneumomediastinum. Diagnosis is confirmed by bronchoscopy.

HOT

KEY

A persistent large air leak after chest tube placement suggests a tracheobronchial tree injury.

---

4. **Blunt cardiac injury** can result in myocardial contusion, cardiac chamber rupture, or valvular disruption. Patients present with an elevated central venous pressure (CVP), hypotension, conduction abnormalities [e.g., multiple premature ventricular contractions (PVCs), unexplained sinus tachycardia, atrial fibrillation, right bundle branch block, ST segment changes], and wall motion abnormalities (on echocardiography). The major differential diagnosis is myocardial infarction.
5. **Traumatic aortic disruption.** Patients who survive this injury usually have incomplete tears near the ligamentum arteriosum; patients with free rupture usually die in minutes.
   a. This injury is suspected in patients when there is a history of decelerating force (e.g., motor vehicle collisions, falls from great heights).
   b. The diagnosis often is made radiographically. Aortic disruption is suggested by mediastinal widening, depression of the left main stem bronchus, and a widened paratracheal stripe.
6. **Traumatic diaphragmatic injury**
   a. **Causes.** Sudden forceful trauma to the chest or abdomen may cause this injury; lap-belts are often the culprit.

HOT

KEY

Left-sided ruptures are more commonly diagnosed because the liver offers some protection to the diaphragm on the right side and can obliterate radiographic evidence of right-sided defects.

---

   b. **Signs** include respiratory distress and a scaphoid abdomen.
   c. **Diagnosis.** A nasogastric tube is inserted, and a chest radiograph is obtained. The tip of the tube should be looked for in the lung fields. Appearance of peritoneal lavage fluid in the chest tube also is diagnostic. An upper gastrointestinal study should be ordered if the diagnosis is unclear.

7. **Rib, sternum, and scapular fractures.** Pain results in splinting, which impairs ventilation and causes atelectasis and pneumonia.

   a. **Fractures of ribs 1–3, the sternum, or the scapula** are associated with a high mortality rate because these fractures are often accompanied by blunt cardiac injury or injuries to the head, neck, spinal cord, lungs, or great vessels. Posterior sternoclavicular dislocation results in superior vena cava obstruction and requires immediate reduction.

   b. **Fractures of ribs 4–9** are the most common type of rib fractures. Patients must be monitored for the development of pneumothorax.

   c. **Fractures of ribs 10–12** often are associated with hepato-splenic injury.

8. **Esophageal rupture** should be considered in patients with:

   a. A left-sided pneumothorax or hemothorax without rib fracture

   b. A history of a severe blow to the lower sternum or epigastrium with pain and shock out of proportion to the apparent injury

   c. Particulate matter in the chest tube after the blood begins to clear

   d. Air in the mediastinum

   e. Radiographic evidence of the nasogastric tube in the chest

III APPROACH TO THE PATIENT

A. **Primary assessment.** Airway, breathing, and circulation should be assessed (see Chapter 102 I).

B. **Secondary assessment.** During the secondary assessment, an attempt is made to define the extent and the nature of the patient's injuries.

   1. Patient history

   2. Physical examination

      a. Inspection

      b. Palpation

      c. Percussion

      d. Auscultation

   3. **Laboratory studies.** Arterial blood gases (ABGs) should be obtained. Alternatively, pulse oximetry can be used for continuous monitoring of oxygen saturation.

   4. **Imaging studies**

      a. **Chest radiography.** Anterior-posterior and lateral films should be obtained if possible. Notable findings are summarized in Table 106–2.

      b. **Chest computed tomography (CT)** may be more sensitive than radiography for detecting pulmonary contusion.

TABLE 106-2. Radiographic Findings in Chest Trauma

Examination	Findings
Bones	Vertebral fractures or misalignment, rib fractures (greenstick fractures, old fractures, and especially first or second rib fractures), clavicular fractures, scapular fractures, shoulder dislocations or fractures
Lungs and pleural space	Contusion, atelectasis, consolidation, hemothorax, apical capping; note the position of any chest drains that have been inserted
Airway	Shifts in position, foreign bodies (teeth); note position of the endotracheal tube
Mediastinum	Shift to one side (tension pneumothorax), widening (aortic trauma—may be hard to assess in the young child with a large thymus), pneumomediastinum, pneumopericardium; note the size and shape of the heart, and the shape and position of the aortic arch
Diaphragm	Rupture, traumatic herniation of abdominal viscera, elevation, paralysis
Soft tissues	Swelling, subcutaneous air, foreign bodies

Reprinted with permission from Blair GK: Chest trauma. In *Handbook of Pediatric Emergencies,* 2nd ed. Edited by Baldwin GA. Boston, Little, Brown, 1994, p 414.

  c. **Electrocardiography.** Continuous heart monitoring should be established. A 12-lead electrocardiogram (ECG) may be indicated, depending on the child's injuries (e.g., cardiac tamponade, blunt cardiac injury).

IV TREATMENT

A. **Laryngeal fractures.** An otolaryngologist should be called immediately.
   1. **Airway.** Orotracheal intubation should be attempted, but endoscopic guided intubation, emergency tracheostomy, or cricothyroidotomy (needle cricothyroidotomy if the patient is younger than 11 years) also should be considered.
   2. **Oxygenation.** Jet insufflation is indicated until a definitive surgical airway can be placed. A large-caliber cannula is inserted and connected to 15 L/min wall oxygen. It is insufflated (1 second on, 4 seconds off) by placing the thumb over the open end of the Y-connector. This technique can provide

adequate oxygenation for 30–45 minutes, as long as there is no associated chest injury. Hypercarbia may occur with prolonged use.

B. Pneumothorax

   1. Simple pneumothorax. A chest tube is placed in the intercostal space between ribs 4 and 5, anterior to the midaxillary line.

HOT KEY Because a simple pneumothorax can develop into a tension pneumothorax, never give positive-pressure ventilation to a patient who has sustained a traumatic pneumothorax unless a chest tube has been placed first!

---

   2. Tension pneumothorax is managed with immediate decompression. A large-bore needle is inserted at the second intercostal space on the midcostal line. Then a chest tube is inserted at the fifth intercostal space between the anterior and midaxillary lines.

   3. Open pneumothorax. A flutter-type valve is created by placing an occlusive dressing taped on three sides over the defect; during inhalation, the dressing will block air entry; during exhalation, air will exit the open end of the dressing. A chest tube is placed, remote from the wound, as soon as possible. Definitive surgical closure ultimately is needed.

C. Flail chest. Patients should receive humidified oxygen, fluids, and analgesics.

HOT KEY In patients who are in shock, injured lung segments are susceptible to underresuscitation; however, in the absence of hypotension, prevent overhydration because the injured lung is sensitive to fluid overload.

D. Hemothorax

   1. Simple hemothorax. If not completely evacuated, a simple hemothorax may develop into a clotted hemothorax with lung entrapment, empyema, or both.

     a. Placement of a large-caliber chest tube will evacuate blood, prevent a clotted hemothorax, and monitor blood loss.

     b. Patients who are unstable as a result of blood loss require surgery.

   2. Massive hemothorax. The sudden drainage of a massive hemothorax may relieve a tamponade and allow for additional hemorrhage. An autotransfusion and early thoracotomy will be needed if large amounts of blood are immediately evacuated.

E. Cardiac tamponade
   1. Pericardiocentesis is a definitive life-saving measure. The needle is inserted below the xiphoid process at a 30° angle, aiming toward the left nipple. When the needle touches the epicardium, increased T-wave voltage is seen on the ECG.
   2. Intravenous fluids increase the CVP, leading to an improvement in the patient's status.
F. Pulmonary contusion. Patients must be monitored over time. Patients who develop significant hypoxia within 1 hour of injury must be intubated.
G. Tracheobronchial tree injury. More than one chest tube may be needed to overcome the leak. Opposite main stem intubation may be temporarily required. Operative correction is required for unstable patients.
H. Blunt cardiac injury. Patients should be monitored for at least 24 hours, and a cardiologist should be consulted.
I. Traumatic diaphragmatic injury is treated with direct surgical repair.
J. Rib fractures. Pain should be controlled with intercostal blocks, epidural anesthesia, or systemic analgesics. The goal is aggressive pain control without respiratory depression.
K. Esophageal rupture requires prompt surgical repair.

 PROGNOSIS. The prognosis for patients with thoracic trauma varies according to the location and severity of the injury.

References
Advanced Trauma Life Support (ATLS), 6th ed. Chicago, American College of Surgeons, 1997.

107. Hemorrhagic Shock

I. INTRODUCTION

A. Classes of hemorrhage are given in Table 107–1. Fatal life-threatening hemorrhage usually is not a diagnostic dilemma. Recognizing early shock is more challenging, and requires keen attention to a variety of signs and symptoms.

TABLE 107-1. Classes of Hemorrhage

Class	Blood Loss (%)	Clinical Manifestations	Fluid for Resuscitation
I	< 15%	Minimal tachycardia; no changes in blood pressure, pulse pressure, or respiratory rate; capillary refill time < 2 seconds	Crystalloid
II	15%–30%	Tachycardia; decreased pulse pressure; cool, mottled skin, anxiety, delayed capillary refill time (>2 seconds); normal urine output	Crystalloid
III	30%–40%	Measurably decreased systolic blood pressure, tachypnea, worsening tachycardia, mental status changes; decreased urine output	Blood
IV	> 40%	Significantly decreased systolic blood pressure; immeasurable pulse pressure; marked tachycardia; depressed mental status; cold, ashen skin; negligible urine output	Blood Death may occur within minutes

> **HOT KEY**
>
> Any injured patient who is cool and tachycardic is in shock until proven otherwise.

B. Special concerns in pediatrics
1. In children, the first sign of hemorrhage is tachycardia. Decreased systolic blood pressure is a **late** finding.
2. In children, the blood volume is 8%–9% of the total body weight (i.e., 80 ml/kg).
3. Formulas for systolic blood pressure values are listed below:

50th percentile = 80 + (2 × the child's age in years)

Lower limit of normal = 70 + the child's age in years

II DIFFERENTIAL DIAGNOSIS. A nonhemorrhagic cause for shock is suspected when the patient does not respond to fluid boluses.

A. Septic shock sometimes is difficult to distinguish from hemorrhagic shock. Sepsis does not occur immediately, so it is suspected in the hours after the initial injury.
1. In early sepsis, signs include modest tachycardia; warm, pink skin; a normal systolic blood pressure; and a wide pulse pressure.
2. In late sepsis, signs include tachycardia, cutaneous vasoconstriction (evidenced by cool, mottled skin), impaired urinary output, a decreased systolic blood pressure, and a narrow pulse pressure.
B. Neurogenic shock. Impairment of sympathetic pathways causes a loss of vasomotor tone, pooling of blood in the extremities, and hypotension. Patients with neurogenic shock are bradycardic and have warm extremities; those with hypovolemic shock are tachycardic and have cool extremities.
C. Spinal shock is seen after spinal cord injury and is associated with flaccidity and the loss of segmental reflexes.

III APPROACH TO THE PATIENT

A. Initial management focuses on immediate stabilization of the patient.
1. **Airway, Breathing, and Circulation (ABCs)**

a. **Airway and breathing.** The patient is given 100% oxygen. The target oxygen saturation is 95% or greater.

b. **Circulation.** The bleeding is controlled by applying direct pressure. Vasopressors should not be given.

c. **Disability.** Depressed mental status may be the result of inadequate perfusion, head trauma, or both.

d. **Exposure.** The patient is examined for associated injuries. Care is taken to prevent hypothermia because low core temperatures exacerbate shock.

2. **Gastric decompression** prevents aspiration and subsequent vagal stimulation, which can cause bradycardia and exacerbate shock. A nasogastric or orogastric tube should be used.

3. **Foley catheter placement.** A Foley catheter should be placed to assess for hematuria and to monitor urine output.

4. **Establishment of intravenous (IV) access.** The more access the better! At least two large-bore IV lines should be established. Blood is sent for type and crossmatch, arterial blood gas, a complete blood count, and a serum electrolyte panel.

HOT **KEY**   An intraosseous line can be placed if a peripheral IV is not established within 90 seconds. Do not use an intraosseous line if the patient is older than age 6 years.

---

5. **Fluid resuscitation.** The **"3 for 1" rule** applies: to compensate for fluid shifts out of the intravascular space, 3 ml of crystalloid are needed to replace each 1 ml of blood loss.

a. **Lactated Ringer solution is** preferred, or normal saline is administered as rapidly as possible in a bolus of 20 ml/kg. All fluids should be warmed.

b. **The patient should not be flooded indiscriminately with fluids!** The patient must be re-evaluated after receiving the initial bolus. End-organ perfusion, vital signs, urine output, level of consciousness, and peripheral perfusion are assessed.

(1) **Rapid response.** The patient's clinical condition improves, and vital signs remain normal. A rapid response suggests that the blood loss was less than 20% of the total volume. No additional treatment is required; however, a blood type and crossmatch should be obtained in case the patient's clinical condition deteriorates.

(2) **Transient response.** The patient responds to the initial bolus, but the clinical status deteriorates as the fluid rate is slowed.

       (a) These patients require additional crystalloid bolus.

       (b) If the patient remains in shock after the two crystalloid boluses, 10 ml/kg packed red blood cells (PRBCs) are transfused. If PRBCs are unavailable, 20 ml/kg of 5% albumin may be used.

    (3) No response. If the patient does not respond to crystalloid and blood administration, surgical intervention is needed immediately. A nonhemorrhagic cause of shock also should be considered.

B. Ongoing management

1. Hematocrit. Although an initially low hematocrit is worrisome for blood loss, an initially normal hematocrit does not rule out blood loss; therefore, repeat hematocrits usually are indicated.

2. Urine output is a good indicator of end-organ perfusion. Adequate volume replacement should result in a urine output of 1 ml/kg/h (in children older than age 1 year) 2 ml/kg/h (in children younger than age 1 year).

3. ABGs

    a. Early hemorrhagic shock. Patients with early hemorrhagic shock have a low carbon dioxide tension ($PaCO_2$) and respiratory alkalosis secondary to carbon dioxide elimination.

    b. Late hemorrhagic shock. Metabolic acidosis as a result of inadequate tissue perfusion is seen if the shock persists. These patients require aggressive fluid resuscitation and surgical intervention; bicarbonate is not used routinely.

4. Central venous pressure (CVP) monitoring. The CVP is a measure of the right atrial pressure (filling pressure) and is not related to cardiac output.

    a. A minimal increase in an initially low CVP after fluid therapy indicates the need for additional volume.

    b. A decreasing CVP indicates ongoing fluid loss.

    c. An abrupt or persistent increase in the CVP indicates that volume replacement is adequate or too rapid, or that cardiac function is compromised.

    d. The initial CVP and the actual blood volume may not be related. The CVP may be elevated in patients with pulmonary disease or vasoconstriction, or after rapid fluid replacement.

    e. CVP monitoring is useful in cases of neurogenic shock.

5. Coagulation studies. Coagulopathies can be caused by massive transfusions, massive closed head injuries, or hypothermia. Coagulopathies should be treated with fresh frozen plasma or whole blood. Patients with low fibrinogen levels require cryoprecipitate.

References
Advanced Trauma Life Support (ATLS), 6th ed. Chicago, American College of Sur-
    geons, 1997.
Waisman Y, Eichelberger MR: Hypovolemic shock. In *Pediatric Trauma: Prevention,
    Acute Care, Rehabilitation.* Edited by Eichelberger MR. St. Louis, Mosby-Year
    Book, 1993.

108. Spinal Cord Injury

I | INTRODUCTION

A. **Special concerns in pediatrics.** The relative hypermobility of the child's spine protects it from injury; however, when an injury does occur, it usually is severe.

1. Children are more susceptible to cervical spine injury.
2. Children are more likely to have spinal cord injury without radiographic abnormality (SCIWRA Syndrome).
3. Children are more likely to suffer dislocation injuries without fracture.

B. **Severity**

1. **Complete injuries.** Patients experience a total loss of sensation and motor function below a certain level.

HOT KEY

Deep tendon reflexes may be preserved in complete injuries and therefore are not helpful in the acute setting.

---

2. **Incomplete injuries.** Sensation (including position sense) and voluntary movement are preserved in the lower extremities. Sacral sparing is evidenced by perianal sensation, voluntary sphincter contraction, or voluntary toe flexion.

II | SPECIFIC INJURIES

A. **Central cord syndrome** often is seen in association with hyperextension injuries resulting from a forward fall. This injury is characterized by greater motor loss in the upper extremities (compared with the lower extremities), with varying degrees of sensory loss.

B. **Anterior cord syndrome** usually is caused by an infarction in the distribution of the anterior spinal artery, and carries a poor prognosis. Symptoms include paraplegia and a loss of pain and temperature sensation. Posterior column function (i.e., position sense, vibration, deep pressure) is preserved.

C. **Brown-Séquard syndrome.** Hemisection of the spinal cord results in ipsilateral motor loss and ipsilateral loss of position sense. Additionally, there is associated contralateral dissociated sensory loss that begins one or two levels below the level of injury.

D. Cervical spine injuries
   1. **Atlanto-occipital dislocation.** Most patients die as a result of brain stem dysfunction.
   2. **Vertebra C1 (atlas) fracture. Atlas rotary subluxation** is a common injury in children. The patient's head may be persistently twisted to the side. **Jefferson, or "burst," fractures** usually are caused by axial loading and are not commonly associated with spinal cord injury.
   3. **Vertebra C2 (axis) fractures**
      a. **Odontoid fractures**. Three types are seen:
         (1) **Type I.** The tip of the odontoid is fractured.
         (2) **Type II.** The fracture occurs through the base of the dens.
         (3) **Type III**. The fracture occurs through the dens and into the body of the axis.
      b. **Posterior element fractures (hangman fractures)** usually are caused by an extension injury.
   4. **Vertebrae C3–C7 fractures and dislocations**
      a. **Vertebra C5 fractures** are the most common type.
      b. **Subluxation** is most common at the C5–C6 junction.
E. Thoracic spine fractures (T1–T10)
   1. **Anterior wedge compression injuries** result from axial loading with flexion.
   2. **Burst injuries** result from true vertical compression.
   3. **Fracture-dislocations** are rare, but usually cause complete deficits because the spinal canal in this region is narrow.
F. Thoracolumbar junction and lumbar fracture
   1. **Thoracolumbar junction fractures** are caused by acute hyperflexion and rotation, and often are seen in patients with a history of a fall or unrestrained motor vehicle collision. Injuries at this level can cause bowel and bladder dysfunction attributable to cauda equina compromise.
   2. **Lumbar fractures.** Computed tomography (CT) scans often are necessary to define canal compromise.

III **APPROACH TO THE PATIENT.** Evaluation of the spine can be deferred, especially in a patient with hemodynamic instability, as long as the spine is protected using a cervical collar, head immobilization, and backboard. Immobilization is essential until spinal cord injury is ruled out by clinical examination, negative plain film results, or both. If there is no spinal cord injury, the patient should be taken off the backboard within 2 hours to reduce the risk of developing decubitus ulcers.

A. Sensory and motor examinations. Spinal cord injury can be described clinically on the basis of the sensory and motor examinations. The level at which injury occurs is crucial. Complete injuries above vertebra T1 result in quadriplegia, and injuries below vertebra T1 result in paraplegia.

HOT KEY It is essential to repeat the sensory and motor examinations over time because the patient's clinical status may improve as trauma-related swelling (which can compromise the cord) resolves.

1. **Sensory examination.** Sensation to light touch and pinprick is assessed, and the level at which sensation is lost is recorded. The **sensory level** is the most caudal (inferior) segment with normal sensory function (Table 108–1).
2. **Motor examination.** The motor level is defined as the lowest muscle with a grade of at least 3/5 on the muscle strength grading scale (Tables 108–2 and 108–3).

HOT KEY Keep in mind that spinal nerves C3–C5 innervate the diaphragm; therefore, patients with a high cervical injury are susceptible to respiratory failure.

TABLE 108-1. Sensory Levels

Sensory Distribution	Sensory Level
Deltoid	C5*
Thumb	C6
Middle finger	C7
Little finger	C8
Nipple	T4
Xiphisternum	T8
Umbilicus	T10
Symphysis	T12
Medial aspect of the leg	L4
First interdigital space of the foot	L5
Lateral border of the foot	S1
Ischial tuberosity	S3
Perianal region	S4–S5

*The sensory distribution for C2–C4 is variable (the "cervical cape").

TABLE 108-2. Muscle Strength Grading Scale	
Grade	**Equivalent Patient Ability**
5/5	Normal ability
4/5	Ability to overcome gravity and some resistance imposed by the examiner
3/5	Ability to overcome gravity only
2/5	Ability to move perpendicular to gravity
1/5	Palpable contraction only
0/5	Complete inability to move

B. The patient is assessed for **pain** by palpation of the spinous processes of the cervical vertebrae, and the need for **cervical radiographs** is determined.

    1. If the patient is alert, awake, has no focal findings and no reproducible focal neck pain, and can move the head from side to side and flex and extend the neck without pain, then cervical spine films are not needed. Do not force the neck into any position!

    2. If the patient is awake, alert, and normal neurologically, but has neck pain, a full cervical spine film series should be obtained.

        a. If the initial cervical film results are negative, flexion-extension cervical spine films can be obtained to rule out a subluxation. If flexion-extension films cannot be obtained because of stiffness or pain, the patient is placed in a semirigid collar and films are obtained in 2–3 weeks.

TABLE 108-3. Motor Levels	
Muscle	**Motor Level**
Deltoid	C5
Wrist extensors	C6
Elbow extensors	C7
Finger flexors (to third finger)	C8
Small finger abductors	T1
Hip flexors	L2
Knee extensors	L3
Ankle dorsiflexors	L4
First toe extensors	L5
Ankle plantar flexors	S1

    b. If any film results are suspicious for fracture, a CT scan
    should be obtained to define the anatomy completely.

HOT

KEY

Patients with fractures of vertebrae C1 or C2 usually require a
CT scan to delineate the fracture completely.

---

    3. If the patient has an altered level of consciousness, is coma-
    tose, or is too young to describe his or her symptoms, a full
    cervical spine film series should be obtained.
C. Imaging studies. Anteroposterior and lateral radiographs of the
    cervical and thoracic spine should be obtained while maintain-
    ing immobilization with a cervical collar and backboard. The
    radiographs are assessed for:
    1. Bony deformity
    2. Fractures of the spinous processes and bodies
    3. Alignment of the vertebral bodies
    4. The distances between the spinous processes
    5. Narrowing of the vertebral canal
    6. Widening of the prevertebral soft tissue space (> 5 mm op-
    posite vertebra C3)

HOT

KEY

Children are more likely to have spinal cord injury without
radiographic abnormality, so trust your examination findings.

IV **TREATMENT** depends on the injury. Supportive measures
    include the following:

A. Methylprednisolone (30 mg/kg intravenously as a loading dose,
    followed by 5.4 mg/kg/h for the next 23 hours) should be ad-
    ministered within 8 hours of injury to patients with neurologic
    deficits to decrease cord swelling. This drug should always be
    used in consultation with a neurosurgeon.
B. Phenylephrine (50 mg diluted in 250 ml of D5W to run at a rate
    of 50–100 μg/kg/h) should be considered for patients in neuro-
    genic shock.

References
Advanced Trauma Life Support (ATLS), 6th ed. Chicago, American College of Sur-
    geons, 1997.

109. Burn Injuries

I INTRODUCTION

A. **Types of burns.** Burns can be **thermal, electrical,** or **chemical** in origin.

   1. **Thermal burns** result from contact with flames, hot liquids, or hot surfaces, and may be associated with **inhalation injury,** especially if the child was trapped in a closed space with a fire. Possible components of inhalation injury include thermal injury to the airway and lungs, carbon monoxide poisoning, or poisoning by other toxic fumes; signs and symptoms are given in Table 109–1.

   2. **Electrical burns** result from contact with an electrical current and may be associated with significant **deep tissue injury,** even when the external manifestations are rather minimal.

   3. **Chemical burns** are caused by contact with alkaline or acidic substances. Alkali burns penetrate more deeply than acid burns.

TABLE 109-1. Signs of inhalation injury		
Pulmonary	**CNS**	**Sign**
Tachypnea	Confusion	Facial Burns
Stridor	Dizziness	Singed nasal hairs
Macrocysts	Headace	Cyanosis
Rales	Hallucinations	Cherry-red color
Wheezing	Restlessness	
Cough	Coma	
Retractions	Seizures	
Nasal flaring		
Carbonaceous sputum		

CNS = central nervous system.
   (Reprinted with permission from Gorelick MH: Thermal injury. In *Clinical Handbook of Pediatrics*, 2nd ed. Edited by Schwartz MW. Baltimore, Williams & Wilkins, 1999, p 663.)

B. Classification of burns. Burns are classified according to their **depth** and **extent** (Table 109–2).

C. Criteria for transfer to a burn center include:

    1. Partial- or full-thickness burns covering more than 10% of the total body surface area in patients younger than age 10

TABLE 109-2. Classification of Burns

Type of Burn	Affected Skin Layer	Depth	Clinical Manifestations
First degree	Epidermis	Superficial	Erythema, pain, no blisters
Second degree			
Superficial	Papillary dermis	Partial thickness	Erythema, blistering, intact hairs, exquisite pain
Deep	Reticular dermis	Full thickness	Skin may be white or mottled and non-blanching, or blistered and moist; pain may or may not be present; hairs easily pulled
Third degree	Entire dermis	Full thickness	Dry, white, or charred skin with a leathery appearance; no pain; no hair
Fourth degree	Subcutaneous tissue	Full thickness	Same as third degree; may have exposed muscle and bone

Adapted with permission from Gorelick MH: Thermal injury. In *Clinical Handbook of Pediatrics*, 2nd ed. Edited by Schwartz MW. Baltimore, Williams & Wilkins, 1999, p 662.

years (20% of the total body surface area in children older than age 10 years and in adolescents)

2. **Full-thickness burns** covering more than 5% of the total body surface area, regardless of the age of the patient
3. Burns involving the face, eyes, ears, hands, feet, genitalia, perineum, or skin over major joints
4. Significant electrical burns
5. Significant chemical burns
6. Inhalation injury
7. The presence of a potentially complicating preexisting illness
8. Suspected child abuse or neglect

II THERMAL BURNS

A. Approach to the patient

1. **The burning process is stopped** (e.g., burning clothing is removed), and the burns are covered with a dry sheet (the covering does not need to be sterile).
2. **Airway, breathing, circulation (ABCs)**
   a. **Airway.** The supraglottic airway is sensitive to inhalation injury. Although manifestations of inhalation injury may not develop for 24 or more hours, the need for aggressive airway management should be anticipated if there are signs of inhalation injury (see Table 109–1) or a history of closed space confinement.
      (1) Patients with stridor require immediate intubation.
      (2) Intubation should also be considered for patients who are being transferred to a burn center to protect the airway during transport.
   b. **Breathing.** Carbon monoxide poisoning (Table 109–3) should be assumed in patients with a history of closed-space confinement. Administration of 100% oxygen can diminish carbon monoxide levels by 50% each hour. Hyperbaric oxygen therapy can further hasten the elimination of carbon monoxide.

TABLE 109-3. Signs and Symptoms of Carbon Monoxide Poisoning	
Carbon Monoxide Level	**Clinical Manifestations**
< 20%	None
20%–30%	Headache and nausea
30%–40%	Confusion
40%–60%	Coma
> 60%	Death

    c. Circulation. Two large-bore intravenous lines should be placed for patients with burns affecting more than 15% of the total body surface area.

      (1) Lines can be placed through burned skin if no other site is available.

      (2) Upper extremity access is preferred over lower extremity access because of the high incidence of phlebitis and septic phlebitis in the saphenous veins.

3. Order appropriate laboratory and imaging studies.

    a. Laboratory studies include a complete blood count, a blood type and crossmatch, a serum electrolyte panel, a serum glucose level, and a human chorionic gonadotropin (hCG) level.

    b. If there is a history of closed-space confinement or suspicion of inhalation injury, arterial blood gas (ABG), carboxyhemoglobin level, and a chest radiograph are obtained.

    c. The percentage of the body surface area that has been burned is estimated. The **rule of nines** divides the total body surface area into regions equalling approximately 9% (or some multiple thereof) each, thereby allowing an examiner to quickly estimate the percentage of the body surface area that is involved (Figure 109–1).

B. Treatment

1. Fluid resuscitation

    a. The volume of resuscitation fluid needed to compensate for the burn injury (i.e., the volume that should be given to the patient in addition to maintenance fluid requirements) is calculated.

      (1) The **Parkland formula** can be used for older or adult-sized patients:

Resuscitation fluid requirement = 2–4 ml/kg/% burn

      (2) Body surface area–based formula. Smaller patients have a larger body surface area in relation to their weight; therefore, formulas based on weight (e.g., the Parkland formula) may underestimate the fluid required to compensate for small injuries in small children or overestimate the fluid required for large injuries in large children. Using the body surface area–based method, the required resuscitation fluid volume can be estimated as 5000 ml/m^2 burned body surface area, where the total body surface area =

$$\text{Total body surface area (m}^2\text{)} = \sqrt{\frac{\text{Height (cm)} \times \text{Weight (kg)}}{3600}}$$

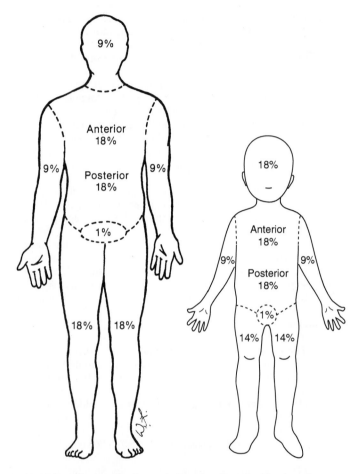

FIGURE 109-1. The rule of nines for estimating involved body surface area in **(A)** adults and **(B)** children with burns. Note that in children, the head accounts for a larger percentage of the body surface area, whereas the legs account for a smaller percentage. (Part A is reprinted with permission from Jarrell BE, Carabasi RA III: *NMS Surgery,* 3rd ed. Baltimore, Williams & Wilkins, 1996, p 404.)

   b. The calculated volume of resuscitation fluid (usually lac-
      tated Ringer solution) is administered as follows: one half
      of the total volume during the first 8 hours, followed by
      the remainder over the next 16 hours.

      c. A Foley catheter is placed and fluids are given to maintain a urine output of 1 ml/kg/h. For children who weigh less than 30 kg, glucose-containing maintenance fluids (see II B 1) are administered in addition to resuscitation fluids to maintain the urine output.

  2. Analgesia. Narcotics should be administered intravenously in small, frequent doses. Opioid use should be avoided in hypovolemic patients.

  3. Adjunctive therapies

    a. Infection prophylaxis. Tetanus toxoid is administered to all patients who have not been immunized within the past 6 months. Prophylactic antibiotics are not indicated.

    b. Nasogastric tube placement may be indicated for patients with nausea, vomiting, or abdominal distension, or burns over more than 20% of the total body surface area.

    c. Albumin replacement. Albumin losses must be anticipated, especially in patients with burns over more than 20% of the total body surface area.

    d. Full-thickness burns and circumferential burns may cause a constricting eschar, which can compromise circulation.

      (1) Escharotomy or fasciotomy may be required, especially if the patient has prolonged capillary refill time, absent or diminished pulses, or paresthesia.

      (2) Fasciotomy may be needed to restore circulation in patients with burns accompanied by a crush injury, electrical burns, or burns deep enough to reach the fascial layer.

III ELECTRICAL BURNS. Electrical burns may be more serious than they appear on the skin. The possibility of internal injuries without external manifestations must be considered. In addition to performing the ABCs, an electrocardiogram (ECG) is obtained and intravenous fluids are administered to promote diuresis.

A. Rhabdomyolysis may lead to acute renal failure. If the urine is dark, a brisk urine output (e.g., > 100 ml/h in adults or > 2 ml/kg/h in children) must be established. If the urine does not clear, mannitol is administered to maintain urine output.

B. If metabolic acidosis occurs, it is important to alkalinize the urine and maintain the diuresis.

C. Be aware of the possibility of myocardial damage and arrhythmias, especially in high-voltage injuries.

IV ALKALI BURNS. Alkali injuries penetrate more deeply than acid burns. They may be full-thickness injuries.

A. Alkali burns must be irrigated continuously for 24 hours, beginning within 1 hour of the time the injury occurred.

B. Alkali burns to the eye require continuous irrigation during the first 8 hours using a small-caliber cannula fixed in the palpebral sulcus. Consultation with an ophthalmologist is required.

V **ACID BURNS.** **Acid burns** also require aggressive lavage; the area should be flushed with water for 20–30 minutes. If hydrofluoric acid was the cause of the burn, 10% calcium gluconate is administered subcutaneously.

VI **DRY CHEMICAL BURNS.** Any dry powder that remains on the skin must be brushed away before irrigating with water. Chemical burns must not be immersed.

References
Advanced Trauma Life Support (ATLS), 6th ed. Chicago, American College of Surgeons, 1997.

Appendix I: Drug Formulary

(Adapted with permission from select drug entries that appear in *Hand-book of Pediatric Drug Therapy,* 2ed. Baltimore, Lippincott Williams & Wilkins, 2000.)

Acetaminophen (Tempra, Tylenol)
►**Indications & Dosage**

MILD PAIN; FEVER

►**Infants and children:** 10 to 15 mg/kg/dose P.O. or P.R. q 4 to 6 hours, p.r.n., up to 5 doses/day.

►**Children ages 12 years and older and adults:** 325 to 650 mg P.O. or P.R. q 4 to 6 hours p.r.n. Maximum daily dose is 4 g. Maximum daily dose for long-term therapy is 2.6 g.

►**Contraindications & Precautions:** Contraindicated in patients with G-6-PD deficiency or hypersensitivity to the drug. Use cautiously in patients with hepatic disease.

Acetylcysteine (Mucomyst, Mucosil)
►**Indications & Dosage**

ACETAMINOPHEN TOXICITY

►**Children and adults:** Initially, 140 mg/kg P.O., followed by 70 mg/kg q 4 hours for 17 doses (a total of 1,330 mg/kg) or until acetaminophen assay reveals nontoxic level.

►**Contraindications & Precautions:** Use cautiously in patients with severe respiratory insufficiency.

Activated Charcoal (Actidose-Aqua, Insta-Char Pediatric)
►**Indications & Dosage**

POISONING

►**Children ages 1 to 12 years:** 1 to 2 g/kg (15 to 30 g) P.O. dispersed in 120 to 240 ml (4 to 8 oz) of water to make a slurry.

►**Adolescents and adults:** Five to ten times the estimated weight of drug or chemical ingested. Dose is 30 to 100 g in 240 ml water to make a slurry.

►**Contraindications & Precautions:** Ineffective for poisoning or overdose of mineral-acids and alkalis. Although not contraindicated, activated charcoal is ineffective in ethanol, methanol, and iron salts poisoning.

Acyclovir (Acycloguanosine) Acyclovir Sodium (Zovirax)
►Indications & Dosage

INITIAL AND RECURRENT MUCOCUTANEOUS HERPES SIMPLEX VIRUS (HSV TYPE I AND HSV TYPE 2) OR SEVERE INITIAL GENITAL HERPES OR HERPES SIMPLEX IN IMMUNOCOMPROMISED PATIENT

►**Neonates and infants up to age 3 months:** 10 mg/kg I.V. q 8 hours for 10 to 14 days.

►**Children younger than age 12 years:** 250 mg/m^2 given at a constant rate over 1 hour by I.V. infusion q 8 hours for 7 days (5 days for genital herpes).

►**Children ages 12 years and older and adults:** 5 mg/kg, given at a constant rate over 1 hour by I.V. infusion q 8 hours for 7 days (5 days for genital herpes).

TREATMENT OF DISSEMINATED HERPES ZOSTER

►**Adults:** 10 mg/kg I.V. q 8 hours for 7 days. Infuse over at least 1 hour.

TREATMENT OF INITIAL GENITAL HERPES

►**Adults:** 200 mg P.O. q 4 hours while awake (total of 5 capsules/day). Continue treatment for 10 days.

TREATMENT OF ACUTE HERPES ZOSTER INFECTIONS

►**Adults:** 800 mg P.O. five times daily for 7 to 10 days. Initiate therapy within 48 hours of rash onset.

INTERMITTENT THERAPY FOR RECURRENT GENITAL HERPES

►**Adults:** 200 mg P.O. q 4 hours while awake (total of five capsules/day). Continue treatment for 5 days. Initiate therapy at first sign of recurrence.

CHRONIC SUPPRESSIVE THERAPY FOR RECURRENT GENITAL HERPES

►**Adults:** 400 mg P.O. b.i.d. for up to 1 year. Followed by reevaluation.

GENITAL HERPES; NON-LIFE-THREATENING HERPES SIMPLEX INFECTION IN IMMUNOCOMPROMISED PATIENTS

►**Children and adults:** Cover lesions with ointment q 3 hours six times daily for 7 days.

TREATMENT OF ACUTE VARICELLA (CHICKENPOX) INFECTIONS

►**Children ages 2 years and older weighing less than 40 kg (88 lb):** 20 mg/kg P.O. q.i.d. for 5 days.

►**Children ages 2 years and older weighing more than 40 kg and adults:** 800 mg P.O. q.i.d. for 5 days.

TREATMENT OF VARICELLA-ZOSTER INFECTIONS IN IMMUNOCOMPROMISED PATIENTS

▶**Children younger than age 12 years:** 500 mg/m^2 I.V. over 1 hour q 8 hours for 7 days.

▶**Children ages 12 years and older and adults:** 10 mg/kg I.V. over 1 hour q 8 hours for 7 days.

HERPES SIMPLEX ENCEPHALITIS

▶**Children ages 3 months to 11 years:** 500 mg/m^2 I.V. every 8 hours for 10 days. Infuse over at least 1 hour.

▶**Children ages 12 years and older and adults:** 10 mg/kg I.V. q 8 hours for 10 days; usual daily dose is 30 mg/kg.

▶**Contraindications & Precautions:** Use cautiously in patients with underlying neurologic problems, renal disease, or dehydration and in those receiving nephrotoxic drugs.

Adenosine (Adenocard)

▶**Indications & Dosage**

CONVERSION OF PAROXYSMAL SUPRAVENTRICULAR TACHYCARDIA (PSVT) TO SINUS RHYTHM

▶**Neonates, infants, and children:** 0.05 mg/kg for the initial dose. Dosage may be increased by 0.05 mg/kg by rapid I.V. bolus q 2 minutes to a maximum dose of 0.25 mg/kg or until termination of PSVT; don't exceed 12 mg/dose.

▶**Adults:** 6 mg I.V. by rapid bolus injection (over 1 to 2 seconds). If PSVT isn't eliminated in 1 to 2 minutes, give 12 mg by rapid I.V. push. Repeat 12-mg dose if necessary. Don't give single doses over 12 mg.

▶**Contraindications & Precautions:** Contraindicated in patients with hypersensitivity to drug and in those with second- or third-degree heart block or sick sinus syndrome. Patients in whom significant heart block develops after a dose of adenosine shouldn't receive additional doses. Use cautiously in patients with asthma because bronchoconstriction may occur.

Albumin (Albuminar, Plasbumin)

▶**Indications & Dosage**

SHOCK

▶**Children:** 10 to 20 ml/kg of 5% solution I.V., at a rate up to 5 to 10 ml/minute.

▶**Adults:** Initially, 500 ml of 5% solution I.V.; may repeat after 30 minutes. Don't exceed 250 g/48 hours.

HYPOPROTEINEMIA

▶**Adults:** 1,000 to 1,500 ml of 5% solution I.V. daily, to a maximum rate of 5 to 10 ml/minute. Or 200 to 300 ml of 25% solution I.V. daily, to a maximum rate 3 ml/minute.

BURNS

▶**Children and adults:** Dosage varies based on extent of burn and patient's condition. Maintain plasma albumin level at 2 to 3 g/dl.

▶**Contraindications & Precautions:** Contraindicated in patients with hypersensitivity to drug. Use with extreme caution in patients with hypertension, cardiac disease, severe pulmonary infection, severe chronic anemia, or hypoalbuminemia with peripheral edema. Rapid administration may cause pulmonary edema, vascular overload or cardiac failure.

Albuterol Sulfate (Proventil, Ventolin)

▶**Indications & Dosage**

TO PREVENT AND TREAT BRONCHOSPASM IN PATIENTS WITH REVERSIBLE OBSTRUCTIVE AIRWAY DISEASE

▶**Children ages 2 to 5 years:** Administer 0.1 mg/kg P.O. t.i.d., not to exceed 2 mg (syrup or immediate-release tablets) t.i.d. Alternatively, in children ages 2 and older, 0.1 to 0.15 mg/kg (maximum dosage is 12 mg/day) t.i.d. or q.i.d. by nebulizer.

▶**Children ages 6 to 11 years:** Administer 2 mg P.O. (syrup or immediate-release tablets) t.i.d. or q.i.d. or 4 mg (sustained-release tablets) P.O. q 12 hours. Alternatively, in children ages 4 and older, 1 or 2 inhalations q 4 to 6 hours using a spacer; or 200 mcg inhaled q 4 to 6 hours using a Rotahaler inhalation device.

▶**Children ages 12 years and older and adults:**

▶**Tablets:** 2 to 4 mg (immediate release) P.O. t.i.d. or q.i.d.; maximum dosage, 8 mg q.i.d. Alternatively, 4 mg (sustained release) P.O. q 12 hours. Increase to 8 mg q 12 hours if patient fails to respond. Cautiously increase stepwise as needed and tolerated to maximum of 16 g q 12 hours.

▶**Syrup:** 2 to 4 mg (1 to 2 tsp) P.O. t.i.d. or q.i.d.

▶**Aerosol inhalation:** 1 or 2 inhalations q 4 to 6 hours.

▶**Solution for inhalation:** 2.5 mg t.i.d. or q.i.d. by nebulizer.

▶**Capsules for inhalation:** 200 mcg inhaled q 4 to 6 hours using a Rotahaler inhalation device.

TO PREVENT EXERCISE-INDUCED BRONCHOSPASM

▶**Children ages 4 years and older and adults:** 2 inhalations 15 minutes before exercise.

▶**Contraindications & Precautions:** Contraindicated in patients with hypersensitivity to drug. Use cautiously in patients with coronary insufficiency, hypertension, hyperthyroidism, diabetes mellitus, cardiac arrhythmias associated with tachycardia, angle-closure glaucoma, shock, and organic brain damage.

Alprostadil (Prostin VR Pediatric)
▶**Indications & Dosage**

TEMPORARY MAINTENANCE OF PATENCY OF DUCTUS ARTERIOSUS UNTIL SURGERY CAN BE PERFORMED

▶**Infants:** Initial I.V. infusion of 0.05 to 0.1 mcg/kg/minute via infusion pump. Doses as high as 0.4 mcg/kg/minute may be used if necessary, although higher infusion rates don't produce greater effects. After satisfactory response is achieved, reduce infusion rate to the lowest dosage that will maintain response. Maintenance doses vary. Infusion rate should be the lowest possible dose and is usually achieved by progressively halving the initial dose. Rates as low as 0.002 to 0.005 mcg/kg/minute have been effective.

▶**Contraindications & Precautions:** Contraindicated in neonates with respiratory distress syndrome. Use cautiously in neonates with bleeding disorders.

Amoxicillin/Clavulanate Potassium (Augmentin)
▶**Indications & Dosage**

▶**Neonates and infants younger than 3 months:** 30 mg (amoxicillin component)/kg P.O. daily in divided doses q 12 hours.

▶**Infants and children 3 months or older and weighing less than 40 kg (for treatment of otitis media, sinusitis, lower respiratory tract infections or severe infections):** 45 mg (amoxicillin component)/kg P.O. daily in divided doses q 12 hours. For less severe infections, 25 mg (amoxicillin component)/kg daily in divided doses q 12 hours

▶**Children weighing more than 40 kg and adults:** 250 mg P.O. q 8 hours or 500 mg q 12 hours. For more severe infections, 500 mg q 8 hours or 875 mg q 12 hours.

▶**Contraindications & Precautions:** Contraindicated in patients with hypersensitivity to drug or other penicillins and in those with a previous history of amoxicillin-associated cholestatic jaundice or hepatic dysfunction.

Amoxicillin Trihydrate (Amoxil, Trimox)
▶**Indications & Dosage**

SYSTEMIC INFECTIONS, ACUTE AND CHRONIC URINARY OR RESPIRATORY TRACT

INFECTIONS CAUSED BY SUSCEPTIBLE ORGANISMS, UNCOMPLICATED URINARY TRACT INFECTIONS CAUSED BY SUSCEPTIBLE ORGANISMS

▸**Neonates and infants younger than age 3 months:** 30 mg/kg P.O. daily, divided into doses given q 12 hours.

▸**Infants and children older than age 3 months:** 20 to 40 mg/kg P.O. daily, divided into doses given q 8 hours.

▸**Adults:** 250 mg P.O. q 8 hours. For adults and children weighing more than 20 kg, 500 mg q 8 hours.

UNCOMPLICATED GONORRHEA

▸**Children older than age 2 years:** 50 mg/kg given with 25 mg/kg probenecid as a single dose.

▸**Adults:** 3 g P.O. as a single dose.

ENDOCARDITIS PROPHYLAXIS FOR DENTAL PROCEDURES

▸**Children:** 50 mg/kg 1 hour before procedure.

▸**Adults:** 2 g 1 hour before procedure.

▸**Contraindications & Precautions:** Contraindicated in patients with hypersensitivity to drug or other penicillins. Use with caution in patients with mononucleosis.

Amphotericin B (Abelcet (lipid complex), Fungizone)

▸**Indications & Dosage**

SYSTEMIC (POTENTIALLY FATAL) FUNGAL INFECTIONS, CAUSED BY SUSCEPTIBLE ORGANISMS; FUNGAL ENDOCARDITIS; FUNGAL SEPTICEMIA

▸**Children and adults:** Give an initial dose of 1 mg in 20 ml D_5W infused over 20 minutes. If test dose is tolerated, then give daily doses of 0.25 to 0.30 mg/kg, gradually increasing by 5 to 10 mg/day until daily dose is 1 mg/kg/day or 1.5 mg/kg q alternate day.

▸**Amphotericin B lipid complex:** 5 mg/kg given as a single infusion, administered at a rate of 2.5 mg/kg/hour. If infusion lasts longer than 2 hours, mix bag q 2 hours by shaking it.

▸**Liposomal amphotericin:** 3 to 5 mg/kg/day I.V. delivered initially over 2 hours. Infusion time may be reduced to 1 hour if well tolerated or extended for patient comfort.

FUNGAL MENINGITIS

▸**Adults:** Intrathecal injection of 25 mcg/0.1 ml diluted with 10 to 20 ml of CSF two or three times weekly. Initial dose shouldn't exceed 50 mcg.

CANDIDAL CYSTITIS

▸**Adults:** Bladder irrigations in concentrations of 5 to 50 mcg/ml instilled periodically or continuously for 5 to 7 days.

CUTANEOUS OR MUCOCUTANEOUS CANDIDAL INFECTIONS

▶**Children and adults:** Apply topical product b.i.d., t.i.d., or q.i.d. for 1 to 3 weeks; apply up to several months for interdigital or paronychial lesions.

▶**Contraindications & Precautions:** Contraindicated in patients with hypersensitivity to drug. Use cautiously in patients with renal impairment and patients receiving other nephrotoxic drugs.

Ampicillin (Omnipen)
▶**Indications & Dosage**

SYSTEMIC INFECTIONS

▶**Neonates** <7 days: 100–150 mg/kg/day divided q 12

▶**Neonates** >7 days: 150–300 mg/kg/day divided q 6–8

▶**Children:** 50 to 100 mg/kg P.O. daily, divided into doses given q 6 hours; or 200 to 400 mg/kg I.M. or I.V. daily, divided into doses given q 4–6 hours.

▶**Adults:** 250 to 500 mg P.O. q 6 hours.

▶severe renal impairment (creatinine clearance 10 ml/minute or less).

PROPHYLAXIS FOR BACTERIAL ENDOCARDITIS BEFORE DENTAL OR MINOR RESPIRATORY PROCEDURES

▶**Children:** 50 mg/kg I.V. or I.M. 30 minutes before procedure.

▶**Adults:** 2 g I.V. or I.M. 30 minutes before procedure

▶**Contraindications & Precautions:** Contraindicated in patients with hypersensitivity to drug or other penicillins.

Ampicillin Sodium/Sulbactam Sodium (Unasyn)
▶**Indications & Dosage**

SKIN AND SOFT-TISSUE INFECTIONS, INTRA-ABDOMINAL AND GYNECOLOGIC INFECTIONS

▶**Infants and children ages 1 month and older for the treatment of mild to moderate infections:** 100 to 150 mg/kg/day divided q 6 hours.

▶**Infants and children ages 1 month and older for the treatment of severe infections:** 200 to 300 mg/kg/day divided q 6 hours.

▶**Children ages 1 year and older for the treatment of skin and soft-tissue infections only:** 30 mg/kg/day (200 mg of ampicillin and 100 mg of sulbactam) I.V. divided q 6 hours for a maximum of 14 days.

▶**Children weighing 40 kg or more and adults:** 1.5 to 3 g I.M. or I.V. q 6 hours.

▶Maximum 4 g/day

Aspirin (A.S.A.)

►**Indications & Dosage**

MILD PAIN OR FEVER

►**Children ages 2 to 11 years:** 1.5 g/m^2 P.O. or P.R. daily or 65 mg/kg P.O. or P.R. daily divided q 4 to 6 hours, p.r.n. Don't exceed 5 doses/day. Total daily rectal dose shouldn't exceed 2.5 g/m^2.

►**Children ages 11 years or older and adults:** 325–1000 mg every 4–6 hours P.O. or P.R. q 4 hours, p.r.n., but shouldn't exceed 4 g daily.

TREATMENT OF KAWASAKI (MUCOCUTANEOUS LYMPH NODE) SYNDROME

►**Adults:** 80 to 100 mg/kg P.O. daily in four divided doses. Some patients may require up to 120 mg/kg daily to maintain acceptable serum salicylate levels of over 200 μg/ml during the febrile phase. After the fever subsides, reduce dosage to 3 to 8 mg/kg once daily. Therapy usually continues for 6 to 10 weeks.

SYMPTOMATIC TREATMENT OF JUVENILE RHEUMATOID ARTHRITIS

►**Children weighing 25 kg or less:** Initially, 60 to 130 mg/kg/day P.O. given in divided doses.

►**Children weighing more than 25 kg:** Initially 2.4 to 3.6 daily given in divided doses. May increase by 10 mg/kg/day q 7 days p.r.n. Usual maintenance dosage is 80 to 100 mg/kg/day.

RHEUMATIC FEVER

►**Children:** Initial: 100 mg/kg/day in 3–6 doses × 2wks, then 75 mg/kg/day × 4–6 wks.

►**Adults:** 4.9 to 7.8 g P.O. daily divided q 4 to 6 hours for 1 to 2 weeks; then decrease to 60 to 70 mg/kg daily for 1 to 6 weeks; then gradually withdraw over 1 to 2 weeks.

►**Contraindications & Precautions:** Contraindicated in patients with hypersensitivity to NSAIDs or salicylates, G6PD deficiency, bleeding disorders such as hemophilia, von Willebrand's disease, or telangiectasia, NSAID-induced sensitivity reactions or in children with chickenpox or flu-like syndrome. Use cautiously in patients with GI lesions, impaired renal function, hypoprothrombinemia, vitamin K deficiency, thrombotic thrombocytopenic purpura, or hepatic impairment.

Atropine Sulfate

►**Indications & Dosage**

SYMPTOMATIC BRADYCARDIA, BRADYARRHYTHMIA (JUNCTIONAL OR ESCAPE RHYTHM)

►**Children:** 0.02 mg/kg I.V. up to maximum 1 mg; or 0.3 mg/m^2; may repeat q 5 minutes.

▶**Adults:** Usually 0.5 to 1 mg by I.V. push; repeat q 3 to 5 minutes, to maximum of 2 mg. Lower doses (less than 0.5 mg) may cause bradycardia.

ANTIDOTE FOR ANTICHOLINESTERASE INSECTICIDE POISONING

▶**Children:** 0.05 mg/kg I.M. or I.V. q 10 to 30 minutes until muscarinic symptoms disappear.

▶**Adults:** 1 to 2 mg I.M. or preferably I.V. Additional 2 mg may be administered q 5 to 60 minutes until muscarinic symptoms disappear.

ACUTE IRITIS, UVEITIS

▶**Adults:** 1 or 2 gtt (0.5% or 1% solution) into the eye q.i.d. (in children use 0.5% solution) or a small amount of ointment in the conjunctiva sac t.i.d.

CYCLOPLEGIC REFRACTION

▶**Children:** 1 or 2 gtt (0.5% solution) into each eye b.i.d. for 1 to 3 days before eye examination and 1 hour before examination.

▶**Adults:** 1 or 2 gtt (1% solution) 1 hour before refraction.

▶**Contraindications & Precautions:** Contraindicated in patients with hypersensitivity to drug or sodium metabisulfite, acute angle-closure glaucoma, obstructive uropathy, obstructive disease of GI tract, paralytic ileus, toxic megacolon, intestinal atony, unstable CV status in acute hemorrhage, asthma, and myasthenia gravis.

Azithromycin (Zithromax)
▶**Indications & Dosage**
COMMUNITY-ACQUIRED PNEUMONIA

▶**Children ages 6 months and older:** 10 mg/kg (maximum 500 mg/day) P.O. on day 1; then 5 mg/kg on days 2 through 5 (not to exceed 250 mg/day).

▶**Adolescents ages 16 and older and adults:** 500 mg P.O. as a single dose on day 1, followed by 250 mg P.O. daily on days 2 to 5. For I.V. therapy, 500 mg I.V. as a single daily dose for 2 days, followed by 500 mg P.O. as a single daily dose to complete a 7- to 10-day course of therapy.

NONGONOCOCCAL URETHRITIS OR CERVICITIS CAUSED BY *CHLAMYDIA TRACHOMATIS*

▶**Adolescents ages 16 years and older and adults:** 1 g P.O. as a single dose.

PELVIC INFLAMMATORY DISEASE CAUSED BY *C. TRACHOMATIS, NEISSERIA GONORRHOEAE,* OR *MYCOPLASMA HOMINIS* IN PATIENTS REQUIRING INITIAL I.V. THERAPY

▶**Adults:** 500 mg I.V. as a single daily dose for 1 to 2 days, followed by 250 mg P.O. daily to complete a 7-day course of therapy.

OTITIS MEDIA

▶**Children older than age 6 months:** 10 mg/kg (maximum 500 mg/day) P.O. on day 1; then 5 mg/kg (maximum 250 mg/day) on days 2 to 5.

TONSILLITIS

▶**Children ages 2 years and older:** 12 mg/kg (maximum 500 mg/day) P.O. daily for 5 days.

CHANCROID

▶**Infants and children:** 20 mg/kg P.O. (maximum 1 g) as a single dose
▶**Adults:** 1 g P.O. as a single dose.

UNCOMPLICATED CHLAMYDIAL INFECTIONS

▶**Children ages 8 years and older weighing 45 kg (99 lb) or more:** 1 g P.O. as a single dose.

▶**Contraindications & Precautions:** Contraindicated in patients with hypersensitivity to erythromycin or other macrolides. Use cautiously in patients with impaired hepatic function.

Bacitracin
▶**Indications & Dosage**

TOPICAL INFECTIONS, IMPETIGO, ABRASIONS, CUTS, AND MINOR WOUNDS

▶**Children and adults:** Apply thin film to clean area once daily to t.i.d. for no more than 7 days.

TREATMENT OF ANTIBIOTIC-RELATED PSEUDOMEMBRANOUS COLITIS CAUSED BY *CLOSTRIDIUM DIFFICILE*

▶**Adults:** 20,000 to 25,000 U P.O. q 6 hours for 7 to 10 days.

▶**Contraindications & Precautions:** Contraindicated in patients hypersensitive to drug and in atopic patients. Use cautiously in patients with myasthenia gravis and neuromuscular disease.

Beclomethasone Dipropionate
▶**Indications & Dosage**

CORTICOSTEROID DEPENDENT ASTHMA

ORAL INHALATION

▶**Children ages 6 to 12 years:** For regular strength: 1 or 2 inhalations t.i.d. or q.i.d. to a maximum of 10 inhalations daily. For double strength: 2 inhalations b.i.d. Don't exceed 5 inhalations/day.

▶**Children older than age 12 years and adults:** For regular strength: 2 inhalations t.i.d. or q.i.d. or 4 inhalations b.i.d. to a maximum of 20 inhalations daily. For double strength: 2 inhalations b.i.d.; for patients with severe asthma, start with 6 to 8 inhalations/day and adjust down. Don't exceed 10 inhalations per day.

PERENNIAL OR SEASONAL RHINITIS, PREVENTION OF RECURRENCE OF NASAL POLYPS AFTER SURGICAL REMOVAL

NASAL INHALATION

▶**Children ages 6 to 12 years:** 1 spray in each nostril t.i.d. (252 mcg daily).

▶**Children older than age 12 years and adults:** 1 spray (42 mcg) in each nostril b.i.d. to q.i.d. Usual total daily dose is 168 to 336 mcg.

NASAL SPRAY

▶**Children ages 6 to 12 years:** Start with 1 spray in each nostril b.i.d. (168 mcg daily). If response is inadequate or symptoms more severe, dose can be increased to 2 sprays/nostril b.i.d. (336 mcg daily).

▶**Children older than age 12 years and adults:** One or two sprays (42 to 84 mcg) in each nostril b.i.d. Usual total daily dose is 168 to 336 mcg.

▶**Contraindications & Precautions:** Contraindicated in patients hypersensitive. Use cautiously in patients with tuberculosis, fungal or bacterial infection, herpes, or systemic viral infection.

Beractant (Natural Lung Surfactant) (Survanta)
▶**Indications & Dosage**

PREVENTION AND TREATMENT (RESCUE) OF RESPIRATORY DISTRESS SYNDROME (RDS; HYALINE MEMBRANE DISEASE) IN PREMATURE NEONATES

▶**Neonates:** 100 mg of phospholipids/kg of birth weight (4 ml/kg) administered by intratracheal instillation through a 5 French end-hole catheter inserted into the infant's endotracheal tube with the tip of the catheter protruding just beyond the end of the tube above the carina.

▶**Contraindications & Precautions:** Use with caution in patients with pulmonary hemorrhage.

Bisacodyl (Bisco-Lax, Fleet Laxative)
▶**Indications & Dosage**

CONSTIPATION; PREPARATION FOR DELIVERY, SURGERY, OR RECTAL OR BOWEL EXAMINATION

▶**Children ages 6 to 12 years:** 5 mg P.O. daily. Alternatively, give one-half of suppository (5 mg) P.R. daily.

▶**Adults:** 10 to 15 mg P.O. daily. Up to 30 mg may be used for thorough evacuation needed for examination or surgery. Alternatively, give one suppository (10 mg) P.R. daily.

►Contraindications & Precautions: Contraindicated in patients with hypersensitivity to drug, abdominal pain, nausea, vomiting, or other symptoms of appendicitis or acute surgical abdomen and in those with rectal bleeding, gastroenteritis, or intestinal obstruction.

Bretylium Tosylate (Bretylate, Bretylol)
►Indications & Dosage

VENTRICULAR FIBRILLATION AND HEMODYNAMICALLY UNSTABLE VENTRICULAR TACHYCARDIA

►Adults: 5 mg/kg undiluted by rapid I.V. injection. If ventricular fibrillation persists, increase dose to 10 mg/kg and repeat p.r.n. For continuous suppression, administer diluted solution by continuous I.V. infusion at 1 to 2 mg/minute, or infuse diluted solution at 5 to 10 mg/kg over more than 8 minutes q 6 hours.

OTHER VENTRICULAR ARRHYTHMIAS

►Children: For acute ventricular fibrillation, initially 5 mg/kg I.V., followed by 10 mg/kg q 15 to 30 minutes, with a maximum total dose of 30 mg/kg; maintenance dose, 5 to 10 mg/kg q 6 hours. For other ventricular arrhythmias, 5 to 10 mg/kg q 6 hours.

►Adults: Initially, 5 to 10 mg/kg I.M., undiluted, or I.V., diluted. Repeat in 1 to 2 hours if necessary. Maintenance dose is 5 to 10 mg/kg q 6 hours I.M. or I.V. or 1 to 2 mg/minute I.V. infusion.

►Contraindications & Precautions: Contraindicated in digitalized patients unless the arrhythmia is life-threatening, not caused by a cardiac glycoside, and unresponsive to other antiarrhythmics. Use with caution in patients with aortic stenosis and pulmonary hypertension.

Budesonide (Pulmicort, Rhinocort)
►Indications & Dosage

MANAGEMENT OF SEASONAL OR PERENNIAL ALLERGIC RHINITIS OR NONALLERGIC PERENNIAL RHINITIS

►Children older than age 6 years and adults: 2 sprays in each nostril in the morning and evening or 4 sprays in each nostril in the morning. Maintenance dose should be the fewest number of sprays needed to control symptoms. Doses exceeding 256 mcg/day (4 sprays/nostril) aren't recommended.

►Note: If patient shows no improvement within 3 weeks, discontinue treatment.

CHRONIC ASTHMA

►Children age 6 years or older: Initially 200 mcg via oral inhalation b.i.d. Maximum dosage is 400 mg b.i.d.

▶**Adults:** 200 to 400 mcg via oral inhalation b.i.d. when previously used bronchodilators alone or inhaled corticosteroids; 400 to 800 mcg oral inhalation b.i.d. when previously used oral corticosteroids.

▶**Contraindications & Precautions:** Contraindicated in patients hypersensitivity to drug and in those who have had recent septal ulcers, nasal surgery, or nasal trauma until total healing has occurred. Use cautiously in patients with tuberculosis infections; untreated fungal, bacterial, or systemic viral infections; or ocular herpes simplex.

Caffeine
▶**Indications & Dosage**

NEONATAL APNEA

▶**Neonates:** 5 to 10 mg/kg (base) I.V., I.M., or P.O. as a loading dose, followed by 2.5 to 5 mg/kg I.V., I.M., or P.O. daily. Adjust dosage according to patient tolerance and plasma caffeine levels. For control of neonatal apnea, maintain plasma caffeine level at 5 to 20 μg/ml.

▶**Contraindications & Precautions:** Contraindicated in patients with hypersensitivity to drug. Use cautiously in patients with history of peptic ulcer, symptomatic arrhythmias, or palpitations and after an acute MI.

Captopril (Capoten)
▶**Indications & Dosage**

MILD TO SEVERE HYPERTENSION, HEART FAILURE

▶**Neonates:** 0.01 to 0.05 mg/kg P.O. q 8 to 12 hours. Adjust dose and interval based on response.

▶**Infants:** 0.05 to 0.1 mg/kg P.O. q 8 to 24 hours. Adjust dose and interval based on response.

▶**Children:** 0.3 mg/kg P.O. q 6 to 12 hours. Adjust dose and interval based on response; up to a maximum of 6 mg/kg/day in divided doses.

▶**Adolescents and adults:** Initially, 12.5 to 25 mg P.O. b.i.d. or t.i.d.; if necessary, dosage may be increased to 50 mg b.i.d. or t.i.d. after 1 to 2 weeks; if control is still inadequate after 1 to 2 weeks more, consider adding a diuretic. Maximum dosage is 150 mg t.i.d. (450 mg/day) while continuing the diuretic. Daily dose may be given b.i.d.

▶**Contraindications & Precautions:** Contraindicated in patients with hypersensitivity to drug or other ACE inhibitors. Use cautiously in patients with impaired renal function, renal artery stenosis, or serious autoimmune diseases (especially lupus erythematosus) and in those taking drugs that affect WBC counts or immune response.

Carbamazepine (Tegretol)
▶**Indications & Dosage**

GENERALIZED TONIC-CLONIC, COMPLEX-PARTIAL, MIXED SEIZURE PATTERNS

▶**Children younger than age 6 years:** initially, 10 to 20 mg/kg P.O. daily in two to three divided doses as tablets or four divided doses as suspension. Increase at weekly intervals based on patient response; up to a maximum of 35 mg/kg in a 24-hour period.

▶**Children ages 6 to 12 years:** Initially, 100 mg P.O. b.i.d. as tablets or 50 mg P.O. q.i.d. as suspension. Increase at weekly intervals by adding 100 mg P.O. daily, first using a t.i.d. schedule and then q.i.d. if necessary. Adjust dosage based on patient response. Generally, daily dose shouldn't exceed 1,000 mg. Children taking 400 mg or more of immediate-release form daily may be converted to same total daily dose of extended-release capsules using a b.i.d. regimen.

▶**Children older than age 12 years and adults:** 200 mg P.O. b.i.d. as tablets or 100 mg P.O. q.i.d. as suspension on day 1. May increase by 200 mg/day P.O. at weekly intervals, in divided doses at 6- to 8-hour intervals. Adjust to minimum effective level when control is achieved; don't exceed 1,000 mg/day in children ages 13 to 15, or 1,200 mg/day in those older than age 15. In rare instances, doses up to 1,600 mg/day have been used in adults.

ORAL LOADING DOSE FOR RAPID SEIZURE CONTROL

▶**Children younger than age 12 years:** 10 mg/kg of oral suspension as a single dose.

▶**Children ages 12 years and older and adults:** 8 mg/kg of oral suspension as a single dose.

Cefaclor (Ceclor)
▶**Indications & Dosage**

▶**Infants and children age 1 month or older:** 20 mg/kg P.O. daily (40 mg/kg for severe infections and otitis media) in divided doses q 8 hours (or 12 hours for the treatment of otitis media or pharyngitis), not to exceed 1 g/day.

▶**Adolescents and adults:** 250 to 500 mg P.O. q 8 hours. Total daily dose shouldn't exceed 4 g. For pharyngitis or otitis media, daily dose may be given in two equally divided doses q 12 hours. For pharyngitis and tonsillitis or skin and soft-tissue infections, 375 mg P.O. q 12 hours for 10 days and 7 to 10 days, respectively.

▶**Contraindications & Precautions:** Contraindicated in patients with hypersensitivity to other cephalosporins. Use cautiously in patients with impaired renal function or penicillin allergy and in patients who are breast-feeding.

Cefadroxil (Duricef)
►**Indications & Dosage**
►**Children:** 30 mg/kg daily in two divided doses q 12 hours.
►**Adolescents and adults:** 1 to 2 g P.O. daily, depending on the infection treated. Usually given once or twice daily.
►**Contraindications & Precautions:** Contraindicated in patients with hypersensitivity to drug or other cephalosporins. Use cautiously in patients with impaired renal function or penicillin allergy and in patients who are breast-feeding.

Cefazolin Sodium (Ancef, Kefzol)
►**Indications & Dosage**
►**Neonates 1 week old or younger:** 40 mg/kg I.M. or I.V. daily in divided doses q 12 hours.
►**Neonates older than 1 week and weighing 2 kg or less:** 40 mg/kg I.M. or I.V. daily in divided doses q 12 hours.
►**Neonates older than 1 week and weighing more than 2 kg (4.4 lb):** 60 mg/kg I.M. or I.V. daily in divided doses q 8 hours.
►**Infants and children older than age 1 month:** 25 to 100 mg/kg/day I.M. or I.V. in divided doses q 6 to 8 hours.
►**Adolescents and adults:** 250 mg I.M. or I.V. q 8 hours to 1.5 g q 6 hours. Maximum dosage is 12 g/day.
►**Contraindications & Precautions:** Contraindicated in patients with hypersensitivity to other cephalosporins. Use cautiously in patients with impaired renal function or penicillin allergy.

Cefixime (Suprax)
►**Indications & Dosage**
OTITIS MEDIA; PHARYNGITIS, TONSILLITIS; UNCOMPLICATED UTIS
►**Infants and children older than ages 6 months to 12 years:** 8 mg/kg P.O. daily in one or two divided doses.
►**Adolescents and adults:** 400 mg P.O. daily in one or two divided doses; for uncomplicated gonorrhea, 400 mg P.O. as a single dose.
►**Contraindications & Precautions:** Contraindicated in patients with hypersensitivity to drug or other cephalosporins. Use cautiously in patients with impaired renal function.

Cefotaxime Sodium (Claforan)
►**Indications & Dosage**
SERIOUS LOWER RESPIRATORY TRACT, URINARY TRACT, CNS, BONE AND JOINT, INTRA-ABDOMINAL, GYNECOLOGIC, AND SKIN INFECTIONS; SEPTICEMIA
►**Neonates up to age 1 week:** 100 mg/kg I.V. q 12 hours.

►**Neonates ages 1 to 4 weeks:** 150 mg/kg I.V. q 8 hours.

►**Infants and children ages 1 month to 12 years weighing less than 50 kg (110 lb):** 50 to 180 mg/kg I.V. daily in four or six equally divided doses. Higher doses are reserved for serious infections (such as meningitis).

►**Children weighing more than 50 kg and adults:** Usual dose is 1 g I.V. or I.M. q 6 to 12 hours. Up to 12 g daily can be administered

UNCOMPLICATED GONORRHEA

►**Adolescents and adults:** 1 g I.M. as a single dose.

DISSEMINATED GONOCOCCAL INFECTION

►**Adolescents and adults:** 1 g I.V. q 8 hours.

GONOCOCCAL OPHTHALMIA; DISSEMINATED GONOCOCCAL INFECTION

►**Neonates and infants:** 25 to 50 mg/kg I.V. q 8 to 12 hours for 7 days or 50 to 100 mg/kg I.M. or I.V. q 12 hours for 7 days.

GONORRHEAL MENINGITIS OR ARTHRITIS

►**Neonates and infants:** 25 to 50 mg/kg I.V. q 8 to 12 hours for 10 to 14 days or 50 to 100 mg/kg I.M. or I.V. q 12 hours for 10 to 14 days.

►**Contraindications & Precautions:** Contraindicated in patients with hypersensitivity to drug or other cephalosporins. Use cautiously in patients with impaired renal function or penicillin allergies and in breast-feeding women.

Cefoxitin Sodium (Mefoxin)
►**Indications & Dosage**

SERIOUS RESPIRATORY TRACT, GU, GYNECOLOGIC, SKIN, SOFT TISSUE, BONE AND JOINT, BLOOD, AND INTRA-ABDOMINAL INFECTIONS.

►**Infants less than 7 days:** 40 mg/kg/d divided q 12

►**Infants >7 days and Children:**

►**Mild to Moderate infection:** 80–100 mg/kg/d divided q 6

►**Severe infection:** 100–160 mg/kg/d divided q 6

►**Adolescents and adults:** 1 to 2 g q 6 to 8 hours for uncomplicated forms of infection. Up to 12 g daily.

PELVIC INFLAMMATORY DISEASE

►**Adolescents and adults:** 2 g I.V. q 6 hours.

►**Contraindications & Precautions:** Contraindicated in patients with hypersensitivity to drug or other cephalosporins. Use cautiously in patients with impaired renal function or penicillin allergy and in breast-feeding women.

Cefpodoxime Proxetil (Vantin)
▶**Indications & Dosage**

ACUTE, COMMUNITY-ACQUIRED PNEUMONIA CAUSED BY NON-BETA-LACTAMASE—PRODUCING STRAINS OF *HAEMOPHILUS INFLUENZAE* **OR** *STREPTOCOCCUS PNEUMONIAE*

▶**Adolescents and adults:** 200 mg P.O. q 12 hours for 14 days.

UNCOMPLICATED GONORRHEA IN MEN AND WOMEN; RECTAL GONOCOCCAL INFECTIONS IN WOMEN

▶**Adolescents and adults:** 200 mg P.O. as a single dose. Follow with doxycycline 100 mg P.O. b.i.d. for 7 days.

UNCOMPLICATED SKIN AND SOFT-TISSUE INFECTIONS CAUSED BY *STAPHYLO-COCCUS AUREUS* **OR** *STREPTOCOCCUS PYOGENES*

▶**Adolescents and adults:** 400 mg P.O. q 12 hours for 7 to 14 days.

UNCOMPLICATED UTIS CAUSED BY *ESCHERICHIA COLI, KLEBSIELLA PNEUMONIAE, PROTEUS MIRABILIS,* **OR** *STAPHYLOCOCCUS SAPROPHYTICUS*

▶**Adolescents and adults:** 100 mg P.O. q 12 hours for 7 days.

ACUTE OTITIS MEDIA CAUSED BY *S. PNEUMONIAE, H. INFLUENZAE,* **OR** *M. CATARRHALIS*

▶**Infants and children ages 5 months to 12 years:** 5 mg/kg (not to exceed 200 mg) P.O. q 12 hours for 10 days.

▶**Contraindications & Precautions:** Contraindicated in patients with hypersensitivity to drug or other cephalosporins. Use cautiously in patients with impaired renal function or penicillin allergy and in breast-feeding women.

Cefprozil (Cefzil)
▶**Indications & Dosage**

PHARYNGITIS OR TONSILLITIS CAUSED BY *STREPTOCOCCUS PYOGENES*

▶**Children ages 2 to 12 years:** 7.5 mg/kg q 12 hours for 10 days.

▶**Adolescents and adults:** 500 mg P.O. daily for 10 days.

OTITIS MEDIA CAUSED BY *STREPTOCOCCUS PNEUMONIAE, HAEMOPHILUS INFLUENZAE,* **AND** *MORAXELLA (BRANHAMELLA) CATARRHALIS*

▶**Infants and children ages 6 months to 12 years:** 15 mg/kg P.O. q 12 hours for 10 days.

ACUTE SINUSITIS CAUSED BY *S. PNEUMONIAE, H. INFLUENZAE,* **AND** *S. PYOGENES*

▶**Infants and children ages 6 months to 12 years:** 7.5 mg/kg P.O. q 12 hours for 10 days; for moderate to severe infection, 15 mg/kg P.O. q 12 hours for 10 days.

►Adolescents and adults: 250 mg P.O. q 12 hours for 10 days; for moderate to severe infection, 500 mg P.O. q 12 hours for 10 days.

UNCOMPLICATED SKIN AND SKIN STRUCTURE INFECTIONS CAUSED BY
STAPHYLOCOCCUS AUREUS* AND *S. PYOGENES

►Children ages 2 to 12 years: 20 mg/kg P.O. q 24 hours for 10 days.

►Adolescents and adults: 250 mg P.O. b.i.d., or 500 mg daily to b.i.d. for 10 days.

►**Contraindications & Precautions:** Contraindicated in patients with hypersensitivity to drug or other cephalosporins. Use cautiously in patients with impaired renal function or penicillin allergy and in breast-feeding women.

Ceftazidime (Fortaz)
►**Indications & Dosage**

►Neonates younger than 1 week old and weighing 2 kg (4.4 lb) or less: 50 mg/kg I.V. q 12 hours.

►Neonates younger than 1 week old and weighing more than 2 kg: 50 mg/kg I.V. q 8 to 12 hours.

►Neonates ages 1 to 4 weeks: 30 to 50 mg/kg I.V. q 12 hours (Fortaz, Tazicef, and Tazidime only).

►Infants and children ages 1 month to 12 years: 30 to 50 mg/kg I.V. q 8 hours to a maximum of 6 g/day.

►Adolescents and adults: 1 g I.V. or I.M. q 8 to 12 hours; up to 6 g daily in life-threatening infections.

►**Contraindications & Precautions:** Contraindicated in patients with hypersensitivity to drug or other cephalosporins. Use cautiously in breast-feeding women and in patients with impaired renal function or penicillin allergy.

Ceftriaxone Sodium (Rocephin)
►**Indications & Dosage**

BACTEREMIA, SEPTICEMIA, AND SERIOUS RESPIRATORY TRACT, BONE, JOINT, URINARY TRACT, GYNECOLOGIC, INTRA-ABDOMINAL, AND SKIN INFECTIONS

►Infants and children: 75 mg/kg I.V. or I.M. daily given in divided doses q 12 hours.

►Adolescents and adults: 1 to 2 g I.M. or I.V. once daily or in equally divided doses b.i.d. Max dose 4 g.

MENINGITIS, ENDOCARDITIS

►Neonates, infants, and children: 100 mg/kg (maximum daily dose is 4 g) I.V. or I.M. divided q 12 hours

►Adolescents and adults: 1 to 2 g I.V. or I.M. q 12 hours

UNCOMPLICATED GONORRHEA

▶**Children weighing less than 45 kg (99 lb):** 125 mg I.M. as a single dose.

▶**Children weighing 45 kg and more, adolescents, and adults:** 125 to 250 mg I.M. given as a single dose; 1 to 2 g I.M. or I.V. daily until improvement occurs.

SEXUALLY TRANSMITTED EPIDIDYMITIS, PELVIC INFLAMMATORY DISEASE

▶**Adolescents and adults:** 250 mg I.M. as a single dose; follow up with other antibiotics.

ANTI-INFECTIVES FOR SEXUAL ASSAULT VICTIMS

▶**Adolescents and adults:** 125 mg I.M. as a single dose with other antibiotics.

LYME DISEASE

▶**Children:** 75 to 100 mg/kg I.M. or I.V. once daily for 14 to 30 days.

▶**Adults:** 2 g I.M. or I.V. daily for 14 to 30 days.

ACUTE BACTERIAL OTITIS MEDIA

▶**Children:** 50 mg/kg I.M. (not to exceed 1 g) as a single dose.

▶**Contraindications & Precautions:** Contraindicated in patients with hypersensitivity to drug or other cephalosporins. Use cautiously in breast-feeding women and in patients with penicillin allergy and those patients with preexisting gallbladder, biliary tract, liver, or pancreas disease.

Cefuroxime Axetil (Ceftin)

▶**Indications & Dosage**

SERIOUS LOWER RESPIRATORY TRACT, URINARY TRACT, SKIN AND SOFT-TISSUE INFECTIONS; SEPTICEMIA

▶**Infants and children older than 3 months:** 50 to 100 mg/kg/day I.M. or I.V. in divided doses q 6 to 8 hours. Some health care providers give 100 to 150 mg/kg/day.

▶**Adolescents and adults:** Usual dosage is 750 mg to 1.5 g I.M. or I.V. q 8 hours, usually for 5 to 10 days.

PHARYNGITIS, TONSILLITIS, LOWER RESPIRATORY TRACT INFECTION, UTI

▶**Infants and children ages 3 months to 12 years:** 20 mg/kg/day in divided doses b.i.d. (oral suspension) to maximum dose of 500 mg/day for 10 days.

▶**Children younger than age 12 who can swallow pills:** 125 mg P.O. b.i.d. (tablets) for 10 days.

▶**Adolescents and adults:** 125 to 250 mg P.O. b.i.d. for 10 days.

OTITIS MEDIA, IMPETIGO

▶Infants and children ages 3 months to 12 years: 30 mg/kg/day P.O. oral suspension divided into two doses (maximum dose, 1 g) for 10 days.

▶Children who can swallow pills: 250 mg P.O. b.i.d. for 10 days.

LYME DISEASE (ERYTHEMA MIGRANS) CAUSED BY *BORRELIA BURGDORFERI*

▶Adolescents ages 13 and older and adults: 500 mg P.O. b.i.d. for 20 days.

▶**Contraindications & Precautions:** Contraindicated in patients with hypersensitivity to drug or other cephalosporins. Use cautiously in breast-feeding women and in those with impaired renal function or penicillin allergy.

Cephalexin Hydrochloride (Keftab)
▶**Indications & Dosage**

RESPIRATORY TRACT, GU, SKIN AND SOFT-TISSUE, OR BONE AND JOINT INFECTIONS CAUSED BY SUSCEPTIBLE ORGANISMS

▶Children: 25 to 50 mg/kg P.O. daily divided into four doses. In patients older than age 1 with streptococcal pharyngitis or skin and soft-tissue infections, dose may be administered q 12 hours.

▶Adults: 250 mg to 1 g P.O. q 6 hours. For streptococcal pharyngitis, skin and soft-tissue infection, or uncomplicated cystitis in patients older than age 15, 500 mg P.O. q 12 hours.

OTITIS MEDIA

▶Children: 75 to 100 mg/kg P.O. daily divided into four doses.

▶**Contraindications & Precautions:** Contraindicated in patients with hypersensitivity to cephalosporins. Use cautiously in patients with impaired renal function or penicillin allergy and in breast-feeding women.

Cetirizine Hydrochloride (Zyrtec)
▶**Indications & Dosage**

SEASONAL ALLERGIC RHINITIS, PERENNIAL ALLERGIC RHINITIS, CHRONIC URTICARIA

▶Children ages 2 to 5 years: 2.5 to 5 mg P.O. daily.

▶Children ages 6 years and older and adults: 5 or 10 mg P.O. daily.

▶**Contraindications & Precautions:** Contraindicated in patients with hypersensitivity to drug or hydroxyzine. Use cautiously in patients with impaired renal function.

Chloral Hydrate (Aquachloral, Noctec)
►**Indications & Dosage**

SEDATION

►**Children:** 8 mg/kg P.O. or P.R. t.i.d. Maximum dosage is 500 mg t.i.d.

►**Adults:** 250 mg P.O. or P.R. t.i.d. after meals.

►**Contraindications & Precautions:** Contraindicated in patients with impaired hepatic or renal function, severe cardiac disease, or hypersensitivity to drug. Oral administration contraindicated in patients with gastric disorders. Use with extreme caution in patients with mental depression, suicidal tendencies, or history of drug abuse.

Cimetidine (Tagamet)
►**Indications & Dosage**

DUODENAL ULCER (SHORT-TERM TREATMENT)

►**Children:** 20 to 40 mg/kg I.V. or P.O. daily in divided doses.

►**Adults:** 800 mg P.O. h.s. for maximum of 8 weeks. Alternatively, give 400 mg P.O. b.i.d. or 300 mg P.O. q.i.d. with meals and h.s. When healing occurs, stop treatment or give h.s. dose only to control nocturnal hypersecretion. For parenteral therapy, 300 mg diluted to 20 ml with normal saline solution or other compatible I.V. solution by I.V. push over 5 minutes q 6 hours. Or 300 mg diluted in 50 ml D_5W solution or other compatible I.V. solution by I.V. infusion over 15 to 20 minutes q 6 to 8 hours. Or 300 mg I.M. q 6 to 8 hours (no dilution necessary). To increase dose, give more frequently to maximum daily dose of 2,400 mg.

HEARTBURN AND ACID INDIGESTION

►**Children ages 12 years and older and adults:** 200 mg (Tagamet HB only) P.O. daily, or up to a maximum of b.i.d. (400 mg). Maximum daily dose is 400 mg; patient shouldn't take drug daily for longer than 2 weeks.

ACTIVE BENIGN GASTRIC ULCER

►**Children:** 20 to 40 mg/kg I.V. or P.O. daily in divided doses.

►**Adults:** 800 mg P.O. h.s., or 300 mg q.i.d. (with meals and h.s.) for up to 8 weeks.

SYMPTOMATIC RELIEF OF GASTROESOPHAGEAL REFLUX

►**Adults:** 800 mg P.O. b.i.d. or 400 mg P.O. q.i.d. (before meals and h.s.), for up to 12 weeks.

►**Contraindications & Precautions:** Contraindicated in patients hypersensitive to drug.

Clarithromycin (Biaxin)
►**Indications & Dosage**
PHARYNGITIS OR TONSILLITIS
►**Infants and children ages 6 months and older:** 15 mg/kg P.O. divided q 12 hours for 10 days.
►**Adults:** 250 mg P.O. q 12 hours for 10 days.

ACUTE MAXILLARY SINUSITIS
►**Infants and children ages 6 months and older:** 7.5 mg/kg P.O. divided q 12 hours for 10 days.
►**Adults:** 500 mg P.O. q 12 hours for 14 days.

UNCOMPLICATED SKIN AND SOFT TISSUE INFECTIONS CAUSED BY *STAPHYLO-COCCUS AUREUS* OR *STREPTOCOCCUS PYOGENES*
►**Infants and children ages 6 months and older:** 7.5 mg P.O. q 12 hours.
►**Adults:** 250 mg P.O. q 12 hours for 7 to 14 days.

PROPHYLAXIS AND TREATMENT OF DISSEMINATED INFECTION CAUSED BY *MYCOBACTERIUM AVIUM* COMPLEX
►**Children older than 20 months:** 7.5 mg/kg b.i.d. up to 500 mg b.i.d.
►**Adults:** 500 mg P.O. b.i.d.

ACUTE OTITIS MEDIA
►**Infants and children ages 6 months and older:** 7.5 mg/kg P.O. b.i.d. up to 500 mg b.i.d.

***HELICOBACTER PYLORI* INFECTION**
►**Adults:** 500 mg P.O. b.i.d. to t.i.d. for 14 days with a combination drug.
►**Contraindications & Precautions:** Contraindicated in patients with hypersensitivity to erythromycin or other macrolides and in those receiving cisapride or pimozide. Use cautiously in patients with impaired renal or hepatic function.

Clindamycin Hydrochloride (Cleocin)
►**Indications & Dosage**
INFECTIONS CAUSED BY SENSITIVE ORGANISMS
►**Neonates:** 15 to 20 mg/kg/day I.V. divided into three or four equal doses. The lower dose may be adequate for small premature infants.
►**Infants and children older than age 1 month:** 8 to 20 mg/kg/day P.O.

divided into 3 or 4 equal doses or 20 to 40 mg/kg/day I.V.
divided into 3 or 4 equal doses.

▶**Adults:** 150 to 450 mg P.O. q 6 hours; or 600 to 2,700 mg/day
I.M. or I.V. divided into 2–4 equal doses.

▶**Contraindications & Precautions:** Contraindicated in patients with
hypersensitivity to the antibiotic congener lincomycin; in those with a
history of ulcerative colitis, regional enteritis, or antibiotic-associated
colitis; and in those with a history of atopic reactions. Use cautiously
in patients with asthma, impaired renal or hepatic function, or
history of GI diseases or significant allergies.

Clonazepam (Klonopin)
▶**Indications & Dosage**

SEIZURES

▶**Children up to age 10 or weighing 30 kg (66 lb) or less:** 0.01 to 0.03
mg/kg P.O. daily (not to exceed 0.05 mg/kg daily), divided q 8
hours. Increase dose by 0.25 to 0.5 mg q third day to a maximum
maintenance dose of 0.2 mg/kg/day.

▶**Adults:** Initial dosage shouldn't exceed 1.5 mg P.O. daily, divided
into three doses, but may be increased by 0.5 to 1 mg q 3 days
until seizures are controlled. Maximum daily dose is 20 mg.

▶**Contraindications & Precautions:** Contraindicated in patients with
significant hepatic disease; in those with sensitivity to benzodiazepines; and in patients with acute angle-closure glaucoma.
Use cautiously in children and in patients with mixed-type seizures,
respiratory disease, or glaucoma.

Clotrimazole (Lotrimin, Mycelex)
▶**Indications & Dosage**

TINEA PEDIS, TINEA CRURIS, TINEA VERSICOLOR, TINEA CORPORIS, CUTANEOUS
CANDIDIASIS

▶**Children and adults:** Apply thinly and massage into cleaned affected
and surrounding area, morning and evening, for prescribed period
(usually 1 to 4 weeks; however, therapy may take up to 8 weeks).

VULVOVAGINAL CANDIDIASIS

▶**Adults:** Insert 1 tablet intravaginally h.s. for 7 consecutive days. If
vaginal cream is used, insert 1 applicator intravaginally, h.s. for
7 to 14 consecutive days. Nonpregnant females may also insert 2,
100-mg tablets intravaginally for 3 days or a single dose of 500
mg for less complicated cases.

▶**Contraindications & Precautions:** Contraindicated in patients hypersensitive to drug.

Codeine Phosphate
►**Indications & Dosage**

MILD TO MODERATE PAIN

►**Children:** 0.5 mg/kg (or 15 mg/m^2) q 4 to 6 hours S.C., P.O., I.M. (Don't use I.V.)

►**Adults:** 15 to 60 mg P.O. or 15 to 60 mg (phosphate) S.C. or I.M. q 4 to 6 hours, p.r.n., or around-the-clock.

NONPRODUCTIVE COUGH

►**Children ages 2 to 6 years:** 1 mg/kg daily divided into four equal doses, administered q 4 to 6 hours, not to exceed 30 mg in 24 hours.

►**Children ages 6 to 11 years:** 5 to 10 mg q 4 to 6 hours, not to exceed 60 mg daily.

►**Children age 12 years and older and adults:** 10 to 20 mg P.O. q 4 to 6 hours. Maximum dose is 120 mg/day.

►**Contraindications & Precautions:** Contraindicated in patients with hypersensitivity to drug. Use cautiously in patients with impaired renal or hepatic function, head injuries, increased intracranial pressure, increased CSF pressure, hypothyroidism, Addison's disease, acute alcoholism, CNS depression, bronchial asthma, COPD, respiratory depression.

Colfosceril Palmitate (EXOSURF Neonatal)
►**Indications & Dosage**

PREVENTION AND TREATMENT (RESCUE) OF RESPIRATORY DISTRESS SYNDROME (RDS) IN PREMATURE INFANTS

►**Prophylaxis:** 5 ml/kg of body weight intratracheally for the first dose, administered as soon as possible after birth; second and third doses should be administered about 12 and 24 hours later to all infants remaining on mechanical ventilation at those times.

►**Rescue:** Initially, give 5 ml/kg of body weight intratracheally, administer as soon as possible after confirming diagnosis of RDS; second dose of 5 ml/kg, about 12 hours after the first, provided the infant remains on mechanical ventilation.

►Administer using endotracheal tube adapter supplied by manufacturer. Suction infant before administration; don't suction for 2 hours after administration except when necessary.

Cortisone Acetate
►**Indications & Dosage**

ADRENAL INSUFFICIENCY, ALLERGY, INFLAMMATION

►**Children:** 20 to 200 mg/m^2 P.O. daily in four divided doses or 7 to

37.5 mg/m^2 I.M. once or twice daily. Dose must be highly individualized.

►**Adults:** 25 to 300 mg P.O. or 20 to 300 mg I.M. daily or on alternate days. Doses highly individualized, depending on severity of disease.

►**Contraindications & Precautions:** Contraindicated in patients with hypersensitivity to drug or systemic fungal infections. Use cautiously in patients with renal disease, a recent MI, GI ulcer, hypertension, osteoporosis, diabetes mellitus, hypothyroidism, cirrhosis, diverticulitis, ulcerative colitis, recent intestinal anastomosis, thromboembolic disorders, seizures, myasthenia gravis, heart failure, tuberculosis, ocular herpes.

Co-trimoxazole (Trimethoprim-sulfamethoxazole)
►**Indications & Dosage**
URINARY TRACT INFECTION AND SHIGELLOSIS

►**Infants and children older than 2 months:** 8 mg/kg of trimethoprim and 40 mg/kg of sulfamethoxazole P.O. daily in two divided doses q 12 hours (10 days for UTIs; 5 days for shigellosis).

►**Adults:** 1 double-strength or 2 regular-strength tablets P.O. q 12 hours for 10 to 14 days or 5 days for shigellosis. Or, 8 to 10 mg/kg (based on trimethoprim) I.V. daily given in 2 to 4 equally divided doses for up to 14 days (5 days for shigellosis). Maximum daily dose is 960 mg.

OTITIS MEDIA

►**Infants and children older than 2 months:** 8 mg/kg of trimethoprim and 40 mg/kg of sulfamethoxazole P.O. daily, in two divided doses q 12 hours for 10 days.

TRAVELER'S DIARRHEA

►**Adults:** 1 double-strength or 2 regular-strength tablets q 12 hours for 5 days.

PERTUSIS

►**Children:** 40 mg/kg/day P.O. in two divided doses.

►Contraindicated in patients with hypersensitivity to trimethoprim or sulfonamides, severe renal impairment, or porphyria; in those with megaloblastic anemia caused by folate deficiency; in pregnant women at term; in breast-feeding women; and in children younger than 2 months. Use cautiously in patients with impaired renal or hepatic function, severe allergies, severe bronchial asthma, G6PD deficiency, or blood dyscrasia.

Cromolyn Sodium (Intal)
▶**Indications & Dosage**

ADJUNCT IN TREATMENT OF SEVERE PERENNIAL BRONCHIAL ASTHMA

▶**Children older than age 5 years and adults:** 2 inhalations q.i.d. at regular intervals; aqueous solution administered through a nebulizer, 1 ampule q.i.d.; or 1 capsule (20 mg) of powder for inhalation q.i.d.

PREVENTION AND TREATMENT OF ALLERGIC RHINITIS

▶**Children age 6 years and older and adults:** 1 spray (5.2 mg) of nasal solution in each nostril t.i.d. or q.i.d. May give up to six times daily.

▶**Contraindications & Precautions:** Contraindicated in patients experiencing acute asthma attacks or status asthmaticus and in patients with hypersensitivity to drug. Use inhalation form cautiously in patients with cardiac disease or arrhythmias.

Deferoxamine Mesylate (Desferal)
▶**Indications & Dosage**

ACUTE IRON INTOXICATION

▶**Children older than age 3 years and adults:** 1 g I.M. or I.V. (I.M. injection is preferred route for all patients in shock), followed by 500 mg I.M. or I.V. q 4 hours for two doses; then 500 mg I.M. or I.V. q 4 to 12 hours if needed. I.V. infusion rate shouldn't exceed 15 mg/kg/hour. Don't exceed 6 g in 24 hours. (I.V. infusion should be reserved for patients in CV collapse.) Alternatively, children can be given 20 mg/kg (or 600 mg/ m^2) I.M. or slow I.V. followed by 10 mg/kg (or 300 mg/m^2) q 4 hours for 2 doses, then 10 mg/kg (or 300 mg/m^2) q 4 to 12 hours as needed.

▶**Contraindications & Precautions:** Contraindicated in patients with severe renal disease or anuria. Use cautiously in patients with impaired renal function or pyelonephritis.

Dexamethasone (Systemic) (Decadron)
▶**Indications & Dosage**

CEREBRAL EDEMA

DEXAMETHASONE SODIUM PHOSPHATE

▶**Adults:** Initially, 10 mg I.V., then 4 mg I.M. q 6 hours for 2 to 4 days, then taper over 5 to 7 days.

INFLAMMATORY CONDITIONS, ALLERGIC REACTIONS, NEOPLASIAS

▶**Children:** 0.024 to 0.34 mg/kg P.O. daily in four divided doses.

▶**Adults:** 0.75 to 9 mg P.O. daily divided b.i.d., t.i.d., or q.i.d.

DEXAMETHASONE ACETATE
▶**Adults:** 4 to 16 mg intra-articularly or into soft tissue q 1 to 3 weeks; 0.8 to 1.6 mg into lesions q 1 to 3 weeks; or 8 to 16 mg I.M. q 1 to 3 weeks, p.r.n.

DEXAMETHASONE SODIUM PHOSPHATE
▶**Adults:** 0.2 to 6 mg intra-articularly, intralesionally, or into soft tissue; or 0.5 to 9 mg I.M.

SHOCK (OTHER THAN ADRENAL CRISIS)
DEXAMETHASONE SODIUM PHOSPHATE
▶**Adults:** 1 to 6 mg/kg I.V. daily as a single dose; or 40 mg I.V. q 2 to 6 hours, p.r.n.; such high doses should only be used until the patient's condition is stabilized, usually not longer than 48 to 72 hours.

DEXAMETHASONE SUPPRESSION TEST FOR CUSHING'S SYNDROME
▶**Adults:** 0.5 mg P.O. q 6 hours for 48 hours.

ADRENAL INSUFFICIENCY
▶**Children:** 0.024 to 0.34 mg/kg P.O. daily in four divided doses.
▶**Adults:** 0.75 to 9 mg P.O. daily in divided doses.

DEXAMETHASONE SODIUM PHOSPHATE
▶**Children:** 0.235 to 1.25 mg/m^2 I.M. or I.V. once daily or b.i.d.
▶**Adults:** 0.5 to 9 mg I.M. or I.V. daily.

ADJUNCTIVE THERAPY IN BACTERIAL MENINGITIS
DEXAMETHASONE SODIUM PHOSPHATE
▶**Infants and children older than 2 months and adults: 0.15 mg/kg I.V. q 6 hours for the first 2 to 4 days of anti-infective therapy.**

PREVENTION OF HYALINE MEMBRANE DISEASE IN PREMATURE INFANTS
▶**Adults:** 5 mg (phosphate) I.M. t.i.d. to mother for 2 days before delivery.

▶**Contraindications & Precautions:** Contraindicated in patients hypersensitive to any component of drug and in those with systemic fungal infections. Use cautiously in patients with a recent MI, GI ulcer, renal disease, hypertension, osteoporosis, diabetes mellitus, hypothyroidism, cirrhosis, diverticulitis, non-specific ulcerative colitis, recent intestinal anastomoses, thrombo-embolic disorders, seizures, myasthenia gravis, heart failure, tuberculosis, ocular herpes simplex

Dextroamphetamine Sulfate (Dexedrine)

▶**Indications & Dosage**

ATTENTION DEFICIT HYPERACTIVITY DISORDER

▶**Children ages 3 to 5 years:** 2.5 mg P.O. daily, with 2.5-mg increments weekly, p.r.n.; not recommended for children younger than age 3.

▶**Children ages 6 years and older:** 5 mg P.O. once daily or b.i.d., increase in 5-mg increments weekly, p.r.n. Total daily dose should rarely exceed 40 mg.

▶**Contraindications & Precautions:** Contraindicated in patients who have taken an MAO inhibitor within the past 2 weeks and in those with hypersensitivity or idiosyncrasy to the sympathomimetic amines, hyperthyroidism, moderate to severe hypertension, symptomatic CV disease, glaucoma, advanced arteriosclerosis, and history of drug abuse. Use cautiously in patients with motor and phonic tics, Tourette syndrome.

Diazepam (Valium)

▶**Indications & Dosage**

ANXIETY

▶**Infants and children ages 6 months and older:** 1 to 2.5 mg P.O. t.i.d. or q.i.d.; increase dose gradually, as needed and tolerated. Alternatively, 0.04 to 0.2 mg/kg I.V. q 3 to 4 hours, p.r.n., to a maximum of 0.6 mg/kg within an 8-hour period.

▶**Adults:** Depending on severity, 2 to 10 mg P.O. b.i.d. to q.i.d. or 15 to 30 mg extended-release capsules P.O. once daily. Alternatively, 2 to 10 mg I.M. or I.V. q 3 to 4 hours, p.r.n.

STATUS EPILEPTICUS

▶**Infants older than 30 days to children age 5 years:** 0.2 to 0.5 mg I.V. q 2 to 5 minutes up to a maximum total of 5 mg.

▶**Children ages 5 years and older:** 1 mg I.V. q 2 to 5 minutes up to a maximum total of 10 mg; repeat in 2 to 4 hours, p.r.n.

▶**Adults:** 5 to 10 mg I.V. (preferred) or I.M. initially, repeated at 10- to 15-minute intervals up to a maximum total of 30 mg. Repeat q 2 to 4 hours, p.r.n.

▶**Contraindications & Precautions:** Contraindicated in patients with hypersensitivity or angle-closure glaucoma; in patients experiencing shock, coma, or acute alcohol intoxication (parenteral form); and in children younger than 6 months (oral form). Use cautiously in debilitated patients and in those with impaired hepatic or renal function, depression, or chronic open-angle glaucoma. Avoid use in pregnant patients, especially during the first trimester.

Dicloxacillin Sodium (Dynapen)
►**Indications & Dosage**

►**Infants and children older than 1 month weighing less than 40 kg (88 lb):**
12.5 to 50 mg/kg P.O. daily, divided into doses given q 6 hours.
Serious infection may require higher dose (75 to 100 mg/kg/day
in divided doses q 6 hours).

►**Children and adults weighing 40 kg or more:** 125 to 250 mg P.O.
q 6 hours.

►**Contraindications & Precautions:** Contraindicated in patients with
hypersensitivity to drug or other penicillins. Use cautiously in
patients with other drug allergies, especially to cephalosporins,
and in those with mononucleosis.

Digoxin (Lanoxin)
►**Indications & Dosage**

**HEART FAILURE, ATRIAL FIBRILLATION AND FLUTTER, PAROXYSMAL ATRIAL
TACHYCARDIA**

►**Premature neonates:** 20 to 30 mcg/kg P.O. over 24 hours in two or
more divided doses q 6 to 8 hours. Maintenance dose is 20% to
30% of total digitalizing dose.

►**Neonates (full-term):** 25 to 35 mcg/kg P.O. over 24 hours in two or
more divided doses q 6 to 8 hours. Maintenance dose is 25% to
35% of total digitalizing dose.

►**Infants and children ages 1 month to 2 years:** 35 to 60 mcg/kg P.O. over
24 hours in two or more divided doses q 6 to 8 hours. Maintenance
dose is 25% to 35% of total digitalizing dose.

►**Children ages 2 to 5 years:** 30 to 40 mcg/kg P.O. over 24 hours in two
or more divided doses q 6 to 8 hours. Maintenance dose is 25% to
35% of total digitalizing dose.

►**Children ages 5 to 10 years:** 20 to 35 mcg/kg P.O. over 24 hours in
two or more divided doses q 6 to 8 hours. Maintenance dose is
25% to 35% of total digitalizing dose.

►**Children ages 10 years and older:** 10 to 15 mcg/kg P.O. over 24 hours
in two or more divided doses q 6 to 8 hours. Maintenance dose is
25% to 35% of total digitalizing dose.

►**Adults:** For rapid digitalization, give 0.75 to 1.25 mg P.O. over
24 hours in two or more divided doses q 6 to 8 hours. For slow
digitalization, give 0.125 to 0.5 mg P.O. daily for 5 to 7 days.
Maintenance dose is 0.125 to 0.5 mg daily.

CAPSULES

►**Children ages 2 to 5 years:** For rapid digitalization, give 25 to 35
mcg/kg P.O. over 24 hours, divided as above. Maintenance dose

is 25% to 35% of total digitalizing dose, divided and given in two or three equal portions daily.

▶**Children ages 5 to 10 years:** For rapid digitalization, give 15 to 30 mcg/kg P.O. over 24 hours, divided as above. Maintenance dose is 25% to 35% of total digitalizing dose, divided and given in two or three equal portions daily.

▶**Children ages 10 years and older:** For rapid digitalization, give 8 to 12 mcg/kg P.O. over 24 hours, divided as above. Maintenance dose is 25% to 35% of total digitalizing dose, divided and given daily as a single dose.

▶**Adults:** For rapid digitalization, give 0.4 to 0.6 mcg/kg P.O. initially, followed by 0.1 to 0.3 mg q 6 to 8 hours, as needed and tolerated, for 24 hours. For slow digitalization, give 0.05 to 0.35 mg daily in two divided doses for 7 to 22 days, p.r.n., until therapeutic serum levels are reached. Maintenance dose is 0.05 to 0.35 mg daily in one or two divided doses.

INJECTION

▶**Premature neonates:** For rapid digitalization, give 15 to 25 mcg/kg I.V. over 24 hours, divided as above. Maintenance dose is 20% to 30% of total digitalizing dose, divided and given in two or three equal portions daily.

▶**Neonates (full term):** For rapid digitalization, give 20 to 30 mcg/kg I.V. over 24 hours, divided as above. Maintenance dose is 25% to 35% of total digitalizing dose, divided and given in two or three equal portions daily.

▶**Infants and children ages 1 month to 2 years:** For rapid digitalization, give 30 to 50 mcg/kg I.V. over 24 hours, divided as above. Maintenance dose is 25% to 35% of total digitalizing dose, divided and given in two or three equal portions daily.

▶**Children ages 2 to 5 years:** For rapid digitalization, give 25 to 35 mcg/kg I.V. over 24 hours, divided as above. Maintenance dose is 25% to 35% of total digitalizing dose, divided and given in two or three equal portions daily.

▶**Children ages 5 to 10 years:** For rapid digitalization, give 15 to 30 mcg/kg I.V. over 24 hours, divided as above. Maintenance dose is 25% to 35% of total digitalizing dose, divided and given in two or three equal portions daily.

▶**Children ages 10 years and older:** For rapid digitalization, give 8 to 12 mcg/kg I.V. over 24 hours, divided as above. Maintenance dose is 25% to 35% of total digitalizing dose, given daily as a single dose.

▶**Adult:** For rapid digitalization, give 0.4 to 0.6 mcg/kg I.V. initially, followed by 0.1 to 0.3 mg I.V. q 4 to 8 hours, as needed and tolerated, for 24 hours. For slow digitalization, give appropriate daily maintenance dose for 7 to 22 days as needed until therapeutic serum levels are reached. Maintenance dose is 0.125 to 0.5 mg I.V. daily in one or two divided doses.

▶**Contraindications & Precautions:** Contraindicated in patients with hypersensitivity to drug, digitalis-induced toxicity, ventricular fibrillation, or ventricular tachycardia unless caused by heart failure. Use very cautiously in patients with an acute MI, incomplete AV block, sinus bradycardia, PVCs, chronic constrictive pericarditis, hypertrophic cardiomyopathy, renal insufficiency, severe pulmonary disease, or hypothyroidism.

Diphenhydramine Hydrochloride (Benadryl)
▶**Indications & Dosage**

RHINITIS, ALLERGY SYMPTOMS, MOTION SICKNESS

▶**Children ages 2 to 5 years:** 6.25 mg P.O. q 4 to 6 hours. Maximum P.O. dose is 37.5 mg daily. Alternatively, 1.25 mg/kg I.V. or deep I.M. q 6 hours. Maximum I.M. or I.V. dose is 300 mg daily.

▶**Children ages 6 to 11 years:** 12.5 to 25 mg P.O. q 4 to 6 hours. Maximum P.O. dose is 150 mg daily. Alternatively, 1.25 mg/kg I.V. or deep I.M. q 6 hours. Maximum I.M. or I.V. dose is 300 mg daily.

▶**Children ages 12 years and older and adults:** 25 to 50 mg P.O. t.i.d. or q.i.d.; or 10 to 50 mg I.V. or deep I.M. Maximum I.M. or I.V. dose is 400 mg daily.

NONPRODUCTIVE COUGH

▶**Children ages 2 to 5 years:** 6.25 mg P.O. q 4 hours. Maximum dose is 37.5 mg daily.

▶**Children ages 6 to 11 years:** 12.5 mg P.O. q 4 hours. Maximum dose is 75 mg daily.

▶**Adults and children ages 12 years and older:** 25 mg P.O. q 4 to 6 hours. Maximum dose is 150 mg daily.

INSOMNIA

▶**Children ages 2 to 11 years:** 1 mg/kg (up to a maximum dose of 50 mg) P.O. 30 minutes before h.s.

▶**Children ages 12 years and older and adults:** 50 mg P.O. 30 minutes before h.s.

▶**Contraindications & Precautions:** Contraindicated in patients with hypersensitivity to drug, during acute asthma attacks, and in newborns, premature neonates, or breast-feeding patients. Use with extreme caution in patients with angle-closure glaucoma, pyloroduodenal and bladder neck obstruction, asthma or COPD, increased intraocular pressure, hyperthyroidism, CV disease, hypertension, and stenosing peptic ulcer.

Dobutamine Hydrochloride (Dobutrex)

►**Indications & Dosage**

TO INCREASE CARDIAC OUTPUT IN SHORT-TERM TREATMENT OF CARDIAC DECOMPENSATION CAUSED BY DEPRESSED CONTRACTILITY

►**Neonates, infants, and children:** 2 to 20 mcg/kg/minute as an I.V. infusion. Begin at a low dose and titrate to desired response.

►**Adults:** 2.5 to 15 mcg/kg/minute as an I.V. infusion. Rarely, infusion rates up to 40 mcg/kg/minute may be needed. Titrate dose carefully to patient response.

►**Contraindications & Precautions:** Contraindicated in patients with hypersensitivity to drug or its formulation and in those with hypertrophic cardiomyopathy. Use cautiously in patients with a history of hypertension or after a recent MI. Drug may precipitate an exaggerated pressor response.

Dolasetron Mesylate (Anzemet)

►**Indications & Dosage**

PREVENTION OF NAUSEA AND VOMITING ASSOCIATED WITH CANCER CHEMOTHERAPY

►**Children ages 2 to 16 years:** 1.8 mg/kg P.O. given 1 hour before chemotherapy, or 1.8 mg/kg as a single I.V. dose given 30 minutes before chemotherapy. Injectable form can be mixed with apple or apple-grape juice and administered P.O. 1 hour before chemotherapy. Maximum daily dose of 100 mg.

►**Adults:** 100 mg P.O. given as a single dose 1 hour before chemotherapy, or 1.8 mg/kg as a single I.V. dose given 30 minutes before chemotherapy, or a fixed dose of 100 mg I.V. given 30 minutes before chemotherapy.

TREATMENT OF POSTOPERATIVE NAUSEA AND VOMITING (I.V. FORM ONLY)

►**Children ages 2 to 16 years:** 0.35 mg/kg, up to a maximum dose of 12.5 mg, given as a single I.V. dose as soon as nausea or vomiting occurs.

►**Adults:** 12.5 mg as a single I.V. dose as soon as nausea or vomiting develops.

►**Contraindications & Precautions:** Contraindicated in patients hypersensitive to drug. Use drug cautiously in patients with or at risk for developing prolonged cardiac conduction intervals, particularly QTc interval. These include patients taking antiarrhythmics drugs or other drugs which lead to QT-interval prolongation; hypokalemia or hypomagnesemia; a potential for electrolyte abnormalities, including those receiving diuretics; congenital QT-interval syndrome; and those who have received cumulative high-dose anthracycline therapy.

Dopamine Hydrochloride (Intropin)
►**Indications & Dosage**

ADJUNCT IN SHOCK TO INCREASE CARDIAC OUTPUT, BLOOD PRESSURE, AND URINE FLOW

►**Neonates:** 0.5 to 20 mcg/kg/minute continuous I.V. infusion. Begin at a low dose and titrate according to response.

►**Infants and children:** 1 to 20 mcg/kg/minute by continuous I.V. infusion. Titrate according to response.

►**Adults:** 1 to 5 mcg/kg/minute I.V. infusion, to 20 to 50 mcg/kg/minute. Infusion rate may be increased by 1 to 4 mcg/kg/minute every 10 to 30 minutes until optimum response is achieved. In severely ill patients, infusion may begin at 5 mcg/kg/minute and gradually increase by increments of 5 to 10 mcg/kg/minute until optimum response is achieved.

SHORT-TERM TREATMENT OF SEVERE, REFRACTORY, CHRONIC HEART FAILURE

►**Adults:** Initially, 0.5 to 2 mcg/kg/minute I.V. infusion. Dosage may be increased until desired renal response occurs. Average dose is 1 to 3 mcg/kg/minute.

►**Contraindications & Precautions:** Contraindicated in patients with uncorrected tachyarrhythmias, pheochromocytoma, or ventricular fibrillation. Use cautiously in patients with occlusive vascular disease, cold injuries, diabetic endarteritis, and arterial embolism; in those taking MAO inhibitors; and in pregnant women.

Dornase Alfa (Pulmozyme)
►**Indications & Dosage**

►**Children ages 5 years and older and adults:** 1 ampule (2.5 mg/2.5 ml) inhaled once daily. Treatment usually takes 10 to 15 minutes. Use drug only with an approved nebulizer. Patients older than age 21 and those with a baseline forced vital capacity greater than 85% may require twice-daily dosing.

►**Contraindications & Precautions:** Contraindicated in patients hypersensitive to drug or Chinese hamster ovary cell-derived products.

Doxycycline (Vibramycin)
►**Indications & Dosage**

INFECTIONS CAUSED BY SENSITIVE ORGANISMS

►**Children older than age 8 years and weighing 45 kg (99 lb) or less:** 4.4 mg/kg P.O. or I.V. daily, divided q 12 hours day 1, then 2.2 to 4.4 mg/kg P.O. or I.V. daily as a single or divided dose.

▶**Children older than age 8 years and weighing more than 45 kg and adults:**
100 mg P.O. q 12 hours on day 1, then 100 mg P.O. daily; or 200
mg I.V. on day 1 in one or two infusions, then 100 to 200 mg I.V.
daily.

▶Give I.V. infusion slowly (minimum 1 hour). Infusion must be completed within 12 hours (within 6 hours in lactated Ringer's solution
or D_5W in lactated Ringer's solution).

CHLAMYDIA TRACHOMATIS, **NONGONOCOCCAL URETHRITIS, AND
UNCOMPLICATED URETHRAL, ENDOCERVICAL, OR RECTAL INFECTIONS**

▶**Adolescents and adults:** 100 mg P.O. b.i.d. for at least 7 days.

ACUTE PELVIC INFLAMMATORY DISEASE

▶**Adolescents and adults:** 250 mg I.M. ceftriaxone, followed by 100 mg
doxycycline P.O. b.i.d. for 10 to 14 days.

▶**Contraindications & Precautions:** Contraindicated in patients with
hypersensitivity to drug or other tetracyclines. Use cautiously in
patients with impaired renal or hepatic function. Use during last
half of pregnancy and in children younger than age 8 may
permanently discolor teeth, cause enamel defects, and retard
bone growth.

Epinephrine
▶**Indications & Dosage**

BRONCHOSPASM, HYPERSENSITIVITY REACTIONS, ANAPHYLAXIS

▶**Children:** 0.01 mg/kg (0.01 ml/kg of a 1:1,000 solution) or 0.3
mg/m^2 (0.3 ml/m^2) of a 1:1,000 solution) S.C. Dose shouldn't
exceed 0.5 mg. May be repeated at 20-minute to 4-hour intervals,
p.r.n. Alternatively, 0.02 to 0.025 mg/kg (0.004 to 0.005 ml/kg)
or 0.625 mg/m^2 (0.125 ml/m^2) of a 1:200 solution. May be
repeated but not more often than q 6 hours. Alternatively, 0.1 mg
(10 ml of a 1:100,000 dilution) I.V. slowly over 5 to 10 minutes,
followed by a 0.1 to 1.5 mcg/kg/minute I.V. infusion.

▶**Adults:** Initially, 0.1 to 0.5 mg (0.1 to 0.5 ml of a 1:1,000 solution)
S.C. or I.M.; may be repeated at 10- to 15-minute intervals, p.r.n.
Alternatively, 0.1 to 0.25 mg (1 to 2.5 ml of a 1:10,000 solution)
I.V. slowly over 5 to 10 minutes. May be repeated q 5 to 15
minutes if needed or followed by a 1 to 4 mcg/minute I.V. infusion.

TO RESTORE CARDIAC RHYTHM IN CARDIAC ARREST

▶**Infants:** Initially, 0.01 to 0.03 mg/kg (0.1 to 0.3 ml/kg of a
1:10,000 solution) I.V. bolus or by intratracheal injection. May
be repeated q 5 minutes, p.r.n.

▶**Children:** Initially, 0.01 mg/kg (0.1 ml/kg of a 1:10,000 solution)
I.V. bolus or intratracheally; may be repeated q 5 minutes, p.r.n.
Alternatively, initially 0.1 mcg/kg/minute; may increase in

increments of 0.1 mcg/kg/minute to a maximum of 1 mcg/kg/minute. Alternatively, 0.005 to 0.01 mg/kg (0.05 to 0.1 ml/kg of a 1:10,000 solution) by intracardiac injection.

▶**Adults:** Initially, 0.5 to 1 mg (range, 0.1 to 1 mg usually as 1 to 10 ml of a 1:10,000 solution) I.V. bolus; may be repeated q 3 to 5 minutes, p.r.n. Alternatively, initial dose followed by 0.3 mg S.C. or 1 to 4 mcg/minute I.V. infusion. Alternatively, 1 mg (10 ml of a 1:10,000 solution) intratracheally, or 0.1 to 1 mg (1 to 10 ml of a 1:10,000 solution) by intracardiac injection.

Erythromycin Base (Ery-Tab)
▶**Indications & Dosage**
MILD TO MODERATELY SEVERE RESPIRATORY TRACT, SKIN, AND SOFT-TISSUE INFECTIONS CAUSED BY SUSCEPTIBLE ORGANISMS

▶**Children:** 30 mg/kg to 50 mg/kg (oral erythromycin salts) P.O. daily, in divided doses q 6 hours; or 15 to 20 mg/kg I.V. daily, in divided doses q 4 to 6 hours.

▶**Adults:** 250 to 500 mg (base, estolate, stearate) P.O. q 6 hours; or 400 to 800 mg (ethylsuccinate) P.O. q 6 hours; or 15 to 20 mg/kg (gluceptate, lactobionate) I.V. daily, in divided doses q 6 hours.

CONJUNCTIVITIS CAUSED BY *CHLAMYDIA TRACHOMATIS* IN NEONATES

▶**Neonates:** 50 mg/kg/day P.O. in four divided doses for at least 2 weeks.

PNEUMONIA OF INFANCY CAUSED BY *C. TRACHOMATIS*

▶**Infants:** 50 mg/kg/day P.O. in four divided doses for at least 3 weeks.

TOPICAL TREATMENT OF ACNE VULGARIS

▶**Children and adults:** apply to the affected area b.i.d.

ACUTE AND CHRONIC CONJUNCTIVITIS, TRACHOMA, OTHER EYE INFECTIONS

▶**Children and adults:** Apply 1-cm long ribbon ointment directly into infected eye up to six times daily, depending on severity of infection.

Ethosuximide (Zarontin)
▶**Indications & Dosage**
ABSENCE SEIZURES

▶**Children ages 3 to 6 years:** 250 mg P.O. daily. Optimal dose for most children is 20 mg/kg/day.

▶**Children ages 6 years and older and adults:** Initially, 250 mg P.O. b.i.d. May increase by 250 mg q 4 to 7 days up to 1.5 g daily.

▶**Contraindications & Precautions:** Contraindicated in patients with hypersensitivity to succinimide derivatives. Use with extreme caution in patients with hepatic or renal disease.

Fentanyl Citrate
►**Indications & Dosage**

►**Children ages 2 years and older, weighing 15 to 39 kg (33 to 86 lb):**
5 mcg/kg P.O. as a lozenge. May need 10 to 15 mcg/kg.
(Maximum dose is 400 mcg.)

►**Children ages 2 years and older, weighing 40 kg (88 lb) or more:** 5 mcg/kg
(maximum dose is 400 mcg) P.O. as a lozenge.

►**Adults:** 50 to 100 mcg I.M. 30 to 60 minutes before surgery. Or one
oralet unit containing 100 mcg, 200 mcg, 300 mcg, or 400 mcg
P.O. 20 to 40 minutes before surgery for patient to suck until
dissolved.

►**Contraindications & Precautions:** Contraindicated in patients with
known intolerance to drug. Fentanyl should not be given to a patient
who has received an MAO inhibitor within the past 14 days. Use
cautiously in debilitated patients and in those with head injuries,
increased CSF pressure, COPD, decreased respiratory reserve,
compromised respirations, arrhythmias, or hepatic, renal, or
cardiac disease.

Ferrous Sulfate
►**Indications & Dosage**

IRON DEFICIENCY ANEMIA

►**Infants:** 10 to 25 mg/day P.O. divided into three or four doses.

►**Infants and children ages 6 months to 2 years:** Up to 6 mg/kg/day P.O.
divided into three or four doses.

►**Children ages 2 to 12 years:** 3 mg/kg/day P.O. divided into three or
four doses.

►**Adults:** 300 mg P.O. b.i.d., gradually increased to 300 mg q.i.d. as
needed and tolerated. For extended-release capsules, 150 to 250
mg P.O. once or twice daily; for extended-release tablets, 160 to
525 mg once or twice daily.

►**Contraindications & Precautions:** Contraindicated in patients receiving
repeated blood transfusions and those with peptic ulceration, regional
enteritis, ulcerative colitis, hemosiderosis, primary hemochromatosis,
or hemolytic anemia unless iron deficiency anemia is also present.
Give long-term therapy cautiously.

Fexofenadine Hydrochloride (Allegra)
►**Indications & Dosage**

SEASONAL ALLERGIC RHINITIS

►**Children ages 12 years and older and adults:** 60 mg P.O. b.i.d.

▶**Contraindications & Precautions:** Contraindicated in patients with hypersensitivity to drug or its components. Use cautiously in patients with impaired renal function.

Fluconazole (Diflucan)
▶**Indications & Dosage**
OROPHARYNGEAL AND ESOPHAGEAL CANDIDIASIS

▶**Neonates older than 14 days, infants, and children:** 6 mg/kg P.O. or I.V. on day 1, followed by 3 mg/kg for at least 2 weeks.

▶**Adults:** 200 mg P.O. or I.V. on day 1, followed by 100 mg P.O. or I.V. once daily. Up to 400 mg daily has been used for esophageal disease. Treatment should continue for at least 2 weeks after symptoms resolve.

SYSTEMIC CANDIDIASIS

▶**Neonates older than 14 days, infants, and children:** 6 to 12 mg/kg/day P.O. or I.V.

▶**Adults:** Up to 400 mg P.O. or I.V. once daily. Treatment should continue for at least 2 weeks after symptoms resolve.

CRYPTOCOCCAL MENINGITIS

▶**Infants and children:** 12 mg/kg P.O. or I.V. on day 1, followed by 6 mg/kg once daily for 10 to 12 weeks after CSF culture becomes negative. To suppress relapse in patients with AIDS, give 6 mg/kg once daily.

▶**Adults:** 400 mg I.V. or P.O. on day 1, followed by 200 mg once daily. Continue treatment for 10 to 12 weeks after CSF culture becomes negative. To suppress relapse in patients with AIDS, give 200 mg once daily.

VAGINAL CANDIDIASIS

▶**Adults:** 150 mg P.O. as a single dose.

▶**Contraindications & Precautions:** Contraindicated in patients hypersensitive to drug and other drugs in the same classification.

Flumazenil (Romazicon)
▶**Indications & Dosage**
MANAGEMENT OF SUSPECTED BENZODIAZEPINE OVERDOSE

▶**Children:** 0.01 mg/kg (maximum 0.2 mg) I.V. over 15 seconds. May repeat q 1 minute to a total cumulative dose of 1 mg.

▶**Adults:** Initially, 0.2 mg I.V. over 30 seconds. If patient fails to reach desired level of consciousness after 30 seconds, administer 0.3 mg over 30 seconds. If patient still fails to respond adequately, give

0.5 mg over 30 seconds; then repeat 0.5-mg doses at 1-minute intervals until a cumulative dose of 3 mg has been given

▶**Contraindications & Precautions:** Contraindicated in patients hypersensitive to drug; in patients who show evidence of serious tricyclic antidepressant overdose; and in those who received a benzodiazepine to treat a potentially life-threatening condition (such as status epilepticus).

▶Use cautiously in alcohol-dependent or psychiatric patients, in those at high risk for seizures, or in those with head injuries, signs of seizures, or a recent high intake of benzodiazepines.

Fluticasone Propionate (Flovent)
▶**Indications & Dosage**

ALLERGIC RHINITIS

▶**Children ages 12 years and older:** 1 spray in each nostril daily. May increase to 2 sprays in each nostril for severe symptoms; depending on patient's response

▶**Adults:** 2 sprays in each nostril once daily or 1 spray b.i.d.

MAINTENANCE TREATMENT OF ASTHMA AS PROPHYLACTIC THERAPY

▶**Children ages 4 to 11 years:** 50 mcg inhalation powder b.i.d. (Maximum 100 mcg inhalation powder b.i.d.)

▶**Children ages 12 years and older and adults:** 88 to 220 mcg inhalation aerosol b.i.d. (Maximum 440 mcg inhalation aerosol b.i.d.)

▶**Adolescents and adults:** 100 mcg inhalation powder b.i.d. (Maximum 500 mcg inhalation powder b.i.d.)

▶**Contraindications & Precautions:** Contraindicated in patients hypersensitive to drug or its components and in patients with viral, fungal, herpetic, or tubercular skin lesions.

Folic Acid
▶**Indications & Dosage**

MEGALOBLASTIC OR MACROCYTIC ANEMIA CAUSED BY FOLIC ACID DEFICIENCY, HEPATIC DISEASE, ALCOHOLISM, INTESTINAL OBSTRUCTION, EXCESSIVE HEMOLYSIS

▶**Infants:** 0.05 mg P.O., S.C., or I.M. daily.

▶**Children younger than age 4 years:** up to 0.3 mg P.O., S.C., or I.M. daily.

▶**Children ages 4 years and older and adults:** 0.4 mg P.O., S.C., or I.M. daily for 4 to 5 days.

▶**Pregnant and breast-feeding patients:** 0.8 mg P.O., S.C., or I.M. daily.

PREVENTION OF MEGALOBLASTIC ANEMIA CAUSED BY PREGNANCY AND FETAL DAMAGE

▶**Adults:** 1 mg P.O., S.C., or I.M. daily during pregnancy.

▶**Contraindications & Precautions:** Contraindicated in patients with vitamin B_{12} deficiency and with undiagnosed anemia, because it may mask pernicious anemia.

Furosemide (Lasix)
▶**Indications & Dosage**

ACUTE PULMONARY EDEMA

▶**Infants and children:** 1 mg/kg I.M. or I.V. q 2 hours until response is achieved. (Maximum 6 mg/kg.)

▶**Adults:** 40 mg I.V. injected slowly; then 80 mg I.V. within 1 hour, p.r.n.

EDEMA

▶**Infants and children:** 2 mg/kg/day P.O., increased by 1 to 2 mg/kg in 6 to 8 hours, p.r.n. Don't exceed 6 mg/kg/day.

▶**Adults:** 20 to 80 mg P.O. daily in morning, with second dose given in 6 to 8 hours, carefully adjusted up to 600 mg daily, p.r.n. or 20 to 40 mg I.M. or I.V. Increase by 20 mg q 2 hours until desired response is achieved. I.V. dose should be given slowly over 1 to 2 minutes.

HYPERTENSION

▶**Adults:** 40 mg P.O. b.i.d., adjusted according to response.

▶**Contraindications & Precautions:** Contraindicated in patients with anuria or history of hypersensitivity to drug. Use cautiously in pregnant patients and those with hepatic cirrhosis.

Gabapentin (Neurontin)
▶**Indications & Dosage**

ADJUNCTIVE TREATMENT OF PARTIAL SEIZURES WITH AND WITHOUT SECONDARY GENERALIZATION

▶**Children older than age 12 years and adults:** 300 mg P.O. on day 1, 300 mg P.O. b.i.d. on day 2, and 300 mg P.O. t.i.d. on day 3. Increase dosage as needed and tolerated to 1,800 mg daily, in three divided doses. Usual dosage is 300 to 600 mg P.O. t.i.d., although dosages up to 3,600 mg/day have been well tolerated.

▶**Contraindications & Precautions:** Contraindicated in patients hypersensitive to drug.

Ganciclovir (DHPG) (Cytovene)
▶**Indications & Dosage**
TREATMENT OF CMV RETINITIS
▶**Infants and children older than 3 months and adults:** Initially, 5 mg/kg I.V.
   (given at a constant rate over 1 hour) q 12 hours for 14 to 21 days;
   followed by a maintenance dose of 5 mg/kg I.V. once daily for
   7 days weekly; or 6 mg/kg I.V. once daily for 5 days weekly.
   These I.V. infusions should be given at a constant rate over 1 hour.
   Alternatively, give a maintenance dose of 1,000 mg P.O. t.i.d. or
   500 mg P.O. q 3 hours while patient is awake, or six times daily.

PREVENTION OF CMV IN HIV-INFECTED PATIENTS
▶**Infants and children:** 5 mg/kg I.V. daily.
▶**Adolescents and adults:** 5 to 6 mg/kg I.V. daily for 5 to 7 days each
   week or 1 g P.O. t.i.d. with meals.

OTHER CMV INFECTIONS
▶**Children and adults:** 5 mg/kg I.V. over 1 hour q 12 hours for 14 to 21
   days; or 2.5 mg/kg I.V. q 8 hours for 14 to 21 days.
▶**Contraindications & Precautions:** Contraindicated in patients hypersensitive to drug and with an absolute neutrophil count below
   500/mm^3 or a platelet count below 25,000/mm^3. Use cautiously
   in patients with impaired renal function.

Gentamicin Sulfate (Cidomycin, Garamycin)
▶**Indications & Dosage**
SERIOUS INFECTION CAUSED BY SUSCEPTIBLE ORGANISM
▶**Neonates younger than age 1 week:** 2.5 mg/kg I.M. or I.V. infusion
   q 12 hours. For I.V. infusion, dilute in normal saline solution or
   D_5W and infuse over 30 minutes to 2 hours.
▶**Neonates older than age 1 week with normal renal function and infants:**
   2.5 mg/kg I.M. or I.V. infusion q 8 to 12 hours.
▶**Children with normal renal function:** 2 to 2.5 mg/kg I.M. or I.V. infusion
   q 8 hours.
▶**Adults with normal renal function:** 3 mg/kg/day I.M. or I.V. infusion (in
   50 to 100 ml of normal saline solution or D_5W infused over 30
   minutes to 2 hours) daily in divided doses q 8 hours. May be given
   by direct I.V. push if necessary. For life-threatening infections, patient
   may receive up to 5 mg/kg/day divided into three to four doses.

MENINGITIS
▶**Children:** systemic therapy as above; may also use 1 to 2 mg
   intrathecally daily.

▶**Adults:** systemic therapy as above; may also use 4 to 8 mg intra-thecally daily.

ENDOCARDITIS PROPHYLAXIS FOR GI OR GU PROCEDURE OR SURGERY

▶**Children:** 2 mg/kg I.M. or I.V. 30 to 60 minutes before procedure and q 8 hours after, for two doses. Given separately with aqueous penicillin g or ampicillin.

▶**Adults:** 1.5 mg/kg I.M. or I.V. 30 to 60 minutes before procedure and q 8 hours after, for two doses. Given separately with aqueous penicillin g or ampicillin.

EXTERNAL OCULAR INFECTION CAUSED BY SUSCEPTIBLE ORGANISM

▶**Children and adults:** Instill 1 or 2 gtt in eye q 4 hours. In severe infections, may use up to 2 gtt q hour. Apply ointment to lower conjunctival sac b.i.d. or t.i.d.

▶**Contraindications & Precautions:** Contraindicated in patients hyper-sensitive to drug and in those sensitive to other aminoglycosides, such as neomycin. Use systemic treatment cautiously in neonates, infants, and patients with renal or neuromuscular disorders.

Griseofulvin Microsize

▶**Indications & Dosage**

TINEA CORPORIS, TINEA CAPITIS, TINEA BARBAE, OR TINEA CRURIS INFECTION

▶**Children older than age 2 years:** 3.3 mg/lb ultramicrosize P.O. daily; or 125 to 250 mg microsize P.O. daily for children weighing 30 to 50 lb (14 to 23 kg) or 250 to 500 mg microsize P.O. daily for children weighing over 50 lb.

▶**Adolescents and adults:** 330 mg ultramicrosize P.O. daily, or 500 mg microsize P.O. daily.

TINEA PEDIS OR TINEA UNGUIUM INFECTION

▶**Children older than age 2 years:** 3.3 mg/lb ultramicrosize P.O. daily; or 125 to 250 mg microsize P.O. daily for children weighing 30 to 50 lb, or 250 to 500 mg microsize P.O. daily for children weighing over 50 lb.

▶**Adolescents and adults:** 660 mg ultramicrosize P.O. daily or 1 g micro-size P.O. daily.

▶**Contraindications & Precautions:** Contraindicated in patients hyper-sensitive to drug and in those with porphyria or hepatocellular failure. Use cautiously in penicillin-sensitive patients.

Heparin Sodium

▶**Indications & Dosage**

▶Heparin dosing is highly individualized according to patient's dis-ease, age, and renal and hepatic status.

DIC

►**Children:** 25 to 50 U/kg I.V. q 4 hours as a single injection or constant infusion. Discontinue if no improvement in 4 to 8 hours.

►**Adults:** 50 to 100 U/kg I.V. q 4 hours as a single injection or constant infusion. Discontinue if no improvement in 4 to 8 hours.

DEEP VEIN THROMBOSIS, PULMONARY EMBOLISM

►**Children:** 50 U/kg I.V. bolus, then maintenance at 50 to 100 U/kg I.V. drip q 4 hours. Constant infusion: 20,000 U/m^2 daily. Adjust dosage based on partial thromboplastin time (PTT).

►**Adults:** 5,000 to 10,000 U I.V. push, then adjust dose according to PTT results and give dose I.V. q 4 hours (usually 4,000 to 5,000 U); or 5,000 U I.V. bolus, then 20,000 to 40,000 U in 24 hours by I.V. infusion pump. Wait 4 to 6 hours after bolus dose and adjust hourly rate based on PTT.

TO MAINTAIN PATENCY OF I.V. INDWELLING CATHETERS

►**Children and adults:** 10 to 100 U as an I.V. flush (not intended for therapeutic use).

►**Contraindications & Precautions:** Contraindicated in patients hypersensitive to drug. Conditionally contraindicated in patients with active bleeding, hemophilia, thrombocytopenia, or hepatic disease with hypoprothrombinemia; suspected intracranial hemorrhage; suppurative thrombophlebitis; inaccessible ulcerative lesions (especially of the GI tract); extensive denudation of skin; ascorbic acid deficiency.

►Also conditionally contraindicated during or after brain, eye, or spinal cord surgery; during spinal tap or spinal anesthesia; or in subacute bacterial endocarditis, shock, advanced renal disease, threatened abortion, or severe hypertension.

Hydralazine Hydrochloride (Apresoline)
►**Indications & Dosage**

MODERATE TO SEVERE HYPERTENSION

►**Children:** 0.75 mg/kg P.O. daily in four divided doses (25 mg/m^2 daily); may increase gradually over 3 to 4 weeks to 7.5 mg/kg daily. I.M. or I.V. dosage is 0.4 to 1.2 mg/kg daily or 50 to 100 mg/m^2 daily in four to six divided doses. Initial parenteral dose should not exceed 20 mg.

►**Adults:** 10 mg P.O. q.i.d. for 2 to 4 days, then increased to 25 mg q.i.d. for remainder of week. If necessary, increase to 50 mg q.i.d. Maximum recommended dosage is 200 mg daily, but some patients may require 300 to 400 mg daily. For severe hypertension, 10 to 50 mg I.M. or 10 to 20 mg I.V. repeated p.r.n. Switch to oral antihypertensives as soon as possible. For hypertensive crisis during pregnancy, 5 mg I.V., followed by 5 to 10 mg I.V. q 20 to 30 minutes until blood pressure reduced (usual range, 5 to 20 mg).

▶**Contraindications & Precautions:** Contraindicated in patients hypersensitive to drug and in patients with coronary artery disease or mitral valvular rheumatic heart disease. Use cautiously in patients with suspected cardiac disease, CVA, or severe renal impairment and in those receiving other antihypertensives.

Hydrochlorothiazide (Apo-Hydro, Aquazide-H, Diuchlor H, Esidrix, Hydro-chlor, Hydro-D, HydroDIURIL, Mictrin, Neo-Codema, Novo-Hydrazide, Oretic, Urozide)

▶**Indications & Dosage**

EDEMA

▶**Infants younger than age 6 months:** up to 3 mg/kg P.O. daily divided b.i.d.

▶**Infants and children older than age 6 months:** 1 to 2 mg/kg P.O. daily divided b.i.d.

▶**Adults:** 25 to 200 mg P.O. daily for several days or until dry weight is attained. Maintenance dose is 25 to 100 mg P.O. daily or intermittently. A few refractory patients may require up to 200 mg daily.

HYPERTENSION

▶**Adults:** 25 to 50 mg P.O. once daily or in divided doses. Dose increased or decreased based on blood pressure.

▶**Contraindications & Precautions:** Contraindicated in patients with anuria or hypersensitivity to thiazides or other sulfonamide derivatives. Use cautiously in patients with severely impaired renal or hepatic function or progressive hepatic disease.

Hydrocortisone (Systemic) (Cortef, Cortenema, Hycort, Hydrocortone)

▶**Indications & Dosage**

SEVERE INFLAMMATION, ADRENAL INSUFFICIENCY
HYDROCORTISONE

▶**Children:** 0.56 to 8 mg/kg P.O. daily or 16 to 240 mg/m^2 P.O. daily divided into 3 or 4 doses.

▶**Adults:** 5 to 30 mg P.O. b.i.d., t.i.d., or q.i.d. (as much as 80 mg P.O. q.i.d. may be given in acute situations).

HYDROCORTISONE ACETATE

▶**Adults:** 10 to 75 mg into joints or soft tissue at 2- or 3-week intervals.

Dose varies with size of joint. In many cases, local anesthetics are injected with dose.

HYDROCORTISONE SODIUM PHOSPHATE
▶**Adults:** 15 to 240 mg S.C., I.M., or I.V. daily in divided doses q 12 hours.

HYDROCORTISONE SODIUM SUCCINATE
▶**Adults:** 100 to 500 mg I.M. or I.V., then 50 to 100 mg I.M. as indicated

SHOCK (OTHER THAN ADRENAL CRISIS)
HYDROCORTISONE SODIUM PHOSPHATE
▶**Children:** 0.16 to 1 mg/kg or 6 to 30 mg/m^2 I.M. daily or b.i.d.

HYDROCORTISONE SODIUM SUCCINATE
▶**Children:** 0.16 to 1 mg/kg or 6 to 30 mg m^2 I.M. or I.V. daily to b.i.d.
▶**Adults:** 100 to 500 mg I.M. or I.V. q 2 to 6 hours.

LIFE-THREATENING SHOCK
HYDROCORTISONE SODIUM SUCCINATE
▶**Adults:** 0.5 to 2 g I.V., repeated at 2- to 6-hour intervals, p.r.n. High-dose therapy should be continued only until patient's condition has stabilized. Therapy shouldn't be continued beyond 72 hours.

ADJUNCTIVE TREATMENT OF ULCERATIVE COLITIS AND PROCTITIS
HYDROCORTISONE
▶**Adults:** one enema (100 mg) nightly for 21 days.

HYDROCORTISONE ACETATE (RECTAL FOAM)
▶**Adults:** 90 mg (1 applicatorful) once or twice daily for 2 or 3 weeks; decrease frequency to every other day thereafter.

▶**Contraindications & Precautions:** Contraindicated in patients hypersensitive to any component of the formulation, in those with systemic fungal infections.

▶Use hydrocortisone sodium phosphate or succinate cautiously in patients with a recent MI, GI ulcer, renal disease, hypertension, osteoporosis, diabetes mellitus, hypothyroidism, cirrhosis, diverticulitis, ulcerative colitis, recent intestinal anastomosis, thromboembolic disorders, seizures, myasthenia gravis, heart failure, tuberculosis, ocular herpes simplex.

Hydromorphone Hydrochloride (Dilaudid)
▶**Indications & Dosage**
MODERATE TO SEVERE PAIN
▶**Adults:** 2 to 10 mg P.O. q 3 to 6 hours, p.r.n. or around the clock; or

2 to 4 mg I.M., S.C., or I.V. q 4 to 6 hours, p.r.n. or around the clock (I.V. dose should be given over 3 to 5 minutes); or 3 mg rectal suppository q 6 to 8 hours, p.r.n. or around the clock. (Give 1 to 14 mg Dilaudid-HP S.C. or I.M. q 4 to 6 hours.)

▶**Contraindications & Precautions:** Contraindicated in patients hypersensitive to drug, those with intracranial lesions from increased intracranial pressure, and those with conditions that depress ventilator function, such as status asthmaticus, COPD, cor pulmonale, emphysema, and kyphoscoliosis.

▶Use cautiously in debilitated patients and in those with hepatic or renal disease, Addison's disease, hypothyroidism, prostatic hyperplasia, or urethral strictures.

Hydroxyzine Hydrochloride (Atarax)
▶**Indications & Dosage**

ANXIETY; TENSION, HYPERKINESIA

▶**Children younger than age 6 years:** 50 mg P.O. daily in divided doses.

▶**Children older than age 6 years:** 50 to 100 mg P.O. daily in divided doses.

▶**Adults:** 50 to 100 mg P.O. q.i.d.

PRURITUS CAUSED BY ALLERGIC CONDITIONS

▶**Children younger than age 6 years:** 50 mg P.O. daily in divided doses.

▶**Children ages 6 years and older:** 50 to 100 mg P.O. daily in divided doses.

▶**Adults:** 25 mg P.O. t.i.d. or q.i.d.

▶**Contraindications & Precautions:** Contraindicated in patients hypersensitive to drug and during early pregnancy.

Ibuprofen (Advil, Motrin)
▶**Indications & Dosage**

MILD TO MODERATE PAIN

▶**Children:** 10 mg/kg P.O. q 6 to 8 hours. Maximum 40 mg/kg.

▶**Adults:** 400 mg P.O. q 4 to 6 hours.

JUVENILE ARTHRITIS

▶**Children:** 20 to 40 mg/kg/day P.O., divided into three or four doses. For mild disease, 20 mg/kg/day in divided doses.

FEVER REDUCTION

▶**Infants and children ages 6 months to 12 years:** 5 mg/kg P.O. q 6 to 8 hours p.r.n. if baseline temperature is 102.5° F (39.2° C) or below;

10 mg/kg P.O. if baseline temperature is over 102.5° F. Recommended maximum 40 mg/kg daily.

▶**Adults:** 200 to 400 mg P.O. q 4 to 6 hours, p.r.n. Don't exceed 1,200 mg/day or take for more than 3 days.

▶**Contraindications & Precautions:** Contraindicated in patients hypersensitive to drug and in those who have the syndrome of nasal polyps, angioedema, and bronchospastic reaction to aspirin or other NSAIDs.

▶Use cautiously in patients with impaired renal or hepatic function, GI disorders, peptic ulcer disease, cardiac decompensation, hypertension, or known coagulation defects. Chewable tablets contain aspartame; use cautiously in patients with phenylketonuria.

Imipenem and Cilastatin (Primaxin)
▶**Indications & Dosage**

MILD TO MODERATE LOWER RESPIRATORY TRACT, SKIN AND SKIN-STRUCTURE, OR GYNECOLOGIC INFECTION

▶**Adults weighing at least 70 kg:** 500 to 750 mg I.M. q 12 hours.

MILD TO MODERATE INTRA-ABDOMINAL INFECTION

▶**Adults weighing at least 70 kg:** 750 mg I.M. q 12 hours.

SERIOUS RESPIRATORY OR URINARY TRACT INFECTION; INTRA-ABDOMINAL, GYNECOLOGIC, BONE, JOINT, OR SKIN INFECTION; BACTERIAL SEPTICEMIA; ENDOCARDITIS

▶**Neonates younger than 1 week and weighing 1.5 kg (3.3 lb) or more:** 25 mg/kg I.V. q 12 hours.

▶**Neonates ages 1 to 4 weeks and weighing 1.5 kg or more:** 25 mg/kg I.V. q 8 hours.

▶**Infants ages 4 weeks to 3 months and weighing 1.5 kg or more:** 25 mg/kg I.V. q 6 hours.

▶**Infants and children ages 3 months and older:** 15 to 25 mg/kg I.V. q 6 hours. Maximum daily dose in pediatric patients is 2 g daily in infections by fully susceptible bacteria or 4 g daily in infections by moderately susceptible bacteria.

▶**Adults weighing at least 70 kg:** 250 mg to 1 g by I.V. infusion q 6 to 8 hours. Maximum 50 mg/kg/day or 4 g/day, whichever is less.

▶**Contraindications & Precautions:** Contraindicated in patients hypersensitive to drug. Imipenem and cilastatin sodium reconstituted with lidocaine hydrochloride for I.M. injection is contraindicated in patients hypersensitive to local anesthetics of the amide type and in patients with severe shock or heart block.

▶Use cautiously in patients with impaired renal function, seizure disorders, or allergy to penicillins or cephalosporins.

Immune Globulin (Gamma Globulin, Ig, Immune Serum Globulin, ISG) (IGIV, Sandoglobulin, Venoglobulin)

▶Indications & Dosage

AGAMMAGLOBULINEMIA, HYPOGAMMAGLOBULINEMIA, IMMUNE DEFICIENCY (IGIV)

▶**Children and adults:** For Gamimune N, 100 to 200 mg/kg or 2 to 4 ml/kg I.V. infusion monthly. Infusion rate is 0.01 to 0.02 ml/kg/minute for 30 minutes. Rate can then be increased to maximum of 0.08 ml/kg/minute for remainder of infusion.

▶For Gammagard S/D, 200 to 400 mg/kg I.V., followed by 100 mg/kg monthly. Start infusion at 0.5 ml/kg/hour, gradually increasing to maximum of 4 ml/kg/hour.

▶For Gammar-P I.V., 200 to 400 mg/kg q 3 to 4 weeks. Infusion rate is 0.01 ml/kg/minute, increasing to 0.02 ml/kg/minute after 15 to 30 minutes, with gradual increase to 0.06 ml/kg/minute.

▶For Iveegam, 200 mg/kg I.V. monthly. If response is inadequate, doses may be increased up to 800 mg/kg or drug may be given more frequently. Infuse at 1 to 2 ml/minute.

▶For Polygam S/D, 100 mg/kg I.V. monthly. A first dose of 200 to 400 mg/kg may be given. Start infusion at 0.5 ml/kg/hour, gradually increasing to maximum of 4 ml/kg/hour.

▶For Sandoglobulin, 200 mg/kg I.V. monthly. Start with 0.5 to 1 ml/minute of a 3% solution; increase up to 2.5 ml/minute gradually after 15 to 30 minutes.

▶For Venoglobulin-I, 200 mg/kg I.V. monthly; may be increased to 300 to 400 mg/kg and may be repeated more often than once monthly. Infuse at 0.01 to 0.02 ml/kg/minute for 30 minutes, then increase to 0.04 ml/kg/minute or higher if tolerated.

▶For Venoglobulin-S, 200 mg/kg I.V. monthly. Increase to 300 to 400 mg/kg monthly or give more often if adequate IgI levels aren't achieved. Start infusion at 0.01 to 0.02 ml/kg/minute for 30 minutes, then increase 5% solutions to 0.04 ml/kg/minute and 10% solutions to 0.05 ml/kg/minute if tolerated.

HEPATITIS A EXPOSURE (IGIM)

▶**Children and adults:** 0.02 to 0.04 ml/kg I.M. as soon as possible after exposure. Up to 0.1 ml/kg may be given after prolonged or intense exposure.

MEASLES EXPOSURE (IGIM)

▶**Children and adults:** 0.25 ml/kg within 6 days after exposure.

POSTEXPOSURE PROPHYLAXIS OF MEASLES (IGIM)

▶**Children and adults:** 0.5 ml/kg I.M. within 6 days after exposure.

CHICKENPOX EXPOSURE (IGIM)
►**Children and adults:** 0.6 to 1.2 ml/kg I.M. as soon as exposed.

RUBELLA EXPOSURE IN FIRST TRIMESTER OF PREGNANCY (IGIM)
►**Women:** 0.55 ml/kg I.M. as soon as exposed.

IDIOPATHIC THROMBOCYTOPENIC PURPURA (IGIV)
►**Children and adults:** 400 mg/kg Sandoglobulin I.V. for 2 to 5 consecutive days; or 400 mg/kg Gamimune N 5% for 5 days or 1,000 mg/kg Gamimune N 10% for 1 to 2 days. Maintenance dose is 400 to 1,000 mg/kg I.V. of Gamimune N 10% as a single infusion to maintain a platelet count greater than 30,000/mm^3.

►**Contraindications & Precautions:** Contraindicated in patients hypersensitive to drug.

Indomethacin (Indocin)
►**Indications & Dosages**

TO CLOSE A HEMODYNAMICALLY SIGNIFICANT PATENT DUCTUS ARTERIOSUS IN A PREMATURE INFANT (I.V. FORM ONLY)
►**Neonates younger than 48 hours:** 0.2 mg/kg I.V. followed by 2 doses of 0.1 mg/kg at 12- to 24-hour intervals.

►**Neonates ages 2 to 7 days:** 0.2 mg/kg I.V. followed by 2 doses of 0.2 mg/kg at 12- to 24-hour intervals.

►**Neonates older than 7 days:** 0.2 mg/kg I.V. followed by 2 doses of 0.25 mg/kg at 12- to 24-hour intervals.

MODERATE TO SEVERE ARTHRITIS, ANKYLOSING SPONDYLITIS, JUVENILE RHEUMATOID ARTHRITIS
►**Children ages 2 to 14 years:** 2 mg/kg P.O. daily in divided doses using conventional capsules. Dosage may be increased to 4 mg/kg daily in divided doses but don't exceed 200 mg daily. As symptoms subside, reduce dosage to lowest effective level until drug is discontinued.

►**Adults:** 25 mg P.O. b.i.d. or t.i.d. with food or antacid; may increase dose by 25 to 50 mg daily q 7 days up to 200 mg daily; or 50 mg P.R. q.i.d. Alternatively, sustained-release capsules may be given: 75 mg to start, in the morning or h.s., followed, if necessary, by 75 mg b.i.d.

►**Contraindications & Precautions:** Contraindicated in patients hypersensitive to drug and patient with a history of aspirin- or NSAID-induced asthma, rhinitis, or urticaria. Also contraindicated in pregnancy and while breast-feeding. Also contraindicated in infants with active bleeding, coagulation defects, thrombocytopenia, congenital heart disease in whom patency of the ductus arteriosus is needed for satisfactory pulmonary or systemic blood flow, necrotizing enterocolitis, or impaired renal function.

Insulin (Regular)
▶**Indications & Dosage**
▶*See Chapter 93*

Ipratropium Bromide (Atrovent)
▶**Indications & Dosage**
BRONCHOSPASM

▶**Children ages 5 to 12 years:** 125 to 250 mcg nebulizer solution dissolved in normal saline solution q 4 to 6 hours via nebulizer.

▶**Children ages 12 years and older and adults:** Usually, 2 inhalations (36 mcg) q.i.d.; patient may take additional inhalations, p.r.n., but shouldn't exceed 12 inhalations in 24 hours or 500 mcg q 6 to 8 hours via oral nebulizer.

▶**Contraindications & Precautions:** Contraindicated in patients hypersensitive to drug, to atropine or its derivatives, or to soya lecithin or related food products, such as soybeans and peanuts. Use cautiously in patients with angle-closure glaucoma or bladder-neck obstruction.

Isoniazid (INH)
▶**Indications & Dosage**
PRIMARY TREATMENT FOR ACTIVE TB

▶**Infants and children:** 10 to 20 mg/kg P.O. or I.M. daily in a single dose up to 300 to 500 mg/day, continued for 18 months to 2 years.

▶**Adults:** 5 mg/kg P.O. or I.M. daily in a single dose, up to 300 mg/day, continued for 9 months to 2 years.

▶Administration of at least one other effective antituberculotic is recommended.

PRIMARY TREATMENT FOR ACTIVE TB IN COMBINATION WITH OTHER ANTITUBERCULOTICS (EXCEPT RIFAMPIN)

▶**Children:** 20 to 40 mg/kg 2 or 3 times weekly, up to 900 mg/dose.

▶**Adults:** 15 mg/kg two or three times weekly, up to 900 mg/dose.

PROPHYLAXIS FOR THOSE CLOSELY EXPOSED OR WITH POSITIVE SKIN TEST

▶**Infants and children:** 10 to 15 mg/kg P.O. as daily single dose, up to 300 mg/day, continued for 6 months to 1 year.

▶**Adults:** 300 mg P.O. as daily single dose, continued for 6 months to 1 year.

▶**Contraindications & Precautions:** Contraindicated in patients with acute hepatic disease. Use cautiously in patients with seizure disorders (especially those taking phenytoin), severe renal impairment.

Ketoconazole (Nizoral)

►**Indications & Dosage**

SEVERE FUNGAL INFECTION CAUSED BY SUSCEPTIBLE ORGANISM

►**Children older than age 2 years:** 3.3 to 6.6 mg/kg P.O. daily as a single dose.

►**Adults:** 200 mg P.O. daily as a single dose. May be increased to 400 mg once daily in patients who do not respond to lower dosage.

TOPICAL TREATMENT OF TINEA CORPORIS, TINEA CRURIS, TINEA VERSICOLOR, AND TINEA PEDIS

►**Adolescents and adults:** Apply once daily or b.i.d. for about 2 weeks; for tinea pedis apply for 6 weeks.

►**Contraindications & Precautions:** Contraindicated in patients hypersensitive to drug and in those taking cisapride because of possible serious adverse CV effects. Use oral form cautiously in patients with hepatic disease.

Levalbuterol Hydrochloride (Xopenex)

►**Indications & Dosage**

TO PREVENT OR TREAT BRONCHOSPASM IN PATIENTS WITH REVERSIBLE OBSTRUCTIVE AIRWAY DISEASE

►**Children ages 12 years and older and adults:** 0.63 mg t.i.d. q 6 to 8 hours, by oral inhalation via a nebulizer. Patients with more severe asthma who don't respond adequately to 0.63 mg may benefit from 1.25 mg t.i.d.

►**Contraindications & Precautions:** Contraindicated in patients hypersensitive to the drug.

►Use cautiously in patients with cardiovascular disorders, especially coronary insufficiency, hypertension, and arrhythmias. Also use cautiously in patients with seizure disorders, hyperthyroidism, or diabetes mellitus.

Levothyroxine Sodium (T_4 L-thyroxine sodium) (Eltroxin, Levo-T, Levothroid, Levoxine, Levoxyl, Synthroid)

►**Indications & Dosage**

CONGENITAL HYPOTHYROIDISM

►**Children younger than age 1 year:** 25 to 50 mcg P.O. daily, increased to 50 mcg in 4 to 6 weeks.

►**Contraindications & Precautions:** Contraindicated in patients hypersensitive to drug; in patients with acute MI or in patients with untreated or uncorrected adrenal insufficiency. Use cautiously in patients with renal impairment, angina, hypertension, ischemia, or other CV disorders.

Lidocaine (Xylocaine)

▶**Indications & Dosage**

VENTRICULAR ARRHYTHMIAS FROM MI, CARDIAC MANIPULATION, OR CARDIAC GLYCOSIDES

▶**Children:** 0.5 to 1 mg/kg by I.V. bolus, followed by infusion of 20 to 50 mcg/kg/minute.

▶**Adults:** 50 to 100 mg (1 to 1.5 mg/kg) by I.V. bolus at 25 to 50 mg/minute. Repeat bolus q 3 to 5 minutes until arrhythmias subside or adverse effects develop. Don't exceed 300-mg total bolus during a 1-hour period. Simultaneously, begin constant infusion of 1 to 4 mg/minute. If single bolus has been given, repeat smaller bolus (usually 1/2 initial bolus) 5 to 10 minutes after start of infusion to maintain therapeutic serum level. After 24 hours of continuous infusion, decrease rate by half.

▶**Contraindications & Precautions:** Contraindicated in patients hypersensitive to amide-type local anesthetics and in patients with Stokes-Adams syndrome, Wolff-Parkinson-White syndrome, and severe SA, AV, or intraventricular block (without an artificial pacemaker). Also contraindicated in patients with septicemia, severe hypertension, spinal deformities, and neurologic disorders.

▶Use cautiously in patients with renal or hepatic disease, complete or second-degree heart block, sinus bradycardia, or heart failure; and in those weighing less than 110 lb.

Lindane (Gamma Benzene Hexachloride) (G-well, Kwell, Scabene)

▶**Indications & Dosage**

▶**Note:** In no case should more than 2 oz be used by one person in one application.

SCABIES

▶**Children and adults:** After bathing with soap and water, apply a thin layer of cream or lotion and gently massage it on all skin surfaces, moving from the neck to the toes. After 8 to 12 hours, remove drug by bathing and scrubbing well. Treatment may be repeated after 1 week if needed.

PEDICULOSIS

▶**Children and adults:** Apply shampoo to dry, affected area and wait 4 minutes. Then add a small amount of water and lather for 4 to 5 minutes; rinse thoroughly. Comb hair to remove nits. Treatment may be repeated after 1 week if needed.

▶**Contraindications & Precautions:** Contraindicated in patients hypersensitive to drug or in patients with seizure disorders. Also contraindicated in premature neonates.

Lorazepam (Ativan)
►**Indications & Dosage**

STATUS EPILEPTICUS

►**Neonates:** 0.05 mg/kg I.V. over 2 to 5 minutes; may repeat dose in
 10 to 15 minutes p.r.n., based on clinical response.

►**Infants and children:** 0.1 mg/kg I.V. over 2 to 5 minutes; may give a
 second dose of 0.05 mg/kg I.V. in 10 to 15 minutes p.r.n. Do not
 exceed 4 mg/dose.

►**Adults:** 4 mg I.V. over 2 to 5 minutes; may give a second dose of
 4 mg I.V. in 10 to 15 minutes p.r.n.

**ANXIETY, TENSION, AGITATION, IRRITABILITY, ESPECIALLY IN ANXIETY NEUROSES
OR ORGANIC (ESPECIALLY GI OR CV) DISORDERS**

►**Adolescents and adults:** 2 to 6 mg P.O. daily in divided doses;
 maximum 10 mg/day.

►**Contraindications & Precautions:** Contraindicated in patients hypersensitive to drug or other benzodiazepines. Also contraindicated
 in patients with acute angle-closure glaucoma. Use cautiously in
 patients with pulmonary, renal, or hepatic impairment and in
 acutely ill or debilitated patients. Don't give to pregnant patients,
 especially during the first trimester.

Mannitol
►**Indications & Dosage**

TREATMENT OF OLIGURIA

►**Children younger than age 12 years:** 2 g/kg or 60 g/m^2 I.V.

►**Children older than age 12 years and adults:** 50 to 100 g as a 15% to
 20% solution I.V. over 90 minutes to several hours.

PREVENTION OF OLIGURIA OR ACUTE RENAL FAILURE

►**Children older than age 12 years and adults:** 50 to 100 g followed by a
 5% to 10% solution I.V. Exact concentration is determined by fluid
 requirements.

TREATMENT OF EDEMA AND ASCITES

►**Children younger than age 12 years:** 2 g/kg over 60 g/m^2 I.V. as a
 15% to 20% solution over 2 to 6 hours.

►**Children older than age 12 years and adults:** 100 g as a 10% to 20%
 solution I.V. over 2 to 6 hours.

TO REDUCE INTRAOCULAR PRESSURE OR INTRACRANIAL PRESSURE

►**Children younger than age 12 years:** 2 g/kg or 60 g/m^2 I.V. as a 15%
 to 20% solution over 30 to 60 minutes.

►Children older than age 12 years and adults: 1.5 to 2 g/kg as a 15% to 25% solution I.V. over 30 to 60 minutes administered 60 to 90 minutes before surgery.

►**Contraindications & Precautions:** Contraindicated in patients with hypersensitivity to drug and in those with anuria, severe pulmonary congestion, frank pulmonary edema, severe heart failure, severe dehydration, metabolic edema, progressive renal disease or dysfunction, or active intracranial bleeding except during craniotomy. Use cautiously in pregnant patients.

Mebendazole (Vermox)
►**Indications & Dosage**

PINWORM INFESTATIONS

►Children older than age 2 years and adults: 100 mg P.O. as a single dose. If infection persists 3 weeks later, repeat treatment.

OTHER ROUNDWORM, WHIPWORM, AND HOOKWORM INFESTATIONS

►Children older than age 2 years and adults: 100 mg P.O. b.i.d. for 3 days. If infection persists 3 weeks later, repeat treatment.

CAPILLARIASIS

►Children and adults: 200 mg b.i.d. for 20 days.

TOXOCARIASIS

►Children and adults: 100 to 200 mg b.i.d. for 5 days.

DRACUNCULIASIS

►Adults: 400 to 800 mg daily for 6 days.

MANSONELLA PERSTANS INFESTATIONS

►Adults: 100 mg b.i.d. for 30 days.

ANGIOSTRONGYLUS CANTONENSIS INFESTATIONS

►Children and adults: 100 mg b.i.d. for 5 days.

ANGIOSTRONGYLUS COSTARI CENSIS

►Children and adults: 200 to 400 mg P.O. t.i.d. for 10 days.

►**Contraindications and Precautions:** Contraindicated in patients with hypersensitivity to drug.

Meperidine Hydrochloride (Pethidine Hydrochloride) (Demerol)
►**Indications & Dosage**

MODERATE TO SEVERE PAIN

►Children: 1.1 to 1.8 mg/kg P.O., I.M., or S.C. q 3 to 4 hours p.r.n., or 175 mg/m^2 daily in six divided doses. Maximum single dose for children shouldn't exceed 100 mg.

▶**Adults:** 50 to 150 mg P.O., I.M., or S.C. q 3 to 4 hours.

PREOPERATIVELY

▶**Children:** 0.5–1 mg/kg I.M. or S.C., 30 to 90 minutes before surgery. Don't exceed adult dose.

▶**Adults:** 50 to 100 mg I.M. or S.C., 30 to 90 minutes before surgery.

▶**Contraindications & Precautions:** Contraindicated in patients with hypersensitivity to drug and in those who have received MAO inhibitors within the past 14 days. Use cautiously in debilitated patients and in those with increased intracranial pressure, head injury, asthma, other respiratory conditions, supraventricular tachycardia, seizures, acute abdominal conditions, renal or hepatic disease, hypothyroidism, Addison's disease, and urethral stricture.

Meropenem (Merrem)
▶**Indications & Dosage**

COMPLICATED APPENDICITIS AND PERITONITIS; BACTERIAL MENINGITIS

▶**Infants and children ages 3 months and older weighing less than 50 kg (110 lb):** Give 20 mg/kg (intra-abdominal infection) or 40 mg/kg (bacterial meningitis) q 8 hours over 15 to 30 minutes as I.V. infusion or over about 3 to 5 minutes as I.V. bolus injection.

▶**Children weighing more than 50 kg:** 1 g I.V. q 8 hours for treating intra-abdominal infections and 2 g I.V. q 8 hours for treating meningitis.

▶**Adolescents and adults:** Administer 1 g I.V. q 8 hours over 15 to 30 minutes as I.V. infusion or over about 3 to 5 minutes as I.V. bolus injection.

▶**Contraindications & Precautions:** Contraindicated in patients with hypersensitivity to any component of drug or other drugs in the same class and in those who have demonstrated anaphylactic reactions to beta-lactams. Use cautiously in patients with history of seizure disorders or impaired renal function.

Methylphenidate Hydrochloride (Ritalin)
▶**Indications & Dosage**

ATTENTION DEFICIT HYPERACTIVITY DISORDER (ADHD)

▶**Children ages 6 years and older:** Initially, 5 to 10 mg P.O. daily before breakfast and lunch, increased in 5- to 10-mg increments weekly p.r.n. until an optimum daily dose of 2 mg/kg is reached, not to exceed 60 mg/day. Usual effective daily dose, 20 to 30 mg.

NARCOLEPSY

▶**Adults:** 10 mg P.O. b.i.d. or t.i.d. 30 to 45 minutes before meals. Dose varies with patient needs; average dose is 40 to 60 mg/day. When using sustained-release tablets, calculate regular dose in q 8-hour intervals and administer as such.

▶**Contraindications & Precautions:** Contraindicated in patients with hypersensitivity to drug, glaucoma, motor tics, family history of or diagnosis of Tourette syndrome, or history of marked anxiety, tension, or agitation. Use cautiously in patients with history of seizures, drug abuse, hypertension, or EEG abnormalities.

Methylprednisolone (Systemic) (Solu-Medrol)

ANTI-INFLAMMATORY OR IMMUNOSUPPRESSIVE

▶**Oral, IM, IV:** 0.5–1.7 mg/kg/day or 5–25 mg/m^2/day in divided doses every 6–12 hours

▶**"Pulse Therapy":** 15–30 mg/kg/dose over >30 minutes given once daily for 3 days

▶**Status Asthmaticus IV:** 2 mg/kg/dose given one time followed by 0.5–1 mg/kg/dose IV q 6 hrs for 5 days

TREATMENT OR MINIMIZATION OF MOTOR AND SENSORY DEFECTS CAUSED BY ACUTE SPINAL CORD INJURY

▶**Adults:** Initially, 30 mg/kg I.V. over 15 minutes followed in 45 minutes by I.V. infusion of 5.4 mg/kg/hour for 23 hours.

▶**Contraindications & Precautions:** Contraindications: Administration of live virus vaccines, systemic fungal infections

▶Use cautiously in patients with hypothyroidism, cirrhosis, hypertension, congestive heart failure, ulcerative colitis, thromboembolic disorders.

Metoclopramide Hydrochloride (Reglan)

▶**Indications & Dosage**

PREVENTION OR REDUCTION OF NAUSEA AND VOMITING INDUCED BY HIGHLY EMETOGENIC CHEMOTHERAPY

▶**Children:** 1 mg/kg I.V. as a single dose. May be repeated one time after 1 hour.

▶**Adolescents and adults:** 1 to 2 mg/kg I.V. q 2 hours for two doses, beginning 30 minutes before emetogenic chemotherapy drug administration, then q 3 hours for three doses.

DELAYED GASTRIC EMPTYING SECONDARY TO DIABETIC GASTROPARESIS

▶**Adolescents and adults:** 10 mg P.O. 30 minutes before meals and h.s. for 2 to 8 weeks, depending on response; or 10 mg I.V. over 2 minutes.

GASTROESOPHAGEAL REFLUX

►**Adolescents and adults:** 10 to 15 mg P.O. q.i.d., p.r.n., taken 30 minutes before meals and h.s.

POSTOPERATIVE NAUSEA AND VOMITING

►**Adolescents and adults:** 10 to 20 mg I.M. near end of surgical procedure, repeated q 4 to 6 hours p.r.n.

►**Contraindications & Precautions:** Contraindicated in patients with GI obstruction and in those with hypersensitivity to drug, pheochromocytoma, or seizure disorders. Use cautiously in patients with history of depression or hypertension.

Metronidazole (Flagyl)
►**Indications & Dosage**

BACTERIAL INFECTIONS CAUSED BY ANAEROBIC MICROORGANISMS

►**Neonates up to 4 weeks of age weighing less than 1.2 kg (2.6 lb):** 7.5 mg/kg P.O. or I.V. q 48 hours.

►**Neonates 1 week old or younger weighing 1.2 to 2 kg (2.6 to 4.4 lb):** 7.5 mg/kg P.O. or I.V. q 24 hours.

►**Neonates 1 week old or younger weighing more than 2 kg:** 7.5 mg/kg P.O. or I.V. q 12 hours.

►**Neonates older than 1 week weighing 1.2 to 2 kg:** 7.5 mg/kg P.O. or I.V. q 12 hours.

►**Neonates older than 1 week weighing more than 2 kg:** 15 mg/kg P.O. or I.V. q 12 hours.

►**Infants and children:** 7.5 mg/kg P.O. or I.V. q 6 hours. Maximum dose 4 g/day.

►**Adults:** Loading dose is 15 mg/kg I.V. infused over 1 hour (about 1 g for a 70-kg [154-lb] adult). Maintenance dose is 7.5 mg/kg I.V. or P.O. q 6 hours (about 500 mg for a 70-kg adult). First maintenance dose should be administered 6 hours after the loading dose. Maximum dose shouldn't exceed 4 g daily.

AMEBIC HEPATIC ABSCESS

►**Children:** 30 to 50 mg/kg P.O. daily (in three divided doses) for 10 days, or 1.3 g/m^2 P.O. daily in three divided doses for 5 to 10 days.

►**Adults:** 500 to 750 mg P.O. t.i.d. for 5 to 10 days.

TRICHOMONIASIS

►**Children:** 15 mg/kg P.O. daily (in three divided doses) for 7 to 10 days, or 40 mg/kg P.O. as a single dose. Maximum dose 2 g.

►**Adults (both males and females):** 375-mg capsule P.O. b.i.d. for 7 days, or 500-mg tablet P.O. b.i.d. for 7 days or a single dose of 2 g P.O. or divided into two doses given on same day.

GIARDIASIS

▶**Children:** 15 mg/kg P.O. daily in three divided doses for 5 to 7 days.

▶**Adults:** 250 mg P.O. t.i.d. for 5 days, or 2 g once daily for 3 days.

CLOSTRIDIUM DIFFICILE

▶**Children:** 30 to 50 mg/kg P.O. daily in three to four divided doses for 7 to 10 days. Don't exceed adult dose.

▶**Adults:** 750 mg to 2 g P.O. daily, in three to four divided doses for 7 to 14 days.

***HELICOBACTER PYLORI* ASSOCIATED WITH PEPTIC ULCER DISEASE**

▶**Children:** 15 to 20 mg/kg P.O. daily, divided in two doses for 4 weeks (in combination with amoxicillin and/or bismuth subsalicylate).

▶**Adults:** 250 to 500 mg P.O. t.i.d. (in combination with at least one other drug active against *H. pylori*).

BACTERIAL VAGINOSIS

▶**Adults:** 500 mg P.O. b.i.d. for 7 days; or 2 g P.O. as a single dose.

PELVIC INFLAMMATORY DISEASE

▶**Adults:** 500 mg P.O. b.i.d. for 14 days (given with 400 mg b.i.d. of ofloxacin).

▶**Contraindications & Precautions:** Contraindicated in patients with hypersensitivity to drug or other nitroimidazole derivatives. Use cautiously in patients with history of blood dyscrasia or alcoholism, hepatic disease, retinal or visual field changes, or CNS disorders and in those receiving hepatotoxic drugs.

Mezlocillin Sodium (Mezlin)
▶**Indications & Dosage**
INFECTIONS CAUSED BY SUSCEPTIBLE ORGANISMS

▶**Neonates 7 days old or younger:** 75 mg/kg I.V. every 12 hours.

▶**Neonates older than 7 days weighing 2 kg (4.4 lb) or less:** 75 mg/kg I.V. every 8 hours.

▶**Neonates older than 7 days weighing more than 2 kg:** 75 mg/kg I.V. every 6 hours.

▶**Infants and children 1 month to 12 years:** 50 to 75 mg/kg I.M. or I.V. q 4 to 6 hours; or for mild to moderate infections 50 to 100 mg/kg daily in four divided doses; for severe infections, 200 to 300 mg/kg daily in four to six divided doses.

▶**Adults:** 200 to 300 mg/kg I.V. or I.M. daily given in four to six divided doses. Usual dose is 3 g q 4 hours or 4 g q 6 hours. For serious infections, up to 24 g daily may be administered.

▶**Contraindications & Precautions:** Contraindicated in patients with hypersensitivity to drug or other penicillins. Use cautiously in patients with bleeding tendencies, uremia, hypokalemia, or allergy to cephalosporins.

Midazolam Hydrochloride (Versed)
▶**Indications & Dosage**

CONTINUOUS INFUSION FOR SEDATION OF INTUBATED AND MECHANICALLY VENTILATED PATIENTS AS A COMPONENT OF ANESTHESIA OR DURING TREATMENT IN THE CRITICAL CARE SETTING

▶**Preterm neonates (born less than 32 weeks' gestation):** 0.03 mg/kg/hour (0.5 mcg/kg/minute) I.V. Adjust rate p.r.n., using lowest possible rate.

▶**Term neonates (born at 32 weeks' gestation or later):** 0.06 mg/kg/hour (1 mcg/kg/minute) I.V. Adjust rate p.r.n., using lowest possible rate.

▶**Children:** 0.05 to 0.2 mg/kg I.V. over 2 to 3 minutes followed by continuous I.V. infusion at rate of 0.06 to 0.12 mg/kg/hour (1 to 2 mcg/kg/minute). Dose may be titrated up or down by 25% of the initial or subsequent infusion rate to obtain optimal sedation.

▶**Adults:** If a loading dose is necessary to rapidly initiate sedation, give 0.01 to 0.05 mg/kg I.V. over several minutes, repeated at 10- to 15-minute intervals until adequate sedation is achieved. For maintenance of sedation, usual infusion rate is 0.02 to 0.10 mg/kg/hour (1 to 7 mg/hour). Infusion rate should be titrated to the desired amount of sedation. Drug can be titrated up or down by 25% to 50% of the initial infusion rate to achieve optimal sedation.

PREOPERATIVE SEDATION (TO INDUCE SLEEPINESS OR DROWSINESS AND RELIEVE APPREHENSION)

▶**Adults younger than age 60 years:** 0.07 to 0.08 mg/kg I.M. about 1 hour before surgery. May be administered with atropine or scopolamine and reduced doses of narcotics.

PREOPERATIVE OR PROCEDURAL SEDATION (TO INDUCE SLEEPINESS OR DROWSINESS AND RELIEVE APPREHENSION) IN PEDIATRIC PATIENTS

I.M.

▶**Children:** 0.1 to 0.15 mg/kg I.M.; doses up to 0.5 mg/kg have been used in anxious patients.

I.V.

▶**Infants and children ages 6 months to 5 years:** 0.05 to 0.1 mg/kg I.V. over 2 to 3 minutes. Additional doses may be given in small increments after 2 to 3 minutes. A total dose of up to 0.6 mg/kg, but not exceeding 6 mg, may be used.

▶**Children ages 6 to 12 years:** 0.025 to 0.05 mg/kg I.V. over 2 to 3 minutes. Additional doses may be given in small increments after 2 to 3 minutes, up to 0.4 mg/kg, but not exceeding 10 mg, may be used.

▶**Children and adolescents 12 to 16 years:** Dose as adults, with total dose not exceeding 10 mg.

CONSCIOUS SEDATION

▶**Young adults:** Initially, 1 to 2.5 mg I.V. administered over at least 2 minutes; repeat in 2 minutes, if needed, in small increments of initial dose over at least 2 minutes to achieve desired effect. Total dose up to 5 mg may be used. Additional doses to maintain desired level of sedation may be given by slow titration in increments of 25% of dose used to reach the sedation endpoint.

▶**Contraindications & Precautions:** Contraindicated in patients with hypersensitivity to drug or acute angle-closure glaucoma and in those experiencing shock, coma, or acute alcohol intoxication. Use cautiously in patients with uncompensated acute illnesses and in debilitated patients.

Mineral Oil
▶**Indications & Dosage**

CONSTIPATION, PREPARATION FOR BOWEL STUDIES OR SURGERY

▶**Children ages 2 to 6 years:** 30- to 60-ml enema.

▶**Children ages 6 to 11 years:** 5 to 15 ml P.O. daily as a single dose or in divided doses, or 30- to 60-ml enema.

▶**Adults and children ages 12 years and older:** 15 to 45 ml P.O. as a single dose or in divided doses, or 120-ml enema.

▶**Contraindications & Precautions:** Contraindicated in patients with abdominal pain, nausea, vomiting, or other symptoms of appendicitis or acute surgical abdomen, and in those with fecal impaction or intestinal obstruction or perforation. Contraindicated in patients with colostomy, ileostomy, ulcerative colitis, and diverticulitis. Use cautiously in debilitated patients and in the young.

Morphine Hydrochloride (morphine sulfate)
SEVERE PAIN

▶**Children:** 0.1 to 0.2 mg/kg S.C. or I.M. q 4 hours. Maximum dose is 15 mg. Alternatively, give 0.05 to 0.1 mg/kg I.V. slowly.

▶**Adults:** 10 mg q 4 hours S.C. or I.M. or 10 to 30 mg P.O., or 10 to 20 mg P.R. q 4 hours, p.r.n. or around the clock. May be injected slow I.V. (over 4 to 5 minutes) 2.5 to 15 mg diluted in 4 to 5 ml water for injection. May also administer controlled-release tablets 30 mg q 8 to 12 hours. As an epidural injection, 5 mg via an epidural catheter q 24 hours.

SEVERE CHRONIC PAIN ASSOCIATED WITH SICKLE CELL CRISIS
▶**Children:** 0.03 to 0.15 mg/kg/hour by continuous I.V. infusion.

PREOPERATIVE SEDATION AND ADJUNCT TO ANESTHESIA
▶**Adults:** 8 to 10 mg I.M., S.C., or I.V.

▶**Contraindications & Precautions:** Contraindicated in patients with hypersensitivity to drug or conditions that would preclude administration of opioids by I.V. route (acute bronchial asthma or upper airway obstruction). Use cautiously in debilitated patients and in those with head injury, increased intracranial pressure, seizures, pulmonary disease, prostatic hyperplasia, hepatic or renal disease, acute abdominal conditions, hypothyroidism, Addison's disease, or urethral strictures.

Mupirocin (Bactroban, Bactroban Nasal)
▶**Indications & Dosage**

TOPICAL TREATMENT OF IMPETIGO DUE TO *STAPHYLOCOCCUS AUREUS*, BETA-HEMOLYTIC *STREPTOCOCCUS*, AND *STREPTOCOCCUS PYOGENES*
▶**Children and adults:** Apply a small amount to affected area, t.i.d. The area treated may be covered with a gauze dressing if desired.

ERADICATION OF NASAL COLONIZATION OF METHICILLIN-RESISTANT *S. AUREUS*
▶**Adults:** Apply one-half of a single-use tube to each nostril b.i.d. for 5 days.

▶**Contraindications & Precautions:** Contraindicated in patients hypersensitive to drug. Use cautiously in patients with burns or impaired renal function.

Nafcillin Sodium (Unipen)
▶**Indications & Dosage**

SYSTEMIC INFECTIONS CAUSED BY SUSCEPTIBLE ORGANISMS (METHICILLIN-SENSITIVE *STAPHYLOCOCCUS AUREUS*)
▶**Neonates 1 week old and younger weighing less than 1.2 kg (2.6 lb):** 25 mg/kg I.M. or I.V. q 12 hours.

▶**Neonates 1 week old and younger weighing between 1.2 and 2 kg (2.6 and 4.4 lb):** 25 mg/kg I.M. or I.V. q 12 hours.

▶**Neonates 1 week old and younger weighing more than 2 kg:** 25 mg/kg I.M. or I.V. q 8 hours.

▶**Neonates older than 1 week old weighing between 1.2 and 2 kg:** 25 mg/kg I.M. or I.V. q 8 hours.

▶**Neonates older than 1 week old weighing more than 2 kg:** 25 mg/kg I.M. or I.V. q 6 hours.

▶**Infants and children older than 1 month:** 50 to 100 mg/kg P.O. daily, divided into doses given q 6 hours; or for mild to moderate infections 50 to 100 mg/kg I.M. or I.V. daily in equally divided doses every 6 hours; for severe infections 100 to 200 mg/kg I.M. or I.V. daily in equally divided doses every 4 to 6 hours.

▶**Adults:** 2 to 4 g P.O. daily, divided into doses given q 6 hours; 2 to 12 g I.M. or I.V. daily, divided into doses given q 4 to 6 hours.

MENINGITIS

▶**Neonates younger than age 7 days:** 50 mg/kg I.V. every 8 hours (for weights of more than 2 kg) or every 12 hours (for weights of 2 kg or less).

▶**Neonates ages 7 to 28 days:** 50 mg/kg I.V. every 6 hours (for weights of more than 2 kg) or every 8 hours (for weights of 2 kg or less).

▶**Contraindications & Precautions:** Contraindicated in patients with hypersensitivity to drug or other penicillins. Use cautiously in patients with GI distress or sensitivity to cephalosporins.

Naloxone Hydrochloride (Narcan)
▶**Indications & Dosage**
KNOWN OR SUSPECTED OPIATE-INDUCED RESPIRATORY DEPRESSION, INCLUDING THAT CAUSED BY NATURAL AND SYNTHETIC NARCOTICS, METHADONE, NALBUPHINE, PENTAZOCINE, AND PROPOXYPHENE

▶**Children:** 0.01 mg/kg I.V.; give a subsequent dose of 0.1 mg/kg if needed. Dose for continuous infusion is 0.024 to 0.16 mg/kg/hour. If I.V. route not available, dose may be given I.M. or S.C. in divided doses.

▶**Adults:** 0.4 to 2 mg I.V., S.C., or I.M., repeated q 2 to 3 minutes p.r.n. If no response is observed after 10 mg have been administered, diagnosis of narcotic-induced toxicity should be questioned.

POSTOPERATIVE OPIATE DEPRESSION

▶**Neonates (asphyxia neonatorum):** 0.01 mg/kg I.V. into umbilical vein repeated q 2 to 3 minutes until desired response is obtained.

▶**Children:** 0.005 to 0.01 mg/kg dose I.M., I.V., or S.C., repeated q 2 to 3 minutes p.r.n. until desired degree of reversal is obtained.

▶Concentration for use in neonates and children is 0.02 mg/ml.

►**Adults:** 0.1 to 0.2 mg I.V. q 2 to 3 minutes p.r.n. until desired response is obtained.

►**Contraindications & Precautions:** Contraindicated in patients with hypersensitivity to drug. Use cautiously in patients with cardiac irritability and opiate addiction or dependence.

Naproxen (Naprosyn, Anaprox)
►**Indications & Dosage**

JUVENILE RHEUMATOID ARTHRITIS

NAPROXEN

►**Children older than age 2 years:** 10 mg/kg/day in two divided doses.

MILD TO MODERATELY SEVERE MUSCULOSKELETAL OR SOFT-TISSUE IRRITATION

NAPROXEN

►**Adults:** 250 to 500 mg P.O. b.i.d. Alternatively, 250 mg in the morning and 500 mg in the evening.

NAPROXEN SODIUM

►**Adults:** 275 to 550 mg P.O. b.i.d. Alternatively, 275 mg in the morning and 550 mg in the evening.

MILD TO MODERATE PAIN; PRIMARY DYSMENORRHEA

NAPROXEN

►**Adults:** 500 mg P.O. to start, followed by 250 mg P.O. q 6 to 8 hours, p.r.n. Maximum daily dose shouldn't exceed 1.25 g naproxen.

NAPROXEN SODIUM

►**Adults:** 550 mg P.O. to start, followed by 275 mg P.O. q 6 to 8 hours p.r.n. Maximum daily dose is 1.375 g naproxen sodium.

►**Self-medication:** 220 mg q 8 to 12 hours. Maximum daily dose is 440 mg for adults ages 65 years and older, or three tablets for adults younger than age 65 years. Don't self-medicate for more than 10 days.

NAPROXEN SODIUM

►**Adults:** 825 mg initially, then 275 mg q 8 hours until attack has subsided.

►**Contraindications & Precautions:** Contraindicated in patients with hypersensitivity to drug or asthma, rhinitis, or nasal polyps. Use cautiously in patients with history of peptic ulcer disease or renal, CV, GI, or hepatic disease.

Nifedipine (Adalat, Procardia)
►**Indications & Dosage**
HYPERTENSION

►**Adolescents and adults:** Initially, 30 to 60 mg P.O. once daily (extended-release tablets). Adjust dosage at 7- to 14-day intervals based on patient tolerance and response. Maximum daily dose is 120 mg.

►**Contraindications & Precautions:** Contraindicated in patients with hypersensitivity to drug. Use cautiously in patients with heart failure or hypotension. Use extended-release form cautiously in patients with GI narrowing. Use with caution in patients with unstable angina who aren't currently taking a beta blocker because a higher incidence of MI has been reported. Also use cautiously in patients with hepatic impairment.

Nitrofurantoin (Macrobid, Macrodantin)
►**Indications & Dosage**
INITIAL OR RECURRENT UTI CAUSED BY SUSCEPTIBLE ORGANISMS

►**Infants and children ages 1 month to 12 years:** 5 to 7 mg/kg/24 hours P.O. daily, divided q.i.d.

►**Children older than age 12 years and adults:** 50 to 100 mg P.O. q.i.d. or 100-mg dual-release capsules q 12 hours.

LONG-TERM SUPPRESSION THERAPY

►**Children:** As low as 1 mg/kg/day in a single dose or two divided doses.

►**Contraindications & Precautions:** Contraindicated in patients with a hypersensitivity to the drug. Also contraindicated in pregnant patients at term (38 to 42 weeks' gestation), during labor and delivery, or when the onset of labor is imminent. Contraindicated in children age 1 month and younger and in patients with moderate to severe renal impairment, anuria, oliguria, or creatinine clearance under 60 ml/minute. Use cautiously in patients with impaired renal function, anemia, diabetes mellitus, electrolyte abnormalities, vitamin B deficiency, debilitating disease, or G6PD deficiency.

Nitroprusside Sodium (Nipride)
►**Indications & Dosage**
HYPERTENSIVE EMERGENCIES

►**Children and adults:** I.V. infusion titrated to blood pressure, with a range of 0.3 to 10 mcg/kg/minute. Maximum infusion rate is 10 mcg/kg/minute for 10 minutes.

ACUTE HEART FAILURE

►**Children and adults:** I.V. infusion titrated to cardiac output and systemic blood pressure. Same dose range as for hypertensive emergencies.

►**Contraindications & Precautions:** Contraindicated in patients with hypersensitivity to drug, compensatory hypertension (such as in arteriovenous shunt or coarctation of the aorta), inadequate cerebral circulation, congenital optic atrophy, or tobacco-induced amblyopia. Use cautiously in patients with renal or hepatic disease, increased intracranial pressure, hypothyroidism, hyponatremia, low vitamin B_{12} levels, and anemia.

Nystatin (Mycostatin)
►**Indications & Dosage**

ORAL, VAGINAL, AND INTESTINAL INFECTIONS CAUSED BY SUSCEPTIBLE ORGANISMS

►**Newborn and premature infants:** 100,000 U of oral suspension q.i.d.

►**Infants older than 3 months and children:** 250,000 to 500,000 U of oral suspension q.i.d.

►**Adults:** 500,000 to 1 million U of oral suspension t.i.d. for oral candidiasis. Alternatively, give 200,000 to 400,000 U (lozenges) four to five times daily; allow to dissolve in mouth.

CUTANEOUS OR MUCOCUTANEOUS CANDIDAL INFECTIONS

TOPICAL USE

►**Adolescents and adults:** Apply to affected areas b.i.d. or t.i.d. until healing is complete.

VAGINAL USE

►**Adolescents and adults:** 100,000 U, as vaginal tablets, inserted high into vagina daily or b.i.d. for 14 days.

►**Contraindications & Precautions:** Contraindicated in patients with hypersensitivity to drug.

Ondansetron Hydrochloride (Zofran)
►**Indications & Dosage**

PREVENTION OF NAUSEA AND VOMITING ASSOCIATED WITH INITIAL AND REPEAT COURSES OF EMETOGENIC CANCER CHEMOTHERAPY, INCLUDING HIGH-DOSE CISPLATIN

P.O.

►**Children ages 4 to 12 years:** 4 mg P.O. t.i.d. starting 30 minutes before start of chemotherapy, with subsequent doses 4 to 8 hours after first dose, then 4 mg q 8 hours for 1 to 2 days after completion of chemotherapy.

▶**Children older than age 12 years and adults:** 8 mg P.O. b.i.d. starting 30 minutes before start of chemotherapy, with subsequent dose 8 hours after first dose, then 8 mg q 12 hours for 1 to 2 days after completion of chemotherapy.

I.V.

▶**Children ages 4 years and older and adults:** Three I.V. doses of 0.15 mg/kg with first dose infused over 15 minutes beginning 30 minutes before start of chemotherapy, with subsequent doses of 0.15 mg/kg administered 4 and 8 hours after first dose. May also administer as a single dose of 32 mg infused over 15 minutes, 30 minutes before start of chemotherapy.

PREVENTION OF POSTOPERATIVE NAUSEA AND VOMITING

▶**Children ages 2 to 12 years and weighing 40 kg (88 lb) or less:** 0.1 mg/kg I.V. over 2 to 5 minutes immediately before anesthesia or shortly postoperatively.

▶**Children ages 2 to 12 years and weighing more than 40 kg:** 4 mg I.V. over 2 to 5 minutes immediately before anesthesia or shortly post-operatively.

▶**Adults:** 16 mg P.O. 1 hour before anesthesia or 4 mg I.V. immediately before anesthesia or shortly postoperatively.

▶**Contraindications & Precautions:** Contraindicated in patients hyper-sensitive to drug. Use cautiously in patients with hepatic failure.

Oxacillin Sodium (Bactocill)
▶**Indications & Dosage**

SYSTEMIC INFECTIONS CAUSED BY *STAPHYLOCOCCUS AUREUS*

▶**Neonates 1 week old or younger weighing 2 kg (4.4 lb) or less:** 50 mg/kg I.M. or I.V. daily in divided doses every 12 hours.

▶**Neonates 1 week old or younger weighing over 2 kg:** 75 mg/kg I.M. or I.V. daily in divided doses every 8 hours.

▶**Neonates older than 1 week weighing 2 kg or less:** 75 mg/kg I.M. or I.V. daily in divided doses every 8 hours.

▶**Neonates older than 1 week weighing over 2 kg:** 100 mg/kg I.M. or I.V. daily in divided doses every 6 hours.

MILD TO MODERATE UPPER RESPIRATORY TRACT INFECTIONS OR SKIN AND SKIN STRUCTURE INFECTIONS

▶**Infants and children older than age 1 month weighing less than 40 kg (88 lb):** 50 mg/kg P.O., I.M. or I.V. daily, divided into doses given every 6 hours.

▶**Children weighing more than 40 kg and adults:** 500 mg P.O. every 4 to 6 hours; or 250 to 500 mg I.M. or I.V. every 4 to 6 hours.

SEVERE INFECTIONS, INCLUDING LOWER RESPIRATORY TRACT, DISSEMINATED INFECTIONS, OR OSTEOMYELITIS

▶Infants and children older than age 1 month and weighing less than 40 kg (88 lb): 100 to 200 mg/kg I.M. or I.V. daily, divided into doses given every 4 to 6 hours.

▶Children weighing more than 40 kg and adults: 1 g I.M. or I.V. every 4 to 6 hours.

▶**Contraindications & Precautions:** Contraindicated in patients with hypersensitivity to drug or other penicillins. Use cautiously in patients with other drug allergies (especially to cephalosporins), in neonates, and in infants.

Palivizumab (Synagis)
▶**Indications & Dosage**

PREVENTION OF SERIOUS LOWER RESPIRATORY TRACT DISEASE CAUSED BY RESPIRATORY SYNCYTIAL VIRUS (RSV) IN CHILDREN AT HIGH RISK

▶Infants and children: 15 mg/kg I.M. monthly throughout RSV season. Administer first dose before beginning of RSV season.

▶**Contraindications & Precautions:** Contraindicated in children with a history of severe prior reaction to the drug or its components. Given with caution in patients with thrombocytopenia or any coagulation disorder.

Penicillin G Benzathine (Bicillin L-A)
▶*penicillin G potassium*

▶*penicillin G procaine*

▶Crysticillin A.S.

▶*penicillin G sodium*

▶**Indications & Dosage**

CONGENITAL SYPHILIS

PENICILLIN G BENZATHINE

▶Asymptomatic neonates with normal CSF whose mothers may not have received adequate syphilis therapy during pregnancy: 50,000 U/kg I.M. as a single dose.

▶Children younger than age 2 years: 50,000 U/kg I.M. as a single dose.

PENICILLIN G POTASSIUM, SODIUM

▶Symptomatic neonates and neonates with presumed or proven congenital syphilis: 50,000 U/kg I.V. every 12 hours during the first 7 days of life then every 8 hours for 3 days for a total duration of 10 days.

PENICILLIN G PROCAINE

►Symptomatic neonates and neonates with presumed or proven congenital syphilis: 50,000 U/kg I.M. once daily for 10 to 14 days.

PREVIOUSLY UNTREATED CONGENITAL SYPHILIS

PENICILLIN G POTASSIUM, SODIUM

►Infants: 50,000 U/kg I.V. every 4 to 6 hours for 10 to 14 days.

PENICILLIN G BENZATHINE

►Children older than age 1 year: 50,000 U/kg I.M. weekly for 3 weeks after 10 to 14 days of penicillin G potassium or sodium therapy.

►Note: In symptomatic children with normal CSF and negative CSF VDRL, penicillin G benzathine may be used alone in same dose as above.

GROUP A STREPTOCOCCAL UPPER RESPIRATORY TRACT INFECTIONS

PENICILLIN G BENZATHINE

►Children weighing less than 27 kg (60 lb): 300,000 to 600,000 U I.M. in a single injection.

►Children who weigh 27 kg or more: 900,000 U I.M. in a single injection.

►Adults: 1.2 million U I.M. in a single injection.

TREATMENT OF GROUP A BETA-HEMOLYTIC STREPTOCOCCAL PHARYNGITIS AND PRIMARY PREVENTION OF RHEUMATIC FEVER

PENICILLIN G BENZATHINE

►Children weighing 27 kg (60 lb) or less: 600,000 U I.M. in a single dose.

►Children weighing more than 27 kg and adults: 1.2 million U I.M. in a single dose.

PROPHYLAXIS OF RECURRENT RHEUMATIC FEVER

►Children and adults: 1.2 million U I.M. every 3 to 4 weeks.

PRIMARY AND SECONDARY SYPHILIS

PENICILLIN G BENZATHINE

►Infants and children ages 1 month and older: 50,000 U/kg I.M. in a single injection. Maximum dose 2.4 million U.

►Adolescents and adults: 2.4 million U I.M. in a single dose.

LATENT SYPHILIS AND TERTIARY SYPHILIS

PENICILLIN G BENZATHINE

►Infants and children ages 1 month and older: 50,000 U/kg I.M. in a single injection. Maximum dose 2.4 million U. For late syphilis or latent syphilis of unknown duration, 50,000 U/kg (up to 2.4 million U) I.M. weekly for 3 successive weeks. Maximum total dose, 7.2 million U.

►**Adolescents and adults:** For early latent syphilis, 2.4 million U I.M. in a single dose. For late latent syphilis, latent syphilis of unknown duration, or tertiary syphilis, 2.4 million U I.M. weekly for 3 successive weeks.

MODERATE TO SEVERE SYSTEMIC INFECTIONS

PENICILLIN G POTASSIUM, SODIUM

►**Neonates younger than 1 week weighing 1.2 to 2 kg (2.6 to 4.4 lb):** 25,000 U I.M. or I.V. every 12 hours.

►**Neonates younger than 1 week weighing more than 2 kg:** 25,000 U I.M. or I.V. every 8 hours.

►**Neonates ages 1 to 4 weeks weighing 1.2 to 2 kg:** 25,000 U I.M. or I.V. every 8 hours.

►**Neonates ages 1 to 4 weeks weighing more than 2 kg:** 25,000 U I.M. or I.V. every 6 hours.

►**Neonates 4 weeks old or older weighing less than 1.2 kg:** 25,000 U I.M. or I.V. every 12 hours.

►**Infants and children ages 1 month and older:** 25,000 to 50,000 U/kg daily I.M. or I.V. in 4 divided doses. For the treatment of severe infections give 250,000 to 400,000 U/kg I.M. or I.V. daily, given in divided doses q 4 to 6 hours.

►**Children ages 12 years and older and adults:** 5 to 15 million U I.M. or I.V. daily, given in divided doses q 4 hours.

MENINGITIS CAUSED BY GROUP B STREPTOCOCCI

PENICILLIN G POTASSIUM, SODIUM

►**Neonates 1 week or younger:** 250,000 to 450,000 U/kg I.V. daily in three divided doses.

►**Neonates older than 1 week:** 450,000 U/kg I.V. daily in four divided doses.

►**Infants and children ages 1 month and older:** 250,000 to 400,000 U/kg I.V. daily, given in divided doses q 4 to 6 hours.

MODERATE TO SEVERE SYSTEMIC INFECTIONS, PNEUMOCOCCAL PNEUMONIA

PENICILLIN G PROCAINE

►**Children weighing less than 27 kg (60 lb):** 300,000 U I.M. daily as a single dose.

►**Adults:** 600,000 to 1.2 million U I.M. daily as a single dose or q 6 to 12 hours.

UNCOMPLICATED GONORRHEA

PENICILLIN G PROCAINE

▶**Children older than age 12 years and adults:** 1 g probenecid, then 30 minutes later, 4.8 million U of penicillin G procaine I.M., divided into two injection sites.

▶**Contraindications & Precautions:** Contraindicated in patients with hypersensitivity to drug or other penicillins. Use cautiously in patients with drug allergies (especially to cephalosporins or imipenem). Penicillin G potassium should be used cautiously in patients with renal failure.

Penicillin V Potassium (Pen-Vee K)

▶**Indications & Dosage**

MILD TO MODERATE SUSCEPTIBLE INFECTIONS

▶**Adolescents and adults:** 125 to 250 mg P.O. q 6 to 8 hours, or 500 mg P.O. q 12 hours, for 10 days. For more severe infections, 250 to 500 mg P.O. q 6 hours while patient is afebrile for 2 days.

▶**Infants and children age 1 month to 12 years:** 15 to 62.5 mg/kg (25,000 to 100,000 U/kg) P.O. daily, divided into doses given q 4 to 8 hours.

GROUP A BETA-HEMOLYTIC STREPTOCOCCAL PHARYNGITIS AND PREVENTION OF INITIAL ATTACKS OF RHEUMATIC FEVER

▶**Children:** 250 mg P.O. b.i.d. to t.i.d. for 10 days.

▶**Adolescents and adults:** 500 mg P.O. b.i.d. to t.i.d. for 10 days.

ENDOCARDITIS PROPHYLAXIS FOR DENTAL SURGERY

▶**Children weighing less than 30 kg (66 lb):** Half the adult dose.

▶**Adults:** 2 g P.O. 30 to 60 minutes before procedure, then 1 g 6 hours later.

▶**Contraindications & Precautions:** Contraindicated in patients with hypersensitivity to drug or other penicillins. Use cautiously in patients with drug allergies (especially to cephalosporins or imipenem).

Phenobarbital (Luminal)

▶**Indications & Dosage**

ALL FORMS OF EPILEPSY EXCEPT ABSENCE SEIZURES, FEBRILE SEIZURES IN CHILDREN

▶**Children:** 1 to 6 mg/kg P.O. daily, usually divided q 12 hours. It can, however, be administered once daily. Alternatively, give 4 to 6 mg/kg I.V. or I.M. daily and monitor patient's blood levels.

►**Adults:** 60 to 100 mg P.O. daily, divided t.i.d. or given as single dose h.s. Alternatively, give 200 to 300 mg I.M. or I.V. and repeat q 6 hours p.r.n.

STATUS EPILEPTICUS

►**Children:** 100 to 400 mg I.V. Repeat if necessary, up to a total dose of 20 mg/kg.

►**Adults:** 200 to 600 mg I.V. Repeat if necessary, up to a total dose of 20 mg/kg.

►**Contraindications & Precautions:** Contraindicated in patients with barbiturate hypersensitivity, history of manifest or latent porphyria, hepatic dysfunction, respiratory disease with dyspnea or obstruction, and nephritis. Use cautiously in debilitated patients and in those with acute or chronic pain, depression, suicidal tendencies, history of drug abuse, blood pressure alterations, CV disease, shock, or uremia.

Phenytoin (Dilantin)

►**Indications & Dosage**

GENERALIZED TONIC-CLONIC SEIZURES, STATUS EPILEPTICUS, NONEPILEPTIC SEIZURES (POSTHEAD TRAUMA, REYE'S SYNDROME)

►**Children:** Loading dose is 15 to 20 mg/kg I.V. at a rate not exceeding 1 to 3 mg/kg/minute, or 5 mg/kg P.O. or 250 mg/m^2 P.O. daily, divided q 8 to 12 hours; then start maintenance dose of 4 to 8 mg/kg P.O. or I.V. daily, divided q 12 hours. Total daily dose shouldn't exceed 300 mg.

►**Adults:** Loading dose is 10 to 15 mg/kg I.V. slowly, not to exceed 50 mg/minute; oral loading dosage consists of 1 g divided into three doses (400 mg, 300 mg, 300 mg) given at 2-hour intervals. Maintenance dose once controlled is 300 mg P.O. daily (extended only); initially use a dose divided t.i.d. (extended or prompt).

►**Contraindications & Precautions:** Contraindicated in patients with hydantoin hypersensitivity, sinus bradycardia, SA block, second- or third-degree AV block, or Stokes-Adams syndrome. Use cautiously in debilitated patients; in those with hepatic dysfunction, hypotension, myocardial insufficiency, diabetes, or respiratory depression; and in those receiving hydantoin derivatives.

Piperacillin Sodium (Pipracil)

►**Indications & Dosage**

INFECTIONS CAUSED BY SUSCEPTIBLE ORGANISMS

►**Neonates 1 week old or younger weighing up to 2 kg (4.4 lb):** 50 mg/kg I.M. or I.V. q 12 hours.

►**Neonates 1 week old or younger weighing 2 kg or more:** 50 mg/kg I.M. or I.V. q 8 hours.

▶**Neonates older than 1 week weighing up to 2 kg:** 50 mg/kg I.M. or I.V. q 8 hours.

▶**Neonates older than 1 week weighing 2 kg or more:** 50 mg/kg I.M. or I.V. q 6 hours.

▶**Infants and children ages 1 month to 12 years:** 50 mg/kg I.V. over 30 minutes every 4 hours.

▶**Children ages 3 to 14 years:** 1.5 g/m^2 I.V. over 30 minutes every 4 hours.

▶**Children older than age 12 years and adults:** Serious infection: 12 to 18 g/day I.V. in divided doses q 4 to 6 hours; uncomplicated UTI and community-acquired pneumonia: 6 to 8 g/day I.V. in divided doses q 6 to 12 hours; complicated UTI: 8 to 16 g/day I.V. in divided doses q 6 to 8 hours; and uncomplicated gonorrhea: 2 g I.M. as a single dose. Maximum daily dose, 24 g.

▶**Contraindications & Precautions:** Contraindicated in patients with hypersensitivity to drug or other penicillins. Use cautiously in patients with other drug allergies (especially to cephalosporins), bleeding tendencies, uremia, or hypokalemia.

Polyethylene Glycolelectrolyte Solution (PEG-ES) (GoLYTELY)

▶**Indications & Dosage**

BOWEL PREPARATION BEFORE GI EXAMINATION

▶**Infants and children ages 3 weeks to 18 years:** 25 to 40 ml/kg for 4 to 10 hours.

▶**Adults:** 240 ml P.O. q 10 minutes until 4 L are consumed or the rectal effluent is clear. Typically, administer 4 hours before examination, allowing 3 hours for drinking and 1 hour for bowel evacuation.

MANAGEMENT OF ACUTE IRON OVERDOSE

▶**Children younger than age 3 years:** 0.5 L/hour.

▶**Note:** If a patient experiences severe bloating, distention, or abdominal pain, slow or temporarily discontinue administration until symptoms abate.

▶**Contraindications & Precautions:** Contraindicated in patients with GI obstruction or perforation, gastric retention, toxic colitis, ileus, or megacolon.

Potassium Chloride

▶**Indications & Dosage**

HYPOKALEMIA

▶**Children and adults:** 40- to 100-mEq tablets divided into two to four doses daily. Use I.V. potassium chloride when oral replacement isn't feasible or when hypokalemia is life-threatening. Dose up to 20 mEq/hour in concentration of 60 mEq/L or less. Further dose based on serum potassium determinations. Don't exceed total daily dose of 150 mEq (3 mEq/kg in children).

▶Further doses are based on serum potassium levels and blood pH. I.V. potassium replacement should be carried out only with ECG monitoring and frequent serum potassium determinations.

▶**Contraindications & Precautions:** Contraindicated in patients with severe renal impairment with oliguria, anuria, or azotemia; in those with untreated Addison's disease; and in those with acute dehydration, heat cramps, hyperkalemia, hyperkalemic form of familial periodic paralysis, and conditions associated with extensive tissue breakdown. Use cautiously in patients with cardiac or renal disease.

Prednisolone (Systemic) (Delta-Cortef, Prelone)
▶**Indications & Dosage**
SEVERE INFLAMMATION, IMMUNE MODULATOR
▶**Children:** 0.14 to 2 mg/kg or 4 to 6 mg/m^2 daily in divided doses.
▶**Adults:** 2.5 to 15 mg P.O. b.i.d., t.i.d., or q.i.d.
▶**Contraindications & Precautions:** Contraindicated in patients with hypersensitivity to drug or its ingredients and systemic fungal infections. Use cautiously in patients with a recent MI, GI ulcer, renal disease, hypertension, osteoporosis, diabetes mellitus, hypothyroidism, cirrhosis, diverticulitis, nonspecific ulcerative colitis, recent intestinal anastomoses, thromboembolic disorders, seizures, myasthenia gravis, heart failure, tuberculosis, ocular herpes simplex

Promethazine Hydrochloride (Phenergan)
▶**Indications & Dosage**
MOTION SICKNESS
▶**Children:** 12.5 to 25 mg P.O., I.M., or P.R. b.i.d.
▶**Adults:** 25 mg P.O. b.i.d.

NAUSEA
▶**Children:** 0.25 to 0.5 mg/kg I.M. or P.R. q 4 to 6 hours p.r.n. or 7.2 to 15 mg/m^2 q 4 hours p.r.n.
▶**Adults:** 12.5 to 25 mg P.O., I.M., or P.R. q 4 to 6 hours p.r.n.
▶**Contraindications & Precautions:** Contraindicated in patients with hypersensitivity to drug; in those with intestinal obstruction, prostatic hyperplasia, bladder neck obstruction, seizure disorders, coma,

CNS depression, and stenosing peptic ulcerations; in newborns, premature neonates, and breast-feeding patients; and in acutely ill or dehydrated children. Use cautiously in patients with asthma or cardiac, pulmonary, or hepatic disease.

Propranolol Hydrochloride (Inderal)
►**Indications & Dosage**
HYPERTENSION

►**Children:** 0.5 to 1 mg/kg P.O. daily in two to four divided doses. Maintenance dose is 2 to 4 mg/kg daily in two divided doses. Maximum dose is 16 mg/kg/day.

►**Adults:** Initially, 80 mg P.O. daily in two to four divided doses or sustained-release form once daily. Increase at 3- to 7-day intervals to maximum daily dose of 640 mg. Usual maintenance dose is 160 to 480 mg daily.

PREVENTION OF FREQUENT, SEVERE, UNCONTROLLABLE, OR DISABLING MIGRAINE OR VASCULAR HEADACHE

►**Adults:** Initially, 80 mg daily in divided doses or one sustained-release capsule once daily. Usual maintenance dose is 160 to 240 mg daily, divided t.i.d. or q.i.d.

►**Contraindications & Precautions:** Contraindicated in patients with bronchial asthma, sinus bradycardia and heart block greater than first-degree, cardiogenic shock, and heart failure (unless failure is secondary to a tachyarrhythmia that can be treated with propranolol). Use cautiously in patients with impaired renal or hepatic function, nonallergic bronchospastic diseases, diabetes mellitus, or thyrotoxicosis; and in those receiving other antihypertensives.

Pseudoephedrine Hydrochloride
►**Indications & Dosage**
NASAL AND EUSTACHIAN TUBE DECONGESTANT

►**Children ages 2 to 5 years:** 15 mg P.O. q 4 to 6 hours. Maximum dose, 60 mg/day, or 4 mg/kg or 125 mg/m^2 P.O. divided q.i.d.

►**Children ages 6 to 11 years:** Administer 30 mg P.O. q 4 to 6 hours. Maximum dose, 120 mg daily.

►**Children ages 12 years and older and adults:** 60 mg P.O. q 4 to 6 hours. Maximum dose, 240 mg daily, or 120 mg P.O. extended-release tablet q 12 hours.

►**Contraindications & Precautions:** Contraindicated in patients with severe hypertension or severe coronary artery disease; in those receiving MAO inhibitors, and in breast-feeding patients. Extended-release preparations are contraindicated in children younger than age 12 years. Use cautiously in patients with hypertension, cardiac disease, diabetes, glaucoma, hyperthyroidism, or prostatic hyperplasia.

Psyllium (Metamucil)
►**Indications & Dosage**

CONSTIPATION, BOWEL MANAGEMENT, IRRITABLE BOWEL SYNDROME

►**Children ages 6 years and older:** 1 level tsp P.O. in 1/2 glass of liquid h.s.
►**Adults:** 1 to 2 rounded tsp P.O. in full glass of liquid daily, b.i.d. or t.i.d., followed by second glass of liquid; or 1 packet P.O. dissolved in water daily; or 2 wafers b.i.d. or t.i.d.
►**Contraindications & Precautions:** Contraindicated in patients with hypersensitivity to drug, abdominal pain, nausea, vomiting, or other symptoms of appendicitis and in those with intestinal obstruction.

Pyridoxine Hydrochloride (Vitamin B$_6$)
►**Indications & Dosage**

DIETARY VITAMIN B$_6$ DEFICIENCY

►**Children:** 10 to 100 mg I.M. or I.V. to correct deficiency, then an adequate diet with supplementary RDA doses to prevent recurrence.
►**Adults:** 2.5 to 10 mg P.O., I.M., or I.V. daily for 3 weeks, then 2 to 5 mg daily as a supplement to a proper diet.

SEIZURES RELATED TO VITAMIN B$_6$ DEFICIENCY OR DEPENDENCY

►**Children and adults:** 100 mg I.M. or I.V. in single dose.
►**Contraindications & Precautions:** Contraindicated in patients hypersensitive to pyridoxine.

Respiratory Syncytial Virus Immune Globulin (RespiGam)
►**Indications & Dosage**

PREVENTION OF SERIOUS LOWER RESPIRATORY TRACT INFECTION CAUSED BY RSV IN CHILDREN WITH BRONCHOPULMONARY DYSPLASIA OR PREMATURE BIRTH (35 WEEKS' GESTATION OR LESS)

►**Premature neonates and infants younger than age 2 years:** 1.5 ml/kg/hour I.V. for 15 minutes. If condition allows, increase to 3 ml/kg/hour for 15 minutes, and then to 6 ml/kg/hour until end of infusion once monthly. Maximum 750 mg/kg recommended per monthly infusion.
►**Contraindications & Precautions:** Contraindicated in patients with severe hypersensitivity to drug or other human immunoglobulins and in patients with immunoglobulin A antibodies.

Ribavirin (Virazole)

►**Indications & Dosage**

RSV INFECTION IN HOSPITALIZED INFANTS AND YOUNG CHILDREN

►**Infants and young children:** 20-mg/ml solution delivered via the Viratek Small Particle Aerosol Generator (SPAG-2), which produces a mist of 190 mcg/L. Treat for 12 to 18 hours/day for at least 3 but no more than 7 days at a flow rate of 12.5 L of mist per minute. For a ventilated patient, use the same dose with a pressure- or volume-cycled ventilator and SPAG-2. Suction patient q 1 to 2 hours and check pulmonary pressures q 2 to 4 hours.

►**Contraindications & Precautions:** Contraindicated in patients hypersensitive to drug. Use cautiously in patients with severe anemia.

Rifampin (Rifadin)

►**Indications & Dosage**

PULMONARY TUBERCULOSIS

►**Neonates, infants, and children:** 10 to 20 mg/kg P.O. or I.V. daily as a single dose. (Give P.O. dose 1 hour before or 2 hours after meals.) Maximum 600 mg daily. Usually given with other effective antitubercular drugs for 6 to 9 months.

►**Adolescents and adults:** 600 mg P.O. or I.V. daily as a single dose. (Give P.O. dose 1 hour before or 2 hours after meals.)

ASYMPTOMATIC MENINGOCOCCAL CARRIERS

►**Neonates:** 5 mg/kg P.O. b.i.d. for 2 days.

►**Infants and children older than 1 month:** 10 mg/kg (up to 600 mg) P.O. b.i.d. for 2 days.

►**Adolescents and adults:** 600 mg P.O. b.i.d. for 2 days.

PROPHYLAXIS OF *HAEMOPHILUS INFLUENZAE* TYPE B

►**Neonates:** 10 mg/kg P.O. once daily for 4 consecutive days.

►**Infants, children, and adults:** 20 mg/kg (up to 600 mg) P.O. once daily for 4 consecutive days.

►**Contraindications & Precautions:** Contraindicated in patients hypersensitive to drug. Use cautiously in patients with hepatic disease.

Salmeterol Xinafoate (Serevent)

►**Indications & Dosage**

LONG-TERM MAINTENANCE IN PATIENTS WITH ASTHMA, PREVENTION OF BRONCHOSPASM IN PATIENTS WITH NOCTURNAL ASTHMA OR REVERSIBLE OBSTRUCTIVE AIRWAY DISEASE WHO REGULARLY NEED SHORT-ACTING BETA AGONISTS

►**Children ages 4 years and older and adults:** One inhalation (powder form) b.i.d. in the morning and evening.

▶**Children older than age 12 years and adults:** Two inhalations (aerosol form) b.i.d. in the morning and evening.

PREVENTION OF EXERCISE-INDUCED BRONCHOSPASM

▶**Children ages 4 years and older and adults:** One inhalation (powder form) at least 30 minutes before exercise. Don't give additional doses for 12 hours.

▶**Children older than age 12 years and adults:** Two inhalations (aerosol form) 30 to 60 minutes before exercise. Don't give additional doses for 12 hours.

▶**Contraindications & Precautions:** Contraindicated in patients hypersensitive to drug or its formulation. Use cautiously in patients with coronary insufficiency, arrhythmias, hypertension, other CV disorders, thyrotoxicosis, or seizure disorders, and in those unusually responsive to sympathomimetics.

Senna (Senokot, Senolax)

▶**Indications & Dosage**

ACUTE CONSTIPATION, PREPARATION FOR BOWEL EXAMINATION

SYRUP

▶**Infants and children ages 1 month to 12 months:** 1.25 to 2.5 ml syrup h.s.

▶**Children ages 1 to 5 years:** 2.5 to 5 ml syrup h.s.

OTHER PREPARATIONS

▶**Children ages 2 to 5 years:** 1/2 tablet, 1/4 tsp of granules dissolved in water. Maximum 1 tablet b.i.d. or 1/2 tsp of granules b.i.d.

▶**Children ages 6 to 11 years:** 1 tablet, 1/2 tsp of granules dissolved in water, 1/2 suppository h.s. or 5 to 10 ml syrup. Maximum 2 tablets b.i.d. or 1 tsp of granules b.i.d.

▶**Children ages 12 years and over and adults:** Usual dose is 2 tablets, 1 tsp of granules dissolved in water, 1 suppository, or 10 to 15 ml syrup h.s. Maximum varies with preparation used.

▶**Contraindications & Precautions:** Contraindicated in patients with ulcerative bowel lesions; nausea, vomiting, abdominal pain, or other symptoms of appendicitis or acute surgical abdomen; fecal impaction; or intestinal obstruction or perforation.

Silver Sulfadiazine (Silvadene)

▶**Indications & Dosage**

ADJUNCT IN THE PREVENTION AND TREATMENT OF WOUND INFECTION FOR SECOND- AND THIRD-DEGREE BURNS

▶**Children and adults:** Apply 16 mm (1/16") thickness of ointment to cleansed and debrided burn wound once or twice daily. Reapply if accidentally removed.

▶**Contraindications & Precautions:** Contraindicated in premature and full-term neonates during first 2 months after birth. Drug may increase possibility of kernicterus. Also contraindicated in patients hypersensitive to drug or in pregnant women at or near term. Use cautiously in patients with sulfonamide sensitivity and in those with impaired hepatic or renal function.

Sodium Bicarbonate
▶**Indications & Dosage**

ADJUNCT TO ADVANCED CARDIAC LIFE SUPPORT

▶**Infants and children ages 2 years or younger:** 1 mEq/kg I.V. bolus of a 4.2% solution. Dose may be repeated q 10 minutes depending on blood gas values. Don't exceed 8 mEq/kg daily.

▶**Children older than age 2 years and adults:** Although no longer routinely recommended, inject either 300 to 500 ml of a 5% solution or 200 to 300 mEq of a 7.5% or 8.4% solution as rapidly as possible. Base later doses on subsequent blood gas values.

METABOLIC ACIDOSIS

▶**Children and adults:** Dose depends on blood carbon dioxide content, pH, and patient's clinical condition. Generally, administer 90 to 180 mEq/L I.V. during first hour, then adjust p.r.n.

URINARY ALKALIZATION

▶**Children:** 1 to 10 mEq (84 to 840 mg)/kg daily.

▶**Adults:** 325 mg to 2 g P.O., up to q.i.d. Don't exceed 17 g in patients younger than age 60 years or 8 g in patients older than age 60 years.

▶**Contraindications & Precautions:** Contraindicated in patients with metabolic or respiratory alkalosis; in those who are losing chlorides from vomiting or continuous GI suction; in those receiving diuretics known to produce hypochloremic alkalosis; and in patients with hypocalcemia in which alkalosis may produce tetany, hypertension, seizures, or heart failure. Orally administered sodium bicarbonate is contraindicated in patients with acute ingestion of strong mineral acids.

▶Use with extreme caution in patients with heart failure, renal insufficiency, or other edematous or sodium-retaining conditions.

Succinylcholine Chloride (Suxamethonium Chloride)
▶**Indications & Dosage**

TO INDUCE SKELETAL MUSCLE RELAXATION; FACILITATE INTUBATION, VENTILATION, OR ORTHOPEDIC MANIPULATIONS; AND LESSEN MUSCLE CONTRACTIONS IN INDUCED SEIZURES

▶Dosage depends on the anesthetic used and the patient's needs and response. Doses are representative and must be adjusted. Paralysis is induced after inducing hypnosis with thiopental or other appropriate drug.

▶**Infants:** 2 mg/kg I.V.

▶**Older children and adolescents:** 1 mg/kg I.V. or 3 to 4 mg/kg I.M. (Don't exceed 150 mg.)

▶**Adults:** For short procedures, 0.6 mg/kg (range, 0.3 to 1.1 mg/kg) I.V. over 10 to 30 seconds; additional doses may be given if needed. For long procedures, 2.5 mg/minute (range, 0.5 to 10 mg/minute) by continuous I.V. infusion. Alternatively, 0.3 to 1.1 mg/kg by intermittent I.V. injection, followed by additional doses of 0.04 to 0.07 mg/kg p.r.n.

▶**Contraindications & Precautions:** Contraindicated in patients hypersensitive to drug and in those with abnormally low plasma pseudo-cholinesterase, angle-closure glaucoma, malignant hyperthermia, or penetrating eye injuries.

Sulfasalazine (Azulfidine)
▶**Indications & Dosage**

MILD TO MODERATE ULCERATIVE COLITIS, ADJUNCTIVE THERAPY IN SEVERE ULCERATIVE COLITIS

▶**Children ages 2 years and older:** Initially, 40 to 60 mg/kg P.O. daily, divided into three to six doses; then 30 mg/kg daily in four doses. Maximum 2 g daily. May need to start at lower dose if GI intolerance occurs.

▶**Adults:** Initially, 3 to 4 g P.O. daily in divided doses. Maintenance dose is 2 g P.O. daily in divided doses q 6 hours. May need to start with 1 to 2 g initially, with a gradual increase in dose to minimize adverse reactions.

▶**Contraindications & Precautions:** Contraindicated in patients hypersensitive to salicylates, sulfonamides, or other drugs containing sulfur (such as thiazides, furosemide, or oral sulfonylureas). Also, contraindicated in patients with porphyria or severe renal or hepatic dysfunction; during pregnancy and at term; in breast-feeding patients; and in infants and children younger than age 2 years. Sulfasalazine is also contraindicated in patients with intestinal or urinary tract obstructions because of the risk of local GI irritation and crystalluria. Use cautiously in patients with mild to moderate renal or hepatic dysfunction, severe allergies, asthma, blood dyscrasia, or G6PD deficiency.

Sulfisoxazole (Gantrisin)
▶**Indications & Dosage**

UTIS AND SYSTEMIC INFECTIONS

▶**Infants older than 2 months and children:** Initially, 75 mg/kg (or 2 g/m^2)

P.O. for 1 dose; then 150 mg/kg (or 4 g/m^2) P.O. daily in divided doses q 4 to 6 hours. Maximum 6 g/day.

▶**Adults:** Initially, 2 to 4 g P.O.; then 4 to 8 g P.O. daily in divided doses q 4 to 6 hours. Maximum 6 g/24 hours.

LYMPHOGRANULOMA VENEREUM (GENITAL, INGUINAL, OR ANORECTAL INFECTION)

▶**Adults:** 500 mg to 1 g q.i.d. for 3 weeks.

CONJUNCTIVITIS, CORNEAL ULCER, SUPERFICIAL OCULAR INFECTIONS; ADJUNCT IN SYSTEMIC TREATMENT OF TRACHOMA

▶**Adolescents and adults:** 1 or 2 gtt in the lower conjunctival sac of affected eye daily q 1 to 4 hours.

▶**Contraindications & Precautions:** Contraindicated in patients hypersensitive to sulfonamides, infants younger than age 2 months (except in congenital toxoplasmosis [oral form only]), pregnant patients at term, and patients who are breast-feeding.

▶Use oral form cautiously in patients with impaired renal or hepatic function, severe allergies, bronchial asthma, or G6PD deficiency.

Terbutaline Sulfate (Brethaire, Brethine, Bricanyl)
▶**Indications & Dosage**

BRONCHOSPASM IN PATIENTS WITH REVERSIBLE OBSTRUCTIVE AIRWAY DISEASE

▶**Adolescents ages 12 to 15 years:** 2.5 mg P.O. t.i.d. Maximum 7.5 mg daily. Alternatively, 2 inhalations may be given q 4 to 6 hours with 1 minute between inhalations.

▶**Adolescents ages 15 years or older and adults:** 5 mg P.O. t.i.d. at 6-hour intervals. Maximum 15 mg daily. Decrease to 2.5 mg P.O. t.i.d. if adverse effects occur. Alternatively, 0.25 mg S.C. may be repeated in 15 to 30 minutes; maximum 0.5 mg q 4 hours. Alternatively, 2 inhalations may be given q 4 to 6 hours with 1 minute between inhalations.

▶**IV:**

Loading: 2–10 mcg/kg over 10 min

Maintenance: Start at 0.1 mcg/kg/min, titrate up to 0.4 mcg/kg/min

▶**Contraindications & Precautions:** Contraindicated in patients hypersensitive to drug or to sympathomimetic amines. Use cautiously in patients with CV disorders, hyperthyroidism, diabetes, or seizure disorders.

Tetracycline Hydrochloride
▶**Indications & Dosage**

INFECTIONS CAUSED BY SUSCEPTIBLE ORGANISMS

▶**Children older than age 8 years:** 25 to 50 mg/kg P.O. daily, divided into two to four doses.

►**Adults:** 1 to 2 g P.O. divided into two to four doses.

BRUCELLOSIS

►**Adolescents and adults:** 500 mg P.O. q 6 hours for 3 weeks with streptomycin 1 g I.M. q 12 hours week 1 and daily week 2.

GONORRHEA IN PATIENTS HYPERSENSITIVE TO PENICILLIN

►**Adolescents and adults:** 1.5 g P.O.; then 500 mg q 6 hours for 4 days.

SYPHILIS IN NONPREGNANT PATIENTS HYPERSENSITIVE TO PENICILLIN

►**Adolescents and adults:** 500 mg P.O. q.i.d. for 14 days.

ACNE

►**Adolescents and adults:** 500 to 1,000 mg P.O. divided q.i.d.; then 125 to 500 mg P.O. daily or every other day. Apply topical ointment generously to affected areas b.i.d. until skin is thoroughly wet.

UNCOMPLICATED URETHRAL, ENDOCERVICAL, OR RECTAL INFECTION WITH *CHLAMYDIA TRACHOMATIS*

►**Adults:** 500 mg P.O. q.i.d. for at least 7 days.

►**Contraindications & Precautions:** Contraindicated in patients hypersensitive to tetracyclines. Use cautiously in patients with impaired renal or hepatic function. Use oral form cautiously during last half of pregnancy and in children younger than age 8 years.

Thiabendazole (Mintezol)
►**Indications & Dosage**

SYSTEMIC INFECTIONS WITH PINWORM, ROUNDWORM, THREADWORM, WHIPWORM, VISCERAL LARVA MIGRANS, TRICHINOSIS

►**Children and adults weighing less than 70 kg (154 lb):** 25 mg/kg P.O. q 12 hours for 2 successive days.

►**Children and adults weighing over 70 kg:** 1.5 g P.O. q 12 hours for 2 successive days. Maximum 3 g daily.

►**Contraindications & Precautions:** Contraindicated in patients hypersensitive to drug. Use cautiously in patients with renal or hepatic dysfunction, severe malnutrition, or anemia, and in those who are vomiting.

Ticarcillin Disodium (Ticar)
►**Indications & Dosage**

SERIOUS INFECTIONS CAUSED BY SUSCEPTIBLE ORGANISMS

►**Neonates 1 week old or younger weighing less than 2 kg (4.4 lb):** 75 mg/kg I.M. or I.V. q 12 hours.

►**Neonates 1 week old or younger weighing more than 2 kg:** 75 mg/kg I.M. or I.V. q 8 hours.

►**Neonates older than 1 week weighing less than 2 kg:** 75 mg/kg I.M. or I.V. q 8 hours.

►**Neonates older than 1 week weighing more than 2 kg:** 100 mg/kg I.M. or I.V. q 8 hours.

►**Infants and children older than 1 month weighing less than 40 kg (88 lb):** 200 to 300 mg/kg daily I.V. in divided doses q 4 to 6 hours.

►**Children weighing more than 40 kg and adults:** 200 to 300 mg/kg I.V. daily in divided doses q 3, 4, or 6 hours.

UTI

►**Infants and children older than 1 month weighing less than 40 kg (88 lb):** For complicated infections, 150 to 200 mg/kg daily I.V. in divided doses every 4 or 6 hours. For uncomplicated infections, 50 to 100 mg/kg daily I.V. or I.M. in divided doses every 6 or 8 hours. Total daily doses in children should not exceed adult doses.

►**Children weighing 40 kg or more and adults:** For patients with complicated infection, give 150 to 200 mg/kg I.V. daily, divided into doses q 4 to 6 hours; for treating uncomplicated infections, give 1 g I.V. or I.M. q 6 hours.

►**Contraindications & Precautions:** Contraindicated in patients hypersensitive to drug or other penicillins. Use cautiously in patients with other drug allergies (especially to cephalosporins), impaired renal function, hemorrhagic conditions, hypokalemia, and sodium restrictions.

Ticarcillin Disodium/Clavulanate Potassium (Timentin)
►**Indications & Dosage**
MILD TO MODERATE INFECTIONS

►**Infants and children ages 3 months to 16 years weighing less than 60 kg (132 lb):** 200 mg of ticarcillin component/kg I.V. daily in divided doses every 6 hours.

►**Infants and children ages 3 months to 16 years weighing 60 kg or more:** 3.1 g (contains 3 g ticarcillin and 0.1 g clavulanate potassium) I.V. every 6 hours.

SEVERE INFECTIONS

►**Infants and children ages 3 months to 16 years weighing less than 60 kg:** 300 mg of ticarcillin component/kg I.V. daily in divided doses every 4 hours.

►**Infants and children ages 3 months to 16 years weighing 60 kg or more:** 3.1 g (contains 3 g ticarcillin and 0.1 g clavulanate potassium) I.V. every 4 hours.

INFECTIONS OF THE LOWER RESPIRATORY TRACT, URINARY TRACT, BONES AND JOINTS, SKIN AND SKIN STRUCTURE, AND SEPTICEMIA

▶**Adults:** 3.1 g (contains 3 g ticarcillin and 0.1 g clavulanate potassium) diluted in 50 to 100 ml D_5W, saline solution, or lactated Ringer's injection and administered by I.V. infusion over 30 minutes q 4 to 6 hours.

▶**Contraindications & Precautions:** Contraindicated in patients with hypersensitivity to drug or other penicillins. Use cautiously in patients with other drug allergies, especially to cephalosporins, impaired renal function, hemorrhagic conditions, hypokalemia, or sodium restrictions.

Tobramycin (Tobramycin Ophthalmic) (Tobrex)
▶**Indications & Dosage**

SERIOUS INFECTIONS CAUSED BY SUSCEPTIBLE *ESCHERICHIA COLI, PROTEUS, KLEBSIELLA, ENTEROBACTER, SERRATIA, STAPHYLOCOCCUS AUREUS, PSEUDOMONAS, CITROBACTER,* OR *PROVIDENCIA*

▶**Neonates younger than age 1 week:** Up to 4 mg/kg I.M. or I.V. daily, divided q 12 hours. For I.V. use, dilute in 50 to 100 ml normal saline solution or D_5W for adults and in less volume for children. Infuse over 20 to 60 minutes.

▶**Children and adults with normal renal function:** 3 mg/kg I.M. or I.V. daily, divided q 8 hours. Up to 5 mg/kg I.M. or I.V. daily, divided q 6 to 8 hours for life-threatening infections.

CYSTIC FIBROSIS WITH *PSEUDOMONAS AERUGINOSA*

▶**Children older than age 6 years and adults:** 1 single-use ampule (300 mg) administered q 12 hours for 28 days, then off for 28 days, then on for 28 days as advised by health care provider. There is no dosage adjustment for age or renal failure.

EXTERNAL OCULAR INFECTION CAUSED BY SUSCEPTIBLE GRAM-NEGATIVE BACTERIA

▶**Children and adults:** For mild to moderate infection, 1 or 2 gtt in affected eye q 4 to 6 hours. For severe infection, 2 gtt in the affected eye hourly or a small amount of ointment in conjunctival sac t.i.d. or q.i.d.

▶**Contraindications & Precautions:** Contraindicated in patients hypersensitive to drug or other aminoglycosides. Use injectable form cautiously in patients with impaired renal function or neuromuscular disorders.

Tretinoin (Topical) (Retin-A)
▶**Indications & Dosage**

ACNE VULGARIS (ESPECIALLY GRADES I, II, AND III)

▶**Children and adults:** Clean affected area and lightly apply solution once daily h.s. or as directed.

►**Contraindications & Precautions:** Contraindicated in patients hypersensitive to vitamin A or retinoic acid. Use cautiously in patients with eczema. Avoid getting drug in eyes, mouth, angles of the nose, mucous membranes, or open wounds. Avoid use of topical substances that contain high levels of alcohol, menthol, spices, or lime because they may cause skin irritation. Avoid use of medicated cosmetics on treated skin.

Valproic Acid (Depakote)
►**Indications & Dosage**

SIMPLE AND COMPLEX ABSENCE SEIZURES AND MIXED SEIZURE TYPES, TONIC-CLONIC SEIZURES

►**Children and adults:** 15 mg/kg P.O. daily, divided b.i.d. or t.i.d.; may increase by 5 to 10 mg/kg daily at weekly intervals to a maximum of 60 mg/kg daily, divided b.i.d. or t.i.d. The b.i.d. dosage is recommended for the enteric-coated tablets; or 10 to 15 mg/kg/day as a 60-minute I.V. infusion (20 mg/minute or less); may increase by 5 to 10 mg/kg daily at weekly intervals to a maximum of 60 mg/kg daily. Drug should be diluted in at least 50 ml of compatible diluent. Use of valproate sodium injection for periods of more than 14 days hasn't been studied. Patient should be switched to oral route as soon as clinically feasible.

►**Contraindications & Precautions:** Contraindicated in patients hypersensitive to drug. Use cautiously in patients with history of hepatic dysfunction. Don't give valproate sodium injection to patients with hepatic disease or significant hepatic dysfunction.

Vancomycin Hydrochloride (Vancocin)
►**Indications & Dosage**

SEVERE STAPHYLOCOCCAL INFECTIONS WHEN OTHER ANTIBIOTICS ARE INEFFECTIVE OR CONTRAINDICATED

►**Neonates younger than 1 week and weighing 2 kg (4.4 lb) or less:** 10 to 15 mg/kg I.V. q 12 to 18 hours.

►**Neonates younger than 1 week and weighing more than 2 kg:** 10 to 15 mg/kg I.V. q 8 to 12 hours.

►**Neonates 1 week or older and weighing 2 kg or less:** 10 to 15 mg/kg I.V. q 8 to 12 hours.

►**Neonates 1 week or older and weighing more than 2 kg:** 15 to 20 mg/kg I.V. q 8 hours.

►**Neonates 4 weeks or younger and weighing less than 1.2 kg (2.6 lb):** 15 mg/kg I.V. every 24 hours.

►**Infants and children:** 40 mg/kg I.V. daily, divided q 6 hours or 1.2 g/m^2 daily given in divided doses or for severe infections, 40 to 60 mg/kg daily, given in four divided doses. Maximum dose 2 g daily.

►**Adults:** 500 mg I.V. q 6 hours, or 1 g q 12 hours.

ANTIBIOTIC-ASSOCIATED PSEUDOMEMBRANOUS AND STAPHYLOCOCCAL ENTEROCOLITIS

►**Children:** 40 mg/kg P.O. daily, divided q 6 to 8 hours for 7 to 10 days. Don't exceed 2 g/day.

►**Adults:** 125 to 500 mg P.O. q 6 hours for 7 to 10 days.

►**Contraindications & Precautions:** Contraindicated in patients hypersensitive to drug. Use cautiously in patients with impaired renal or hepatic function, hearing loss, or allergies to other antibiotics and in those receiving other neurotoxic, nephrotoxic, or ototoxic drugs.

Vecuronium Bromide (Norcuron)

►**Indications & Dosage**

ADJUNCT TO ANESTHESIA, TO FACILITATE INTUBATION, AND TO RELAX SKELETAL MUSCLES DURING SURGERY OR TO INCREASE COMPLIANCE DURING ASSISTED VENTILATION

►Dose depends on anesthetic used and patient's needs and response. Doses are representative and must be adjusted.

►**Children ages 10 years and over and adults:** Initially, 0.08 to 0.1 mg/kg by I.V. bolus. Higher initial doses (up to 0.3 mg/kg) may be used for rapid onset. Maintenance doses of 0.01 to 0.015 mg/kg within 25 to 40 minutes of initial dose should be administered during prolonged surgical procedures. Maintenance doses may be given q 12 to 15 minutes in patients receiving balanced anesthetic.

►**Contraindications & Precautions:** Contraindicated in patients with hypersensitivity to vecuronium and bromides. Use cautiously in patients with altered circulation caused by CV disease, edema, hepatic disease, severe obesity, bronchogenic carcinoma, electrolyte disturbances, or neuromuscular diseases.

Verapamil Hydrochloride

►**Indications & Dosage**

SUPRAVENTRICULAR TACHYARRHYTHMIAS

►**Infants younger than age 1 year:** 0.1 to 0.2 mg/kg (0.75 to 2 mg) as I.V. bolus over 2 minutes. May repeat in 30 minutes if no response occurs.

►**Children ages 1 to 15 years:** 0.1 to 0.3 mg/kg (2 to 5 mg) as I.V. bolus over 2 minutes. Don't exceed 5 mg. May repeat in 30 minutes if no response occurs; don't exceed 10 mg.

►**Adults:** 0.075 to 0.15 mg/kg (5 to 10 mg) I.V. push over 2 minutes. If no response occurs, give a second dose of 10 mg (0.15 mg/kg) 15 to 30 minutes after the first dose.

CONTROL OF VENTRICULAR RATE IN DIGITALIZED PATIENTS WITH CHRONIC ATRIAL FLUTTER OR FIBRILLATION

►**Adults:** 240 to 320 mg P.O. daily in three to four divided doses.

HYPERTENSION

►**Adults:** Initially, 80 mg P.O. t.i.d., possibly increased to 360 to 480 mg. Most patients respond to 240 mg daily. Start with sustained-release capsules at 180 mg (240 mg for Verelan) daily in the morning. A starting dose of 120 mg may be indicated in people who may have an increased response to verapamil. Adjust dosage based on clinical effectiveness 24 hours after dosing. Increase by 120 mg daily until a maximum of 480 mg daily is given. Give sustained-release capsules only once daily. Antihypertensive effects are usually seen within the first week of therapy.

►**Contraindications & Precautions:** Contraindicated in patients hypersensitive to drug and in those with severe left ventricular dysfunction, cardiogenic shock, second- or third-degree AV block or sick sinus syndrome (unless patient has a functioning pacemaker), atrial flutter or fibrillation and accessory bypass tract syndrome, severe heart failure (unless secondary to verapamil therapy), and severe hypotension. In addition, I.V. verapamil is contraindicated in patients receiving I.V. beta blockers and in those with ventricular tachycardia. Use cautiously in patients with impaired renal or hepatic function or increased intracranial pressure.

Warfarin Sodium (Coumadin, Panwarfin)

►**Indications & Dosage**

►**Adolescents and adults:** 2 to 5 mg P.O. or I.V.; then use daily PT and INR to establish optimal dose. Usual maintenance is 2 to 10 mg P.O. daily. Use I.V. only when patient can't tolerate P.O. Give over 1 to 2 minutes into peripheral vein.

►**Contraindications & Precautions:** Contraindicated in pregnant patients and in patients with bleeding disorders, GI ulcerations, severe hepatic or renal disease, severe uncontrolled hypertension, subacute bacterial endocarditis, aneurysm, ascorbic acid deficiency, history of warfarin-induced necrosis, threatened abortion, eclampsia, preeclampsia, regional or lumbar block anesthesia, polycythemia vera, and vitamin K deficiency.

Appendix II: Pediatric Codes

PEDIATRIC BRADYCARDIA ALGORITHM

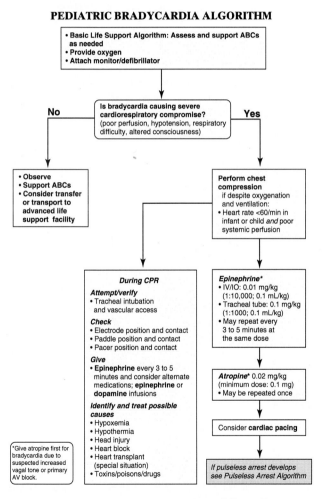

Mary Fran Hazinski, Senior Science Editor. PALS Provider Manual, American Heart Association, Dallas, 2002.

PEDIATRIC PULSELESS ARREST ALGORITHM

- **Basic Life Support Algorithm: Assess and support ABCs as needed**
- **Provide oxygen**
- **Attach monitor/defibrillator**

↓

Assess rhythm (ECG)

VF/VT ← | → **Not VF/VT (includes PEA and asystole)**

Attempt defibrillation
- Up to 3 times if needed
- Initially 2 J/kg, 2 to 4 J/kg, 4 J/kg*

During CPR

Attempt/verify
- Tracheal intubation and vascular access

Check
- Electrode position and contact
- Paddle position and contact

Give
- **Epinephrine** every 3 to 5 minutes (consider higher doses for second and subsequent doses)

Epinephrine
- IV/IO: 0.01 mg/kg (1:10,000; 0.1 mL/kg)
- Tracheal tube: 0.1 mg/kg (1:1000; 0.1 mL/kg)

Epinephrine
- IV/IO: 0.01 mg/kg (1:10,000; 0.1 mL/kg)
- Tracheal tube: 0.1 mg/kg (1:1000; 0.1 mL/kg)

Attempt defibrillation with 4 J/kg* within 30 to 60 seconds after each medication
- Pattern should be CPR-drug-shock (repeat) or CPR-drug-shock-shock-shock (repeat)

Antiarrhythmic
- *Amiodarone:* 5 mg/kg bolus IV/IO *or*
- *Lidocaine:* 1 mg/kg bolus IV/IO/TT *or*
- *Magnesium:* 25 to 50 mg/kg IV/IO for torsades de pointes or hypomagnesemia (maximum: 2 g)

Consider alternative medications
- Vasopressors
- Antiarrhythmics (see box at left)
- Buffers

Identify and treat causes
- Hypoxemia
- Hypovolemia
- Hypothermia
- Hyper-/hypokalemia and metabolic disorders
- Tamponade
- Tension pneumothorax
- Toxins/poisons/drugs
- Thromboembolism

- **Continue CPR up to 3 minutes**

Attempt defibrillation with 4 J/kg* within 30 to 60 seconds after each medication
- Pattern should be CPR-drug-shock (repeat) or CPR-drug-shock-shock-shock (repeat)

*Alternative waveforms and higher doses are Class Indeterminate for children.

Mary Fran Hazinski, Senior Science Editor. PALS Provider Manual, American Heart Association, Dallas, 2002.

PEDIATRIC TACHYCARDIA ALGORITHM FOR INFANTS AND CHILDREN WITH RAPID RHYTHM AND POOR PERFUSION

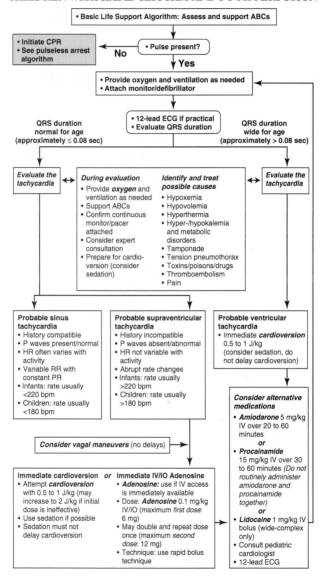

Mary Fran Hazinski, Senior Science Editor. PALS Provider Manual, American Heart Association, Dallas, 2002.

Appendix II: Pediatric Codes

PEDIATRIC TACHYCARDIA ALGORITHM FOR INFANTS AND CHILDREN WITH RAPID RHYTHM AND ADEQUATE PERFUSION

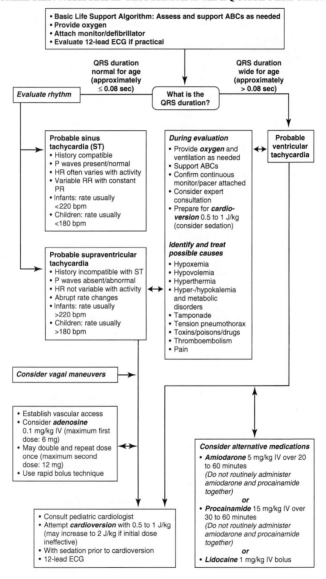

Mary Fran Hazinski, Senior Science Editor. PALS Provider Manual, American Heart Association, Dallas, 2002.

Subject Index

In this index, page numbers in *italics* designate figures; page numbers followed by *t* designate tables; vs. designates differential diagnoses; (*see also*) cross-references designate related topics or more detailed lists of subtopics.

ABCDEFGHI mnemonic, for hematuria, 439
ABCs of emergency care, 566–567
in burns, 610–611
in febrile seizures, 558
in head injury, 582–583
in shock, 599–600
in toxic ingestion, 256–257
Abdominal crisis, sickle-cell vs. acute abdomen, 414*t*
Abdominal distention, in necrotizing enterocolitis, 149
Abdominal examination, in traumatic injury, 586–588
Abdominal free-fluid sign, of splenic injury, 588
Abdominal trauma, 586–589
in child abuse, 42
indicators of serious injury, 586*t*
Abrasion, corneal, 47
Abscess
antimicrobial therapy, 160*t*, 166*t*, 167*t*
brain, 561
dental, 561
parapharyngeal, 160*t*
peritonsillar, 212–216, 213*t*
pharyngeal vs. croup, 69
retropharyngeal, 160*t*, 212–216, 213*t*
Absence seizures, 274, 550, 551, 553*t*
Abuse, 40–44
head injury and, 578
sexual, 235–236
Acetaminophen, 615
toxicity, 258–260, *259*
Acetylcysteine, 615
Acetylsalicylic acid (ASA, aspirin), 622
in Kawasaki disease, 306–307
Reye syndrome and, 50
Acid(s)
acetylsalicylic (ASA), 50, 306–307, 622
folic, 652–653
toxic ingestion, 263

Acid burns, 614
Acidemia
isovaleric, 517*t*
methylmalonic, 517*t*
organic, 518, 517–520*t*
proprionic, 517*t*
Acid-fast bacillus (Ziehl-Nelson) skin test, 191
Acidosis
in mechanical ventilation, 114
metabolic, 445
in necrotizing enterocolitis, 150
organic, 516, 517–520*t*
in renal failure, 445
Aciduria, arginosuccinic, 521*t*
Acquired immunodeficiency disease (AIDS), 237–244 (*see also* AIDS entries; Human immunodeficiency virus)
Activated charcoal, 257, 615
Acute abdomen, vs. sickle-cell crisis, 414*t*
Acute cerebral edema, in diabetic ketoacidosis, 505–506
Acute chest syndrome, in sickle cell disease, 415*t*, 415–416
Acute glaucoma, 47
Acute hematogenous osteomyelitis, 216–220
Acute Illness Observation Scale (AIOS), 154, 155*t*
Acute interstitial nephritis, 445
Acute leukemias, 397–401
acute lymphocytic leukemia (ALL), 397, 399–400
acute myelogenous leukemia (AML), 397, 399–400
Acute renal failure (ARF), 443–448
causes, 443*t*
postrenal causes, 445
prerenal causes, 443–444
renal (intrinsic) causes, 444–445

Acute rheumatic fever, 284
Acute suppurative cervical lymphad-
    enopathy, 305
Acute tubular necrosis, 444
Acyclovir, 616–617
    in chickenpox, 49
    in HSV infection, 232*t*
    in meningitis, 177
ACYC mnemonic, 49
Adenoma sebaceum, 550
Adenosine, 617
Adipose rose sign, 466
ADMIT mnemonic
    in diabetic ketoacidosis, 503
    in pneumonia, 195
Adrenal hyperplasia, congenital, 511
Adrenal leukodystrophy, 527*t*
Adrenal maturation, in normal puberty,
    507
Adrenarche, premature, 511
AEIOU mnemonic, for dialysis indica-
    tions, 448
Aganglionosis, intestinal (Hirschsprung
    disease), 81, 462, 464, 468–470,
    472
Age
    of bruises, 41*t*
    of fractures, 43*t*
Agitation, with mechanical ventilation,
    109
AIDS-defining conditions, 239*t*
Air trapping, in mechanical ventilation,
    115
Airway and surgical spine precautions,
    565–566
Airway, breathing, circulation (*see*
    ABCs of emergency care)
Airway malformations, upper, 387–390
    (*see also* Upper airway mal-
    formations *and specific
    disorders*)
Airway management
    in burns, 610
    in laryngeal fractures, 595
Alagille syndrome (arteriohepatic dys-
    plasia), 145–146, 148
Alanine aminotranferase (ALT) test, in
    abdominal injury, 587
Albumin, 617–618
Albumin replacement, in burn injury,
    613
Albuterol, in anaphylaxis, 268
Albuterol sulfate, 618–619
Alice in Wonderland syndrome, 560
Alkali burns, 613–614

Alkalinization, in persistent pulmonary
    hypertension of newborn, 140
Alkali toxicity, 263
Allergens
    in asthma, 71
    food, 267
Allergic conjunctivitis, 46, 48
Allergic coryza, 66
Allergy
    amoxicillin, 301*t*
    ampicillin, 301*t*
    penicillin, 300*t*
Allopurinol, in tumor lysis syndrome,
    409
Alopecia, in systemic lupus erythema-
    tosus, 545
α-hemolytic streptococci, in bacterial
    endocarditis, 294
α-interferon, in hepatitis, 204
Alport syndrome, 434, 440–441
Alprostadil, 619
ALTEs (apparent life-threatening
    events), 250–255
Amanita poisoning, 266
Ambulatory pediatrics, 7–94
    abuse and neglect, 40–44
    atopic dermatitis (eczema), 86–88
    attention deficit-hyperactivity
        disorder (ADHD), 89–93
    breast-feeding and nutrition, 20–24
    colic, 77–79
    conjunctivitis, 45–48
    constipation, 80–85
    croup, 67–70
    developmental delay and disability,
        25–33
    ear infection, 60–64
    failure to thrive, 34–39
    immunization, 7–16
    infection control measures, 17–18*t*
    pharyngitis, 53–55
    sinusitis, 57–59
    upper respiratory infections, 65–67
    varicella, 49–52
Amenorrhea, in systemic lupus erythe-
    matosus, 544
American College of Rheumatology, di-
    agnostic criteria for systemic lupus
    erythematosus, 544–546
American Diabetes Association (ADA)
    exchange system, 498
Amino acid disorders, 516, 520*t*
Amino acids, in premature infant, 100
Aminoglycosides, in urinary tract infec-
    tions, 452

Aminophylline, in status asthmaticus, 273
5-Aminosalicylates (5-ASA), in inflammatory bowel disease, 474–475
Amitriptyline, in headache, 562
Ammonia metabolism, inborn errors of, 516, 521*t*, 522
Amniotic fluid aspiration, 106
Amoxicillin, 619
  allergy, 301–302*t*
  in urinary tract infections, 452
Amoxicillin-clavulanic acid, in sinusitis, 59
Amoxicillin trihydrate, 619–620
Amphetamine aspartate, in ADHD, 92
Amphotericin B, 620–621
Ampicillin, 621
  allergy, 301–302*t*
  in neonatal sepsis, 130
  in urinary tract infections, 452
Ampicillin sodium/sulbactam sodium, 621
Amputation, traumatic, 576
Anal examination, in gastrointestinal bleeding, 483
Analgesics, in ear infections, 61
Anal stenosis, 80*t*
Anaphylaxis, 267–269 (*see also* Allergy; Hypersensitivity)
Androgens, in puberty, 507
Anemias, 419–428
  aplastic, 425
  approach to patient, 419–423, 420*t*, 421
  hemolytic, 545
  microcytic, 423–425
    anemia of chronic disease, 425
    iron deficiency anemia, 423
    lead poisoning, 424
    thalassemia, 423–424
  normocytic, 425–427
    hemolytic, 425–427
    of underproduction, 425
  pernicious, 427
  in systemic lupus erythematosus, 544, 545
Anesthesia, emergency induction, 566*t*, 567*t*
Aneurysms, in Kawasaki disease, 307–308
Angina, Ludwig, antimicrobial therapy, 163*t*
Angiography, in gastrointestinal bleeding, 486
Animal bites, antimicrobial therapy, 163*t*
Anomalous left pulmonary artery, 390

Anterior cord syndrome, 603
Anthropometric measurement, 36
Antibiotic-associated colitis, antimicrobial therapy, 166*t*
Antibiotic prophylaxis
  in cystic fibrosis, 395
  in Henoch-Schönlein purpura, 532
  intrapartum, 127
  in valvular heart disease, 345, 346
Antibiotic resistance, in tuberculosis, 192
Antibiotics, 158–159–168*t* (*see also specific drugs*)
  in atopic dermatitis, 88
  in bacterial endocarditis, 295
  in bronchiolitis, 186
  in conjunctivitis, 47
  contraindications, 172
  in ear infections, 63–64
  in fractures, 574
  in head injury, 584
  in hyaline membrane disease, 106
  in inflammatory bowel disease, 475
  in malignancy-associated fever, 430–432
  in meningitis, 177
  in meningococcemia, 182, *183*
  in neonatal sepsis, 130
  in osteomyelitis, 217–219, 218*t*
  in pharyngitis, 55
  in septic arthritis, 224
  in sexually transmitted diseases (STDs), 231–235*t*, 235
  in sinusitis, 58–59
  in toxic shock syndrome, 210
  in urinary tract infections, 452–453
Antibody-mediated hemolysis, 427
Antibody tests, in diabetes mellitus, 495
Anticholinergic plants, 266
Anticonvulsants, 551–555*t*
  in headache, 562
  in head injury, 584
  in seizure prophylaxis, 558–559
  side effects, 551
  in status epilepticus, 275
Antidepressants, in ADHD, 92
Antidiuretic hormone (ADH, vasopressin), syndrome of inappropriate secretion (SIADH), 175, 177, 178
Antifungals, in soft-tissue infections, 207
Antihistamines, in sinusitis, 59
Antinuclear antibodies (ANA), in juvenile rheumatoid arthritis, 540
Antipruritic medications, 88

Anti-Smith antibodies, in systemic lupus
    erythematosus, 546
α1-Antitrypsin deficiency, 144
Anuria, 443
Aortic arch malformations, 390
Aortic disruption, traumatic, 593
Aortic ejection click, 339–340, *340*
Aortic ejection murmur, 291
Aortic regurgitation, 341–342, 351
Aortic stenosis, 339–341, *340*
Aortic valve disease, 339–342
Aphthous oral ulcers (stomatitis),
    471–472
Aplastic anemia, 425
Apnea, 250–255
    of infancy (idiopathic ALTE), 250–255
    obstructive sleep, 253
    of prematurity, 253
    prolonged expiratory (breath-holding
      spells), 253, 551
Apparent life-threatening events
    (ALTEs), 250–255
    differential diagnosis, 253
Appendiceal CT scan with rectal
    contrast, 480
Appendicitis, 478–481
    vs. diabetic ketoacidosis, 502
Appendix testis, torsion of, 456–459
Apt-Downey test, 484
Arginosuccinic aciduria, 521*t*
Arterial blood gases (ABGs)
    in asthma, 72
    in hypoplastic left heart syndrome,
      382
    in mechanical ventilation, 114,
      118–119*t*
    in premature infant, 101
    in shock, 601
    in status asthmaticus, 271
Arterial transposition, 372–374
Arteriohepatic dysplasia (Alagille
    syndrome), 145–146, 148
Artery (arteries)
    anomalous left pulmonary, 390
    transposition of great, *372,* 372–374
Arthritis
    juvenile rheumatoid, 284–285, 288,
      533–541 (*see also* Juvenile
      rheumatoid arthritis)
    poststreptococcal reactive, 284
    pyogenic, antimicrobial therapy, 164*t*
    septic, 216, 221–225, 283
    in systemic lupus erythematosus, 544
Arum (dieffenbachia) poisoning, 266
Ash leaf spots, 550

Aspartate aminotransferase (AST) test,
    in abdominal injury, 587
Aspiration
    amniotic fluid, 106
    foreign body, 69
    synovial fluid, 222–224, 223*t,* 288, 533,
      534, 540
Aspirin (*see* Acetylsalicylic acid)
Assessment
    qualitative, 2–3
    quantitative, 3–6
Assist control ventilation, 112
Asthma
    definitions, 71
    management
      acute, 73*t,* 73–74
      ongoing, 74, 75–76*t*
    outpatient treatment, 71–76
    status asthmaticus, 270–273
    symptoms, 71–72
Asymptomatic bacteriuria, 449 (*see also*
    Urinary tract infections)
Athetoid cerebral palsy, 26
Athlete's foot (tinea pedis), 206
Atlanto-occipital dislocation, 604
Atonic seizures, 550, 551
Atopic dermatitis (eczema), 85–88
    differential diagnosis, 87*t*
Atopic triad, 85
Atresia
    cardiovascular
      pulmonary atresia, 364
      tricuspid atresia, 361–364
    choanal, 389–390
    duodenal, 462
    esophageal, 461–462
    extrahepatic biliary, 144–145
    pulmonary, 364
    tricuspid, 361–364, *362, 363*
Atrial fibrillation, 348
Atrial hypertrophy, 347
Atrial septal defect, 354–357, 365, *365,*
    385 (*see also* Tetralogy of Fallot)
    ostium premium, 354, 356, *357*
    ostium secundum, 354, 356
    sinus venous, 354
Atrioventricular canal, complete
    (endocardial cushion defect),
    385–386
Atropine sulfate, 622–623
Attention deficit hyperactivity disorder
    (ADHD), 89–93
    clinical manifestations, 89, 90–91*t*
    comorbidities, 91
Atypical febrile seizures, 557–559

Aura, in migraine, 560
Auralgan, in ear infections, 61
Autoimmune diseases (*see also* Rheumatology)
 juvenile rheumatoid arthritis, 533–541
 systemic lupus erythematosus, 542–548
Autoimmune hepatitis, 200
Axenfeld anomaly, 148
Axonal injury, diffuse, 579–580
Azithromycin, 623–624
 in pharyngitis, 55

Bacitracin, 624
Bacteremia, 293, 450
 occult, 153
 WBC in, 154
Bacterial causes, of otitis media, 61*t*
Bacterial endocarditis, 293–303
 cardiac conditions associated with, 298–299*t*
 microbiology, 294
 prophylaxis, 295, 296–297*t*
Bacterial enteritis, antimicrobial therapy, 165*t*
Bacterial meningitis, antimicrobial therapy, 167*t*
Bacterial pharyngitis, 53–55
Bacterial tracheitis, vs. croup, 69
Bacterial vaginitis, 227–234*t*
Bacteriuria, 452 (*see also* Urinary tract infections)
 asymptomatic, 449
Balloon valvuloplasty, 341, 345
Barbiturates (*see also specific drugs*)
 side effects, 551
 in status epilepticus, 276
Barium (contrast) enema, 467, 469
 in inflammatory bowel disease, 474
Barotrauma, 109
Basilar skull fracture, 578
Beck triad, 592
Beclomethasone dipropionate, 624–625
Behavioral interventions
 in ADHD, 92
 in headache, 562
Behavior patterns
 between ages 1 and 5, 28–30*t*
 first-year, 27–28*t*
Bell's staging criteria, for necrotizing enterocolitis, 150
Benign epilepsy of childhood, 554*t*
Benzodiazepines (*see also specific drugs*)
 in status epilepticus, 276

Beractant, 625–626
β$_2$ agonists
 in asthma, 73
 in status asthmaticus, 271
β-blockers
 in headache, 562
 in tetralogy of Fallot, 367
 toxic ingestion, 260–262
Bicarbonate of soda (*see* Sodium bicarbonate)
Biguanides, 497
Biliary atresia, extrahepatic, 144–145
Bilirubin encephalopathy, 122, 123
Bilirubin physiology, 121
Biofeedback, in headache, 562
Biopsy
 bone marrow, 398
 liver, 148
 rectal, 469
 renal, 447, 531, 546
 skin, 531, 547
Bisacodyl, 85*t*
Biventricular hypertrophy, 332–333, 334, 376
Blalock-Taussig shunt, 361–363, 367
Bleeding (*see* Hemorrhage)
Bleeding scans, 486
Blood cell indices, normal, 420*t*
Blood cultures
 in endocarditis, 295
 in malignancy-associated fever, 430
 in neonatal sepsis, 130
Blood gases (*see* Arterial blood gases)
Blood lead level (BLL), 424
Blood pressure measurement, 315 (*see also* Hypertension)
Blood transfusion
 in gastrointestinal bleeding, 483–484
 in meningococcemia, 182
Blunt cardiac injury, 593, 597
Bone involvement, in acute leukemias, 398–399
Bone marrow biopsy, 398
Bone marrow relapse, in acute leukemias, 400
Bone marrow transplantation, in acute leukemias, 399–400
Bone scan
 in osteomyelitis, 217
 in refusal to bear weight, 288
Bone tumors, 404
Bony enlargement, in anemia, 422
Bowing, traumatic, 571
Brain abscess, 561
 antibiotic therapy, 168*t*

Brain lesions, precocious puberty and, 508
Brain stem herniation, 407
Brain tumors, 402, 561
Breast development
   normal, 507
   premature, 510–511
Breast engorgement, 21–22*t*
Breast-feeding, 20–24 (*see also* Nutrition)
   benefits, 20
   common concerns, 22–23*t*
   medications and, 21*t*
Breast-feeding jaundice, 122
Breast milk jaundice, 122
Breath-holding spells, 253
   vs. seizures, 551
Bretylium tosylate, 626
Bronchiolitis, 185–188
Bronchoconstriction, in mechanical ventilation, 115
Bronchodilators
   in bronchiolitis, 186
   in cystic fibrosis, 394
Brown Séquard syndrome, 603
Brudzinski sign, 174
Bruising, 40–41
   age determination by color, 41*t*
Buccal cellulitis, antimicrobial therapy, 163*t*
Budesonide, 626–627
   in croup, 70
Bulk-forming laxatives, 83*t*
Burns, 608–614
   acid, 614
   alkali, 613–614
   in child abuse, 41
   classification of, 609*t*
   criteria for transfer to burn center, 609–610
   dry chemical, 614
   electrical, 613
   thermal, 610–613
      fluid resuscitation, 611–613
      rule of nines, 611, *612*
   types of, 608*t*, 608–609
Butterfly (malar) rash, 543
Button batteries, ingestion, 262

C-A-BIG-K mnemonic, for hyper-kalemia, 448
Café-au-lait spots, 550
Caffeine, 627
Calcium channel blockers, toxic ingestion, 262

Calculi, renal (nephrolithiasis), 439–440
Caloric insufficiency, failure to thrive and, 35*t*
Cancer, colon, 476–477
Candida albicans, 227–234*t*
Candidiasis, 227–234*t*
Captopril, 627
Carbamazepine, 628
Carbohydrate metabolism, inborn errors of, 522, 523–525*t*
Carbon monoxide poisoning, 262–263
   signs of, 610*t*
Cardiac examination, 325–326, *326* (*see also* Electrocardiography)
   for aortic coarctation, 337
Cardiac infections, antimicrobial therapy, 165*t*
Cardiac injury, blunt, 593, 597
Cardiac output
   impaired, 109
   in renal failure, 444
Cardiac syncope, 277, 279*t*
Cardiac tamponade, 592, 597
Cardiac transplantation, 319
Cardiac trauma, 577–585
Cardiology, 291–386 (*see also individual conditions*)
   congenital heart disease, 321–386
      aortic valve disease, 339–342
      approach to patient, 324–335
      atrial septal defects, 354–357
      coarctation of aorta, 336–338
      complete atrioventricular canal (endocardial cushion defect), 385–386
      Ebstein anomaly, 369–371
      hypoplastic left heart syndrome, 381–386
      mitral valve disease, 346–348
      patent ductus arteriosus, 358–360
      physiology and pathophysiology, 321–322
      pulmonary atresia, 364
      pulmonary valve disease, 343–345
      tetralogy of Fallot, 365–368
      total anomalous pulmonary venous return, 377–380
      transposition of great arteries, 372–374
      tricuspid atresia, 361–364
      truncus arteriosus, 375–376
      types, 322, 323*t*
      ventricular septal defects, 349–353
   general, 291–321
      bacterial endocarditis, 293–303

hypertension, 309–316
  Kawasaki disease, 304–308
  myocarditis, 317–319
  normal murmurs, 291–292
Cardiovascular collapse, in anaphylaxis,
    268
Cardiovascular development, 321–322
Cardiovascular manifestations, in sys-
    temic lupus erythematosus, 543
Cardiovascular stabilization, of prema-
    ture infant, 100–101
Castor bean poisoning, 266
Casts, urinary, 446
Catch-up immunization schedule, 10–11t
Catheterization
  contraindications, 569
  Foley in trauma, 568–569
  urinary in abdominal injury, 589
Cefaclor, 628
Cefadroxil, 629
Cefazolin, in septic arthritis, 224
Cefazolin sodium, 629
Cefixime, 629
Cefotaxime, in neonatal sepsis, 130
Cefotaxime sodium, 629–630
Cefoxitin sodium, 630
Cefpodoxime proxetil, 631
Cefprozil, 631–632
Ceftazidime, 632
  in malignancy-associated fever,
    430–431
Ceftriaxone, in status epilepticus, 276
Ceftriaxone sodium, 632–633
Cefuroxime, in cellulitis, 208
Cefuroxime axetil, 633–634
Celiotomy, in abdominal injury, 589
Cellulitis
  antimicrobial therapy, 160–163t
  buccal, 163t
  orbital or periorbital, 47, 162t, 208
  retropharyngeal, 160t
Central cord syndrome, 603
Central hypoventilation syndrome,
    congenital, 253
Central nervous system (CNS)
  in acute leukemias, 400
  antimicrobial therapy, 167–168t
  herpesvirus infection, 137
  in sickle cell disease, 414–415
Central venous pressure monitoring, in
    shock, 601
Cephalexin hydrochloride, 634
Cephalosporins
  in sinusitis, 59
  in urinary tract infections, 452, 453

Cerebral contusion, 578
Cerebral edema, in diabetic keto-
    acidosis, 502, 505–506
Cerebral hematoma, 561
Cerebral palsy, 25
  athetoid, 26
  risk factors, 32
Cerebral perfusion pressure, 577
Cerebrospinal fluid (CSF) analysis
  in febrile seizures, 558
  in meningitis, 175, 176t
  in meningococcemia, 181–182
  in neonatal sepsis, 130–131
Cerebrovascular accident (stroke), in
    systemic lupus erythematosus,
    544
Cervical lymphadenitis, 207–208
Cervical lymphadenopathy, suppurative,
    305
Cervical spine injuries, 604
Cervicitis (see Sexually transmitted
    diseases)
Cetirizine hydrochloride, 634
Chemical burns, 614
Chemical conjunctivitis, 48
Chemotherapy
  in acute leukemias, 399–400
  tumor lysis syndrome and, 409
Chest auscultation, in pneumonia, 194
Chest examination, for congenital heart
    disease, 324–325
Chest radiography
  in aortic coarctation, 337–338
  in aortic regurgitation, 342
  in aortic stenosis, 340
  in asthma, 72
  in atrial septal defect, 356
  in chest trauma, 594, 595t
  in hypoplastic left heart syndrome,
    382
  in mechanical ventilation, 115
  in mitral regurgitation, 348
  in patent ductus arteriosus, 359
  in tetralogy of Fallot, 367
  in transposition of great arteries, 373
  in upper airway malformations, 390
  in ventricular hypertrophy, 333–334,
    335
  in ventricular septal defect, 353
Chest syndrome, acute, in sickle cell
    disease, 415t, 415–416
Chest trauma, 590–597 (see also
    Thoracic trauma)
Chickenpox (varicella), 49–52
Child abuse, 40–44, 235–236, 578

Childhood, benign epilepsy of, 554*t*
Childhood conjunctivitis (pinkeye),
    45–48
Chlamydial conjunctivitis, 46
Chlamydial infection, 227–234*t*
Chloral hydrate, 635
Choanal atresia, 389–390
Cholangiography, 145
Cholestasis, defined, 145
CHOLESTATIC mnemonic for
    jaundice, 144
Cholesteatoma, 64
Chondrodysplasia punctata, rhizomelic,
    527*t*
Chromosomal studies, in developmental
    delay, 32
Chronic disease, anemia of, 425
Cimetidine, 635
Ciprofloxacin, in inflammatory bowel
    disease, 475
Cisapride, adverse effects, 490
Citrulinemia, 521*t*
Clarithromycin, 636
Clindamycin, in toxic shock syndrome,
    210
Clindamycin hydrochloride, 636–637
Clonazepam, 637
Clonidine
    in ADHD, 92
    toxic ingestion, 262
Clotrimazole, 637
Coagulation abnormalities
    in acute leukemias, 399
    in shock, 601
    in systemic lupus erythematosus, 544,
        545
Coarctation of aorta, *336,* 336–338
    complicated, 338
    simple, 336–338, *339*
Codeine phosphate, 638
4 C's of cyanotic heart disease, 323
Cognitive impairment, in systemic lupus
    erythematosus, 544
Cold anaphylaxis, 267
Colfosceril palmitate, 638
Colic, 77–79
Colitis
    antibiotic-associated, antimicrobial
        therapy, 166*t*
    ulcerative, 471–477 (*see also*
        Inflammatory bowel disease)
Colon cancer, inflammatory bowel
    disease and, 476–477
Colonoscopy, 474
Coma, hyperosmolar nonketotic, 501

Comminuted fracture, 571, *571*
Communication disorder, 26
CO_2 monitoring, 115
    end-tidal, 114
    transcutaneous, 114
Compartment syndromes, 575
Complement tests, in systemic lupus
    erythematosus, 547
Complete atrioventricular canal (endo-
    cardial cushion defect), 385–386
Complete blood count (CBC)
    in acute leukemias, 398
    in apparent life-threatening event
        (ALTE), 252
    in Kawasaki disease, 306
    in neonatal sepsis, 130
    in osteomyelitis, 217
    in pneumonia, 195
    in refusal to bear weight, 287
    in renal failure, 446
Compression
    of esophagus, 390
    of trachea, 390
Computed tomography (CT scan)
    in abdominal injury, 588
    appendiceal with rectal contrast, 480
    in chest trauma, 594
    in child abuse, 43–44
    in developmental delay, 32
    in head injury, 581
    in meningitis, 175, 178
Concussion, 578
Congenital adrenal hyperplasia, 511
Congenital central hypoventilation
    syndrome, 253
Congenital heart disease, 321–386 *(see
        also specific disorders)*
    approach to patient, 324–335
    atresia
        pulmonary, 364
        tricuspid, 361–364
    bacterial endocarditis risk and, 299*t*
    coarctation of aorta, 336–338
    complete atrioventricular canal
        (endocardial cushion defect),
        385–386
    Ebstein anomaly, 369–371
    hypoplastic left heart syndrome,
        381–384
    patent ductus arteriosus, 358–360
    physiology and pathophysiology,
        321–322
    septal defect
        atrial, 354–357
        ventricular, 349–353

tetralogy of Fallot, 365–368
total anomalous pulmonary venous return, 377–380
transposition of great arteries, 372–374
truncus arteriosus, 375–376
types, 322, 323t
valvular disease
  aortic, 339–342
  mitral, 346–348
  pulmonary, 343–345
vs. hyaline membrane disease, 106
Congenital hypothyroidism, 146
Congenital STORCH infection, 132–138, 144, 148
Congenital upper airway malformations, 387–390 (see also Upper airway malformations and specific disorders)
Congenital varicella syndrome, 52
Congestive heart failure, 317, 341
Conjunctivitis, 45–48, 304
  antimicrobial therapy, 162t
Constipation, 80–85
  secondary causes, 80–81t
  therapy, 82, 83–85t
Contact dermatitis, 87t
Continuous positive airway pressure (CPAP), 111
Contraception, emergency, 236
Contrast (barium) enema, 467
  in inflammatory bowel disease, 474
Contrast study, upper gastrointestinal, 489
Contusion
  cerebral, 578
  pulmonary, 592, 597
Coombs test, 422, 546
Cori, Hers disease, 523t
Corneal abrasion, 47
Corneal trauma, 47
Corticosteroids
  in anaphylaxis, 269
  in atopic dermatitis, 87–88
  in bronchiolitis, 186
  in Henoch-Schönlein purpura, 531–532
  hyaline membrane disease and, 106
  in inflammatory bowel disease, 475
  in juvenile rheumatoid arthritis, 540
  in meningococcemia, 182
  myocarditis, 318
  in status asthmaticus, 271–273
Cortisone acetate, 638–639
Coryza (upper respiratory tract infection), 65–67

Co-trimoxazole, 639
Coxa plana (Legg-Calvé-Perthes disease), 285, 289
CPS deficiency, 521t
C-reactive protein test
  in inflammatory bowel disease, 473
  in Kawasaki disease, 306
  in neonatal sepsis, 131
  in osteomyelitis, 217
  in refusal to bear weight, 287–288
  in systemic lupus erythematosus, 545
Creatine kinase, 318
Critical care/emergency medicine, 245–289 (see also individual subtopics)
  anaphylaxis, 267–269
  apparent life-threatening events (ALTEs) and apnea, 250–255
  dehydration, 245–249
  refusal to bear weight, 283–289
  status asthmaticus, 270–273
  status epilepticus, 274–276
  syncope, 274–282
  toxic ingestions, 256–267
Crohn disease (regional enteritis), 471–477 (see also Inflammatory bowel disease)
Cromolyn sodium, 640
Croup, 68–70
  differential diagnosis, 69
Crush injuries, 575–576
Cullen sign, of splenic injury, 587
Currant jelly stool, 465
Cyanide poisoning, 265
Cyanosis, 366
Cyanotic lesions, 322, 323t
Cystic fibrosis, 80t, 391–395
  antimicrobial therapy, 161t
Cystic fibrosis transmembrane regulator (CFTR), 391
Cystitis, 449, 450 (see also Urinary tract infections)
  antimicrobial therapy, 167t
Cystography, radionuclide, 453
Cystourethrography, voiding, 453, 454t
Cytomegalovirus, 133t, 135–136 (see also STORCH infections)
Cytotoxic agents, in systemic lupus erythematosus, 547

Dacrocystitis, 47
Dactylitis, in sickle cell disease, 414
Dawn phenomenon, 498
Decision-making, medical, 2–6 (see also Medical decision-making)

Decongestants
  in coryza, 66
  in sinusitis, 59
Deferoxamine challenge test, 264
Deferoxamine mesylate, 640
Dehydration, 245–249 (*see also*
      Fluid/electrolyte therapy)
  in diabetic ketoacidosis, 501
  evaluation, 503–504, 504*t*
  hypernatremic, 245–246
  hyponatremic, 245, 246–247
Dental abscess, 561
Dental procedures, bacterial endocarditis
      prophylaxis in, 296–297*t*
Dermatitis
  atopic (eczema), 85–88
  contact, 87*t*
  seborrheic, 87*t*
Dermatophyte infections, 206–207
Development, 25–33
  adaptive and visuomotor, 31
  gross motor, 31
  milestones of, 25–28
    age 1 to 5, 29–30*t*
    birth to age 1, 27–28*t*
Developmental delay, terminology,
      25–36
Developmental disability, 25
  treatment, 32–33
Developmental hip dysplasia, 285, 289
Developmental quotient (DQ), 26
Dexamethasone, 640–641
  in croup, 69
  in meningitis, 177
Dextroamphetamine sulfate, 642
Dextrose administration, 505
Diabetes Control and Complication
      Trial, 499
Diabetes mellitus, 493–501 (*see also*
      Diabetic ketoacidosis; Hyper-
      glycemia; Insulin)
  complications, 498–499
  in cystic fibrosis, 393
  diagnosis, 494–495
  epidemiology, 494
  maturity-onset diabetes of the young
      (MODY), 493
  recent advances, 499
  ᵗvpe I (IDDM), 493, 495–497, 496*t*
  ⁻ II (NIDDM), 493, 497–498
    ⁻d pathogenesis, 493
      vention Trial, 499
        ·ᵈosis, 501–506
          ⁻ᵓ2

  vs. appendicitis, 502
  vs. meningitis, 503
Diagnostic approach, 1–2
Diagnostic continuum, 2
Dialysis, AEIOU indications, 448
Diamond-Blackfan anemia, 428
Diaphragm, spinal cord injury and, 605
Diaphragmatic trauma, 593, 597
Diarrhea, in inflammatory bowel
      disease, 474
Diazepam, 642
  in status epilepticus, 275
Dicloxacillin sodium, 643
Diet, in diabetes mellitus, 498
Diffuse axonal injury, 579–580
Digoxin, 643–645
Di-isopropyl iminodiacetic acid
      (DISIDA) scan, 145
Dimethylsuccinic acid (DMSA) scan,
      453–454
Diphenhydramine, 645
Diphtheria/tetanus/pertussis immuni-
      zation, 8*t*, 12–13*t*
Diplegia, spastic, 26
Dipstick tests, urine, 433*t*, 434
Discoid rash, 543
Dislocation, atlanto-occipital, 604
Disseminated herpes infection, 136–137
Disseminated intravascular coagulation
      (DIC), in meningococcemia, 182
Distributive shock, 268–269
Diuretic therapy
  in head injury, 584
  in renal failure, 447
Dobutamine hydrochloride, 646
Docusate sodium, 85*t*
Dolasetron mesylate, 646
Dopamine hydrochloride, 647
Dornase alfa, 647
Down syndrome, 468
Doxycycline, 647–648
Drash syndrome, 434
Drug-induced hematuria, 440
Drug-induced systemic lupus erythe-
      matosus, 542
Drug-related anaphylaxis, 267
Drugs
  causing proteinuria, 434
  constipation-causing, 81*t*
  contraindicated in breast-feeding, 21*t*
Drug sensitivity testing, in tuberculosis,
      192
Duhamel procedure, 469
  Martin modification, 469
Dysplasia, developmental hip, 285, 289

Ear infections
    otitis externa (swimmer's ear), 60t,
        60–61
    otitis media, 61–64, 62t
Ebstein anomaly, 369–371
Echocardiography
    in acute leukemias, 399
    in aortic coarctation, 337
    in endocarditis, 295
    in mitral valve prolapse, 346
    in Romano-Ward syndrome, 282
    in syncope, 281
    in systemic lupus erythematosus, 546
    in transposition of great arteries, 372,
        373
    in ventricular hypertrophy, 335
Eczema (atopic dermatitis), 85–88
Eczema herpeticum, 88
Edema, cerebral, in diabetic keto-
        acidosis, 502, 505–506
Eisenmenger syndrome, 321–322, 349
Ejection click
    aortic, 339–340, 340
    pulmonary, 344, 344
Ejection murmur
    aortic, 291
    pulmonary, 291–292, 366
Electrical burns, 608, 613 (see also
        Burns)
Electrocardiography (ECG)
    in acute leukemias, 399
    in aortic coarctation, 337
    in aortic regurgitation, 342
    in aortic stenosis, 340
    in atrial septal defect, 356, 356, 357
    in congenital heart disease, 326–334,
        327–328t, 329t
    in Ebstein anomaly, 369–370, 370
    in hypoplastic left heart syndrome,
        382
    in Kawasaki disease, 306
    in mitral regurgitation, 347–348, 348
    in mitral valve prolapse, 346
    in myocarditis, 318
    in patent ductus arteriosus, 359
    in pulmonary atresia, 364
    in pulmonary stenosis, 344, 344–345
    in syncope, 280, 281, 282
    in tetralogy of Fallot, 367
    in transposition of great arteries, 373
    in trauma, 568
    in tricuspid atresia, 361, 363
    in ventricular septal defect, 351, 352
    in Wolff-Parkinson-White syndrome,
        281

Electroencephalography (EEG)
    in developmental delay, 32
    in febrile seizures, 558
    in seizures, 550–551
    in syncope, 281
Emergencies, oncologic, 406–411 (see
        also Oncologic emergencies)
Emergency contraception, 236
Emergency medicine, 245–289 (see also
        Critical care/emergency
        medicine)
Empyema, antimicrobial therapy, 161t
Encephalitis
    defined, 173
    herpesvirus, 175
Encephalopathy, bilirubin, 122, 123
Endocardial cushion defect (complete
        atrioventricular canal), 385–386
Endocarditis
    antimicrobial therapy, 165t
    bacterial, 293–303 (see also Bacterial
        endocarditis)
    culture-negative, 294
    fungal, 294
    Libman-Sacks, 543
    in systemic lupus erythematosus, 543
Endocrine manifestations
    of cystic fibrosis, 393
    in systemic lupus erythematosus, 544
Endocrinology, 493–528 (see also
        individual subtopics)
    diabetes mellitus, 493–501
    diabetic ketoacidosis, 501–506
    inborn errors of metabolism, 512–528
        (see also Inborn errors of
        metabolism)
    precocious puberty, 507–512
Endophthalmitis, antimicrobial therapy,
        162t
Endoscopy
    in GERD, 489
    in inflammatory bowel disease, 474
End-tidal CO_2 monitoring, 114
Enema, contrast (barium), 467, 469
    in inflammatory bowel disease, 474
Enteral feedings, in premature infant,
        100
Enterocolitis, necrotizing, 149–151
Enzyme assays, in abdominal injury,
        587
Eosinophilic myocarditis, 318
Epididymitis, 456–459
    antimicrobial therapy, 167t
Epiglottitis, 212–216, 213t
    antimicrobial therapy, 160t

Epilepsy, 274–276 (*see also* Seizures)
   benign of childhood, 554*t*
   juvenile myoclonic, 555*t*
   risk factors for, 559
Epinephrine, 648–649
   in anaphylaxis, 268
   racemic, in croup, 69
   in resuscitation, 98*t*
Epi-Pen, 269
Epiphysis, slipped capital femoral, 285,
   289
Episodic hypoglycemia, 499
Ergot, in headache, 562
Erythroblastopenia, transient of child-
   hood, 425
Erythrocyte sedimentation rate (ESR)
   in inflammatory bowel disease, 473
   in Kawasaki disease, 306
   in osteomyelitis, 217
   in refusal to bear weight, 287
   in systemic lupus erythematosus, 545
Erythromycin, in pharyngitis, 55
Erythromycin base, 649
Esophageal atresia, 461–462
Esophageal causes, of gastrointestinal
   bleeding, 485
Esophageal compression, 390
Esophageal rupture, 594, 597
Esophagoduodenostomy, 474, 484
Esophography, in upper airway mal-
   formations, 390
Estrogen
   in premature thelarche, 510
   in puberty, 507
Ethanol, toxic ingestion, 265
Ethosuximide, 649
   side effects, 551
Exanthem, in chickenpox, 49
Exchange transfusion, 101, 122–123,
   125–126
Exercise, in diabetes mellitus, 498
Exercise-induced anaphylaxis, 267
Exercise-induced hematuria, 440
Expiratory stridor, 387
Expiratory time (T_E), 109
Extracorporeal membrane oxygenation
   (ECMO), 139, 140
Extrahepatic biliary atresia, 144–145
Extubation, 117
Eye conditions, conjunctivitis, 45–48
Eye examination
   in head injury, 583
   in juvenile rheumatoid arthritis, 540
Eye infections, antimicrobial therapy,
   162*t*

Eye inflammation, in juvenile rheumatoid arthritis, 538*t*, 540

Fabry syndrome, 527*t*
Factitious hematochezia, 482
Failure to thrive, 34–39
   approach to patient, 36–38
   causes, 34–36, 35*t*
   prognosis, 38–39
   treatment, 38
Fallot, tetralogy of, 365, 365–368
Familial hematuria, 440–441
Farber syndrome, 527*t*
Fasciitis, necrotizing, 211
   antimicrobial therapy, 163*t*
Fatty acid oxidation, inborn errors of,
   526*t*, 528
Febrile seizures, 557–559
Fecalith, 479
Feeding assessment, 36
Feminization, 510 (*see also* Precocious
   puberty)
Femoral shaft fractures, 575
Fentanyl citrate, 650
Ferritin level test, 422
Ferrous sulfate, 650
Fever
   defined, 153, 429
   without focus, 153–157
   in malignancy, 429–432
   patterns of, 169
   in sickle cell disease, 416
   of unknown origin, 169–173, 170*t*
Fexofenadine hydrochloride, 650–651
Fiber supplementation, contra-
   indications, 82
Fibrillation, atrial, 348
Fibrosis, cystic, 391–395
Figure 3 sign, 337
Fistula, tracheoesophageal, 388–389, 389
Flail chest, 591–592, 596 (*see also*
   Thoracic trauma)
Fluconazole, 651
Fluid deficit, 503–504, 504*t* (*see also*
   Dehydration; Fluid/electrolyte
   therapy)
   calculation of, 246
Fluid/electrolyte therapy, 246–247
   contraindications, 583
   in diabetic ketoacidosis, 503
   in hemorrhagic shock, 600–601
   in meningitis, 177–178
   in prematurity, 97–99, 99*t*
   3-for-1 rule of, 600
Fluid restriction, in renal failure, 447

Fluid resuscitation, in burns, 611–613
Fluids, isotonic, 245
Flumazenil, 651–652
Fluticasone propionate, 652
Folic acid, 427, 652–653
Fontan procedure, 363
  hemi-, 384
  in hypoplastic left heart syndrome, 384
Food allergens, 267
Foreign body aspiration, 69
Foxglove, 266
Fraction of inspiratory oxygen (FIO₂), 109
Fractures, 571–576 *(see also* Trauma)
  in child abuse, 42
  Harris classification, *573*
  laryngeal, 591, 595–596 *(see also* Thoracic trauma)
  lower extremity, 575
  pelvic, 574–575
  rib, 597
  skull, 578
  spinal cord, 603–604 *(see also* Spinal cord injury)
  thoracic, 594
  thoracic spine, 604
  toddler's, 285, 289
  traumatic, 285
  types, *571, 571–575, 573*
  upper extremity, 574
  vertebral, 604
Free water calculation, 248
Fructose intolerance, 525*t*
  hereditary, 146
Fulminant hepatic failure, 198
Fundoplication, gastric (Nissen), in GERD, 490
Fungal endocarditis, 294
Furosemide, 653 *(see also* Diuretic therapy)
  in head injury, 584

Gabapentin, 653
GABHS infection, 54
Gait evaluation, 283, 286
Galactosemia, 146, 524*t*
Gallbladder, hydrops of, 530
Ganciclovir, 654
Gardnerella vaginalis, 227–234*t*
Gas gangrene, antimicrobial therapy, 163*t*
Gastric aspirate culture, in neonatal sepsis, 130
Gastric decompression, in hemorrhagic shock, 600

Gastric (Nissen) fundoplication, in GERD, 490
Gastric lavage
  in suspected tuberculosis, 191
  in toxic ingestions, 257
Gastric tube, pre-peritoneal lavage, 588
Gastroenterology, 461–491 *(see also specific disorders and* Gastrointestinal *entries)*
  appendicitis, 478–481
  constipation, 80–85
  gastroesophageal reflux disease (GERD), 77–79, 250, 463–464, 497–491
  gastrointestinal bleeding, 482–486
  Hirschsprung disease (toxic megacolon), 81, 462, 464, 468–470, 472
  inflammatory bowel disease, 471–477
  intussusception, 464, 465–467
  vomiting, 461–464
Gastroesophageal reflux disease (GERD), 77–79, 250, 463–464, 497–491
  in colic, 77–79
  differential diagnosis, 488*t*
  types, 487
  vs. regurgitation, 487
Gastrointestinal bleeding, 482–486
  nomenclature, 482
  occult, 482
Gastrointestinal manifestations
  of cystic fibrosis, 392
  of systemic lupus erythematosus, 543
Gastrointestinal problems, in Henoch-Schönlein purpura, 530
Gastrointestinal procedures, bacterial endocarditis prophylaxis in, 297*t*, 300–301*t*
Gaucher disease, 527*t*
Genital warts (HPV), 227–234*t*
Genitourinary conditions, swollen scrotum, 456–459
Genitourinary infections, antimicrobial therapy, 167*t*
Genitourinary tract procedures, bacterial endocarditis and, 297*t*, 300–301*t*
Gentamicin, 654–655
  in malignancy-associated fever, 431
  in neonatal sepsis, 130
GERD *(see* Gastroesophageal reflux disease)
Ghon complex, 189
Glasgow Coma Scale, 580, 580*t*

Glasgow Meningococcal Septicemia
    Score, 184, 184*t*
Glaucoma, acute, 47
Glomerulonephritis, 437, 444
    rapidly progressive, 543
Glucose and electrolytes, in premature
    infant, 97
Glucose intolerance, 494–495 (*see also*
    Diabetes mellitus)
Glucose-6-phosphate dehydrogenase
    (G6PD) deficiency, 425
Glucosuria, 494, 495
Gluteal trauma, 587
Glycogen storage disease, type IV, 146
Glycogen storage disorders, 523*t*
Glycosylated hemoglobin (HbA$_{1c}$) test,
    495, 498
Gonadal failure, in systemic lupus
    erythematosus, 544
Gonadotropin-dependent precocious
    puberty, 507–509
Gonadotropin-independent (peripheral)
    precocious puberty, 509–510
Gonadotropin-releasing hormone
    (GnRH) agonists, 509
Gonadotropin-releasing hormone
    (GnRH) stimulation test, 508
Gonococcal conjunctivitis, 46
Gonorrhea, 227–234*t*
Granulocyte colony-stimulating factor,
    in malignancy-associated
    neutropenia, 431
Granulomatous myocarditis, 318
Greenstick fracture, 571
Grey-Turner sign, of splenic injury,
    586–587
Griseofulvin microsize, 655
Growing pains, 287
Growth plate (physeal) fracture, 572,
    573
Guaiac test, 587
Gynecomastia, 512

HACEK organisms, in bacterial
    endocarditis, 294
Haemophilus influenzae, 221
    control measures, 17*t*
    immunization, 8*t*
Haemophilus influenzae meningitis, 175
Hamartoma, hypothalamic, 509
Hand and foot syndrome (dactylitis), in
    sickle cell disease, 414
Harris classification, of fractures, *573*
HBsAg surface antigen, in hepatitis,
    202–203

Headaches, 560–564
    differential diagnosis, 560–561
    migraine, 560
    tension, 560
    types, 560
Head, ears, eyes, nose, and throat
        (HEENT) examination
    in coryza, 66
    in fever of unknown origin, 170–171
    in gastrointestinal bleeding, 483
    in jaundice, 147
    in pharyngitis, 54
    in pneumonia, 194
    for stomatitis, 472
Head injury, 577–585 (*see also* Intra-
        cranial pressure)
    in child abuse, 41–42
    differential diagnosis, 578–580
    Glasgow Coma Scale, 580, 580*t*
    initial management, 581–583
    primary survey, 580*t*, 580–581
    secondary survey, 583
Hearing loss, 64
Heart failure, congestive, 317
Heart rate, in premature infant, 97
Heart sounds, in ventricular septal
        defect, 352
Helicobacter pylori, 484
Hematemesis, 482
Hematochezia, 482
    factitious, 482
Hematocrit, in shock, 601
Hematologic manifestations, in systemic
        lupus erythematosus, 544
Hematology, 412–432
    acute leukemias, 397–401
    anemia, 419–428
    fever and neutropenia, 429–432
    sickle cell disease, 412–418
Hematoma, 578–579
    cerebral, 561
    epidural, 578, *579*
    intracerebral, 578–579
    subdural, 578, *579*
Hematuria, 438–445
    ABCDEFGHI workup, 439
    gross, 438
    in Henoch-Schönlein purpura, 530
    microscopic, 438
    in systemic lupus erythematosus, 543
Hemiplegia, spastic, 25
Hemlock, 266
Hemoglobin, glycosylated (HbA$_{1c}$), 495,
    498
Hemoglobin S, in sickle cell disease, 412

Hemolysis
    antibody-mediated, 427
    mechanical, 427
Hemolytic anemias, 425–427, 545
Hemorrhage
    classes of, 598, 598*t*
    external, 568
    with fracture, 575
    gastrointestinal, 482–486
    intraventricular, 102, 103
    pulmonary, in premature infant, 101
    special concern in pediatrics, 599
Hemorrhagic shock, 598*t*, 598–602
Hemothorax, 592, 596 (*see also* Thoracic
        trauma)
Henoch-Schönlein purpura, 284,
        529–532
Heparin sodium, 655–656
Hepatic failure, fulminant, 198
Hepatic glycogen storage disorders, 523*t*
Hepatitis, 198–205
    A, 18*t*, 200–201, *201*
    autoimmune, 200
    B, 201–203, *202*
    C, 203–204
    D, 204
    differential diagnosis, 198
    fulminant hepatic failure, 198
    idiopathic neonatal, 146–147
    immunization, 8*t*, 236
    viral, 200–204, 201*t*
Hepatobiliary manifestations, of cystic
        fibrosis, 392
Hepatoiminodiacetic (HIDA) scan, in
        jaundice, 148
Hepatosplenomegaly, 171
Hereditary fructose intolerance, 146
Hereditary nephritis, 440–441
Hernia, inguinal, incarcerated, 464
Herniation
    brain stem, 407
    midbrain, 407
    uncal, 407
Herpes
    central nervous system (CNS), 137
    skin, eye, and mouth, 137
Herpes simplex viral conjunctivitis, 46,
        47
Herpes simplex virus, 133*t*, 136–137 (*see
        also* STORCH infections)
Herpesvirus, febrile seizures and, 557
Herpesvirus encephalitis, 175
Herpesvirus I and II, 227–234*t*
High-frequency oscillating (HFOV)
        ventilation, 112, 113*t*, 115–116

Hip dysplasia, developmental, 285, 289
Hip radiography, in septic arthritis, 222
Hirschsprung disease (toxic megacolon),
        81, 462, 464, 468–470, 472
Hirshsprung disease (toxic megacolon),
        constipation in, 80*t*
Holter monitoring, in syncope, 281
Home monitoring, in ALTEs, 254
Homocystinuria, 519*t*
Human immunodeficiency virus (HIV),
        237–244
    AIDS-defining conditions, 239*t*
    clinical categories, 240–242*t*
    pediatric classification, 243*t*
Human leukocyte antigen (HLA), in
        systemic lupus erythematosus,
        542
Human papillomavirus (HPV), 227–234*t*
Humidification therapy, in croup, 70
Hunter syndrome, 527*t*
Hurler syndrome, 527*t*
Hyaline membrane disease (respiratory
        distress syndrome), 103–107, 114
    differential diagnosis, 104–106
Hydralazine hydrochloride, 656–657
Hydrocarbons, toxic ingestion, 263
Hydrocephalus, 561
Hydrochlorothiazide, 657 (*see also*
        Diuretic therapy)
Hydrocortisone (systemic), 657–658
Hydromorphone, 658–659
Hydrops of gallbladder, 530
Hydroxychloroquine, in systemic lupus
        erythematosus, 547
Hydroxyzine hydrochloride, 659
Hyperalimentation, in premature infant,
        99–100
Hyperbilirubinemia
    conjugated (cholestatic jaundice),
        143–148
    in hepatitis, 199
    unconjugated (jaundice), 101, 102*t*,
        121–126
Hypercalcemia
    in acute leukemias, 398
    as oncologic emergency, 409–411, 410*t*
    treatment, 410*t*
Hypercalciuria, 441
Hyperglycemic episodes, in diabetes
        mellitus, 497–498
Hyperkalemia
    C-A-BIG-K mnemonic, 448
    in diabetic ketoacidosis, 505
    in premature infant, 97–99
    in tumor lysis syndrome, 409

Hyperleukocytosis, 408
Hypernatremia, in premature infant, 97
Hypernatremic dehydration, 245–246
Hyperosmolar nonketotic coma, 501
Hyperosmotic laxatives, 83–84*t*
Hyperphosphatemia, in acute
    leukemias, 398
Hyperpigmentation, 550
Hyperplasia, congenital adrenal, 511
Hyperpyrexia, in head injury, 584
Hypersensitivity (*see also* Allergy)
    in asthma, 71
Hypertension, 309–316
    causes, 310*t*
    definitions, 309, 311–314*t*
    evaluation, 315, 316*t*
    in Henoch-Schönlein purpura, 530
    persistent pulmonary of newborn
        (PPHN), 139–142
    pulmonary, 114
    in renal failure, 445, 447
    in systemic lupus erythematosus, 543
    treatment, 315–316
Hypertrophy
    atrial, 347
    ventricular (*see* Ventricular hyper-
        trophy)
Hyperventilation, 109
    in head injury, 582
Hypocalcemia, in premature infant, 99
Hypoglycemia
    episodic, 499
    in premature infant, 97
Hypoglycemic episodes, in diabetes
    mellitus, 497
Hyponatremia, in premature infant, 97
Hyponatremic dehydration, 245
Hypoplasia, right ventricular, 361, *363,*
    364
Hypoplastic left heart syndrome, *381,*
    381–386
Hypotension
    in head injury, 582
    syncope in, 280
Hypothalamic hamartoma, 509
Hypothalamic-pituitary-gonadal axis,
    507
Hypothermia, 568
Hypothyroidism, 509
    congenital, 146
    constipation in, 81*t*
Hypoventilation syndrome, congenital
    central, 253
Hypovolemia, renal failure and,
    443–444

Ibuprofen, 659–660 (*see also* NSAIDs)
    in cystic fibrosis, 395
    toxicity, 260
Icterus (*see* Jaundice)
Idiopathic neonatal hepatitis, 146–147
Idiopathic (constitutional or functional)
    precocious puberty, 508
Ileus, meconium, 462
Imipenem, in malignancy-associated
    fever, 431
Imipenem and cilastatin, 660
Immune globulin (Ig), 661–662
    in Kawasaki disease, 306
    in myocarditis, 318
Immunizations, 7–16
    bacille Calmette-Guérin, tuberculin
        testing and, 191
    catch-up schedule, 10–11*t*
    contraindications and precautions,
        12–15*t*
    hepatitis, 236
    in HIV-positive patients, 244
    immunoglobulin (Ig) therapy and, 307
    indications for nonroutine vaccines,
        16*t*
    schedule, 7, 8–9*t*
    varicella zoster virus, 50
Immunocompromised, antimicrobial
    therapy in, 161*t*
Immunoglobulin A (IgA), in Henoch-
    Schönlein purpura, 529
Immunoglobulin A (IgA) nephropathy,
    441
Immunologic screening, 399
Immunologic studies, in systemic lupus
    erythematosus, 546
Immunosuppressive therapy, in inflam-
    matory bowel disease, 475
Immunotherapy, post-anaphylaxis, 269
Impaired glucose tolerance, 494–495
    (*See also* Diabetes mellitus)
Impetigo, 207
    antimicrobial therapy, 162–163*t*
Inborn errors of metabolism, 512–528
    amino acid disorders, 516, 520*t*
    of ammonia metabolism, 516, 521*t,*
        522
    of carbohydrate metabolism, 522,
        523–525*t*
    of fatty acid oxidation, 526*t,* 528
    lysosomal and peroxisomal disorders,
        527*t,* 528
    organic acidemias/acidosis, 516,
        517–520*t*
    preliminary diagnosis, 514, 515*t*

Incarcerated inguinal hernia, 464
Incomplete (partial) precocious
    puberty, 510–512
Indomethacin, 662
  in patent ductus arteriosus, 359
Infantile spasms (West syndrome), 552t
Infantile syncope (breath-holding
    spells), 253, 551
Infarction
  bone vs. osteomyelitis, 413t
  pulmonary vs. pneumonia, 415t
Infection(s), 153–245
  antibiotic therapy, 158, 159–168t
  bronchiolitis, 185–188
  central nervous system (CNS),
    167–168t
  conjunctival, 304
  ear, 60–64
  epiglottitis, 212–215
  febrile seizures and, 557–559
  fever of unknown origin, 169–173
  fever without focus, 153–157
  gastrointestinal, 165t
  genitourinary, 167t
  headaches in, 561
  hepatitis, 198–205
  human immunodeficiency virus
    (HIV), 237–244
  lower respiratory, antimicrobial
    therapy, 160–162t
  meningitis, 180–184, 561
  meningococcemia, 180–184
  osteomyelitis, 216–220
  peritonsillar abscess, 212–215
  pneumonia, 194–197
  refusal to bear weight in, 284
  retropharyngeal abscess, 212–215
  septic arthritis, 221–225
  sexually transmitted diseases (STDs),
    226–236
  skeletal, antimicrobial therapy, 164t
  soft tissue/toxic shock syndrome,
    206–211
  STORCH, 32, 132–138, 144, 148
  in systemic lupus erythematosus, 544,
    547
  tuberculosis, 189–193
  upper respiratory tract (coryza),
    65–67
    antimicrobial therapy, 159t
  urinary tract (UTIs), 449–455
Infection control measures, 17–18t
Infection prophylaxis, in burn injury,
    613
Inflammation (see also Infections)

myocardial, 317–319
Inflammatory bowel disease (IBD),
    471–477
  extraintestinal manifestations, 473t
Inflammatory causes, in refusal to bear
    weight, 284–285
Infliximab, in inflammatory bowel
    disease, 476
Influenza immunization, 8t, 16t
Inguinal hernia, incarcerated, 464
Inhalation injury, 608t, 609t (see also
    Burns)
Inotropics, in persistent pulmonary
    hypertension of newborn, 140
Inspiratory stridor, 387
Inspiratory time (T_I), 109
Insulin
  continuous infusion (insulin pump),
    499
  conversion from intravenous to
    subcutaneous, in diabetic
    ketoacidosis, 506
  in diabetic ketoacidosis, 504–506
  in head injury, 584
  intravenous infusion, 504–505
  preparations, 495, 496t
  requirements in children, 495
Integumentary system (see Skin
    disorders)
Intermittent mandatory ventilation
    (IMV), 111
Intracranial pressure (ICP), 407–408,
    577, 582, 583–584
  measurement, 577
  Monro-Kellie doctrine, 577
Intrahepatic vaso-occlusive crisis, in
    sickle cell disease, 416
Intralipids, in premature infant, 100
Intrapartum antibiotic prophylaxis, 127
Intravenous access, in hemorrhagic
    shock, 600
Intravenous immunoglobulin (see
    Immunoglobulin)
Intraventricular hemorrhage, 102, 103
Intubation (see also Ventilation)
  emergency, 566, 566t, 567t
  indications for, 109
  in status asthmaticus, 273
  in status epilepticus, 275–276
Intussusception, 464, 465–468, 530
  in Henoch-Schönlein purpura, 530
Ipecac
  indications/contraindications, 257
  in toxic ingestions, 257
Ipratropium bromide, 663

IQ, in developmental delay/disability, 25
Iron binding capacity, total, 423
Iron deficiency anemia, 423
Iron supplementation, 21
Iron toxicity, 263–264
Irrigation, whole-bowel in toxic ingestions, 258
Isoniazid, 663
    in tuberculosis, 192
Isotonic dehydration, 245, 246–247
Isotonic fluids, 245
Isovaleric acidemia, 517t

Jatene (arterial switch) procedure, 373–374
Jaundice
    cholestatic (conjugated hyper-bilirubinemia), 145–148
    defined, 145
    unconjugated hyperbilirubinemia, 101, 102t, 121–126
Jitteriness, vs. seizures, 551
Joint fluid, aspiration of (see Synovial fluid aspiration)
Joint pain, in Henoch-Schönlein purpura, 530
Jones criteria (revised), for rheumatic fever diagnosis, 55t
Juvenile myoclonic epilepsy, 555t
Juvenile rheumatoid arthritis (JRA), 284–285, 288, 533–541
    clinical manifestations, 534–537t, 535–537t
    definitions, 533
    epidemiology, 534t
    morbidity, 541t
    types, 538–539t

Kawasaki disease, 304–308
Kayser-Fleischer rings, 32, 199, 200
Kehr sign, of splenic injury, 586
Kernicterus, 122, 123
Kernig sign, 174
Ketoconazole, 664
Ketonuria, 498
Ketosis, 501
Kidney stones (calculi, nephrolithiasis), 439–440
KOH test, 206
Korotkoff sound, 315
Krabbe syndrome, 527t
Kussmaul sign, 592

Laboratory studies, in failure to thrive, 37–38

Lactose dehydrogenase, in acute leukemias, 398
Lactulose, 83t
Lap-belt trauma, 586
Laryngeal fractures, 591, 595–596 (see also Thoracic trauma)
Laryngeal webs, 388
Laryngomalacia, 387–388
Latching, improper, 22t
Latex agglutination test
    in neonatal sepsis, 131
    in septic arthritis, 224
Lavage
    gastric, 191, 237, 588
    peritoneal diagnostic, 588
Laxatives, 83–84t
LDHAD deficiency, 526t
Lead poisoning, 424
Lead screening, 32
Left ventricular hypertrophy, 326–331, 330, 331t, 347–348, 361, 363, 364
Legal issues, in child abuse, 44
Legg-Calvé-Perthes disease (coxa plana), 285, 289
Lennox-Gastaut syndrome, 552t
LES manometry, in GERD, 489
Leucocoria, 404
Leukemia, 286
Leukemias, acute, 397–401
Leukocyte esterase test, 450
Leukocytosis, in appendicitis, 479
Leukodystrophy
    adrenal, 527t
    metachromatic, 527t
Levobuteral hydrochloride, 664
Levothyroxine sodium, 664
Libman-Sacks endocarditis, 543
Lidocaine, 665
Likelihood ratio, 3–5
Lindane, 665
Lipohypertrophy, in diabetes mellitus, 499
Liver biopsy, in jaundice, 148
Liver enzyme tests, 199
    in myocarditis, 318
Long QT syndrome, 282
Lorazepam, 666
    in status epilepticus, 275
Lower extremity fractures, 575
Lower respiratory infections
    antimicrobial therapy, 160–162t
    pneumonia, 194–197
    tuberculosis, 189–193
Lower respiratory tract disorders, bronchiolitis, 185–188

Lubricant laxatives, 84*t*
Ludwig angina, antimicrobial therapy, 163*t*
Lumbar puncture
 in febrile seizures, 558
 in meningitis, 175, 176*t*
 in meningococcemia, 181–182
 in neonatal sepsis, 130–131
 in status epilepticus, 276
 in systemic lupus erythematosus, 546
Lung transplantation, 395
Lupus erythematosus, systemic (SLE), 542–548 (*see also* Systemic lupus erythematosus)
Lymphadenitis, cervical, 207–208
Lymphadenopathy, 405
 acute suppurative cervical, 305
 in Kawasaki disease, 305
Lymphangiitis, antimicrobial therapy, 163*t*
Lymphocytic myocarditis, 318
Lysosomal congenital disorders, 527*t*, 528

Macrocytic anemias, 427–428 (*see also under* Anemias)
 Diamond-Blackfan anemia, 428
 folic acid deficiency, 427
 vitamin B₁₂ deficiency, 427
Magnesium citrate, 84*t*
Magnesium hydroxide, 84*t*
Magnetic resonance imaging (MRI)
 in meningitis, 178
 in osteomyelitis, 217
Malar (butterfly) rash, 543
Malformations, mechanical ventilation and, 109–110
Malignancy, inflammatory bowel disease and, 476–477
Mallory-Weiss tear, 485
Malrotation (midgut volvulus), 462–463
Mannitol, 666–667
 in head injury, 584
Manometry, in GERD, 489
Maple syrup urine disease, 520*t*
Marcus-Gunn pupils, 583
Martin modification, of Duhamel procedure, 469
Mass lesions (*see* Cancer; Malignancy; Tumors)
Mastoiditis, 64
 antimicrobial therapy, 159*t*
Mauriac syndrome, 499
MCAD deficiency, 526*t*
McBurney point, 478

McCune-Albright syndrome, 510
Mean airway pressure (MAP), 109
Measles/mumps/rubella immunization, 8*t*
Measurement, anthropometric, 36
Mebendazole, 667
Mechanical hemolysis, 427
Mechanical ventilation, 108–120, 140 (*see also* Ventilation)
Meckel scan, 485
Meconium ileus, 80*t,* 462
Medical decision-making, 2–6
 diagnostic continuum, 2
 qualitative assessment, 2–3
 quantitative assessment, 3–6
MedicAlert bracelets, 269
Medications (*see* Drug *entries and specific drugs*)
Megacolon, toxic (Hirschsprung disease), 81, 462, 464, 468–470, 472
Melena, 482
Menarche, premature, 512
Meningitis, 130, 173–179, 561 (*see also* Meningococcemia)
 bacterial, antimicrobial therapy, 167*t*
 defined, 173
 epidemiology, 174*t*
 vs. diabetic ketoacidosis, 503
Meningococcemia, 180–184 (*see also* Meningitis)
 Glasgow Meningococcal Septicemia Score, 184, 184*t*
 management algorithm, *183*
Meningococcus
 control measures, 17*t*
 immunization, 16*t*
Meningoencephalitis, 173, 175
Mental retardation, 25, 31–32
Meperidine hydrochloride, 667–668
Meropenem, 668
Metabolic disorders (*see also* Endocrinology)
 jaundice in, 146
Metabolic manifestations, of cystic fibrosis, 393
Metabolism, inborn errors of, 512–528 (*see also* Inborn errors of metabolism)
Metachromatic leukodystrophy, 527*t*
Methotrexate, in juvenile rheumatoid arthritis, 540
Methylmalonic acidemia, 517*t*
Methylphenidate, 668–669
 in ADHD, 92
Methylprednisolone
 in spinal cord injury, 607

Methylprednisolone—*Continued*
    in status asthmaticus, 271
    systemic administration, 669
    in systemic lupus erythematosus, 547
Metoclopramide hydrochloride,
        669–670
Metronidazole, 670–671
    in inflammatory bowel disease, 475
Mezlocillin sodium, 671–672
Microalbuminuria, 498
Microbiology
    bacterial endocarditis, 294
    cystic fibrosis, 391
    fever without focus, 154
    gastrointestinal bleeding, 486
    urinary tract infections, 449
Microcytic anemias (*see under*
        Anemias)
Microvascular complications, in dia-
        betes mellitus, 498–499
Midazolam hydrochloride, 672–673
Midbrain herniation, 407
Midgut volvulus, 462–463
Migraine headaches, 560
Mineral oil, 84*t*, 673
Minute ventilation (V_M), 109
Mitral regurgitation, 347–348, *348*
Mitral valve disease, 346–348
    prolapse, 346
    regurgitation, 347–348, *348*
Mnemonics (*see also* ABCs of
        emergency care)
    ABCDEFGHI in hematuria, 439
    ACYC, 49
    ADMIT
        in diabetic ketoacidosis, 503
        in pneumonia, 195
    AEIOU indications for dialysis, 448
    C-A-BIG-K for hyperkalemia, 448
    CHOLESTATIC, 144
    CHOPPED MINTS, 1–2, 2*t*
    4 C's of cyanotic heart disease, 323
    MONITOR in bronchiolitis, 186
    NAILED for drugs causing con-
        stipation, 81
    OUTGROW for colic, 78
    PIPE for osteomyelitis, 216
    STARTS HOT in refusal to bear
        weight, 283–284
    STORCH infection, 132
Monitoring, home, 254
MONITOR mnemonic for bronchiolitis,
        186
Monro-Kellie doctrine of intracranial
        pressure, 577

Morphine hydrocloride, 673–674
Morphine sulfate, in tetralogy of Fallot,
        367
Morquio syndrome, 527*t*
Motility, ocular, 583
Motor examination, 604–605, 605*t*, 606*t*
Motor levels, of spinal cord, 606*t*
Mucocutaneous ulcers, in systemic lupus
        erythematosus, 543
Munchausen syndrome by proxy, 253
Mupirocin, 674
Murmurs (*see also* Congenital heart
        disease *and specific diseases*)
    in aortic coarctation, 337, *337*
    aortic ejection, 291
    aortic regurgitation, 342, *342*
    aortic stenosis, 339, *340*
    in atrial septal defect, 355–356, *356*
    examination for, 325–326, *326*
    normal, 291–292
        aortic ejection murmur, 291
        peripheral pulmonary stenosis, 292
        pulmonary ejection murmur,
            291–292, 366
        venous hum, 292
    in patent ductus arteriosus, 359, *359*
    in pulmonary stenosis, 344, *344*
    pulmonic ejection, 291–292, 366
    regurgitant, 376
    systolic ejection, 376
    tricuspid regurgitation, 369
    tricuspid stenosis, 369 (*see also*
        Ebstein anomaly)
    in ventricular septal defect, 350, *351*,
        351–352
Muscle glycogen storage disorders, 523*t*
Muscle strength grading scale, 606*t*
Mushroom poisoning, 266
Mustard procedure, 374
Mycobacterium tuberculosis, 189 (*see
        also* Tuberculosis)
Mycoplasma pneumonia, 196
Myocarditis, 317–319
Myoclonic epilepsy, juvenile, 555*t*
Myoclonic seizures, 550, 551
Myositis
    supporative, antimicrobial therapy,
        163*t*
    in systemic lupus erythematosus, 544

Nafcillin, 674–675
    in malignancy-associated fever, 431
    in neonatal sepsis, 130
    in septic arthritis, 224
    in toxic shock syndrome, 210

NAILED mnemonic for drugs causing constipation, 81
Naloxone, 675–676
  in resuscitation, 98*t*
Naproxen, 676 (*see also* NSAIDs)
Nasal membrane potential difference, in cystic fibrosis, 393
Nasogastric tubes, 568
  in burn injury, 613
Nasolacrimal duct obstruction, 47
Necrosis, acute tubular, 444
Necrotizing enterocolitis, 149–151
Necrotizing fasciitis, 211
  antimicrobial therapy, 163*t*
Necrotizing pneumonia, antimicrobial therapy, 161*t*
Neiman-Pick disease, 527*t*
Neisseria gonorrhoeae, 227–234*t*
  in septic arthritixs, 221, 224
Neisseria meningitides, 175, 180–184
Neonatal conjunctivitis, 45–48
Neonatal hepatitis, idiopathic, 146–147
Neonatal sepsis, 127–131
Neonatology, 95–151 (*see also individual subtopics*)
  enterocolitis, 149–151
  hyaline membrane disease, 103, 104–107
  initial stabilization of premature infant, 95–103
  jaundice
    conjugated hyperbilirubinemia (cholestatic jaundice), 143–148
    unconjugated hyperbilirubinemia, 101, 102*t,* 121–126
  persistent pulmonary hypertension of newborn (PPHN), 139–142
  sepsis, 127–131
  STORCH infections, 32, 132–138, 144, 148
  ventilator management, 108–120
Nephritis (*see also* Glomerulonephritis)
  acute interstitial, 445
  hereditary, 440–441
Nephrolithiasis (kidney stones), 439–440
Nephrology, 433–459 (*see also* Urology)
Nephropathy, immunoglobulin A (IgA), 441
Nephrotic syndrome, 436–437
Neuroblastoma, 403
Neurocardiogenic (vasodepressor) syncope, 278*t,* 282
Neurocutaneous syndromes, 550
Neurofibromatosis, 550
Neurogenic shock, 599

Neurologic examination, 550
Neurologic manifestations
  in acute leukemias, 400
  in Henoch-Schönlein purpura, 530–531
  in systemic lupus erythematosus, 544, 545
Neurologic stabilization, of premature infant, 102
Neurology, 549–564 (*see also* Trauma *and individual subtopics*)
  febrile seizures, 557–559
  headache, 560–564
  seizure disorders, 549–556
Neuropsychiatric syncope, 278*t*
Neuropsychological testing, for ADHD, 92
Neurotoxicity, in lead poisoning, 424
Neutropenia
  defined, 429
  in malignancy, 429–432
Nifedipine, 677
Nines, rule of, 611, *612*
Nipple soreness, 22*t*
Nissen fundoplication, in GERD, 490
Nitric oxide, in persistent pulmonary hypertension of newborn, 140
Nitrite urine tests, 450–452
Nitrofurantoin, 677
Nitroprusside sodium, 677–678
Nonpathogenic (self-resolving) protein-uria, 434
Normocytic anemias, 425–427 (*see also under* Anemias)
  of underproduction, 425
Norwood procedure, in hypoplastic left heart syndrome, *383, 384*
NSAIDs
  contraindicated in myocarditis, 318
  in cystic fibrosis, 395
  in juvenile rheumatoid arthritis, 540
  in systemic lupus erythematosus, 547
Nuclear scintigraphy, in GERD, 489
Nutrition (*see also* Breast-feeding)
  in cystic fibrosis, 393, 394
  in failure to thrive, 38
  failure to thrive and, 35*t*
  in inflammatory bowel disease, 476
  in premature infant, 99–100
  transition to solid foods, 20–21
  vitamin and iron supplementation, 21
Nystatin, 678

Oblique fracture, *571,* 572
Obstruction
  intestinal, 80–81*t*

Obstruction—*Continued*
    nasolacrimal duct, 47
    renal, 445
Obstructive sleep apnea syndrome, 253
Obturator sign, 479
Occult bacteremia, 153
Occult gastrointestinal bleeding, 482
Ocular manifestations, in juvenile
        rheumatoid arthritis, 538*t,* 540
Ocular motility, 583
Oleander, 266
Oliguria, 443
Oncologic emergencies, 406–411
    hypercalcemia, 409–411
    hyperleukocytosis, 408
    intracranial pressure increase,
        407–408
    spinal cord compression, 406–407
    superior vena cava syndrome, 406
    tumor lysis syndrome, 409
Oncology, 397–411 *(see also* Hema-
        tology *and specific subtopics)*
    fever and neutropenia, 429–432
    leukemias, 286, 397–401
    oncologic emergencies, 406–411
    tumors, 402–405
Ondansetron hydrochloride, 678–679
Onychomycosis (tinea unguium), 206
Open pneumothorax, 591, 596
Ophthalmologic examination, in
        jaundice, 148
Oral rehydration, 248–249
Oral ulcers, aphthous, 471–472
Orbital cellulitis, 208
    antimicrobial therapy, 162*t*
Organic acidemias/acidosis, 516,
        517–520*t*
Organic brain lesions, precocious
        puberty and, 508
Organophosphate poisoning, 265
Orthopedics *(see also* Fractures;
        Trauma)
    refusal to bear weight, 285–286
Orthostatic proteinuria, 436
Osgood-Schlatter disease, 285–286, 289
Osmolality, serum, 503–504
Osteochondritis, antimicrobial therapy,
        164*t*
Osteomyelitis, 216–220, 284
    antimicrobial therapy, 164*t*
    vs. bone infarction, 413*t*
    vs. leukemia, 398–399
OTC deficiency, 521*t*
Otitis externa, 60*t,* 60–61
Otitis media, 61–64, 62*t*

OUTGROW mnemonic for colic, 78
Oxacillin sodium, 679–680
Oximetry, pulse, 569
Oxygenation
    extracorporeal membrane (ECMO),
        139, 140
    in laryngeal fractures, 595–596
Oxygenation index, 139
Oxygenation monitoring, 115
Oxygen saturation, pre- and postductal,
        140
Oxygen toxicity, 109

Pain
    in Henoch-Schönlein purpura, 530
    with mechanical ventilation, 109
    refusal to bear weight and, 286
    scrotal, 456–459
    in systemic lupus erythematosus, 543
Pain crises, in sickle cell disease,
        412–413
Pains, growing, 287
Palivizumab, in bronchiolitis, 186
Pallor *(see also* Anemias)
    evaluation, *421*
Palvizumab, 680
Pancreatic enzyme replacement, in
        cystic fibrosis, 394
Pancreatitis, in systemic lupus erythem-
        atosus, 543
Parapharyngeal abscess, antimicrobial
        therapy, 160*t*
Partial seizures, 550
Patent ductus arteriosus (PDA), *358,*
        358–360, 365, *365 (see also*
        Tetralogy of Fallot)
    fluid overload and, 97
    indomethacin prophylaxis, 100–101
Pattern of disease, 1
Peak inspiratory pressure (PIP), 108,
        108
Pediatric trauma score, 570*t*
Pelvic examination, 226
Pelvic fractures, 574–575
Pelvic inflammatory disease (PID), 226,
        227–234*t,* 235–236
Penicillin
    allergy, 300*t*
    in pharyngitis, 55
    resistance, 62
Penicillin G benzathine, 680–683
Penicillin V potassium, 683
Peptic ulcers, 485
Perforation
    small-bowel, 587

tympanic-membrane, 64
Perfusion pressure, cerebral, 577
Pericardiocentesis, in cardiac tamponade, 597
Pericarditis, antimicrobial therapy, 165*t*
Periorbital/orbital cellulitis, 47, 208
Peripheral pulmonary stenosis, 292
Perirectal abscess, antimicrobial therapy, 166*t*
Perirenal or perinephric abscess, antimicrobial therapy, 167*t*
Peritoneal diagnostic lavage, 588
Peritoneal dialysis, antimicrobial therapy in, 166*t*
Peritonitis, 589
   antimicrobial therapy, 166*t*
Peritonsillar abscess, 212–216, 213*t*
   antimicrobial therapy, 160*t*
Pernicious anemia, 427
Peroxisomal congenital disorders, 527*t*, 528
Persistent asymptomatic isolated proteinuria, 435–436
Persistent pulmonary hypertension of newborn (PPHN), 139–142
Pertussis
   antimicrobial therapy, 162*t*
   control measures, 17*t*
   immunization, 8*t*, 12–13*t*
Petechiae, in meningococcemia, 181
Pharyngitis, 53–55
Phenobarbital, 683–684
   side effects, 551
Phenylephrine, in spinal cord injury, 607
Phenylketonuria, 518*t*
Phenytoin, 275, 684
Photosensitivity, in systemic lupus erythematosus, 543
Phototherapy, in jaundice, 101, 102*t*, 122, 125
pH probe testing, 489
Pigments, endogenous in acute tubular necrosis, 444
PIPE mnemonic for osteomyelitis, 216
Piperacillin sodium, 684–685
Plain radiography, in refusal to bear weight, 288
Plants, toxic, 266
Plaques, verrucous, 550
Pneumatosis intestinalis, in necrotizing enterocolitis, 149–150
Pneumococcal immunization, 8*t*, 16*t*
Pneumococcus, penicillin-resistant, 62
Pneumocystis carinii pneumonia, 237, 244

Pneumography, 489
Pneumonia
   antimicrobial therapy
      afebrile pneumonia of infancy, 162*t*
      beta-lactam unresponsive pneumonia, 162*t*
      lobar, 160–161*t*
      necrotizing, 161*t*
   bacterial, 195–196
   mycoplasma, 196
   pneumocystis carinii, 237, 244
   viral, 196
   vs. hyaline membrane disease, 105
   vs. pulmonary infarction, 415*t*
Pneumothorax, 596 (*see also* Thoracic trauma)
   open, 591, 596
   simple, 592, 596
   tension, 567, 591, 596
   vs. hyaline membrane disease, 106
Poisoning, 256–267 (*see also* Toxic ingestions)
   carbon monoxide, signs of, 610*t*
Poliovirus immunization, 8*t*
Polydipsia, 494
Polyethylene glycol electrolyte sodium (PEG-ES), 685
Polymerase chain reaction test, in meningococcemia, 182
Polysomnography (PSG), 252
Polyuria, 494
Pompe disease, 523*t*
Positive end-expiratory pressure (PEEP), 108, *108*
Poststreptococcal reactive arthritis, 284
Posttest probability, 5–6
Potassium, serum level, 502–503, 504
Potassium chloride, 685–686
Pre- and postductal oxygen saturation, 140
Precocious puberty
   gonadotropin-dependent, 507–509
   gonadotropin-independent (peripheral), 509–510
   idiopathic (constitutional or functional), 508
   incomplete (partial), 510–512
Prednisolone, 686
Prednisone
   side effects, 551
   in status asthmaticus, 273
Premature adrenarche, 511
Premature menarche, 512
Premature thelarche, 510–511 (*see also* Precocious puberty)

Prematurity
  antibiotic prophylaxis, 102
  apnea of, 253
  gastrointestinal bleeding in, 486
  initial stabilization, 95–103
    cardiovascular, 100–101
    fluids and electrolytes, 95–97, 99*t*
    jaundice (unconjugated hyper-
      bilirubinemia), 101, 102*t*
    neurologic, 102
    nutrition, 99–100
    pulmonary, 101
    resuscitation in delivery room, 95,
      96
    resuscitation medications, 98*t*
  neonatal sepsis in, 129–130
  patent ductus arteriosus and, 358
  prognosis, 103
Pretest probability, 3
Prevention
  of bacterial endocarditis, 295, 296–297*t*
  of urinary tract infections, 454
Priapism, in sickle cell disease, 416
Probability
  posttest, 5–6
  pretest, 3
Prolapse, mitral valve, 346
Prolonged expiratory apnea (breath-
    holding spells), 253, 551
Promethazine hydrochloride, 686–687
Promotility agents, in GERD, 490
Proprionic acidemia, 517*t*
Prostaglandins *(see also specific drugs)*
  in hypoplastic left heart syndrome,
    384
  in transposition of great arteries, 373
Proteinuria, 433*t*, 433–437, *434*
  glomerulonephritis, 437
  nephrotic syndrome, 436–437
  nonpathogenic (self-resolving), 434
  orthostatic, 436
  persistent asymptomatic isolated,
    435–436
  in systemic lupus erythematosus, 543
Proton pump inhibitors
  adverse effects, 490
  in GERD, 489–490
Pseudoephedrine hydrochloride, 687–688
Pseudotumor cerebri, 561
Psoas sign, 479
Psoriasis, 87*t*
Psychological consequences, in child
    abuse, 42
Psychosocial factors, in failure to thrive,
    36–37

Psyllium, 83*t*, 688
Puberty
  normal, 507
  precocious, 507–512
Pulmonary artery, anomalous left, 390
Pulmonary atresia, 364
Pulmonary contusion, 592, 597
Pulmonary ejection click, 344, *344*
Pulmonary ejection murmur, 291–292,
    366
Pulmonary exacerbations, in cystic
    fibrosis, 393
Pulmonary function tests, in asthma, 73
Pulmonary hemorrhage, in premature
    infant, 101
Pulmonary hypertension, 114
  persistent of newborn (PPHN),
    139–142
Pulmonary infarction, vs. pneumonia,
    415*t*
Pulmonary manifestations, of systemic
    lupus erythematosus, 543
Pulmonary stabilization, in premature
    infant, 101
Pulmonary stenosis, *343,* 343–345, *344*
  peripheral, 292
Pulmonary valve disease, 343–345
Pulmonary vascular bed, development,
    321
Pulmonary venous return, total
    anomalous, 377–380, *378*
Pulmonology, 387–395
  cystic fibrosis, 391–395
  upper airway malformations, 387–390
    (see also specific disorders)
Pulseless electrical activity, 592
Pulse oximetry, 114, 569
Pupillary light response, 583
Purified protein derivative (PPD) skin
    test, 190
Purpura
  Henoch-Schönlein, 284, 529–532
  in meningococcemia, 181
Pyelonephritis, 449, 450 *(see also*
    Urinary tract infections)
  antimicrobial therapy, 167*t*
Pyloric stenosis, 463
Pyloromyotomy, Ramstedt, 463
Pyogenic arthritis, antimicrobial
    therapy, 164*t*
Pyridoxine hydrochloride (vitamin B$_6$),
    688
  in status epilepticus, 276
Pyruvate kinase deficiency, 425
Pyuria, 452

QRS complex, 340 (*see also* Electro-
    cardiography)
Quadriplegia, spastic, 26
Qualitative assessment, 2–3
Quantitative assessment, 3–6

Rabies immunization, 16*t*
Racemic epinephrine, in croup, 69
Radiography (*see also specific
        modalities*)
    in abdominal injury, 587–588
    in appendicitis, 479–480
    chest (*see* Chest radiography)
    in child abuse, 43
    in inflammatory bowel disease, 474
    in leukemia, 398–399
    in refusal to bear weight, 288
    in spinal cord injury, 606–607
    in thoracic trauma, 595*t*
    in trauma, 569
Radionuclide cystography, 453
Radionuclide scans
    bleeding, 486
    dimethylsuccinic acid (DMSA),
        453–454
    in GERD, 489
    Meckel, 485
Ramstedt pyloromyotomy, 463
Range of motion, 287
Rapidly progressive glomerulo-
        nephritis, 543
Rash
    discoid, 543
    in fever of unknown origin, 171
    in Henoch-Schönlein purpura, 530
    in Kawasaki disease, 304–305
    malar (butterfly), 543
    in systemic lupus erythematosus, 543
Ratio, likelihood, 3–5
Raynaud phenomenon, 543
Rectal biopsy, 469
Rectal digital examination, in gastro-
        intestinal bleeding, 483
Refeeding, in failure to thrive, 38
Reflux
    gastroesophageal (GERD), 77–79,
        250, 463–464, 487–491
    vesicoureteral, 453–454, 454*t*
Refusal to bear weight, 283–289
Regional enteritis (Crohn disease),
        471–477 (*see also* Inflammatory
        bowel disease)
Regurgitant murmur, 376
Regurgitation (cardiac)
    aortic, 341–342, 351

    mitral, 347–348, *348*
    tricuspid, 369 (*see also* Ebstein
        anomaly)
Regurgitation (spitting up), 23*t*
    vs. GERD, 487
Rehydration (*see also* Fluid/electrolyte
        therapy)
    intravenous, 246–247
    oral, 248–249
Renal biopsy, 447, 531, 546
Renal disorders (*see* Urology)
Renal failure, acute (ARF), 443–448
        (*see also* Acute renal failure)
Renal manifestations
    in Henoch-Schönlein purpura, 530
    in systemic lupus erythematosus, 543
Renal stones (calculi, nephrolithiasis),
        439–440
Reproductive manifestations, of cystic
        fibrosis, 392–393
Respiratory complications
    of cystic fibrosis, 392
    of GERD, 490
Respiratory compromise, in thoracic
        injuries, 590*t*
Respiratory failure, in spinal cord
        injury, 605
Respiratory support, 108–120 (*see also*
        Ventilation)
    in hyaline membrane disease, 106
Respiratory syncytial virus (RSV), 185
Respiratory syncytial virus immune
        globulin, 688
Respiratory tract procedures, bacterial
        endocarditis prophylaxis in,
        297*t*
Respiratory viral direct fluorescent
        antibody testing, 68
Resuscitation
    in dehydration, 247
    in delivery room, 95, *96*
    medications, 98*t*
Reticulocyte count, 422
Retinoblastoma, 404–405
Retinopathy of prematurity (ROP), 102,
        103
Retropharyngeal abscess, 212–216, 213*t*
    antimicrobial therapy, 160*t*
Retropharyngeal cellulitis, antimicrobial
        therapy, 160*t*
Reverse Trendelenburg position, in
        head injury, 584
Reye syndrome, 50
Rheumatic fever, 55, 284
    Jones criteria (revised), 55*t*

Rheumatic heart disease, 341
Rheumatoid arthritis, juvenile, 284–285,
        288, 533–541 (see also Juvenile
        rheumatoid arthritis)
Rheumatology, 529–548 (see also
        individual disorders)
    Henoch-Schönlein purpura, 284,
        529–532
    juvenile rhuematoid arthritis (JRA),
        284–285, 388, 533–541
    systemic lupus erythematosus (SLE),
        542–548
Rhizomelic chondrodysplasia punctata,
        527t
Ribavirin, 689
    in bronchiolitis, 186
Rib fractures, 594, 597
Rib notching sign, 337
Rifampin, 689
    in meningitis, 177
Right ventricular hypertrophy, 329–331,
        330, 331t, 376
Right ventricular hypoplasia, 361, 363,
        364
Rings, vascular, upper airway, 390
Ringworm (tinea corporis), 206
Risk factors
    for abuse and neglect, 40
    for bacterial endocarditis, 298–299t
    for cerebral palsy, 32
    for diabetes mellitus, 499
    for epilepsy, 559
    for hepatitis, 202
    for HIV, 237
    for hyaline membrane disease, 104
    for intraventricular hemorrhage, 102
    for meningococcemia, 180
    for neonatal sepsis, 127–128
    for pathologic jaundice, 122t
    for seizure recurrence, 559
    for tuberculosis, 189, 190–191
Romano-Ward syndrome, 282
Rovsing sign, 479
Rubella, 133t, 135 (see also STORCH
        infections)
Rupture, esophageal, 594, 597

Salicylate toxicity, 260, 261
Salmeterol xinafoate, 689–690
Sandhoff syndrome, 527t
Sandifer syndrome, 490
Sanfillipo syndrome, 527t
Scabies, 87t
Scalded skin syndrome, antimicrobial
        therapy, 163t

Scans, radionuclide (see Radionuclide
        scans)
Scheie syndrome, 527t
Sclerosis, tuberous, 550
Screening
    developmental, 29–31
    immunologic, 399
    lead, 32
    for sexually transmitted diseases
        (STDs), 226
    urine toxicology in apparent life-
        threatening event (ALTE), 252
Scrotal swelling, 456–459
Seborrheic dermatitis, 87t
Seizures, 274–276, 280, 549–559 (see also
        Epilepsy)
    absence, 553t
    differential diagnosis, 551
    febrile, 557–559
    generalized, 549–550, 551
        absence, 550, 551, 553t
        atonic, 550, 551
        myoclonic, 550, 551
        tonic-clonic, 549, 551
    in head injury, 584
    partial, 549, 550
    prophylaxis, 558–559
    in systemic lupus erythematosus, 544
    treatment, 551, 552–555t
Senna, 85t, 690
Sensory and motor examination,
        604–605, 605t, 606t
Sensory levels, of spinal cord, 605t
Sepsis
    neonatal, 127–131
    in sickle cell disease, 416
    vs. hyaline membrane disease, 105
Septal defects
    atrial, 354–357, 365, 365, 385 (see also
        Tetralogy of Fallot)
    ventricular, 349–353, 385 (see also
        Tetralogy of Fallot)
Septic arthritis, 216, 221–225, 283
Septic shock, 599
Sequestration, splenic, in sickle cell
        disease, 416
Serotonin (5-hydroxytriptamine)
        antagonists, 562
Serum osmolality, 503–504
Serum potassium level, 502–503, 504
Serum sodium calculation, 247
Serum sodium level, 502
Sexual assault, 235–236
Sexually transmitted infections (STIs),
        32, 226–236 (see also Human

immunodeficiency virus *and specific diseases)*
conjunctivitis in, 46
septic arthritis in, 221
Shock
anaphylactic, 267–269
in diabetic ketoacidosis, 505
differential diagnosis, 599
distributive, 268–269
hemorrhagic, 598*t,* 598–602 *(see also* Hemorrhagic shock)
hypothermia and, 568
in meningococcemia, 181
neurogenic, 599
septic, 599
spinal, 599
toxic shock syndrome, 208, 209*t,* 210*t*
Shunt(s)
atrioventricular, 349
bacterial endocarditis risk and, 299*t*
Blalock-Taussig, 361–363, 367
vascular, 322
ventriculoperitoneal, infection, 168*t*
Sickle cell disease, 412–418, 419, 441
differential diagnosis, 413*t,* 414*t,* 415*t*
specific sequelae, 412–413
Sigmoidoscopy, 474, 485
Sign(s)
Beck triad, 592
Brudzinski, 174
of cardiac tamponade, 592
of diaphragmatic trauma, 593
Kernig, 174
Kussmaul, 592
obturator, 479
psoas, 479
Rovsing, 479
of splenic injury
abdominal free-fluid sign, 588
Cullen, 587
Grey-Turner, 586–587
Kehr, 586
Silver sulfadiazine, 690–691
Simple pneumothorax, 592, 596
Sinusitis, 57–59, 561
acute, 57–58
chronic, 58
Skeletal infections, antimicrobial therapy, 164*t*
Skeletal survey radiographs, 43
Skin biopsy, 531, 547
Skin care, in meningococcemia, 181
Skin lesions
antimicrobial therapy, 162–163*t*
atopic dermatitis (eczema), 85–88

in Henoch-Schönlein purpura, 530
skin, eye, and mouth herpes, 137
in systemic lupus erythematosus, 543
Skin signs, in fever of unknown origin, 171
Skull fracture, 578 *(see also* Head injury; Intracranial pressure)
Sleeping position, in GERD, 489
Sleep state, apparent life-threatening events and, 253
Sleepy infant, 24*t*
Slings, vascular, upper airway, 390
Slipped capital femoral epiphysis, 285, 289
Small-bowel perforation, 587
Soave procedure, 470
Sodium, serum level, 502
Sodium bicarbonate, 691
in diabetic ketoacidosis, 505
in persistent pulmonary hypertension of newborn, 140
in resuscitation, 98*t*
Sodium deficit, 247
Soft-tissue infections, 206–211
cervical lymphadenitis, 207–208
dermatophyte, 206–207
impetigo, 207
necrotizing fasciitis, 211
periorbital or orbital cellulitis, 208
toxic shock syndrome, 208, 209*t,* 210*t*
Somogyi phenomenon, 498
Spasms, infantile (West syndrome), 552*t*
Spastic diplegia, 26
Spastic hemiplegia, 25
Spastic quadriplegia, 26
Spinal cord compression, 406–407
Spinal cord injury
differential diagnosis, 603–604
sensory and motor examination, 604–605, 605*t,* 606*t*
Spinal shock, 599
Spinal tumors, 402–403
Spiral fracture, *571,* 572
Splenic injury, 586–587, 588
Splenic sequestration, in sickle cell disease, 416
Splenomegaly, 422
S_2 split, 339
Stabilization, of premature infant, 95–103 *(see also* Prematurity)
Staphylococcal endocarditis, 298*t*
Staphylococcal toxic shock syndrome, 209*t*
Status asthmaticus, 71, 270–273
Status epilepticus, 274–276

Stenosis
    anal, 80*t*
    aortic, 339–341, *340*
    peripheral pulmonary, 292
    pulmonary, *343,* 343–345, *344*
    pyloric, 463
    subglottic, 388
    tricuspid, 369 (*see also* Ebstein
        anomaly)
Sternum, fractured, 594
Stimulant laxatives, 85*t*
Stomatitis, in inflammatory bowel
    disease, 471–472
Stones (calculi), kidney, 439–440
Stool
    bloody, mucous, 466
    currant jelly, 465
Stool culture, 485–486
Stool guaiac test, 483
    in inflammatory bowel disease, 474
Stool softeners, 85*t*
STORCH infections, 32, 132–138,
    144–148
"Strawberry" cervix, 229*t*
Streptococcal endocarditis, 298*t*
Streptococcal toxic shock syndrome, 210*t*
Streptococcus pneumoniae meningitis,
    175
Stress testing
    tilt-table (orthostatic), 281–282
    treadmill, 281
Stridor, 387
ST segment abnormalities (*see* Electro-
    cardiography)
Sturge-Weber syndrome, 550
Subglottic stenosis, 388
Succinylcholine chloride, 691–692
Sudden infant death syndrome (SIDS),
    vs. apparent life-threatening
    event (ALTE), 250, 251
Sulfasalazine, 692
    in inflammatory bowel disease, 475
Sulfonylureas, 497
Sulfisoxazole, 692–693
Sumatriptan, in headache, 562
Superior vena cava syndrome, 406
Suppurative myositis, antimicrobial
    therapy, 163*t*
Suppurative cervical lymphadenopathy,
    305
Surfactant, 104
Surfactant replacement, 106
Sweat chloride testing, in cystic fibrosis,
    393
Swenson procedure, 469

Synchromized intermittent mandatory
    ventilation (SIMV), 111–112
Syncope, 274–282, 277–282
    cardiac, 277, 279*t*
    differential diagnosis, 278–279*t*
    infantile (breath-holding spells), 253,
        551
Syndrome of inappropriate antidiuretic
    hormone secretion (SIADH),
    175, 177, 178
Synovial fluid analysis, 533
    in juvenile rheumatoid arthritis, 534,
        540
    in refusal to bear weight, 288
    in septic arthritis, 222–224, 223*t*
Synovial fluid aspiration, 533
Synovitis, transient (toxic), 284, 289
Syphilis, 133*t,* 133–134, 227–234*t* (*see
    also* STORCH infections)
Systemic lupus erythematosus (SLE),
    542–548
    American College of Rheumatology
        diagnostic criteria, 544–546
Systolic ejection murmur, 376

Tachycardia, in hemorrhage, 599
Tachypnea, transient of newborn, 106
Tamponade, cardiac, 592
Tay-Sachs disease, 527*t*
Tension headaches, 560
Tension pneumothorax, 567, 591, 596
Terbutaline sulfate, 693
Test, polymerase chain reaction, 182
Testicular relapse, in acute leukemias,
    400
Testicular torsion, 456–459
Tethered cord, constipation in, 80*t*
Tetracyline hydrochloride, 693–694
Tetralogy of Fallot, *365,* 365–368
"Tet spells," 366, 367 (*see also* Tetralogy
    of Fallot)
Thalassemia, 419, 423–424
Thelarche, premature, 510–511 (*see also*
    Precocious puberty)
Thermal burns, 610–613 (*see also* Burns)
Thiabendazole, 694
Thoracic spine fractures, 604
Thoracic trauma, 590–597
    differential diagnosis, 591–594
    immediately life-threatening disor-
        ders in, 591–592
    primary assessment, 594
    radiographic findings in, 595*t*
    respiratory compromise in, 590*t*
    secondary assessment, 594, 595*t*

3-for-1 rule, 600
Thrombocytopenia, in systemic lupus
     erythematosus, 544
Thyroiditis, in systemic lupus erythe-
     matosus, 544
Thyroid-stimulating hormone (TSH),
     495
Tibial fractures, 575
Ticarcillin/clavulanate, in malignancy-
     associated fever, 431
Ticarcillin disodium, 695–696
Ticarcillin sodium, 694–695
Tidal volume (V_T), 109
Tilt-table (orthostatic) stress testing,
     281–282
Tinea corporis (ringworm), 206
Tinea pedis (athlete's foot), 206
Tinea unguium (onychomycosis), 206
Tobramycin, 696
Toddler's fracture, 285, 289
Tonic-clonic seizures, 549, 551
Tonsillopharyngitis, antimicrobial
     therapy, 159t
Torsion
     of appendix testis, 456–459
     testicular, 456–459
Torus fractures, 571
Total anomalous pulmonary venous
     return, 377–380, 378
     nonobstructed, 377–379
     obstructed, 379–380
Total body water (TBW), 246
Total iron binding capacity, 423
Toxic ingestion, lead poisoning, 424
Toxic ingestions, 256–267
     acetaminophen, 258–260, 259
     acids, 263
     alkalis, 263
     beta-blockers, 260–262
     button batteries, 262
     calcium channel blockers, 262
     carbon monoxide poisoning, 262–263
     clonidine, 262
     cyanide, 265
     decontamination, 257–258
     ethanol, 265
     hydrocarbons, 263
     ibuprofen, 260
     iron, 263–264
     organophosphates, 265
     plants, 266
     salicylates, 260, 261
     tricyclic antidepressants, 264–265
Toxic megacolon (Hirschsprung dis-
     ease), 81, 462, 464, 468–470, 472

Toxic shock syndrome, 208, 209t, 210t
Toxic (transient) synovitis, 284, 289
Toxoplasmosis, 133t, 134–135 (see also
     STORCH infections)
Tracheal compression, 390
Tracheitis, bacterial, vs. croup, 69
Tracheobroncheal trauma, 593
Tracheobronchial tree injury, 597
Tracheoesophageal fistula, 388–389, 389
     (see also Esophageal atresia)
Transcutaneous CO_2 monitoring, 114
Transfusion, exchange, 101, 122–123,
     125–126
Transient erythroblastopenia of child-
     hood, 425
Transient (toxic) synovitis, 284, 289
Transient tachypnea of newborn, 106
Transplantation
     bone marrow, 399–400
     cardiac, 319, 384
     lung, 395
Transposition of great arteries, 372,
     372–374
Transverse fracture, 571, 571
Trauma, 565–614 (see also Neurology
     and individual subtopics)
     abdominal, 586–589
     burns, 608–614
     cardiac, 577–585
     corneal, 47
     fractures, 571–574
     head, 577–585
     hemorrhagic shock, 698–602
     initial assessment and management,
          565–570
          anesthesia induction, 567t
          pediatric trauma score, 570t
          primary survey, 565–569
          secondary survey, 569–570
     spinal cord injury, 603–607
     thoracic, 590–597
Traumatic amputation, 576
Traumatic aortic disruption, 593
Traumatic bowing, 571
Traumatic fracture, 285
Treponema pallidum, 227–234t
Tretinoin (topical), 696–697
Trichimonas vaginalis, 227–234t
Tricuspid atresia, 361–364, 362, 363
Tricuspid regurgitation, 369 (see also
     Ebstein anomaly)
Tricuspid stenosis (see also Ebstein
     anomaly)
Tricyclic antidepressants, ingestion,
     264–265

Trimethoprim-sulfamethoxazole, in
        urinary tract infections, 452–453
Truncus arteriosus, 375–376
    van Praagh classification, *375*
Tubes
    gastric pre-peritoneal lavage, 588
    nasogastric, 568
        in burn injury, 613
    tympanostomy, 64
Tuberculin skin test, 190, 547
Tuberculosis, 189–193
Tuberous sclerosis, 550
Tumor lysis syndrome, 409
Tumor necrosis factor (TNF), in juve-
        nile rheumatoid arthritis, 540
Tumor necrosis factor (TNF)
        antagonists, in juvenile rheu-
        matoid arthritis, 540
Tumors, 402–405 (*see also* Hematology;
        Oncology)
    bone, 404
    brain, 402, 561
    genitourinary, 434
    lymphadenopathy, 405
    neuroblastoma, 403
    pelvic, 80*t*
    retinoblastoma, 404–405
    spinal, 402–403
    Wilms tumor, 403–404, 440
T wave abnormalities (*see* Electro-
        cardiography)
Tympanic membrane perforation, 64
Tympanocentesis, 63
Tympanometry, 63
Tympanostomy tubes, 64
Type I diabetes mellitus (IDDM), 493,
        495–497, 496*t*
Type II diabetes mellitus (NIDDM),
        493, 497–498
Tyrosinemia, 146, 519*t*

Ulcerative colitis, 471–477 (*see also*
        Inflammatory bowel disease)
Ulcers
    aphthous oral (stomatitis), 471–472
    mucocutaneous, in systemic lupus
        erythematosus, 543
    peptic, 485
Ultrasonography
    abdominal
        in jaundice, 147–148
        in trauma, 588
    in appendicitis, 479
    in precocious puberty, 508–509
    in scrotal swelling, 458

    in urinary tract infections, 453
Uncal herniation, 407
Unconjugated hyperbilirubinemia
        (jaundice), 101, 102*t*, 121–126
Upper airway malformations, 387–390
    choanal atresia, 389–390
    laryngeal webs, 388
    laryngomalacia, 387–388
    subglottic stenosis, 388
    tracheoesophageal fistula, 388–389,
        389 (see also Esophageal atresia)
    vascular rings and slings, 390
Upper extremity fractures, 574
Upper gastrointestinal contrast study,
        489
Upper respiratory infections, 65–67
    antimicrobial therapy, 159*t*
Urea cycle disorders, 521*t*, 522
Uremia, 448
Urethritis, 450 (*see also* Sexually trans-
        mitted diseases; Urinary tract
        infections)
Urethrography, in abdominal injury, 589
Urinalysis, 446, 446*t*, 450–452
    in appendicitis, 479
Urinary tract infections (UTIs), 449–455
    antimicrobial therapy, 452–453
    microbiology, 449
    urinalysis, 446, 446*t*, 450–452
    urine collection methods, 450, 451*t*
    vesicoureteral reflux, 453–454, 454*t*
Urine collection, 450, 451*t*
Urine output, in shock, 601
Urine protein dipstick readings, 433*t*,
        434
Urology, 433–459 (*see also individual
        subtopics*)
    hematuria, 438–445
    proteinuria, 433–437
    renal failure, 443–448
    scrotal swelling, 456–459
    urinary tract infections (UTIs),
        449–455
Urosepsis, 450
Uveitis, in juvenile rheumatoid arthritis,
        538*t*, 540

Vaginitis
    bacterial, 227–234*t*
    fungal, 227–234*t*
Valproic acid, 697
    side effects, 551
Valves, prosthetic heart, 298*t*
Valvular heart disease
    antimicrobial therapy, 165*t*

aortic, 339–342
   aortic regurgitation, 341–342
   aortic stenosis, 339–341, *340*
   mitral valve, 346–348
   pulmonary, 343–345
Valvuloplasty
   in aortic stenosis, 341
   balloon, 341
   in pulmonary valve disorders, 345
Vancomycin hydrochloride, 697–698
Vancomycin plus cefotaxime, in
      neonatal sepsis, 130
Van Praagh classification, of truncus
      arteriosus, *375*
Varicella (chickenpox), 49–52
   congenital varicella syndrome, 52
   immunization, 8*t*
Varicella immune globulin, 49
Varicella zoster virus immunization, 50
Vascular complications, in diabetes
      mellitus, 498–499
Vascular diseases *(see specific disorders)*
Vascular injury, with fracture, 575
Vascular rings and slings, upper airway,
      390
Vasculitic lesions, in Henoch-Schönlein
      purpura, 530
Vasculitis of childhood, 444
Vaso-occlusion, in sickle cell disease,
      412, 413*t*, 413–415
   intrahepatic, 416
Vasovagal syndrome, 278*t*
Vecuronium bromide, 698
Vegetations, endocardial, 293 *(see also*
      Endocarditis)
Venereal Disease Research Laboratory
      (VDRL) criteria, 134
Venous hum, 292
Ventilation
   mechanical, 108–120
      complications, 109–110
      goals, 108, 114
      high-frequency oscillating
         (HGOV), 112, 113*t*, 115–116
      indications, 109
      management, 117–118*t*, 118–119*t*
      modes, *110*, 110–113, 113*t*
      monitoring, 114
      in persistent pulmonary hyper-
         tension of newborn, 140
      setting adjustment, 114–116
      setting guidelines, 113*t*
      types, *108*, 108–109
      weaning, 117, 119
   minute (V_M), 109

Ventricular hypertrophy
   biventricular, 376
   chest radiography in, 333–334, *335*
   left, 326–331, *332, 333,* 347–348, 361,
      363, 364
   right, 329–331, *330, 331*t, 376
Ventricular hypoplasia, right, 361, *363,*
      364
Ventricular septal defect, 349–353, 365,
      365, 385 *(see also* Tetralogy of
      Fallot)
Ventriculoperitoneal shunt infection, 168*t*
Verapamil hydrochloride, 698
Verrucous plaques, 550
Vertebral fractures, 604 *(see also* Spinal
      injury)
Vesicoureteral reflux, 453–454, 454*t*
VICAD deficiency, 526*t*
Viral hepatitis, 200–204, 201*t*
Viral myocarditis, 317
Viral pharyngitis, 53–55
Viral pneumonia, 196
Virilization, 510 *(see also* Precocious
      puberty)
Vitamin B_6 (pyridoxine), 688
   in status epilepticus, 276
Vitamin B_{12} deficiency, 427
Vitamin C, in coryza, 66
Vitamin deficiencies, in cystic fibrosis,
      393
Vitamin supplementation, 21
   in cystic fibrosis, 394
Voiding cystourethrography, 453, 454*t*
Volume expanders
   in persistent pulmonary hypertension
      of newborn, 140
   in resuscitation, 98*t*
Volutrauma, 109
Volvulus, midgut, 462–463
Vomiting, 461–464
   diseases causing, 461*t*
   in first month of life, 463–464
   hematemesis, 482
   in newborn period, 461–463
   projectile, 24*t*
   vs. regurgitation, 23*t*
Von Gierke disease, 523*t*
Vulvovaginitis, 227–234*t*

Warts, genital, 227–234*t*
Water deficit calculation, 248
Weaning, from mechanical ventilation,
      117–119
Webs, laryngeal, 388
Weight, refusal to bear, 283–289

Weight gain, in infancy, 23*t*
West syndrome (infantile spasms), 552*t*
Wheezing, 71–72, 186, 270, 271
White blood cell count (WBC), 154
   in appendicitis, 479
Whole-bowel irrigation, in toxic
   ingestions, 258
Wilms tumor, 403–404, 440

Wilson disease (hepatolenticular
   degeneration), 199–200
Wolff-Parkinson-White syndrome, *281*

Zellweger syndrome, 527*t*
Ziehl-Nelson (acid-fast bacillus skin)
   test, 191
Zinc, 66